NATURAL HEALTH

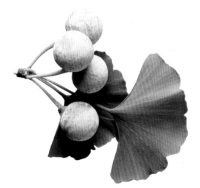

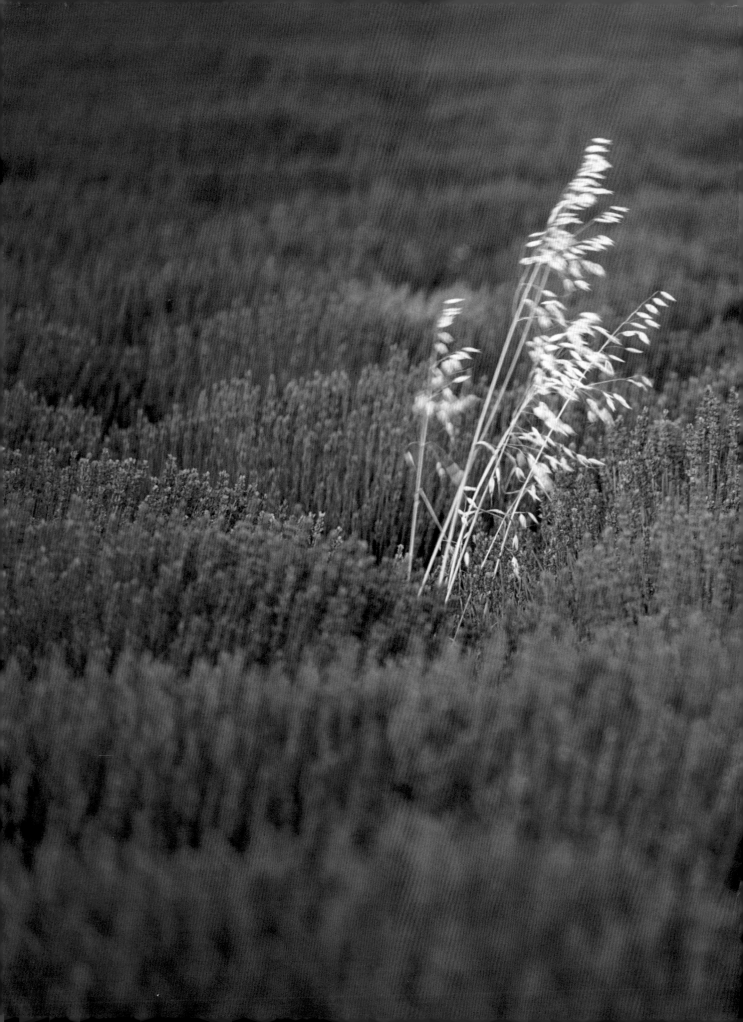

NATURAL HEALTH

NERYS PURCHON

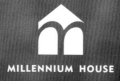

MILLENNIUM HOUSE

First published in 2006 as *The Essential Natural Health Bible* by
Millennium House Pty Ltd
52 Bolwarra Rd, Elanora Heights NSW, 2101, Australia

ISBN 978-1-921209-66-6

SALES
For all sales, please contact:
Millennium House Pty Ltd
52 Bolwarra Rd, Elanora Heights NSW, 2101, Australia
Ph: (612) 9970 6850 Fx: (612) 9970 8136
email rightsmanager@millenniumhouse.com.au

Printed in China
Color separation Pica Digital Pte Ltd, Singapore

Publisher	Gordon Cheers
Associate Publisher	Janet Parker
Project Manager	Carol Jacobson
Art Director	Melanie Feddersen
Text	Nerys Purchon
Editors	Carol Jacobson, Philippa Sandall, James Young
Picture research	Bernard Roberts, Carol Jacobson
Cover design	Melanie Feddersen
Designers	Melanie Feddersen, Warwick Jacobson, Kim Webber
Production	Simone Russell

Photographers are acknowledged on page 524

PHOTOGRAPHERS
Millennium House would like to hear from photographers
interested in supplying photographs

Photographs on preliminary pages:
Pages 2–3, *Stalks of grass in lavender field, Provence, France*
Page 5, *Chamomile tea with honeycomb*
Pages 8–9, Ocimum sanctum *(holy basil)*
Page 10, *Fresh and dried medicinal herbs*

IMPORTANT NOTICE

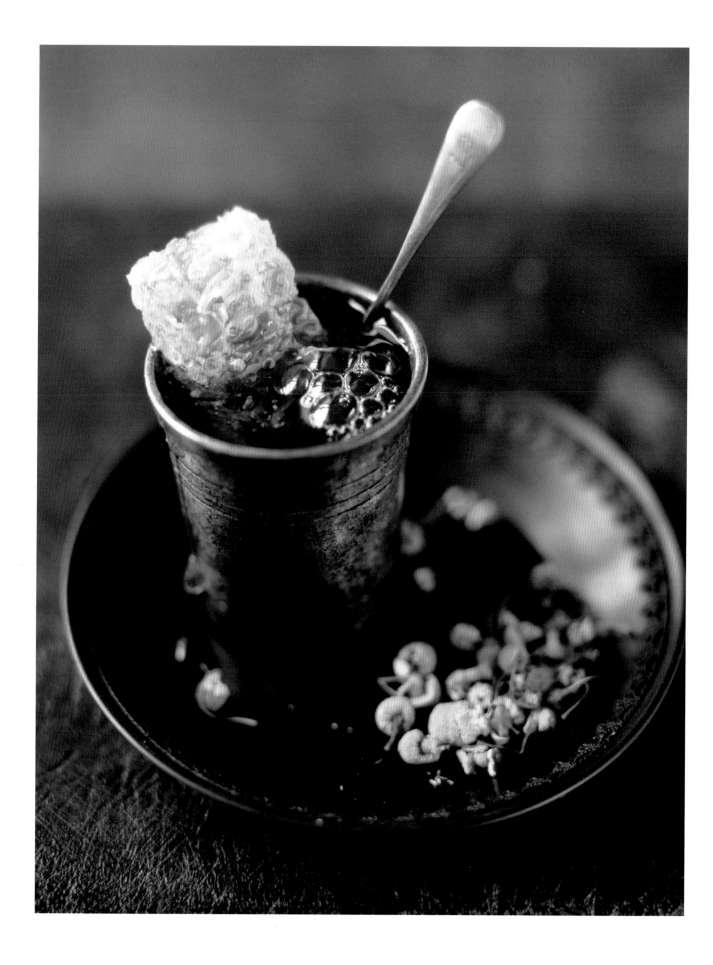

EARTH is an epic publishing feat never to be repeated, proudly created by Millennium House

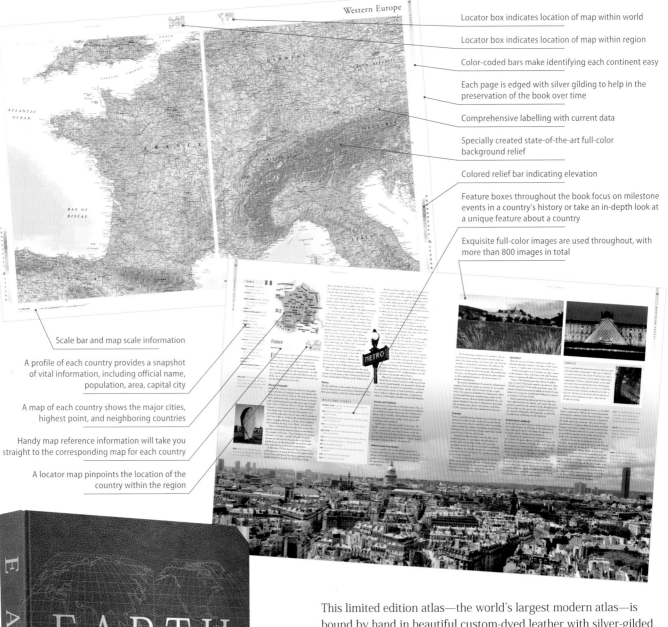

Locator box indicates location of map within world

Locator box indicates location of map within region

Color-coded bars make identifying each continent easy

Each page is edged with silver gilding to help in the preservation of the book over time

Comprehensive labelling with current data

Specially created state-of-the-art full-color background relief

Colored relief bar indicating elevation

Feature boxes throughout the book focus on milestone events in a country's history or take an in-depth look at a unique feature about a country

Exquisite full-color images are used throughout, with more than 800 images in total

Scale bar and map scale information

A profile of each country provides a snapshot of vital information, including official name, population, area, capital city

A map of each country shows the major cities, highest point, and neighboring countries

Handy map reference information will take you straight to the corresponding map for each country

A locator map pinpoints the location of the country within the region

This limited edition atlas—the world's largest modern atlas—is bound by hand in beautiful custom-dyed leather with silver-gilded pages for preservation and silver-plated corners for protection. *Earth* establishes a new benchmark in the world of atlases, with highly detailed mapping and comprehensive country profiles. With 580 pages, including 355 maps of 194 countries, more than 800 images, 4 breathtaking gatefolds, and information on every country, territory and dependency in the world, *Earth* will appeal to book collectors, libraries and institutions, map lovers, and anyone wishing to enjoy now, and preserve for the future, a record of our world today.

Earth can be ordered from all good book stores or contact Millennium House for your nearest supplier

 www.millenniumhouse.com.au

CONTENTS

Introduction 11

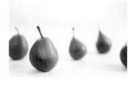

ESSENTIALS 12

NUTURE AND NOURISH 32

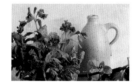

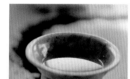

CHERISH 242

PRACTICALITIES 504

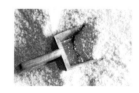

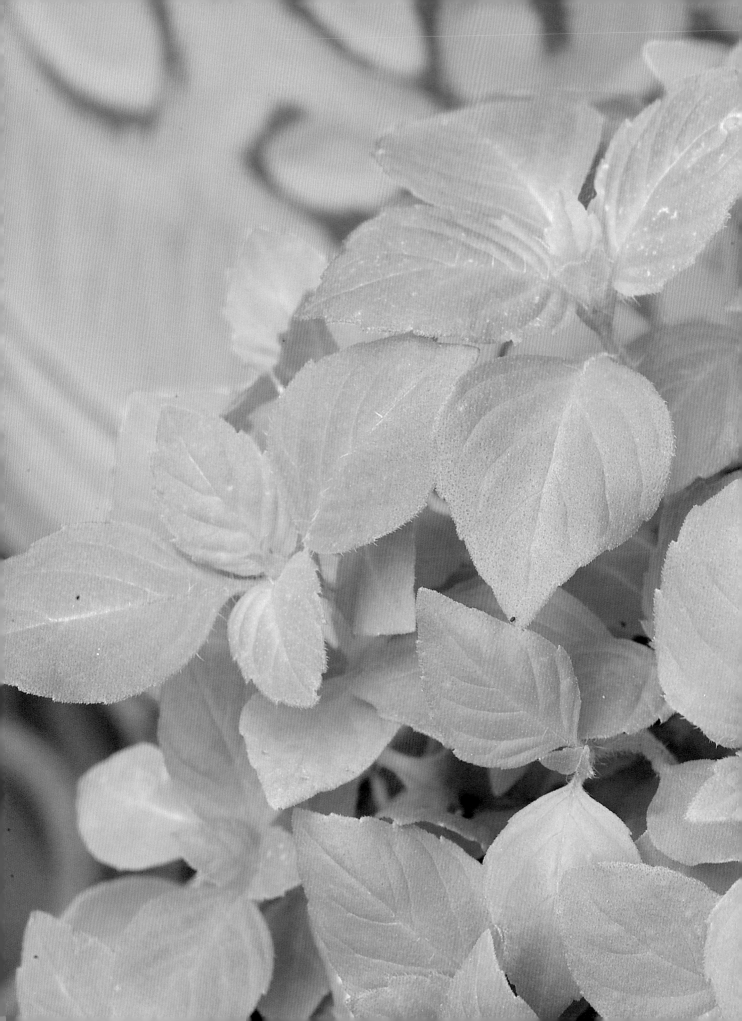

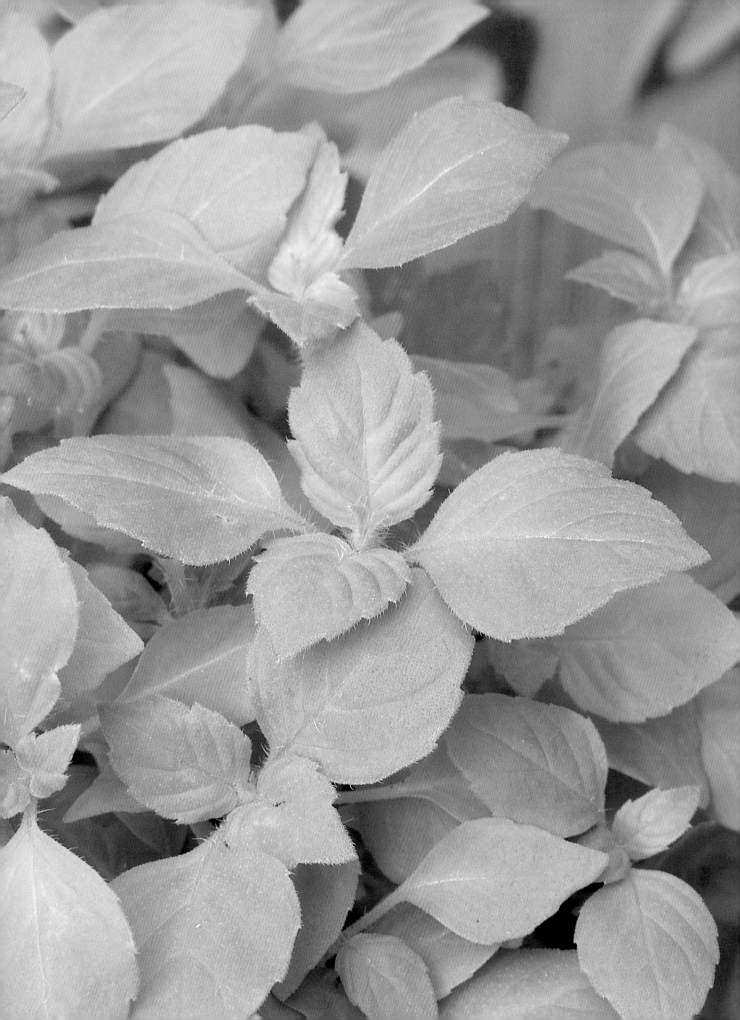

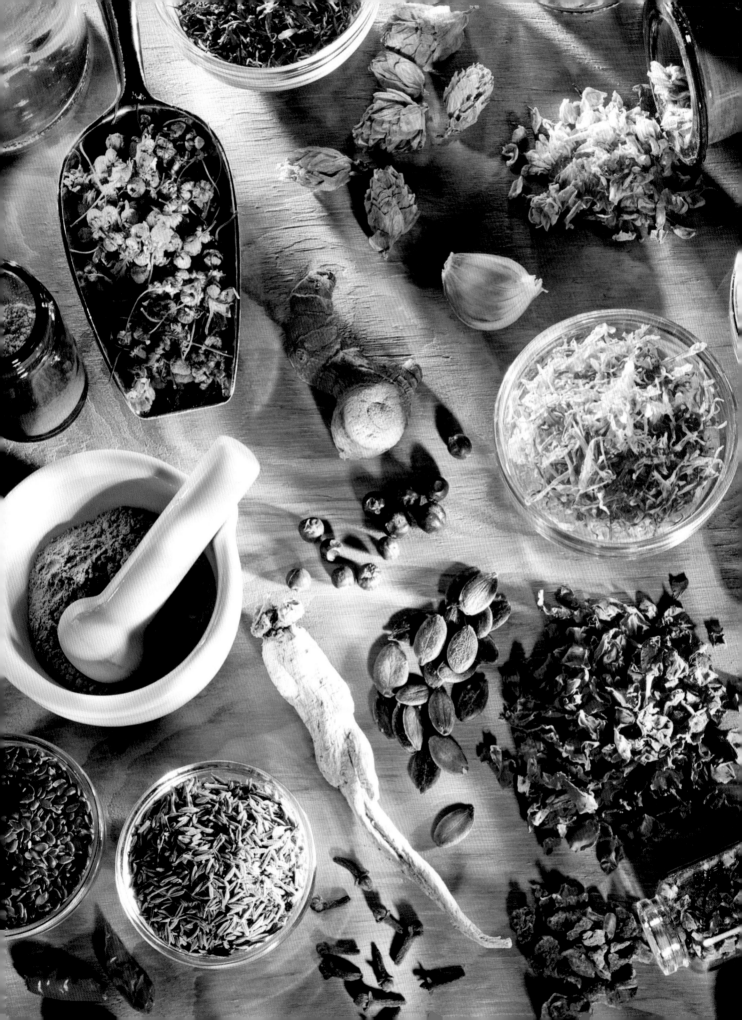

INTRODUCTION

Today we are living longer but we aren't necessarily healthier. Our stress levels keep rising as the pace of life accelerates. Labor-saving devices and convenience foods have given us more time, but in many ways our quality of life hasn't improved.

More and more people want to take control of their own lives and health, and are recognizing the merits of natural remedies as an alternative for popping a pill for every minor ailment. Herbs, herbal teas, vitamins, and essential oils are increasingly a staple of our kitchen shelves and medicine cabinets, and natural skincare and beauty products are finding a place in the bathroom and in the make-up bag.

Not so many years ago, alternative healing methods were regarded with some suspicion. But now there are millions of people preferring to try a cup of peppermint tea rather than take an aspirin to ease a headache, or will try meditation rather than risk becoming addicted to stress-relieving drugs.

Meditation, diet, aromatherapy, and herbs are now recognized as being valuable adjuncts to orthodox medical cancer treatments and sometimes help to alleviate the unpleasant side effects of cancer treatments such as chemotherapy and radio-therapy.

If you want to take responsibility for your health and wellness, then you will treasure the lifetime of experience and wisdom in this practical, down-to-earth guide to herbal remedies, and natural beauty and skincare products. It shows you how to use herbs and oils as potent tools for natural healing for yourself and your family, how you can help to prevent sickness with an overall healthy lifestyle, and how you can create natural personal household products.

The Essential Natural Health Bible includes an A to Z of the important herbs and essential oils and their properties along with practical pointers on buying, storing, and, if appropriate, growing the plants.

Author Nerys Purchon explains how you can treat common ailments safely with herbs and oils, and provides clear and concise instructions on how to make and use syrups, infusions, decoctions, tinctures, tonic wines, capsules, compresses, poultices, hot and cold infused oils, massage oils, ointments, creams, lotions, emulsions, eyewashes, mouthwashes, and more.

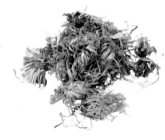

She also shows you how to create natural beauty and skincare products including luscious lotions, creams, toners, and butters for a fraction of the cost of buying from a store, and you will know exactly what you are putting on your skin and your family's.

This book doesn't take the place of professional help. If you have a sudden or severe health problem or a long-term one, then you must consult the health professionals and perhaps you will find they will encourage you to use natural therapies as a complementary treatment.

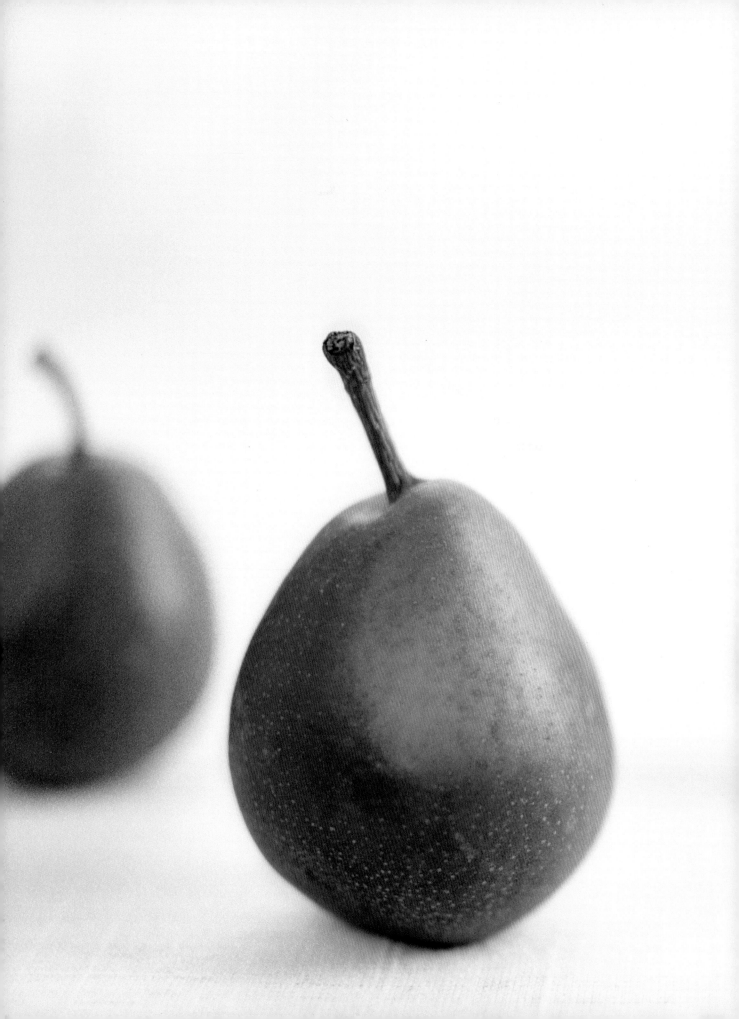

PART ONE

ESSENTIALS

We put more and more demands on our bodies and minds every day, yet we increasingly neglect them, in favor of our heavy life schedules. We need to step back and assess what are the real essentials needed for a healthy and long life. Food, exercise, relaxation, and time alone are fundamental, but we must continually re-examine our choices so we don't slip into a pattern that leaves our bodies tired and our minds stressed. This chapter will get you back on course, naturally, ready to take on the challenges of our fast and furious lives.

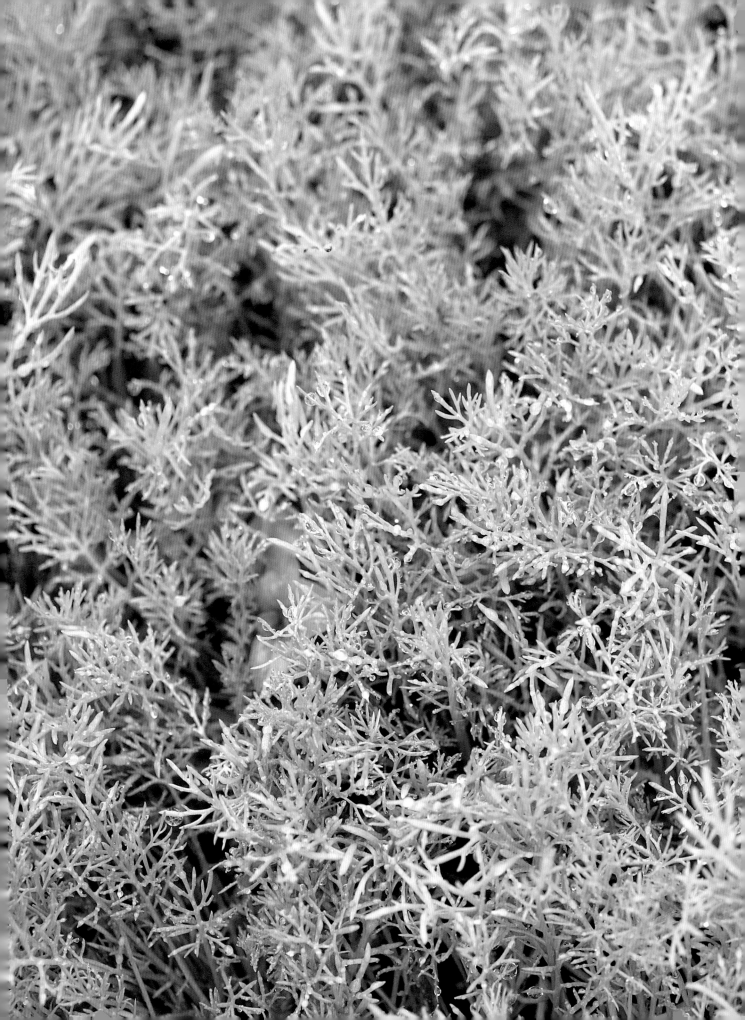

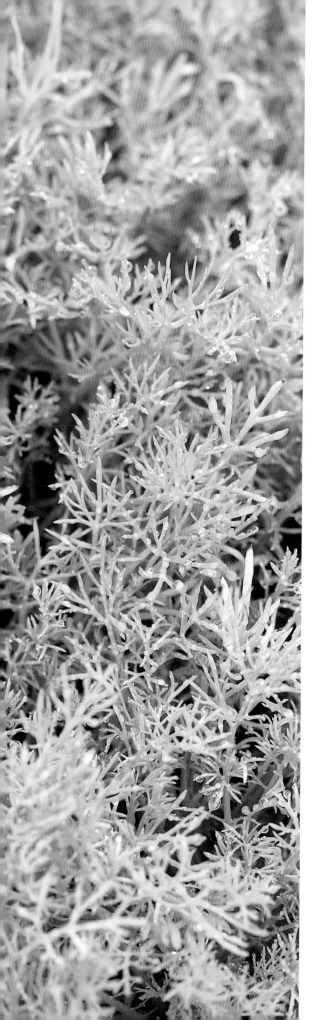

NATURAL
WELL-BEING

This chapter deals with two aspects of our

being: Body and mind. The essentials of

a good eating plan are set out along with

some truths about carbohydrates, fats,

water, and salt. The warnings are there

along with the myths. When to move more

often, and how, are explained. Then, to

complete the essentials of natural health,

there is a section on meditation. These,

then, comprise the simple first steps to

greater well-being.

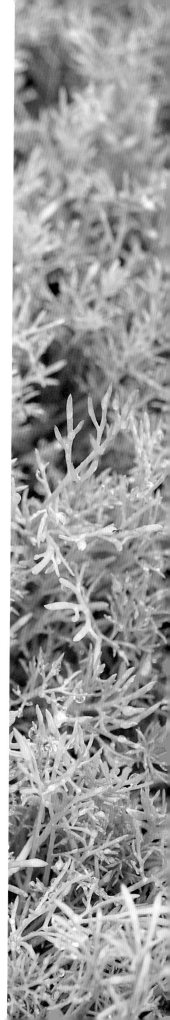

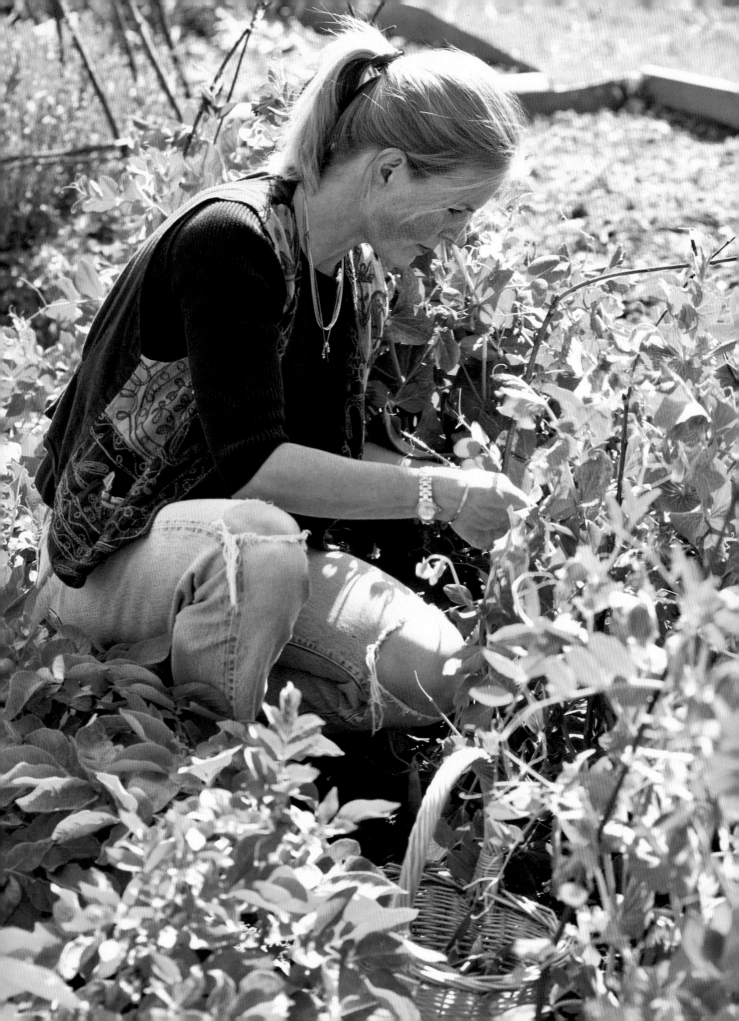

Natural health essentials

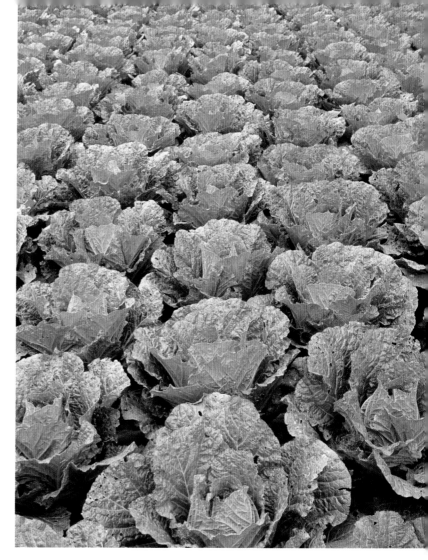

I grew up in North Wales where, for my family, the remedies for health, healing, and beautifying were all around in the fields, streams, and hedgerows. The air and soil were unpolluted where we lived, and the water was pure. The vegetables we ate were grown in the garden, without the use of pesticides or herbicides, and meat and fish we ate had grown naturally to maturity, without being dosed with antibiotics. Houses were cleaned with simple carbolic soap, hot water, and lots of elbow grease. Life was not always easy, but it was wholesome.

These days we have many domestic labor-saving devices unheard of by our grandparents. Sophisticated cleaning chemicals, washing machines, vacuum cleaners, food processors, and juicers, for example, have given us more hours to pursue careers and hobbies, but in many ways our quality of life hasn't improved. People may be better off than their parents and grandparents, but they don't always feel it, as families struggle with two parents working often long hours to pay the mortgage and educate the kids.

Personal stress levels have certainly become much higher with an accelerated pace of life. People live longer without being healthier. In fact many diseases once treatable by antibiotics are now resistant to these drugs, leaving us more vulnerable to some diseases.

Treated with proper respect and care, the human body is naturally equipped to repel disease and invading organisms. We need to build up and enhance the natural defenses of the body, and enable it to heal itself (or not get sick in the first place), with a healthy diet and lifestyle including plenty of exercise and fresh air. We often deny the body its natural function, however, and destroy many of its natural defenses by overeating fat-laden food, by not exercising or making sure we get enough sleep, by smoking

A field of lush green cabbages in a market garden.

cigarettes, or overindulging in alcohol, and by resorting to antibiotics, when a simpler solution would suffice.

We all need to learn to take more responsibility for our own health instead of handing that responsibility to others. We need to look at our lifestyle and make changes, instead of taking medications to mask the underlying problem. We need to adopt lifestyle changes for our long-term health and well-being.

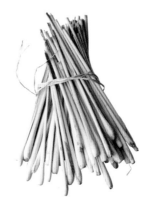

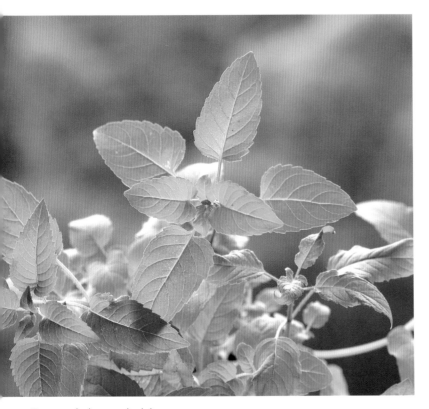

Bergamot, also known as bee balm, can be eaten in salads and fruit dishes or dried to make potpourri.

eat in secret, but our bodies know and will respond. This is not about what others think is right for them, but rather, what we feel is right for us, and us alone.

Begin by keeping a food diary. It's a little tedious at first, but soon a pattern will develop, and it will be easy to seewhen and where we are eating badly. And it's those times that we have to change. Try substituting bad eating habits with some other time-consuming habit. Make it a ritual, and before long you will have forgotten to eat at that time. Try eating different foods. Buy that fresh herb you haven't tried and add it to the everyday vegetables. It's amazing the difference it makes. Be brave with food choices, and try to fill the shopping cart with more fresh than prepared food. The fridge will look fantastic each time it's opened, and everyone will notice how quickly they are eating better. Fresh leafy vegetables, for instance, take only minutes to cook.

Next, it's time to move. Yes, like it or not, we have to move more if we want to stay healthy. Our

These changes have to be complete. There is no use changing our diet, if we do not increase our exercise. And it is no use running the streets, if we return home to a meal of high fats and instant gratification. And it is no use eating well and exercising well, if your mind is stressed.

A healthy life can only be achieved by an all-round approach to lifestyle, beginning with diet, then working through a program of exercise, reducing stress and finally a calm and centered mind through meditation.

Making the necessary changes

We must begin by thinking of everything we eat. Not just the three main meals of the day, but the in-between snacks, the drinks, both alcoholic and sugar, tea, coffee, and anything else we put in our mouths, like cigarettes. They are all adding, or subtracting, from our well-being. We can

The perfect food pyramid, showing the proportions of different foods that we should eat during a day.

bodies were designed to walk, lift, bend, and generally gather and prepare our food from scratch. And now that we don't have to do that, we need to find other reasons to get going. Of course there are gyms, but personally I find it easier to get my exercise in my own way. I clean vigorously. I make sure I carry my own heavy parcels, and call it my weight-bearing exercise. I volunteer to help family members with the big jobs around their homes, and I'm first in the garden, digging and mulching. If you live in an apartment, find other ways to get moving. There are always the stairs, but you should also think about not ordering home delivery and instead walk down and pick it up yourself. And carry that heavy load. It's much nicer to carry home your own food, than spend time in a gym lifting weights.

After we have made the changes to our body, we must also rethink the way our mind handles our modern lifestyle. We cannot allow the pressure of our lives to take over all our thinking. If we do, we will find ourselves slipping back into a lifestyle of fast food and

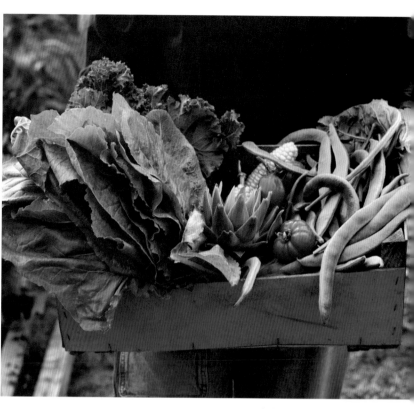

The key to good health begins with good food, preferably fresh from our own garden.

the remote control when we get home, because we don't allow our minds to let go of the day any other way. Remember that it's normal to worry, to feel anxious, and to feel overwhelmed at times. It's the continuation of these feelings that cause damage to the body and mind. Make sure that stress has an end, before moving onto the next one.

The perfect way to alleviate stress is to meditate. Meditation is now a major force in a healthy lifestyle and is being recommended by many health practitioners. It's proven to calm and center the mind, allowing it to focus on what really matters, instead of the many day-to-day occurrences in our lives. It's not hard to meditate, and it costs nothing. The right environment and time are the keys. It's simple and empowering to take such control of our minds.

Don't be put off by thinking this is all too much to take in, or to change. This is not a race. It's a lifestyle, and that can sometimes take a whole lifetime.

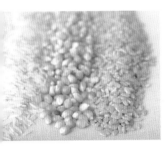

Basmati rice, an Asian staple, is a low GI rice. Corn is an excellent carb along with brown rice.

Achieving a balanced diet

The old saying "You are what you eat" is only partly true. It takes a great deal more than just food to create a holistically healthy person, but food does form a good foundation on which to build.

We hear so much about the "balanced diet," but even though there is plenty of literature available, it's not always easy to translate this into the contents of the shopping cart. In order to get and stay healthy, we need to eat foods from all the food groups: Carbohydrates (including fiber), protein, and fats. We also need vitamins, minerals and trace elements, and water.

Carbohydrates and what they do

Carbohydrates come mainly from plant foods. They are the fuel that provides energy and "staying power" for your body. These nourishing foods also contain fiber, minerals, vitamins, and protein. During digestion, carbs are broken down and absorbed into the bloodstream as glucose, which is the primary fuel for the brain. What we now

Plump ripe blueberries taste so much better straight from the garden.

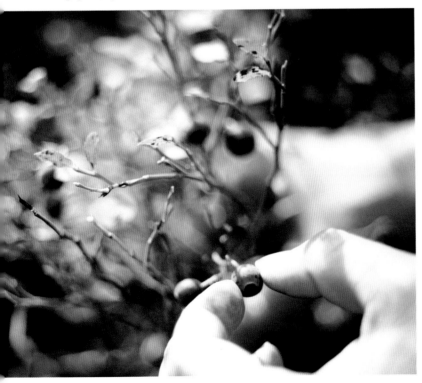

know is that not all carbs were created equal. Different carb foods behave differently in our bodies. Carbs that break down quickly have what are called high GI (glycemic index) values; those that break down slowly, releasing glucose gradually into the bloodstream have lower GI values. For most of us most of the time, low GI foods have advantages over high GI foods, especially for people with diabetes, or heart disease.

Until the last few years, carbohydrates were seen as "fattening." Foods rich in carbs include:

* Grains and grain foods, including rice, wheat, oats, barley, rye, bread, pasta, noodles, flour, and breakfast cereals.
* All fruits from temperate climates: Apples, pears, peaches, plums, apricots, and oranges. And tropical melons, bananas, pineapples, and berries of all kinds.
* Starchy vegetables such as potatoes, sweet potato, sweet corn, yams, and taro.
* Legumes including beans, chickpeas, lentils, and the favorite stand-by, baked beans
* Dairy products including milk, yoghurt, and ice cream. Cheese is not a source of carbohydrate, and foods such as butter and cream are primarily a source of saturated fat.

Fiber

Dietary fiber is a carbohydrate made up of material that forms the cell wall of plants.

* Insoluble fiber such as wheat bran can't be digested by body enzymes and passes as roughage through the body. It works mostly in the bowel where it holds water, creating soft, bulky stools, that are easier to expel. It also helps to control blood sugar and cholesterol levels and is valuable in managing diabetes.
* Soluble fiber, present in oats, legumes, and fruits, is digested by bacteria, and produces valuable acids during the process.

Get an adequate supply of both types of fiber by eating whole grain cereals, washed, unpeeled fruit, salads, and scrubbed, raw or cooked, unpeeled vegetables.

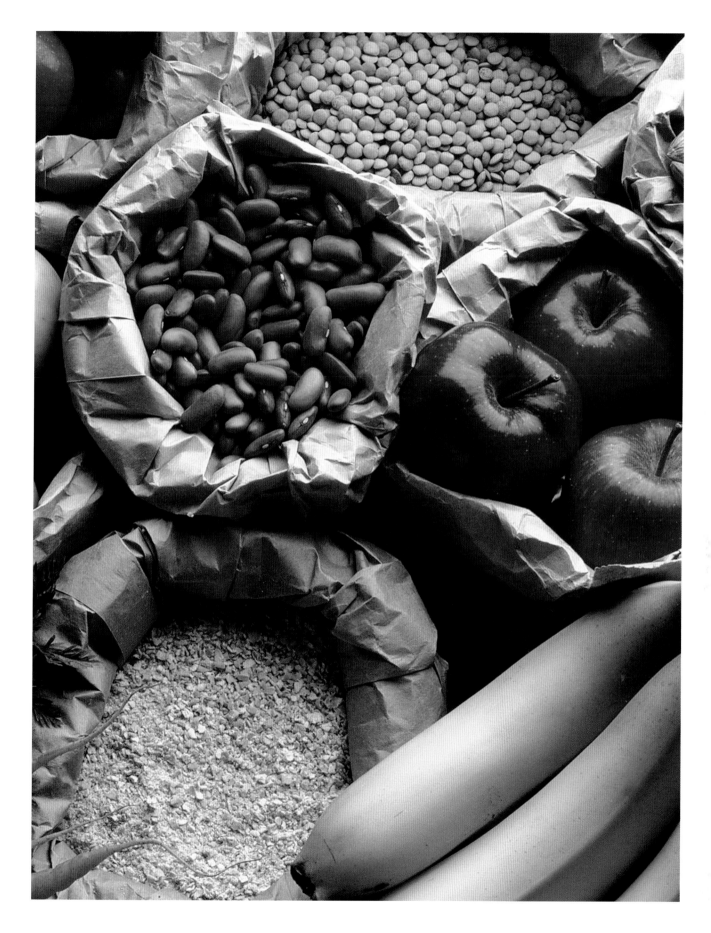

Protein and what it does

Our skin, hair, nails, tendons, muscles, and cartilages form the 20 percent protein of our body's composition. Proteins are needed for building and replacing body cells and for production of hormones and enzymes. The body can't stockpile extra protein, so you need to eat it every day. Keep your protein lean, and eat according to appetite.

Oils and fats

It's not just the quantity of fat in your diet—the type of fat in your diet can make a big difference to your health. It's important to include good fats, and cut back on foods high in saturated fat and trans fatty acids. Focus on monounsaturated and omega-3 fats.

Eat plenty of nuts, seeds, olives, and avocados, to gain unsaturated fats. Other fats, called essential fatty acids, can't be made by the body, so have to be obtained through diet. The best of these healthy fats are from seafood, polyunsaturated oil, linseed, mustard seed oil, and canola oil.

Minimize saturated fats and oils including: Fatty meats, sausages, salami, full-fat dairy products, potato crisps, cakes, cookies, pastries, pizza, and deep-fried foods, such as French fries, and fried chicken. Look for products low in saturated fat, rather than just low fat.

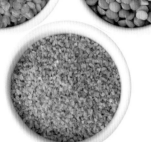

Lentils and crushed wheat can be added to many stews and casseroles to increase fiber and taste.

Rainbow food—eat every color you can find and your body will love you for it.

Vitamins and minerals

Vitamins and minerals are natural substances, present in minute amounts in food. Many people seem to harbor the delusion that if you swallow a handful of vitamin and mineral supplements, then you can eat what you like. The word "supplement" is the key.

We need vitamins and minerals for growth, and good health. These micronutrients play important roles in the body, such as making new cells and promoting healing. Some also act as antioxidants, protecting the body's cells from damage.

The best way to get the vitamins and minerals we need is to eat a balanced diet that includes plenty of fruits, vegetables, whole grains, and legumes.

To make sure your diet contains all the nutrients you need, eat by the rainbow. The pigments that give foods their color can reduce your risk of cancer, and chronic diseases. Fruits and vegetables like carrots, peaches, and apricots, are all rich in beta-carotene. The purple and red pigments (anthocyanins) in blueberries, peppers, and beetroot, function as antioxidants.

The foods with the most "pigment power" are fruits and vegetables; another reason to fill your plate with fiber-filled, fat-free, super foods! Health authorities all agree that we need to eat at least two servings of fruit and five of servings of vegetables every day.

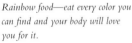

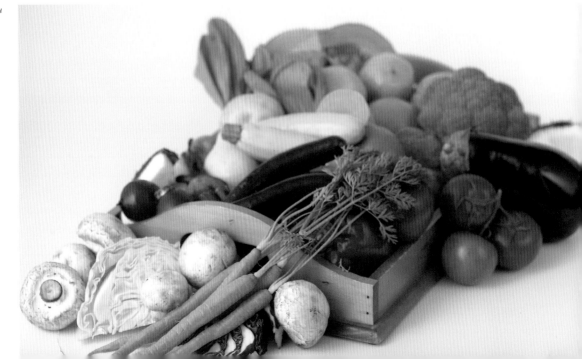

Water

In order to replace water lost through perspiration, digestive, and excretory processes, we should drink six to eight glasses of water a day. A water purifier is great as the water tastes better, and has chlorine and unwanted minerals removed. Change the filters often, or you could end up with a home for bacteria in your purifier.

Salt

Salt has always been an important commodity. The old superstition of throwing salt over your shoulder (the left please note!), if you have accidentally spilt some, dates from times when it was so precious and rare, that it was courting disaster to waste even a grain.

It is often not realized that the amount of salt that the body needs (between 0.5 and 5 grams a day) is contained naturally in fish, meat, vegetables, and grains. Yet on average we eat 8–12 grams a day, hidden in fast foods, or added in cooking, or at the table.

Too much salt may result in retention of liquids in the body, overloaded kidneys struggling to excrete excess salt and water, circulatory problems, and blood pressure.

Ways of reducing salt consumption

* Slowly reduce the amount of salt you use.
* Try using more herbs in cooking.
* Stop putting the shaker on the table.
* Avoid salty foods such as crisps, pretzels.
* Avoid preserved meats and salami.
* Eat "take-out" foods only occasionally.
* Buy only low-salt and salt-free varieties.

Food additives

On one hand we are pressured by advertising presenting convenience foods as desirable to ensure health, happiness, and well-being. On the other hand we have the purists (often uninformed), who condemn all foodstuffs not in their original state. We need to decide in an educated way which, and how much (if any), convenience food we put on our plates.

FOODS RICH IN PROTEIN INCLUDE:

* Meat (beef, pork, lamb)
* Poultry
* Fish and seafood
* Eggs
* Low-fat dairy foods such as curd (cottage) cheese, skim milk, and low-fat yoghurt
* Legumes including beans, chickpeas, and lentils, and soy products, such as tofu, and calcium-enriched soy beverages
* Nuts

If you don't eat meat, plant proteins can provide you with all the essential and non-essential amino acids you need. Eat plenty of legumes (beans, chickpeas, and lentils), foods rich in soy protein. It's even easier if you eat dairy foods and eggs.

Protein foods are excellent sources of micronutrients such as iron, calcium, zinc, vitamin B12, and omega-3 fats.

* Lean red meat is the best source of iron you can get.
* Fish and seafood are important sources of omega-3 fats.
* Dairy foods supply the highest amounts of calcium.
* Eggs are great sources of several essential vitamins and minerals, including vitamins A, D, E, and B-group vitamins, in addition to iron, phosphorus, and zinc.
* Legumes are high in fiber, B vitamins, minerals, and phytochemicals.
* Nuts are one of the richest sources of vitamin E, which, along with the selenium they contain, works as an antioxidant.

Not all additives are synthetic and, in fact, some of the natural additives (such as salt) are the most suspect in that they are dangerous to health, if used excessively. Others, notably benzoic acid, carrageenan and tragacanth can create allergic reactions in sensitive people. Many food sensitivities may be traced to additives (some synthetic colorings seem to be particular culprits).

One way to avoid overuse of canned and packaged foods, and still prepare a meal quickly, is by making and freezing/drying our own "convenience" foods. It's just as easy to make two or three dishes of lasagne, chili con carne, etc., at the weekend. Eat one tonight and freeze the rest.

Fruits and vegetables freeze well and can be bought in bulk when in season. A good food dehydrator is another way to preserve surplus fruit and vegetables.

The word "salary" comes from the Latin *salarium* which was the money allowed to Roman soldiers for the purchase of salt.

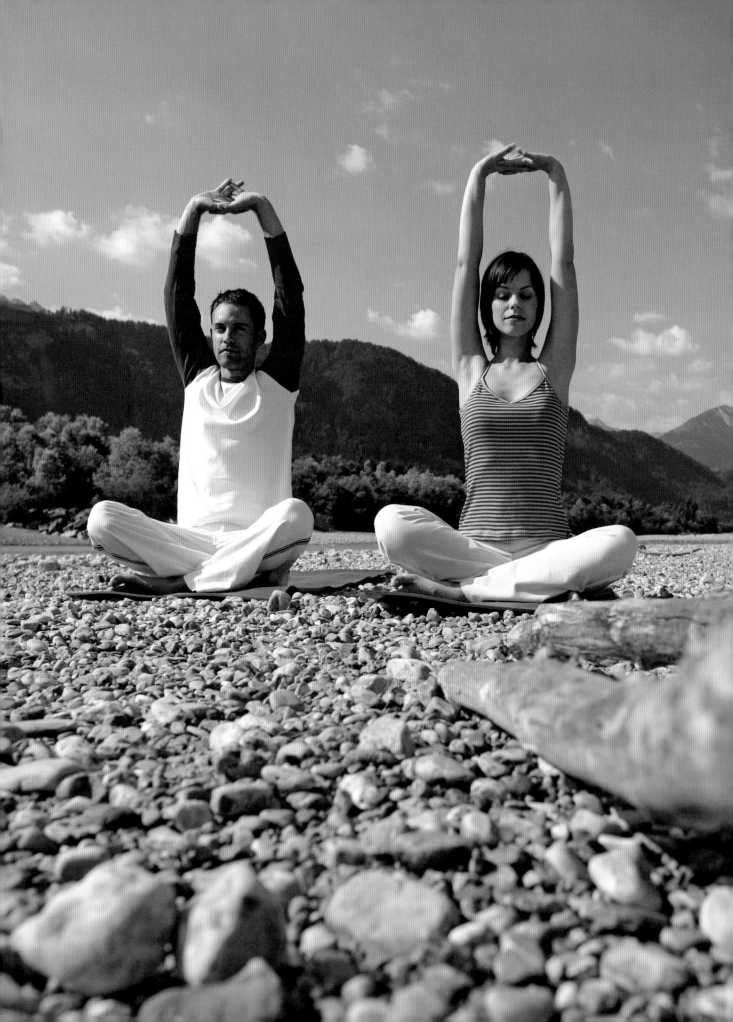

Body and mind

Diet is not the only way to look after our body and mind. We need to exercise and reduce stress, if we are to achieve good health. The body needs a pattern for life if it is to achieve perfect harmony. Excess in any part of the pattern will inhibit the other parts from functioning properly. Thus it is important to exercise in moderation, and keep stress to a minimum.

Exercise

Regular exercise stimulates the metabolic rate (which slows down dramatically if you reduce your calorie [kilojoule] intake and don't exercise). I find that a 30 minute walk in the evening about 30 minutes after dinner makes me feel really good about myself and my body. Choose the same time of day if possible, so that a habit is formed.

The older you are, the more important the exercise becomes. Your metabolic rate slows down and you need fewer calories to maintain your correct weight. Weight-bearing exercise is also needed to help prevent osteoporosis in ageing bones.

The benefits of regular exercise

We were made to move. It is what our bodies were built for. It will:
* Help lower blood pressure
* Cut heart attack, and diabetes risk
* Reduce insulin needs if you have diabetes
* Help you stop smoking
* Control weight
* Increase levels of good HDL cholesterol
* Keep bones and joints strong
* Reduce colon cancer risk
* Improve mood
* Ease depression

We now know that one of the "golden rules" for good health is to accumulate 60 minutes of physical activity every day. That includes incidental activity (the calories we burn in our everyday activities) and planned exercise. To make a real

HOW MANY STEPS?

Research has shown that we need to take every day:
* 7,500 steps to maintain weight
* 10,000 steps to lose weight
* 12,500 steps to stay very active

difference, it must be regular and some of it needs to get the heart pumping. Every single bit counts!

Make it a daily challenge to find ways to move your body. Anything that moves your limbs is not only a fitness tool, it's a stress buster. Think "move" in small increments of time. It doesn't have to be an hour in the gym, or a 45 minute aerobic dance class. That's great when you're up to it. Meanwhile, move more. Thought for the day: Cha, cha, cha...then do it!

And, whenever possible, stay standing instead of sitting. Even standing still will burn more calories than sitting on your butt!

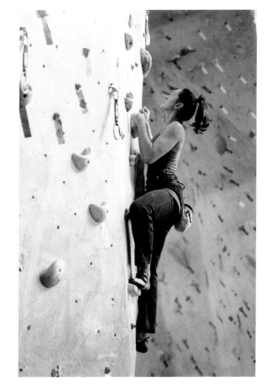

Although usually a young person's sport, climbing in any form is excellent exercise for the whole body.

Try to walk every day. You should accumulate 30 minutes or more, most days.

Planned exercise doesn't mean a gym. The key is to find some activities you enjoy. And do them regularly. Here are some ideas:

* Aerobics, exercise classes, spin sessions
* Dancing
* Exercise bikes
* Weight training is very important
* Paddling, rowing, and kayaking
* Swimming, surfing, and body surfing
* Team sports like baseball and basketball
* Tennis, squash, and other racket sports
* Yoga, Pilates, t'ai chi

Reduce stress

Stress is a constant part of our lives, and without it we would be walking cabbages.

Eustress is the healthy one that adds sparkle to our lives. We need eustress in order to function, and to be alert. It has a beginning, a middle and, most importantly, an end.

Dystress (distress) is unresolved stress that is emotionally and physically exhausting. The chemicals that our bodies produce in stressful situations, such as adrenalin, are not dispersed, and can contribute to such things

Grains, honey, and milk—a perfect and very healthy start to the day.

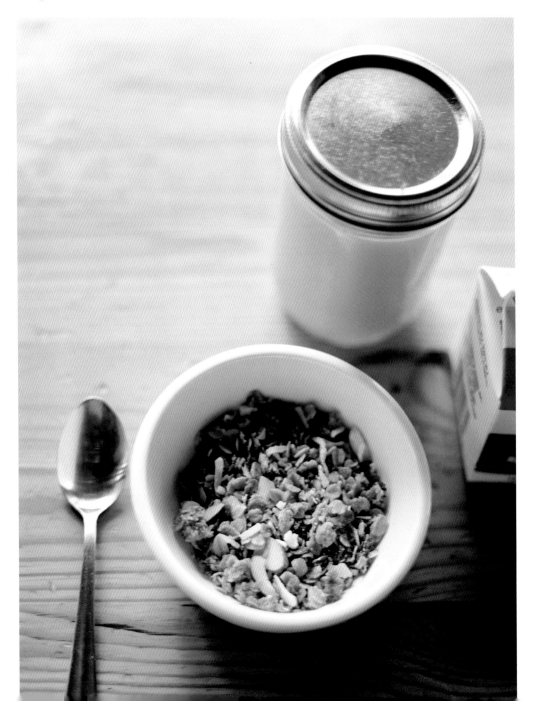

as high blood pressure, heart problems, cancer, migraine, back problems, depression, and nervous breakdowns.

If you have the following symptoms, your stress and tension levels need to be addressed before you "burn out."

* No enthusiasm for work, play, or family.
* Finding it difficult to laugh, and getting upset and irritable easily.
* A feeling of impending doom.
* Constant backaches, headaches, or stomach aches.
* An inability to sleep, or waking up in the morning feeling just as anxious and as tired as when you went to bed.

Stress busters come in many forms. Some techniques recommended by experts are to spend time out doing something you like—walk on the beach, or in a park; read a good book. Get a massage, a facial, or a haircut. Meditate!

Essential oils used in massage and oil burners can help you learn to relax. Aromatic baths are an ideal way of using essential oils to alleviate stress, insomnia, depression, and other stress-related problems. In fact, it is very difficult to lie in warm, beautifully scented water, and remain miserable, or tense! Breathe slowly and gently. As you breathe in, feel the aromatic vapors entering every cell of your body and mind, collecting all negative, tense, tired feelings into a gray mist. As you breathe out, imagine the gray mist being breathed out.

Remain in the bath for at least 30 minutes. After the bath, imagine all the tension running down the drain with the bath water.

If you have depression you really need the help of a trained therapist, especially if the depression is of long duration or is profound and affecting your life.

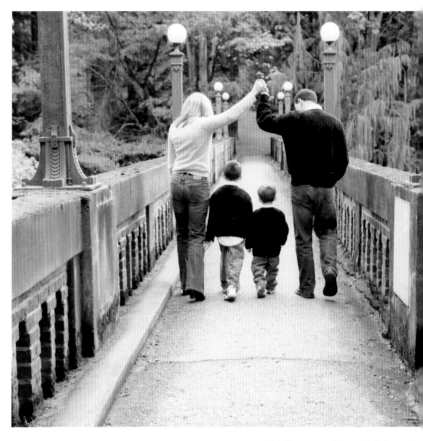

Kids love to go walking with their parents. It gives the whole family easy and enjoyable exercise.

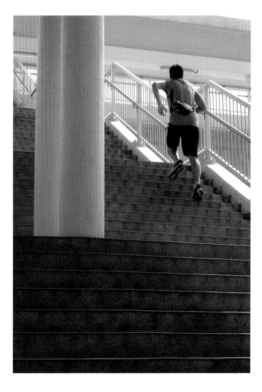

Taking the stairs doesn't have to mean a marathon. Just walking up slowly is very good for you.

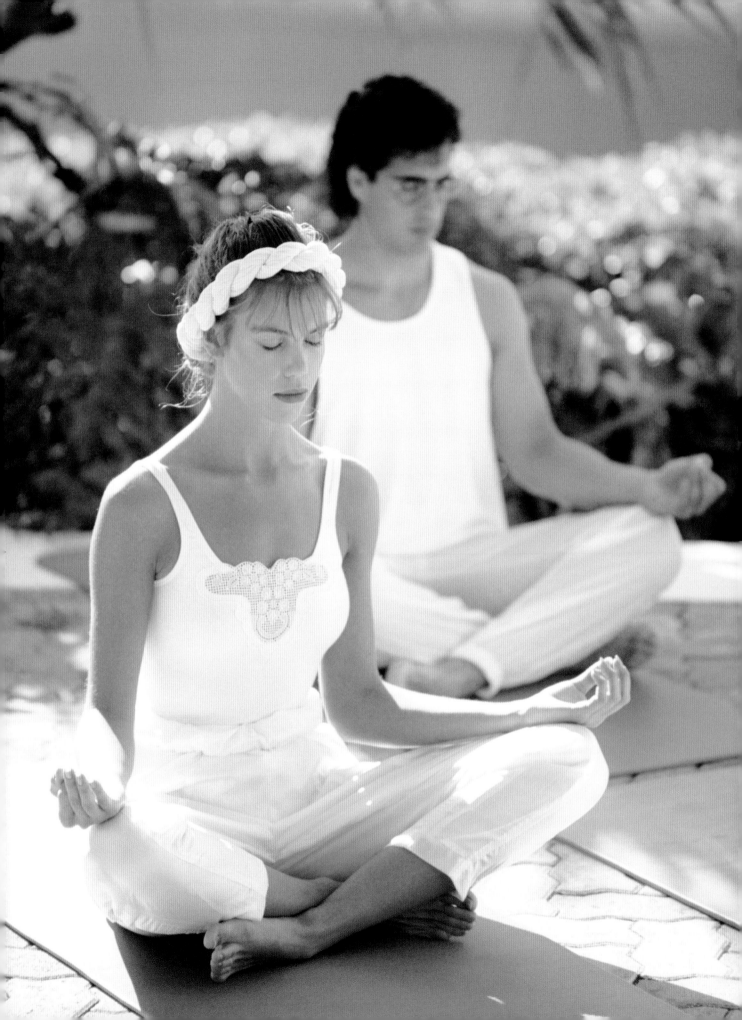

Meditation

Anyone can meditate. In fact you already meditate. It doesn't require special esoteric training, or mysterious secret mantras, but it does require time and patience.

All of us have learned special skills in our lives, such as how to walk and talk, cook, ride a bicycle, operate a computer, to play a guitar, or to speak a foreign language. So many things, all so difficult and requiring time and patience, but once mastered, able to be done intuitively.

Think about driving a car. When you began you had to remember so much: Look in the mirrors, change gears, use the accelerator, adjust the brake, steer, and on and on. You now get into the car and drive away using instinctive actions that have become part of your deep understanding.

Put simplistically, meditation is the art of doing one thing at a time. You meditate if you stop what you are doing and just "be." At first, the process of stopping will feel as difficult as learning any other skill, but slowly it will happen, and you will begin to experience positive changes in your life.

You meditate constantly without being aware of it. You are meditating when you silently, mindlessly watch the flames in the fire; when you watch the sun setting, and there is nothing but the setting sun. When you are alone with your mind drifting, not thinking, you are meditating. Whenever you are totally immersed in an experience in which time stands still, and thought processes stop, you are meditating.

When you are swimming, dancing, drumming your fingers for a long time, the thought process stops and you become the swimming not the swimmer, the dancing not the dancer, the drumming not the drummer. Thought stops and there is just the swimming, the dancing, the drumming.

You are starting on a journey of discovery, where the only thing to expect is the unexpected.

Your mind is tricky; it will resent meditation and will fight to fill your mind. It's very good at "chattering." It's been doing it for many years and won't see any good reason for stopping. Be gentle with it. When thoughts come, move them quietly to one side, tell them "later," and return to meditation. At first you will have to do this every few seconds. Don't give up, don't feel a failure: this is new to both you and your brain, and will need patience.

The idea is implanted in childhood that in order to win approval from other humans, we have to be logical, useful, and busy. We spend our lives trying to please others, and in the process we lose sight of who we are.

If we spend all our waking hours with either people, or fully occupied with work, we allow no time to be with ourselves. Unless we spend time in silence, experiencing our "aloneness," our brains remain like a cluttered attic full of our own, and other people's junk.

Begin today throwing that junk away and experiencing the freedom that comes from meditation. It won't happen overnight—it took a long time to learn to play the guitar or to speak a foreign language, and it will take time to learn to meditate. The benefits will be enormous—not only on a spiritual level, but a physical level also.

Sitting silently on a beach watching the sun begin to set... is a meditation.

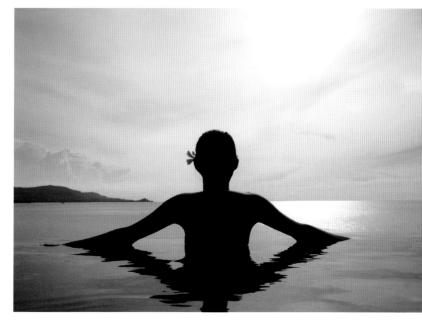

First steps

When you meditate you will find some answers to the question "Who am I?" and feel more in touch with the universe and everyone in it.

Sitting and breathing

From the three choices below, find a comfortable place to sit or lie. If you choose to sit, you need to sit straight—imagine a line from the top of your head to the base of your spine.

1. You can sit on a straight-backed chair with your feet firmly on the floor and a little apart, and your hands resting softly on your knees, palms up, second finger and thumb lightly together.

2. Or use a cushion on the floor, or sit with your back against a wall. Your legs should be folded and crossed but if this is uncomfortable they may be straight, with a cushion under the knees to prevent stress. Hands resting on your knees, palms up, second finger and thumb lightly together.

3. You can lie down with a small pillow under your head, and another under your knees (it's easy to fall asleep like this though!). Hands resting loosely by your sides, palms up, second finger and thumb lightly together.

    Sit or lie quietly for a few moments, hearing sounds far away, not analyzing them, just hearing them. Leave them and find a sound quite close to you, be aware of it without judgment, leave it, and enter your own space.

*   Feel where your body touches the surface it rests on.
*   Feel all the spaces where the body doesn't touch.
*   Feel the clothes touching your body.
*   Feel your heart beating, sending blood around your body to nourish you.
*   Feel the breath easily and lightly entering and leaving your body.

Clearing your mind is easier if you can clear yourself of your normal environment.

Sitting silently on a beach watching the sun begin to set, Feeling the breeze as it touches your skin... Is a meditation. Seeing the changing colors With your heart and not your mind. Feeling the breeze without thinking ... Is a meditation.

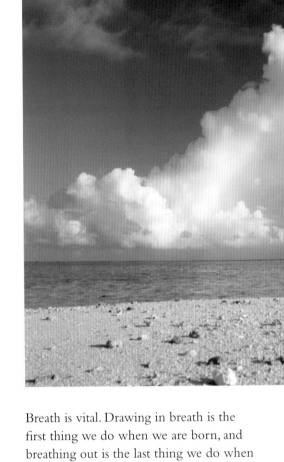

Breath is vital. Drawing in breath is the first thing we do when we are born, and breathing out is the last thing we do when we die. We can live for about four weeks without food, four days without water, and only four minutes without air, and yet we have almost forgotten how to breathe.

Remember, shallow breathing creates tension; deep breathing releases tension.

Take your attention to your breath, keep your shoulders loose and relaxed and forget about your chest. Imagine that in your belly you have a balloon. As you gently breath in through your nose, the balloon inflates until it fills your belly space. As you breath out through your mouth, the balloon slowly deflates, until it's quite flat.

When you are nervous, tense, or angry, STOP, drop your shoulders and take three or four deep "belly breaths." Your tension, will begin to dissipate, leaving you in control once again.

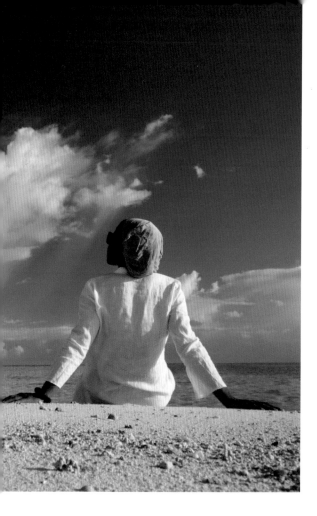

Relaxation

Devote the first few minutes of each meditation time to relaxation. First the breathing.

Take each breath slowly and gently into the dark, secret place deep within you, where you feel at peace.

As you release the breath, release any fear, hostility, anger, or sadness. Experience the feelings flowing out with each breath.

Keep the breathing relaxed and easy, taking peace and tranquility into your body and releasing negativity as breath flows out.

Now that you have relaxed your mind, you are ready to begin relaxing your body. Do all the movements and breathing very slowly, and quietly.

At first, the breathing and relaxing may take up most of your allotted meditation time. Don't worry—this is needed until you are practiced in the technique. After a while you will be able to relax very quickly by breathing deeply.

TIME OUT

"Time Out" is for everyone: Women, men, and children. Somehow the idea of taking time to cherish yourself seems to be confined to women (who rarely do it), but children enjoy pampering and are the best meditators, and men are slowly getting the idea that it's all right to take care of your body and soul.

Budget time in the same way as you budget money. Thirty minutes can be spent on: A facial steam, a pack or scrub, a manicure or pedicure, a walk or swim, a meditation. One hour can be spent on: A deep facial, a hair treatment, a massage, a luxurious bath. Half a day, or even one whole day a month can be spent as follows:

- Do a deal with the family—if each person has a "Time Out" day each month or so, the rest of the family will relieve the family member of chores for this day. You will all feel more appreciative of each other and completely renewed after giving yourself this break. You might like to follow some or all of my suggestions.
- Sleep in as late as you want, have your favorite breakfast in bed, read a book, listen to some music, meditate—whatever.
- Prepare what you need for a facial steam, and put it on to simmer. Prepare a hair rinse at the same time.
- Heat the bathroom if it's cold, and collect everything you will need, including oils or mixtures for the bath, soap, two big fluffy towels, a book, incense.
- Apply a pre-shampoo treatment to your hair.
- Steam the face for 5–10 minutes, splash with cool water.
- Make a face mask.
- Begin to run the bath, adding anything you fancy.
- Make your favorite drink, retire to the bathroom and shut the door.
- Body-brush from head to foot, shower if you like, then climb into a hot bath.
- Spend as long as you like sipping your drink, reading your book, or just enjoying the luxury of allowing yourself to do nothing.
- When you are ready, you can spread the mask on your face and then begin to pay some attention to your hands and feet. Scrub the nails, push the softened cuticles back very gently with an orange stick, pumice any rough patches on soles or heels.
- Time to leave the bath and wash the face mask off in the shower with lukewarm water. Wash your hair with one of the herbal shampoos and rinses and finishes.
- Wrap your head in a towel, and dry your body. Massage some moisture lotion over your entire body and face.
- Time for another drink, and maybe something to eat (my favorite is feta and avocado salad, and my husband's home-made bread).
- Now brush your hair, file the nails on your hands and feet, and massage some hand cream into them.
- This is the point where I dress, then take the dogs for a walk, and call at the video store for a good movie. I must confess that this is also the time when I indulge my tastebuds, and buy some chocolate to go with the movie—an end to a perfect day!

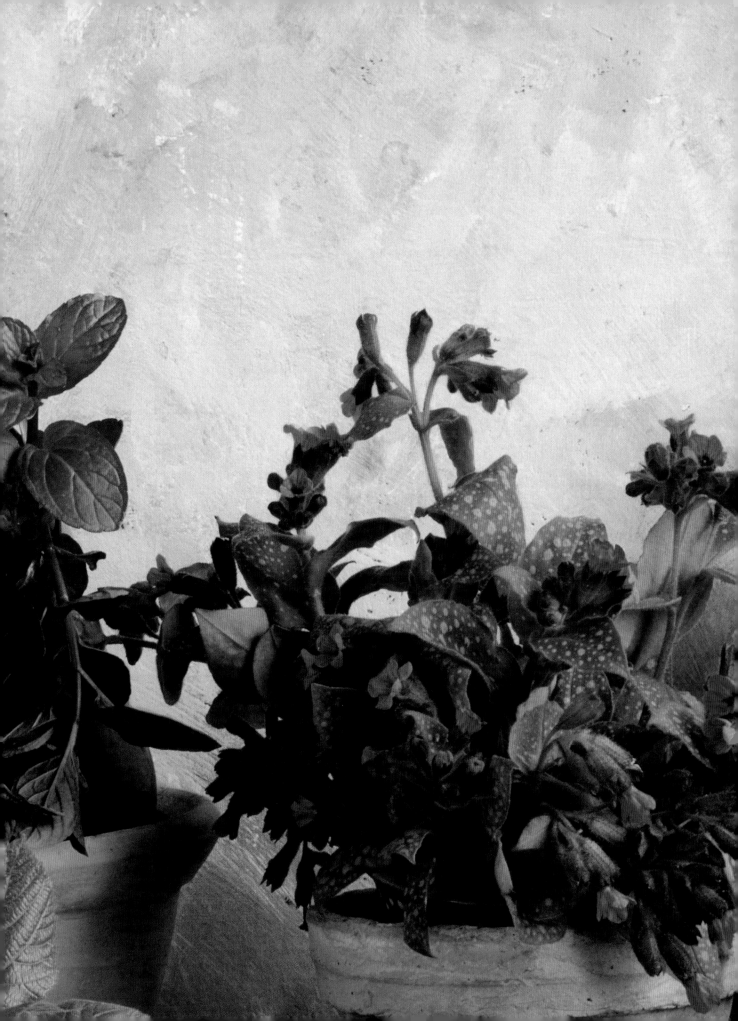

NURTURE
AND
NOURISH

Throughout the ages, herbs have been gathered from the wild or specially cultivated for their unique medicinal and aromatic qualities. They have played a key role in health and well-being, they make all the difference to the food we eat [including wines and liqueurs], and they have long been prized for the aromatic and toning qualities they bring to cosmetics, toiletries, and perfumes.

This book is designed to provide you with an easy way to learn about every aspect of herbs and oils. You can begin your collection in a small way, enlarging it as you become more confident. Buy your herbs, oils, plants, or seeds from reputable sources and only if the label carries the correct botanical name.

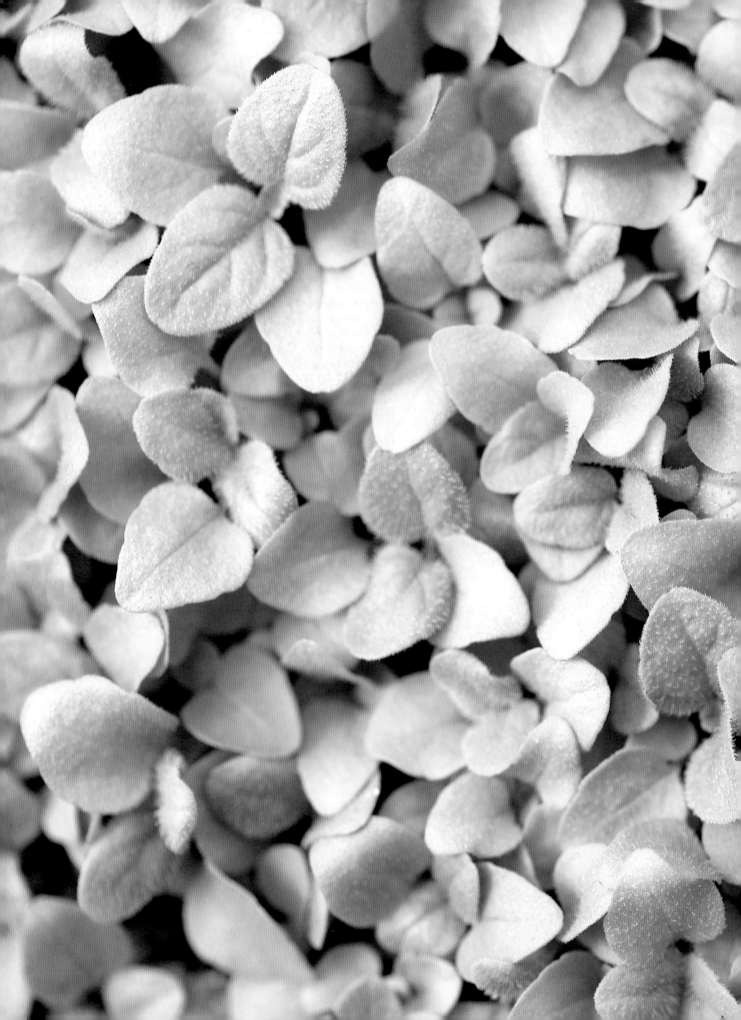

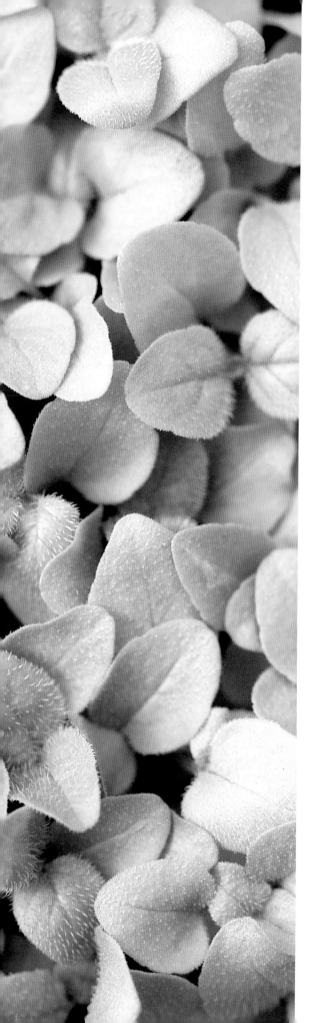

THE NATURAL PHARMACY

What a perfect name to describe this chapter. It's a wealth of knowledge on the herbs and their attributes and how to grow, harvest, and store them. There is no better place to find the remedies we all need than in our own garden, and here is where you start. Not everything can be grown, but you do need the information about the herbs and oils before you buy them. And then, when you're ready, head to the nursery and begin your own natural pharmacy.

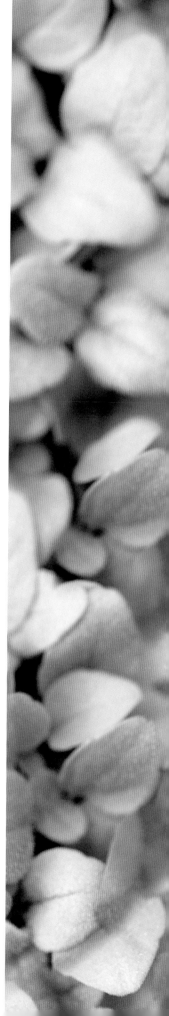

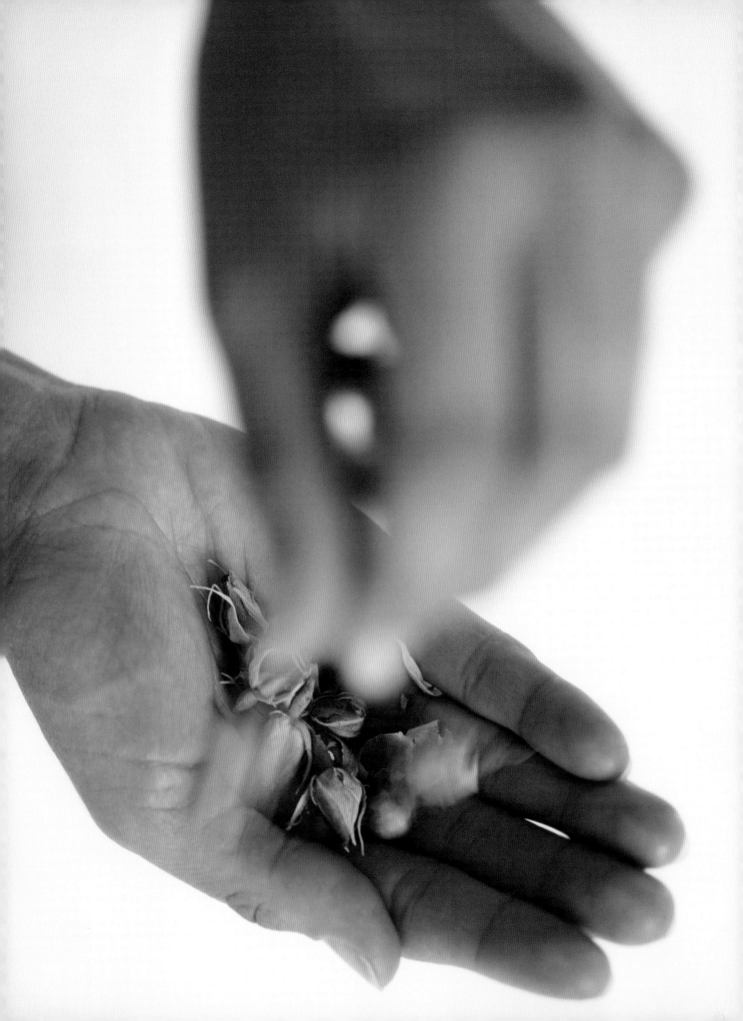

Using herbs and essential oils

Using herbs

What exactly are herbs? If you visit your plant nursery today you'll probably find a special section for herbs packed with punnets of green leafy plants. But this is a very small part of the herb story. In its broadest sense, the term "herbs" encompasses the astonishing diversity of plants from around the world that are valued for their therapeutic or aromatic qualities from tall trees to tiny ground covers, or favorite flowers.

Today, herbs are attracting more attention and emerging as scientifically proven and accepted remedies for treating everyday ailments, strengthening the immune system, fighting bacteria, fungi, and viruses, reducing stress levels and toning, relaxing, and strengthening the muscles. In fact, they are assisting the body to heal itself.

In addition, herbs and essential oils enable us to create cruelty-free toiletries, including soaps, shampoos, and skin-care preparations.

The "Properties of herbs and essential oils" table (pages 45–9) describes the therapeutic properties, gives the technical terms for these properties, and lists the herbs and essential oils that are important in each category.

The plant profiles that follow in the A–Z section will help you become familiar with the herbs, understand their properties, be confident about using them safely, and learn how to grow them in your own garden.

Throughout the book, herbs are referred to by their common name because that's the one we are all most familiar with. However, if you intend to make a serious study of herbs or use them in any of the many ways suggested in this book, you will also need to learn the botanical names (genus and species), as this is the only way to accurately identify the plants. For this reason, the A–Z

WHAT ARE ESSENTIAL OILS?

Essential oils have been variously described as the life force or essence of plants. Pure essential oils are the end products of distillation (or other methods of extraction) of the aromatic substances or essences found in plants. They are widely used in therapeutic massage and in the pharmaceutical, cosmetic, and perfume industries today. The oils are volatile, evaporate on exposure to air, and have a powerful aroma. Essential oils differ from cooking or fixed oils in that they are not oily to the touch, and they evaporate when exposed to air.

The essences are composed of molecules small enough to penetrate the skin and enter the bloodstream, and are employed in many ways including massage oils, fomentations and compresses, antiseptics and tonic waters, creams and healing ointments, beauty and skin-care products, cleansers, and antibacterial sprays, and more.

section is organized alphabetically by the plant's botanical name.

Some words of warning
* This book is not intended to take the place of advice from your health practitioner. Remember that even simple symptoms can mask serious complaints. If symptoms are severe or of long duration, the condition needs to be assessed professionally.
* Just because herbs are "natural" doesn't make them safe. Any herb, whether used internally or externally, can produce unexpected reactions in some people.
* All herbs and essential oils need to be treated with respect. If a recipe or formula calls for one gram or drop, two will **not** be better.

Opposite: *Dried rosebuds can be used to make a rejuvenating tea.*

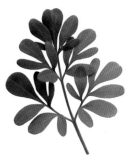

Mrs M. Grieve published *A Modern Herbal* in 1931 with descriptions of over 1,000 herbs covering their medicinal, culinary, and cosmetic uses along with a wealth of information on cultivation and folklore. It is available in paperback [two volumes] and online at www.botanical. com

HOW PLANTS ARE NAMED

Why the botanical name matters

Plants can have numerous common names. I don't know how many plants there are bearing the common name of "all heal." Mrs Grieve who published *A Modern Herbal* in 1931 mentions three. Bruisewort and colic root are other examples of widely used names. I recently saw a punnet of plants in the nursery labeled Queen Anne's lace, but when I looked at the botanical name it was something quite different from the herb used medicinally. Had I not known the botanical name I could have grown and used the plant with possible serious consequences. That's why it is essential to learn the genus and the species names of herbs.

Genus and species

This system of naming is called the binomial system, comprising two parts: *Genus* and *species*. Genus and species are usually written in italic, with a capital letter for the genus. A genus is a group of lower rank than a family, and species are the different varieties within the genus. Family names are usually written in roman type with a capital letter to start, e.g. Umbelliferae. Genus and species names are usually used together, e.g. *Borago officinalis*. There are sometimes disagreements among botanists about these relationships. You will often see the name, shortened name, or initial of the botanist who classified the plant added to the genus and species name, e.g. *Borago officinalis* L. (the L. here means it was classified by Linnaeus). The species name *"officinalis"* means that the plant is recognized in the pharmacopoeia as having medicinal value. The herbs in the plant profiles section are organized by genus.

Family

This is a group of plants having the same characteristics e.g.

Umbelliferae: With hollow stems
Leaves: Alternate, deeply divided
Flowers: Compound terminal or lateral umbels
Stamens: Five, alternating with petals
Examples: Parsley, angelica, anise, caraway

Labiatae: Having quadrangular stems
Leaves: Opposite
Flowers: Axillary cymes, calyx five-toothed, corolla usually forms two lips
Ovary: Four-lobed, each containing one seed
Examples: Catnep, marjoram, oregano

Common name

This is the name by which most people know a plant.

The layout adopted in the A–Z section is:

Genus	Species	Family	Common name
Borago	*officinalis*	Boraginaceae	Borage
Petroselinum	*crispum*	Apiaceae	Parsley

Ways in which herbs can be used

The following list sets out some of the culinary, medicinal, and cosmetic uses of herbs that have natural beauty care or healing recipes in this book. Herbs can be:

* Added fresh or dried to cooking, to make herbal vinegars or oils, to flavor wines and liqueurs, and to combine with fruit and vegetable juices
* Simmered or steeped in hot water to make teas, tisanes, infusions, decoctions, and macerations
* Combined with alcohol or glycerine to make tinctures
* Used fresh or dried to make compresses, poultices, and fomentations
* Combined with oils to make infused oils
* Powdered to make lozenges, pills, capsules, and pastes
* Incorporated in cosmetic creams, lotions, and healing ointments
* Used in shampoos, conditioners, and hair tonics
* Used to strengthen the perfume of potpourris
* Used to add antibacterial and antiviral qualities to room freshener sprays
* Used in preparations for pets, to heal skin conditions, and repel fleas
* Added to floor and furniture cleaners

All the herbs included in the book are basically very safe herbs and many of them are very easy to obtain and grow in your own garden. Even if you don't live in a climate in which these herbs will grow, to use them safely you need information about them. Herbs such as foxglove, aconite, and many others have been omitted as they contain substances called alkaloids, some of which can be toxic in overdose.

As well as describing the more common herbs, I have also included some of the more exotic herbs in the plant profile section, such as cat's claw, as they are gaining in popularity.

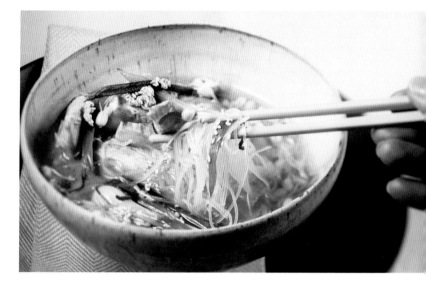

Some herbs can be added to food, often in the last few minutes of cooking so that the active ingredients are not destroyed in the process.

Where care needs to be exercised there is a "caution" in the description.

All herbs need to be treated with respect. If a recipe or formula calls for one gram, two grams will **not** be better.

__Caution__ Many people who do not appreciate the properties of herbs consider them harmless. This is a dangerous misconception. To be of use, any herb needs pharmacological activity. This is the property that can alter the state of the body, and, when used correctly, promote healing and well-being. That's why when you make and use your own preparations, there are a few cautions to be observed.

* Ensure that the herb you are about to use is the correct one. Check, and check again, using the botanical (binomial) name for reference. You will find all the botanical names in the plant profile A–Z section.
* If you intend making a tincture for internal use, make sure that the alcohol you use is safe for consumption. Rubbing alcohol is not suitable.
* Adhere to the dose recommendations.
* If the problem is severe or of long duration seek the help of a medical practitioner. After the nature of the problem is established, you can then suggest that you would like to use herbs as part of your healing process.

Ways in which essential oils can be used

The most wonderful thing about essential oils is that they are available to everyone and, once you understand the basic concepts and observe the appropriate methods and procedures, they are very simple to use. The best-known way to employ the oils is through massage but, as you will see in this book, there are many more ways to use the oils. Essential oils can be:

* Incorporated with carrier oils to make massage oils
* Added to water to be used as fomentations and compresses
* Added in minute quantities to baths
* Added to alcohol to make toilet waters and perfumes
* Incorporated with a carrier to make insect repellents
* Used in shampoos, conditioners, and hair tonics
* Used to strengthen the perfume of potpourri
* Used to add antibacterial and antiviral qualities to room freshener sprays
* Used in preparations for pets, to heal skin conditions, and repel fleas
* Added to floor and furniture cleaners

Blending essential oils

The theory behind blending is that the sum of the whole is greater than the individual parts. If you blend three or four essential oils having the same or very similar therapeutic properties, you have created a synergistic blend that is more powerful than the individual oils used on their own. It's probably best not to use more than three to four essential oils in blends until you are very familiar with all the individual oils, and what each of them can do.

Caution Used externally and in the correct manner and dilution, most oils are perfectly safe but there are a few that have special properties which can cause problems under certain conditions.

* Essential oils should only be used internally on the advice of a qualified aromatherapist or naturopath.
* Keep the essential oils out of the reach of children—they could be lethal if taken,

INFUSED OILS

Basically, infused oils are produced by soaking wilted or well-dried plant material in warm oil over a period of time. It is probably the oldest method of herbal extraction, and was used thousands of years before distillation and other methods were devised. Infused oils have many of the properties of essential oils, and also the benefits of other plant substances not in essential oils. The resulting oil is not as strong. Don't use fresh herbs as their water content could cause bacteria to grow and spoil the oil. One of the main advantages of this method is that it makes it possible to utilize many plants that yield either very little or no essential oil but which are immensely useful.

Neroli, rose, chamomile, jasmine, and melissa are all very expensive essential oils. Beautiful, effective, and inexpensive massage oils can be made from these plants by using the infusion method, see Practicalities page 504.

Neroli
When making infused oil use the flowers.
Rose
When making infused oil use the petals.
Chamomile
When making infused oil use the flowers.
Jasmine
When making infused oil use the flowers.
Melissa
When making infused oil use the leaves and flowers.

PHOTOTOXICITY

Certain chemicals when applied to the skin can cause an excessive reaction to sunlight (or sunlamps) for up to 12 hours (and possibly for much longer) after application. The combination of oil plus sunlight can result in burns that can range from mild to very severe depending on whether the oils are used undiluted or diluted. Even the use of a mere 0.4 percent of some oils can cause the phototoxic effect. Take note of the cautions on the profiles of the individual oils regarding this.

Sensitization

A gradual build-up of an allergic reaction and intolerance to a substance even when used in minuscule amount. This sensitivity may be scarcely apparent on first application, but if the substance is used more often the reaction usually worsens steadily. Take note of the warnings on the label and patch test.

Skin irritants

Unlike sensitization that may develop over a considerable period, irritation and inflammation may occur on the first application of a substance. The severity and reaction is dependent on the amount of substance used, and the "reactiveness" of the person. Some essential oils can produce skin irritation ranging from very severe to mild. If you have sensitive skin, or if you develop allergic reactions frequently, you would be wise to use a patch test before applying any unfamiliar substance to your skin.

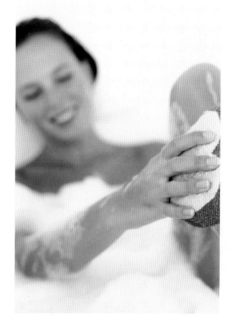

Some herbal preparations need to be patch tested at appropriate concentrations before you immerse yourself in them. Don't ignore warnings or cautions.

even in small quantities (see "First aid procedures," page 422).

* It is essential that you read the cautions associated with the oils provided, as some must be avoided during pregnancy, and others are toxic in large quantities.
* Most of the essential oils should be combined with a carrier oil such as sweet almond oil or olive oil, before using on the skin as they are too strong to use alone.
* Always use the appropriate proportions of the essential oils and the carrier oil. The total amount of essential oils should rarely exceed three or four percent of the total amount, and some oils should be used in far smaller amounts.

* Use only the best quality essential oils—there are many synthetic oils now on the market. Look for the label that states 100 percent pure and natural essential oil. The synthetic oils are usually called fragrant oil, compounded oil. or perfume oil. Descriptions like these mean that the oil is likely to be synthetic and has no therapeutic properties at all.
* The cautions and suggestions for quantities to use need to be carefully observed. The difference in action between one and two drops can be very great.

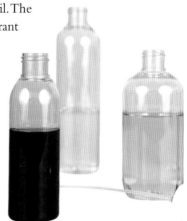

Buying essential oils

Make sure when you choose packaged herbs and essential oils, that the containers are properly labeled with all the information you need. The label should tell you:

* The common or popular name for the herb or oil (such as "tea tree")
* Its botanical name (tea tree is *Melaleuca alternifolia*)
* The instructions for use and any warnings or cautions such as:

> *"For external use only"*
> *"Keep out of reach of children"*
> *"Not to be used at more than three percent (or whatever is applicable, some oils can only be used at 0.5 percent)"*
> *"Not to be used during pregnancy"*

Don't buy any essential oil product that doesn't include the botanical name on the label. The botanical name is essential because many of the oils have the same common name—which could lead to mistakes being made.

For example:
Tagetes (*Tagetes patula, T. minuta, T. erecta*) oil is often sold as calendula or marigold oil. True calendula (*Calendula officinalis*) oil is only produced in very small quantities and is difficult to obtain. Tagetes oil is distilled from French, African, or Mexican marigolds. The two must not be confused, as *Tagetes* spp. oil doesn't have the same therapeutic properties of calendula, and is very phototoxic.

Thuja (*Thuja occidentalis*) is sometimes sold as white cedar oil or cedar leaf oil. This oil is severely toxic due to its high alpha and beta thujone content, and deaths have been reported from its oral use. The oil names "white cedar" should not be confused with Atlas cedar (*Cedrus atlantica*), which is the appropriate aromatherapy oil to use.

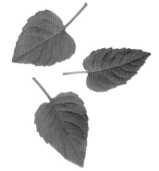

The Chinese have been using herbs for thousands of years and today there are herb pharmacies all over China.

Lemon verbena (*Aloysia tryphilla*) oil is difficult to obtain and the oil sold as lemon verbena is often a blend of citrus oils. However, true lemon verbena oil presents many hazards and it might be safer to use the blend!

Melissa (*Melissa officinalis*) oil is very costly, as huge amounts of plant materials are needed to produce a very small amount of oil. Most of the melissa essential oil offered is adulterated with other lemon-scented oils.

Where to buy your oils?

There is very little regulation regarding the quality or type of essential oils available. This is why I always recommend that you select brands well-known for their quality from reputable outlets.

For example, it is very rare to find essential oils that are inappropriate for home aromatherapy in leading health food stores or aromatherapy specialist outlets. I have, however, occasionally come across them in market stalls.

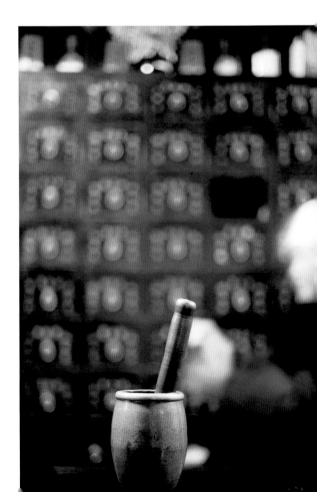

FOR PROFESSIONALS ONLY

The following essential oils are not for the home aromatherapist because they all contain high percentages of toxic, narcotic, abortifacient (capable of producing abortion), or carcinogenic chemicals. Some are safe (used according to the instructions) as infused oils.

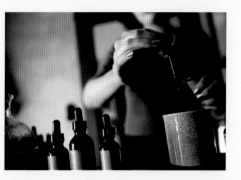

Almond, bitter (unrectified)	*Prunus amygdalus*
Aniseed	*Pimpinella anisum*
Armoise (mugwort)	*Artemisia herba-alba*
Arnica	*Arnica montana*
Birch, sweet	*Betula lenta*
Buchu	*Agathosma betulina*
Calamus	*Acorus calamus*
Camphor, white, brown, yellow	*Cinnamomum camphora*
Cassia	*Cinnamomum cassia*
Costus	*Saussurea costus*
Elecampane	*Inula helenium*
Elemi	*Canarium luzonicum*
Horseradish	*Armoracia rusticana*
Lemon verbena	*Aloysia tryphilla*
Mustard	*Brassica nigra*
Oakmoss	*Evernia prunastri*
Oregano	*Origanum vulgare*
Pennyroyal	*Mentha pulegium*
Sage	*Salvia officinalis*
Sassafras	*Sassafras albidum*
Savin	*Juniperus sabina*
Savory	*Satureja hortensis*
Tansy	*Tanacetum vulgare*
Tarragon	*Artemisia dranunculus*
Thuja and western red cedar	*Thuja occidentalis, T. plicata*
Wintergreen	*Gaultheria procumbens*
Wormseed	*Chenopodium ambrosioides*
Wormwood	*Artemisia absinthium*

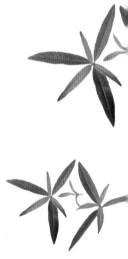

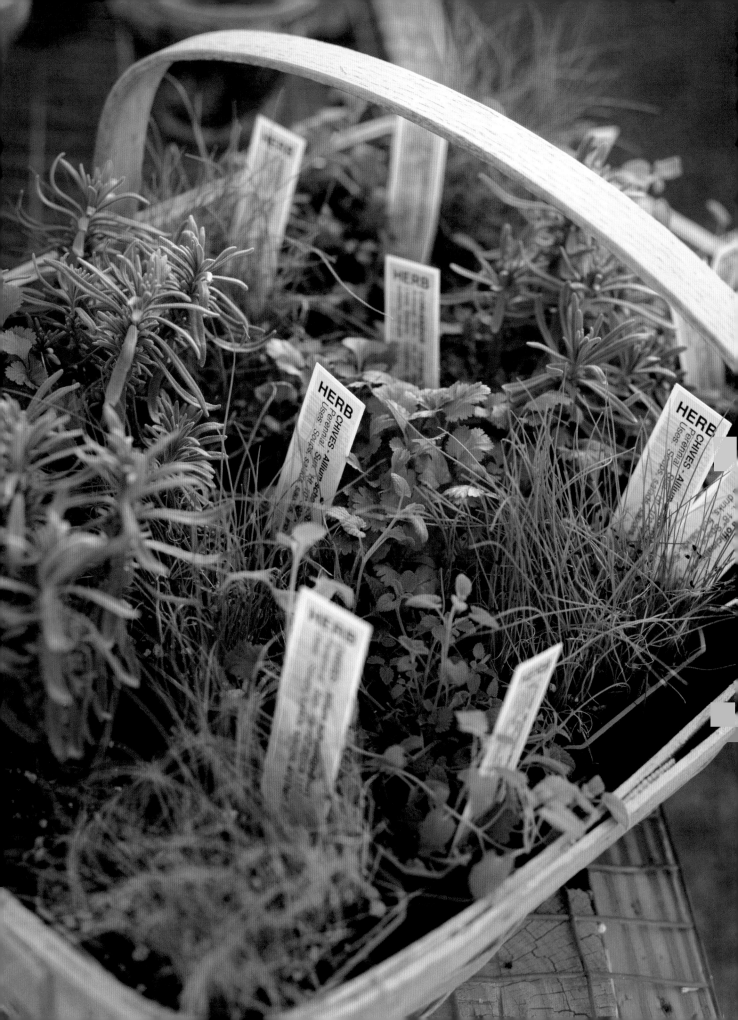

Properties of herbs and essential oils

Following are the medical terms that you will encounter when reading books on the medicinal uses of herbs and essential oils. It is far from being a comprehensive list and it contains only those herbs and essential oils that are included in this book.

If, on consulting a recipe for a particular condition, you find you do not have some of the herbs or essential oils recommended, you can simply choose another from the same category.

Alterant or adaptogen	Gradually produces a beneficial change in bodily functions *Herbs:* Astragalus, burdock, devil's claw, echinacea, garlic, ginseng, goldenseal, meadowsweet, nettle, red clover, violet, yarrow, yellow dock
Analgesic	Relieves or diminishes pain by exerting a nerve-numbing effect *Herbs:* Chamomile, devil's claw, mullein, passionflower, peppermint, skullcap, valerian, willow bank *Essential oils:* Bergamot, chamomile, eucalyptus, lavender, marjoram, peppermint, rosemary
Anaphrodisiac	Reduces sexual response *Essential oils:* Marjoram
Antibiotic	Combats infection in the body *Herbs:* Astragalus, echinacea, garlic, goldenseal, nettle, St John's wort *Essential oils:* Cajuput, garlic, manuka, niaouli, ravensara, tea tree
Antidepressant	Helps to lift the emotions from a depressed state *Herbs:* Ginkgo, lavender, lemon balm, rosemary, passionflower, St John's wort *Essential oils:* Bergamot, clary sage, geranium, grapefruit, jasmine, lavender, lemon grass, mandarin, melissa, neroli, orange, petitgrain, rose, rosemary, sandalwood, ylang-ylang
Anti-emetic	Helps to reduce and control vomiting and nausea *Herbs:* Dill, fennel, ginger, meadowsweet, peppermint *Essential oils:* Star anise, black pepper, chamomile, clove, fennel, ginger, peppermint, spearmint
Anti-inflammatory	Reduces inflammation *Herbs:* Calendula, cat's claw, chamomile, curcumin (extract of tumeric), devil's claw, goldenseal, feverfew, lavender, licorice, meadowsweet, nettle, rue, St John's wort, saw palmetto, turmeric, violet, willow bark, witch hazel *Essential oils:* Bergamot, chamomile, immortelle, lavender, myrrh

Antiseptic	Helps to control or destroy infection-causing bacteria *Herbs:* Calendula, echinacea, eucalyptus, lavender, nasturtium, shepherd's purse, tea tree, thyme, violet, wormwood, yarrow *Essential oils:* Most essential oils have some antiseptic qualities but the following are particularly good—bergamot, eucalyptus, garlic, juniper, lavender, manuka, niaouli, ravensara
Anti-spasmodic	Prevents or relieves cramps and/or spasms in the intestines or uterus *Herbs:* Angelica, anise, catnep, chamomile, cramp bark, dill, fennel, garlic, goldenseal, gotu kola, horehound, hyssop, lavender, lemon balm, licorice, marjoram, peppermint, skullcap, valerian, yarrow *Essential oils:* Chamomile, clary sage, ginger, juniper, lavender, marjoram, orange, peppermint
Anti-sudorific	Reduces sweating *Herbs:* Sage *Essential oils:* Clary sage, cypress
Anti-toxic	Counteracts the effects of a poison *Herbs:* Lavender *Essential oils:* Bergamot, black pepper
Antiviral	Combats or inhibits the growth of viruses *Herbs:* Cat's claw, eucalyptus, garlic, goldenseal, tea tree *Essential oils:* Bergamot, eucalyptus, garlic, lavender, manuka, palmarosa, ravensara, tea tree
Aperient	An opening, laxative agent *Herbs:* Burdock, dandelion root, licorice, psyllium seed, yellow dock
Aphrodisiac	Increases sexual response *Essential oils:* Clary sage, jasmine, neroli, patchouli, rose, rosewood, sandalwood, vetiver, ylang-ylang
Aromatic	Adds pleasant taste and odour to medicines *Herbs:* Anise, angelica, caraway seed, cinnamon, dill, fennel, licorice, rosemary, spearmint
Astringent	Causes contraction of soft tissue *Herbs:* Blackberry root and leaves, blessed thistle, calendula, catnep, comfrey, cramp bark, mallow, meadowsweet, nettle, plantain, raspberry leaf, rue, St John's wort, sage, shepherd's purse, thyme, willow (bark and leaves), yarrow, yellow dock. *Essential oils:* Benzoin, cedarwood, cypress, frankincense, juniper, myrrh, rose, sandalwood
Cardiac toning	Strengthens cardiac action *Herbs:* Dong quai, hawthorn (berries, leaves, and bark)

Carminative	Expels wind and eases gripe pains *Herbs:* Angelica, anise, caraway, catnep, cayenne, chamomile, dill, fennel, ginger, hyssop, lemon balm, parsley, peppermint, spearmint, thyme, valerian *Essential oils:* Angelica, star anise, black pepper, caraway, cardamom, cilantro (coriander), dill, fennel, ginger, peppermint, spearmint
Cholagogue	Stimulates bile production and flow *Herbs:* Calendula, dandelion root, garlic, goldenseal, milk thistle, rosemary, sage, yellow dock *Essential oils:* Chamomile, lavender, peppermint, rosemary, spearmint
Cicatrisant	Promotes the formation of scar tissue *Essential oils:* Bergamot, cypress, eucalyptus, frankincense, immortelle, lavender, neroli, patchouli, petitgrain, rosewood
Demulcent	Softens and lubricates internally *Herbs:* Borage, chickweed, comfrey, fenugreek, licorice, mallow, meadowsweet, milk thistle, mullein, plantain, slippery elm
Deodorant	Reduces odor *Essential oils:* Bergamot, clary sage, cypress, eucalyptus, lavender, lemon grass, litsea cubeba, patchouli, petitgrain
Depurative	Purifies the blood *Herbs:* Dandelion, meadowsweet, thyme *Essential oils:* Carrot seed, clary sage, fennel, garlic, juniper, rose
Diaphoretic	Promotes perspiration *Herbs:* Angelica, black cohosh, blessed thistle, borage, catnep, cayenne, chamomile, elder (berries and flowers), hyssop, garlic, ginger, lemon balm, oregano, pennyroyal, peppermint, yarrow
Digestive	Aids digestion *Herbs:* Angelica, fenugreek, feverfew, ginger, goldenseal, marjoram, parsley, yarrow *Essential oils:* Star anise, black pepper, caraway, cardamom, chamomile, dill, marjoram, rosemary
Diuretic	Increases elimination of urine from the body *Herbs:* Angelica, burdock, dandelion leaf, elder (bark and berries) gotu kola, heartease, mallow, horseradish, nettle, parsley, plantain, shepherd's purse, red clover, violet, yarrow *Essential oils:* Chamomile, cedarwood, fennel, geranium, juniper, parsley
Emmenagogue	Encourages and regulates menstrual flow *Herbs:* Black cohosh, blessed thistle, calendula, chamomile, cramp bark, dong quai, fenugreek, oregano, marjoram, parsley, pennyroyal, yarrow *Essential oils:* Basil, chamomile, clary sage, marjoram

Emollient	Softens and soothes the skin *Herbs:* Calendula, chickweed, comfrey, elder leaves, fenugreek, mallow, mullein, plantain
Expectorant	Helps to expel mucus *Herbs:* Angelica, anise, blessed thistle, borage, comfrey, fennel, fenugreek, ginger, hyssop, licorice, mallow, mullein, nasturtium, oregano, parsley, plantain, red clover, thyme, turmeric, violet *Essential oils:* Benzoin, eucalyptus, frankincense, lavender, marjoram, myrrh, sandalwood, tea tree
Febrifuge	Agent for cooling and reducing fever *Herbs:* Angelica, blessed thistle, borage, calendula, cayenne, elder flower, fenugreek, feverfew, ginger, lemon balm, peppermint, plantain, sage, yarrow *Essential oils:* Bergamot, chamomile, eucalyptus, lavender, peppermint, ravensara, tea tree
Fungicidal	Prevents or destroys fungal infection *Essential oils:* Lavender, myrrh, tea tree *Fixed oil:* Neem
Galactagogue	Encourages the production of breast milk *Herbs:* Blessed thistle, dill, fennel, fenugreek, raspberry *Essential oils:* Star anise, basil, celery seed, litsea cubeba, fennel
Hepatic	Aids the working of the liver *Herbs:* Astragalus, dandelion root, dong quai, milk thistle, goldenseal, wormwood, yarrow, yellow dock *Essential oils:* Angelica, clary sage, grapefruit, immortelle, lemon, peppermint, rose, rosemary
Hypertensive	Raises blood pressure *Essential oils:* Black pepper, clary sage, hyssop, peppermint, rosemary
Hypotensive	Lowers blood pressure *Essential oils:* Garlic, lavender, marjoram, melissa, ylang-ylang
Immuno-stimulant	Strengthens the body's defences to infection *Herbs:* Astragalus, calendula, cat's claw, echinacea, garlic, gotu kola, mallow *Essential oils:* Garlic, lavender, eucalyptus, immortelle, manuka, ravensara, rosewood, tea tree
Nervine	Strengthens and calms the nerves *Herbs:* Catnep, chamomile, ginkgo, ginseng, gotu kola, hyssop, lavender, lemon balm, peppermint, rosemary, St John's wort, skullcap, valerian *Essential oils:* Angelica, basil, clary sage, chamomile, marjoram, melissa

Rubefacient	Produces localized redness and warmth when applied to the skin by increasing the flow of blood to the area *Essential oils:* Black pepper, eucalyptus, ginger, juniper, marjoram, rosemary, thyme
Stomachic	Aids and tones the digestive system *Essential oils:* Angelica, star anise, basil, bergamot, black pepper, carrot seed, chamomile, cinnamon, clary sage, nutmeg, peppermint, rosemary
Styptic	Stops or reduces external bleeding *Herbs:* Plantain *Essential oils:* Benzoin, cypress, lemon
Stimulant	A substance that is energy producing *Herbs:* Angelica, calendula, cayenne, dandelion, feverfew, garlic, ginger, ginseng, horseradish, pennyroyal, peppermint, shepherd's purse, yarrow *Essential oils:* Basil, bergamot, black pepper, cypress, eucalyptus, geranium, peppermint, rosemary
Sudorific	Increases sweating *Essential oils:* Basil, chamomile, juniper, manuka, peppermint, ravensara, rosemary, tea tree
Tonic	Aids in strengthening an organ or the whole body *Herbs:* Alfalfa, angelica, astragalus, borage, blessed thistle, burdock, calendula, cayenne, curcumin (turmeric), dandelion, dong quai, echinacea, fenugreek, feverfew, garlic, ginger, ginseng, goldenseal, gotu kola, hawthorn, nettle, raspberry, red clover, rosemary, skullcap, wormwood *Essential oils:* Angelica, basil, bergamot, black pepper, clove, geranium, ginger, juniper, lavender, lemon, marjoram, myrrh, neroli, rose, rosemary, tea tree, thyme
Uterine	A substance which tones and strengthens the uterus *Herbs:* Cramp bark, dong quai, feverfew, raspberry, yarrow *Essential oils:* Clary sage, frankincense, jasmine, melissa, myrrh, rose
Vasoconstrictor	Causes small blood vessels to contract *Essential oils:* Chamomile, cypress, rose
Vasodilator	Causes small blood vessels to dilate *Essential oils:* Marjoram
Vulnerary	Aids the healing of wounds and inflammations *Herbs:* Aloe, arnica, calendula, cayenne, chamomile, chickweed, comfrey, echinacea, elder leaves, fenugreek, garlic, ginger, goldenseal, lavender, mallow, mullein, nettle, plantain, rosemary, rue, St John's wort, shepherd's purse, thyme, violet, wormwood, yarrow *Essential oils:* Benzoin, bergamot, chamomile, geranium, lavender, myrrh, rosemary, tea tree

TIP SWEET THINGS
HERBS, SUCH AS
ANGELICA, CAN HELP
TO SWEETEN FOOD,
MAKING IT EASIER TO
REDUCE OUR INTAKE OF
SUGAR. THEY CAN ALSO
BE USED AS A SUGAR
SUBSTITUTE FOR THOSE
ON A SUGAR-FREE DIET.

Parts of a herb

There are some herbs that are valuable because the whole plant is used. Others are only useful for individual parts. Plants have many complicated names for their different parts but here we'll deal with the most common.

Flowers

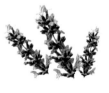

Flowers are the part used extensively for the distilling of essential oils. Some flowers can be added to food. It is from flowers that we usually get the marvelous scents to add to bath salts, shampoos and cosmetics. Usually the whole flower, including the stamens is crushed. Many flowers can also be dried to be used in pot pourri. These include all the roses.

Seeds, berries, and fruits

Seeds, berries, and fruits of many herbs are used in decoctions or dried for use in cooking. Some fruits are used ground in cosmetics and bath products. Many are also ground to make spices for food. This is very common in Asia. The range of citrus fruit are also edible as they come off the tree, but the skin and flesh are also used in cosmetics.

Leaves

One of the most useful parts of most herbs. Leaves can be crushed to add to various recipes for relief from health problems, or added to food. There are few herbs where the leaves are not useful. It's important to filter any recipe made with leaves that bear tiny hairs.

Stems

Stems are the parts of the plant visible above the ground. Some herbs are best known for their stems, such as chives. Soft stems can be included with the leaves but if they are tough, they are often discarded, as with lemongrass. The trunks of some trees are also used in natural medicine. These include cedar and sandalwood.

Roots, rhizomes, tubers and bulbs

Roots are usually the underground parts of a plant. They keep the plant firm in the ground, and absorb nutrients from the soil. These are often the bulk of the plant and take careful removal from the ground. Ginger and horseradish are two plants that are renowned for their roots. The flavor is often strong and so only a little is needed to enhance food. They are often used to make tea. Garlic is probably the most well-known bulb.

HOUSEHOLD HERBAL TIPS

In the Middle Ages, 'strewing herbs' were often used along with rushes or straw as a floor covering in all areas of the home. Herbs were often added to the mix for their aromatic or insect repellent properties – the essential oils would be released as you crushed the herbs underfoot. The use of herbs for their insect, disinfectant and pest repellent properties can still be utilized today. Here are some modern day ways to 'strew' herbs about the house and reap the benefits.

- Make herbal sachets and pop them into drawers with underwear or woolens.
- Make your own home-made potpourri and place in bowls about the house
- Make a pet pillow for your dog (or cat)

Here is Thomas Tusser's list of the top 21 strewing herbs:

Bassell, fine and busht,
  sowe in May.
Bawlme, set in Marche
Camamel
Costemary
Cowsleps and paggles
Daisies of all sorts
Sweet fennell
Germander
Hop, set in Februarie
Lavender
Lavender spike

Lavender cotten
Marjorom, knotted, sow or set,
  at the spring.
Mawdelin
Peny ryall
Roses of all sorts, in January
  and September
Red myntes
Sage
Tansey
Violets
Winter savery

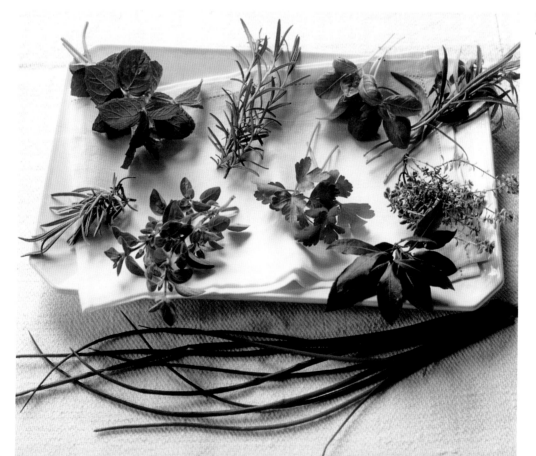

The leaves of herbs come in many different forms.

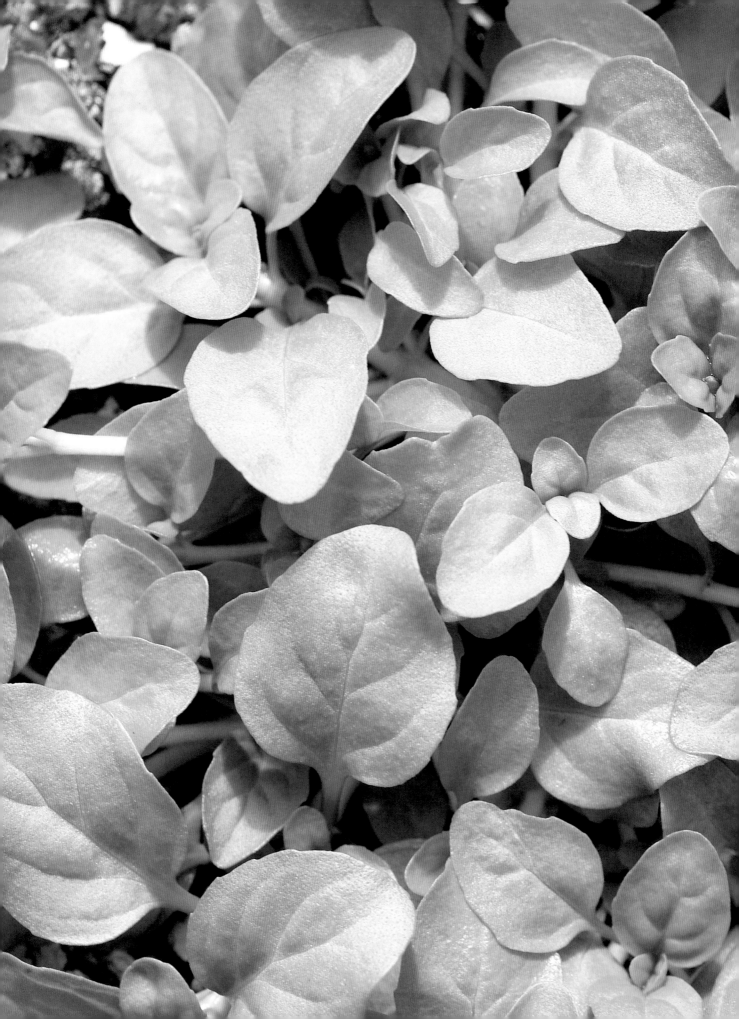

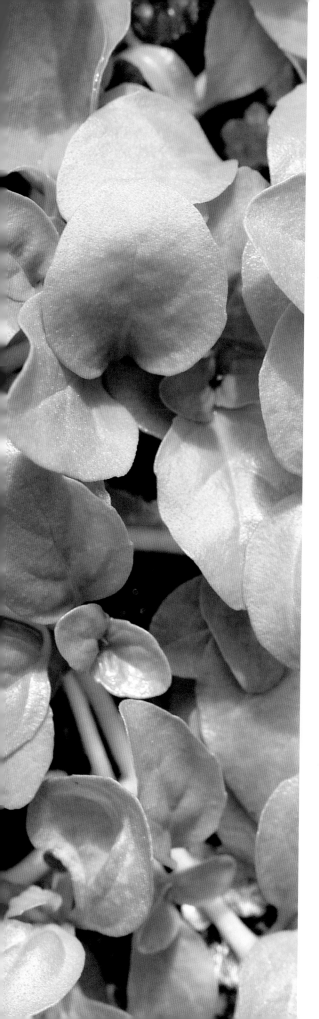

A-Z HERBS AND ESSENTIAL OILS

The plant profiles in this section are arranged in alphabetical order by genus. They provide a brief description of the herbs and their hardiness, information on the parts of the plant used, along with a simple outline of their common culinary, medicinal, and cosmetic uses. Where appropriate, there are warnings about the toxicity and medicinal uses of the herbs. For the home gardener, each entry includes short notes on growing, propagating, and harvesting your herbs.

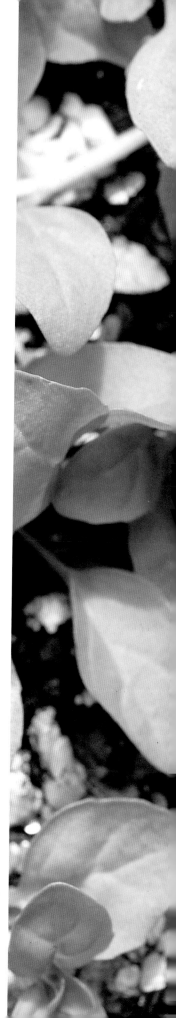

Achillea millefolium

Asteraceae
Yarrow
Also known as milfoil, thousand leaf, nosebleed, soldier's woundwort

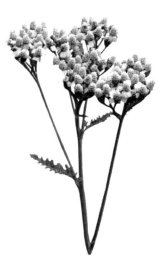

The Herball or *Generall Historie of Plantes* was published by Elizabethan herbalist and gardener, John Gerard, in 1597. It includes descriptions of plants from all over the world.

In *The Herball* (1597), Gerard writes that Achilles used this plant to stem the bleeding from his soldiers' wounds after the siege of Troy, hence *Achillea*.

Summer-flowering yarrow is a hardy, aromatic perennial growing up to 2 ft (60 cm). It has feathery leaves, and long-lasting small, white, and daisy-like flowers in flattened heads. There are also varieties with deep pink, and even reddish flowers. The stiff dried stems are the most authentic way for casting the I Ching.

Uses: HERB
Yarrow tea is useful in treating cystitis, digestive stomach cramps, flatulence, gastritis, and gall bladder and liver complaints.

A classic remedy among herbalists for colds, influenza, and fever is a tea made of yarrow, peppermint, and elder flower to encourage sweating, and reduce fever.

Use in compresses, fomentations, and ointments to help to stop bleeding, and heal wounds.

Yarrow is an insect-attracting herb, and is often planted in butterfly gardens. Add to the compost pile to accelerate decomposition.

Caution: Extended use may make skin light sensitive. Not to be used during pregnancy.

Growing and harvesting
Yarrow likes a sunny spot with room to spread. It doesn't need much water and will tolerate poor soil so long as it is well drained. Propagate by root division in spring or fall. Cut flowering, leafy stems before the sun is too strong but after the dew has evaporated. Hang in bunches in an airy room, spread out on a drying rack, or dry in the oven.

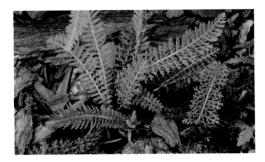

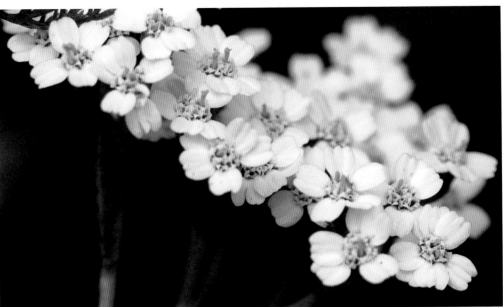

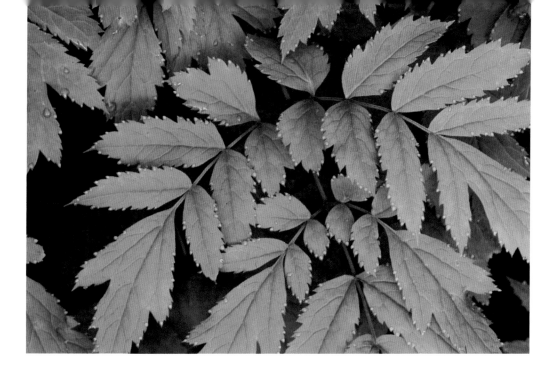

Actaea racemosa
syn. *Cimicifuga racemosa*

Ranunculaceae
Black cohosh
Also known as squaw root, black snake
root, rattle weed

Black cohosh is a North American
woodland plant growing 4–7 ft (1.2–2.2 m)
and bearing long 2 ft (60 cm) bottlebrush
spikes of brilliant, white flowers in
summer. The rhizome, a traditional Native
American remedy for menstrual matters
and menopause, is now regarded as a
valuable herb for problems of the female
reproductive system.

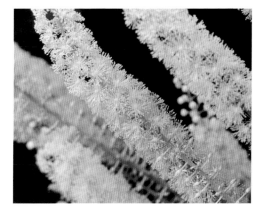

Uses: HERB
Eases cramping in the ovaries or uterus.
It may also be helpful to ease premenstrual
symptoms, painful menstruation, and
menopausal symptoms, such as hot flashes,
especially when combined with St John's
wort (*Hypericum perforatum*).

A decoction or tincture (60 drops of
black cohosh tincture in 2 tablespoons
[40 ml] of water three times a day),
or externally as a liniment can help
relieve neuralgia, rheumatoid arthritis,
osteoarthritis, and muscular pain.

Its relaxing nervine qualities can help
tinnitus sufferers.

*Caution: The dosage should be carefully
adhered to. Not to be used during pregnancy
or while breastfeeding.*

Growing and harvesting
Black cohosh is a woodland plant, so if you
want to grow it in your garden, remember
it prefers cool, moist, semi-shade but will
tolerate other conditions provided it isn't
grown in clay or waterlogged soil. The seed
can take several months to germinate. Lift
rhizomes in the fall for use fresh in tinctures,
or dried, in decoctions and tinctures.

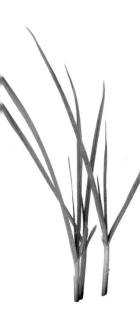

Allium sativum

Alliaceae
Garlic

A hardy perennial, garlic grows to about 12–36 in (30–90 cm), with long, green, strap-like leaves growing from leaf sheaths up the unbranched stem. On top of the stem, a clump of small, white florets is held together by a leaf-shaped skin. The bulb is the most important part of the plant, both for culinary and medicinal purposes. It is made up of a number of cloves or bulbets enclosed in a paper-like skin.

Garlic is one of the most trusted herbs, valued for its flavor and healing powers. It's generally regarded as a preventive measure for colds and influenza, and is an approved remedy in some countries for cardiovascular conditions, especially high cholesterol and high triglyceride levels. Medicinally, it is usually taken in capsule form because of its pungent odor.

The essential oil is distilled from the garlic bulb—a tight papery sheath enclosing numerous cloves. The perfume is strong, pungent, and lingering.

Uses: HERB AND ESSENTIAL OIL
Add garlic to savory dishes with meat, fish, chicken, vegetables, soups, stews, salads, dressing, and vinegars.

It is ideal for respiratory tract infections where it will act as a decongestant, loosening and removing mucus too.

It increases perspiration thereby cooling and reducing fever.

Cystitis sufferers may find garlic capsules an effective treatment (maybe only temporarily until the cause is found and treated). The antibiotic action is such that it doesn't destroy the beneficial flora in the intestine.

Of great benefit to the digestive system, garlic stimulates bile production, tones the entire system, relieves cramps, spasms, and gas in the intestines, and counteracts the effects of overindulgence in food.

Garlic prevents or destroys fungal infections, and the oil can be beneficial dabbed on ringworm, spots, and pimples.

In the garden, it is useful in sprays to repel insect pests, and for pets to repel fleas.

Caution: Garlic (and its odor) may irritate sensitive stomachs. Children need to be introduced to garlic very slowly.

Growing and harvesting
Grow garlic from bulbets in a sunny spot with moderate water. Plant it near apple or peach trees, lettuces, parsnips, and roses, but away from beans, cabbages, and strawberries. To harvest, dig bulbs gently in late summer.

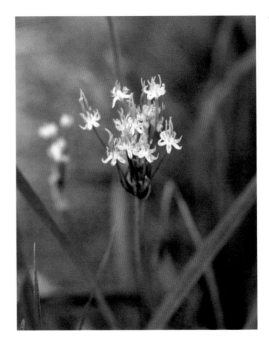

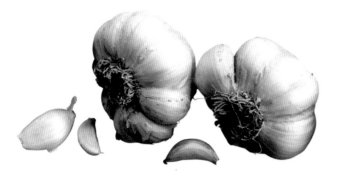

Allium schoenoprasum

Alliaceae
Chives
Also known as onion chives

A hardy perennial growing as a cluster of bulbs, the leaves of onion chives are hollow, cylindrical, green, and spear-like, and the whole plant rarely exceeds 4–24 in (10–60 cm). A cluster of lavender florets grows like a pompom on a single stem. Mature garlic chives (*Allium tuberosum*) have long, flat, broad leaves.

Uses: HERB
Freshly snipped chives aid digestion. Add generous amounts to cheese, eggs, and potato or vegetable dishes, sauces, soups, salads, dressings, juices.

In the garden, chives repel aphids, apple scab, and fungi, and are a good companion to apple trees, carrots, cucumber, and tomatoes.

Growing and harvesting
Grow from seed or bulb division in a sunny position in well-drained soil. Pick the flower buds and the leaves grow much more luxuriantly. Pick leaves from the base with your fingers—using scissors will cause the leaves to die back. Enjoy fresh; drying chives is not satisfactory—they tend to lose their color and flavor.

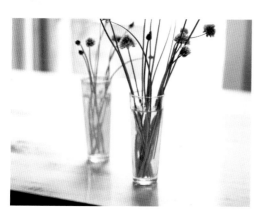

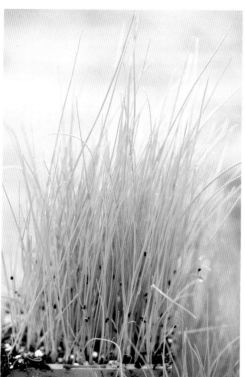

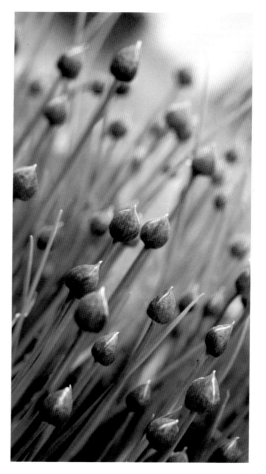

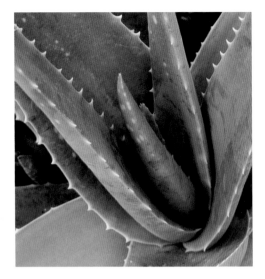
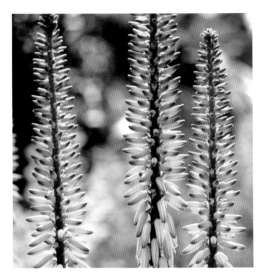

Aloe vera
syn. *Aloe barbadensis*

Aloeaceae
Aloe
Also known as medicinal aloe,
medicine plant, burn plant

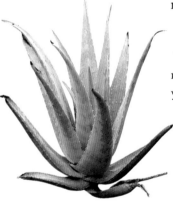

The name comes from the Arabic "alloeh,"
meaning "bitter," because of the bitter
yellow liquid found between the gel and the
leaf skin (once used to paint on the nails
to deter nail biters).

This succulent, clump-forming
perennial reaches 2–3 ft (60–90 cm),
growing straight from the soil as a rosette
of thick, fleshy, spear like, spiny toothed,
gray-green leaves. The tall, annual flower
head bears yellow-orange flowers on
3 ft (90 cm) spikes.

Uses: HERB

The best known use of aloe is the topical
treatment of minor burns and scalds.

Slice open the leaf and apply the clear,
pale green gel for pain relief, and antisepsis.
The gel can heal wounds, soothe irritable
rashes, stings, bites, and ulcers, and help
manage acne and eczema.

Internally, the stabilized juice (bought
from health-food stores) is used to ease
arthritis symptoms, digestive disorders, ulcers,
colitis, constipation, irritable bowel syndrome,
and inflammatory bowel complaint.

The syrupy aloe gel can be applied as a
moisturizing treatment, helping to keep skin
smooth and supple, and delay the effects
of ageing. It's widely used in commercial
toiletries including shampoos, face and hand
creams, and suntan lotions.

*Caution: Not to be used internally during
pregnancy or while breastfeeding; or if you have
diarrhea, loose stools, or abdominal pain.*

Growing and harvesting

Aloe is easily grown. It needs a dry, well-
drained spot, as it will quickly die in wet
soil. It can survive long, hot summers with
little water. It will look a bit sad and thin
by the end of the season, but will become
plump and juicy once the rains come.
Aloe won't tolerate heavy frost, nor the
severe heat of the tropics, unless it is grown
in semi-shade. As the plant grows and
matures, it will form little suckers around
its base that can be gently pulled away
and planted into pots or directly into the
garden, or propagate from stem cuttings.
Cut leaves as required from two- to three-
year-old plants.

Aloysia triphylla

Verbenaceae
Lemon verbena

Deciduous lemon verbena has yellow-green, narrow, and pointed leaves, and in the right spot will reach 10 ft (3 m). The spikes of pink flowers are much loved by bees. The plant can become straggly and needs careful pruning after flowering to promote a bushy shape.

Uses: HERB
A jug of water with a few slices of lemon, a couple of lightly bruised lemon verbena leaves, and a sprig or two of peppermint makes a refreshing drink. It is also delicious hot and sweetened with honey.

Flavor desserts, stuffings, and salads with a couple of lemon verbena leaves.

A tea made with lemon verbena leaves can be used to treat the symptoms of colds, sinus congestion, indigestion, and diarrhea.

Use the aromatic, dried leaves (and flowers) for potpourri.

Growing and harvesting
Plant in a sunny, sheltered spot in loamy, well-drained soil. Propagate by soft tip cuttings in spring. To harvest, cut the branches before midday, and hang in a protected, shady spot to dry completely before stripping off and storing the foliage.

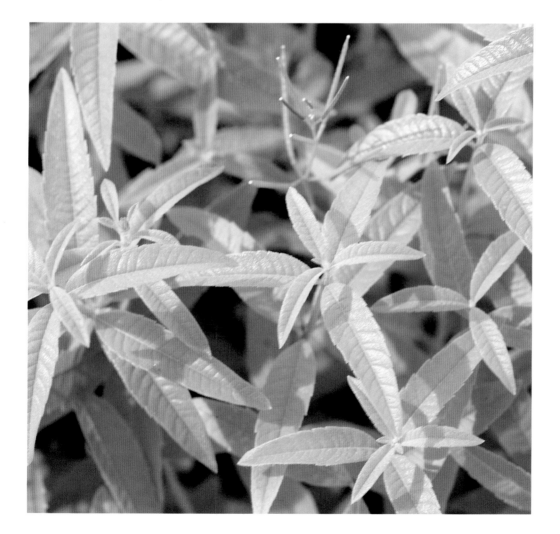

Althaea officinalis

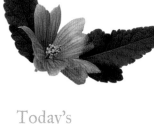

Malvaceae
Mallow
Also known as common mallow, musk mallow, dwarf mallow, marsh mallow

Today's marshmallow confectionery has nothing to do with this herb. It is packed with sugar, gelatine, artificial coloring and flavoring.

Delicious marshmallows were once made from mallow root, and they must have been very beneficial. Pliny said: "Whosoever shall take a spoonful of the Mallows shall that day be free from disease that may come to him."

The common mallow is the one most often used because of its availability. It can be seen almost everywhere, including on roadsides and garbage tips. It is a biennial or perennial of quite straggly habit: branching with coarse, rounded, notched, slightly lobed leaves, and reaching a height of 3–4 ft (1–1.2 m). The flowers are pink to mauve, with dark purple vein-like marking on each heart-shaped petal. The thick and fleshy root is the most important part of the plant.

Uses: HERB

Mallow flowers make a bright addition to salads along with the leaves and seeds. Even chopped mallow root can be added to casseroles and stews.

Use the root, leaves, and flowers for treating wounds, and for their soothing, softening, and cleansing qualities. Mallow can be used as a poultice, an infused oil, or an ointment for burns, sprains, swelling and other inflammations, to ease stings and bites, soothe pain, and heal ulcers.

Soaked in cold water overnight, and then simmered gently for 10 minutes and strained, a drink made with very finely chopped mallow root will soothe stomach and intestinal inflammation, and loosen dry coughs.

Growing and harvesting

Plant seeds in a sunny, sheltered position in well-drained soil. Gather the leaves in summer, and dry for infusions, ointments, and liquid extracts. In the fall, lift the roots, wash thoroughly, and chop and dry quickly. If left too long they become too hard to cut.

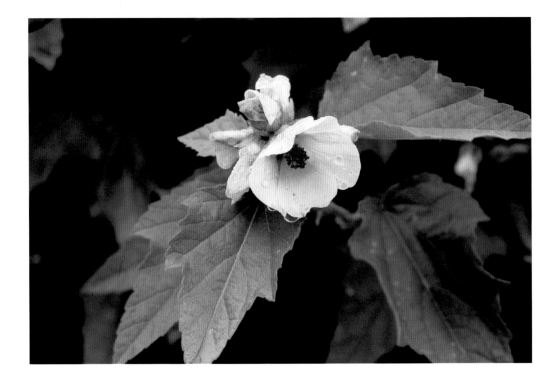

Anethum graveolens

Apiaceae
Dill
Also known as dill seed, benth, dill weed

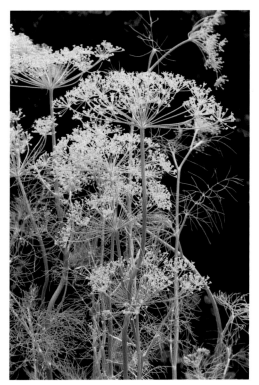

Dill has a long history of culinary and medicinal use. Dill is an annual, growing to about 3 ft (90 cm). The small, yellow flowers are clustered on flat heads from midsummer. The seeds are oval, flat, ribbed, and light brown.

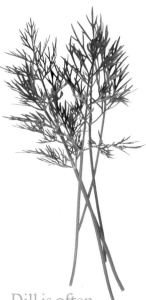

Uses: HERB

With its refreshing, anise flavor, dill seeds and leaves are used in vegetable, egg, lamb, and shellfish dishes, in soups, salads, sandwiches, pickles, dressings, and vinegars.

A tea to ease the discomfort of gripe and wind is made from the leaves and seeds—it's well known to mothers of colicky babies for its ability to bring up wind.

Dill repels cabbage moth, and is a good companion to cabbage, celery, and tomatoes.

Growing and harvesting

Grow from seed in a sheltered, sunny spot in well-drained soil. Cut the feathery green tips, and dry on paper towel in an airy place or in the microwave. To collect the seeds, snip off the flower heads and spread them out on a tray for a few days.

Dill is often confused with fennel, as the leaves, seeds, and flavor are similar—the feathery leaves are darker green, and smaller than fennel's. However, mistakes are not serious, as both are very mild, and have a similar action.

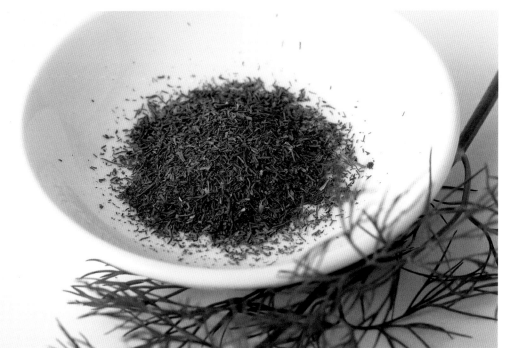

Besides its use as a soothing tea, ground dill is an excellent additive to egg dishes.

Angelica archangelica

Apiaceae
Angelica

Angelica is an aromatic biennial with thick, hollow stems growing to 3–8 ft (1–2.5 m). The lower leaves are very large with deeply serrated edges; the upper leaves are smaller. Large, round flower heads are borne in umbels in the second year. The florets are greenish white, and the seeds that follow are pale brown.

The essential oil distilled from the root and seeds blends well with basil, chamomile, geranium, grapefruit, lavender, lemon, and mandarin. It is used in the perfume industry as a fragrance for soaps, perfumes, and colognes, and for making liqueurs such as chartreuse and Benedictine.

Angelica was once used as a protection against the plague. A well-known story tells of a monk who dreamed an angel visited him and told him to use the herb to cure the plague-smitten people hence "angelica."

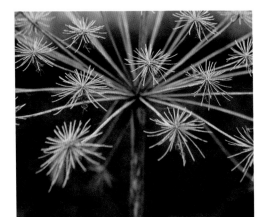

Angelica has eye-catching clusters of white flowers in summer. These are followed by pale brown seeds.

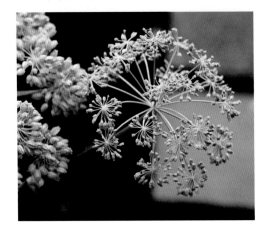

Uses: HERB AND ESSENTIAL OIL

Decorate cakes and puddings with candied young angelica stems. Add finely chopped fresh stems to milk puddings, stewed fruits (especially rhubarb), and jellies.

Use the chopped stems and leaves to flavor cold summer drinks, punches, and liqueurs.

A tea, tasting much like China tea, is infused from fresh or dried leaves.

A decoction of dried angelica root or 40-60 drops of tincture can ease coughs, colds, asthma, and bronchitis; stomach discomfort, heartburn, colic, stimulate lack of appetite, dispel gas, and soothe intestinal cramps.

A fomentation of angelica will help cleanse and heal stubborn skin ulcers.

Angelica can relieve exhaustion and stress, and ease the pain of headache, migraine, and toothache.

Angelica oil is excellent in all skin care preparations both as a tonic, and to soften and smooth, rough, dry skin. It reduces inflammation, and can be useful when applied to irritated skin, and psoriasis.

In baths, massage oils, and compresses, it is a useful urinary antiseptic for cystitis, and urethritis.

Angelica flowers attract beneficial insects to the garden.

Caution: Avoid using on skin that will be exposed to sunlight. Not to be used during pregnancy, if you have diabetes, or if you are taking blood-thinning medication.

Growing and harvesting

The plant can be propagated by seeds or root division, but the seeds are hard to germinate. It's easier to buy seedlings and plant them 18 in (45 cm) apart in a semi-shaded, moist spot. Angelica needs good soil, frequent watering, and weeding. It will grow as a perennial if the flower heads are cut off as they begin to blossom. Lift roots in the fall, gather leaves before flowering, and seeds as they ripen, to dry for decoctions.

Angelica sinensis

Apiaceae
Dong quai

Dong quai is typically found growing in damp mountain ravines, meadows, on riverbanks, and in coastal areas. It is from the same family as *Angelica archangelica*, and the root has been used for centuries in Chinese medicine, often referred to as the "female ginseng" because of its use in herbal remedies to treat muscle cramps associated with menstrual pain.

Uses: HERB

Dong quai is becoming well known for its estrogenic-like activity, making it useful for treating fibrocystic breast disease, painful or difficult menstruation, menopausal symptoms such as hot flashes and vaginal spasms, for premenstrual syndrome, and to help women resume normal menstruation after using birth-control pills.

The herb helps to improve liver function when impaired by hepatitis or cirrhosis.

It is a general tonic for women who are feeling tired and run down.

Caution: *Not to be used during pregnancy or if you are taking blood-thinning medication.*

Growing and harvesting

See *Angelica archangelica*.

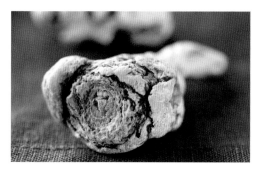

The dried root, dong quai, is essential in all Chinese medicine and is especially beneficial in women's remedies.

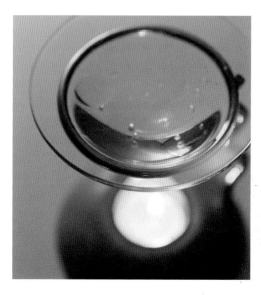

The aroma of rosewood essential oil offers a spicy combination of forest and rose. It is excellent in combination with other essential oils.

Aniba roseaodora

Lauraceae
Rosewood

The rosewood tree is a native of the Amazon basin, and its fragrant heartwood was once used to make fine furniture. Due to indiscriminate felling, this tree is now an endangered species. The essential oil is distilled from heartwood chips, and the perfume is a pleasant blend of wood and flower, with spicy undertones, that blends well with most other essential oils. It is sometimes sold as "bois de rose."

Uses: ESSENTIAL OIL

Rosewood oil assists in cell regeneration, is antiseptic, and can help to treat acne, cuts, dermatitis, eczema, scars, and wounds. A good oil for skin care blends to treat dry, sensitive, and wrinkled skin. It also makes a good deodorant, and insect repellent.

Use in baths and massages as an immune system booster, especially to treat chronic fatigue syndrome, glandular fever, influenza.

It has a calming effect on the nerves and brain and this, combined with some pain-killing quality, makes it a good oil to use in blends for headaches, jet lag, frigidity.

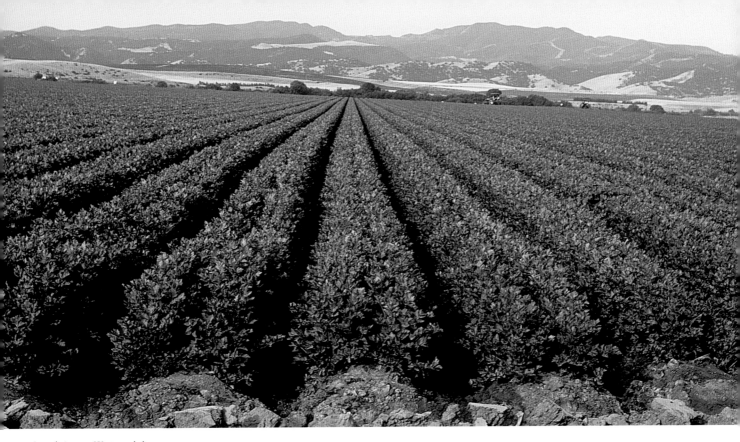

A staple in most Western salads, celery is cultivated throughout the world.

Apium graveolens

Apiaceae
Celery seed

Wild celery is a strong smelling vegetable but has been domesticated for some 2,000 years to produce the popular vegetable (*A. graveolens* var. *dulce*) enjoyed in soups, salads, and crudites. The oil can be extracted from the whole plant but the best oil is steam-distilled almost exclusively these days in

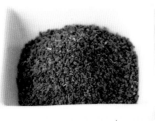

India from wild celery seeds. The perfume is spicy and warm with a long-lasting odor, and it blends well with angelica, basil, chamomile, grapefruit, lemon, orange, palmarosa, and rosemary.

Uses: ESSENTIAL OIL
Include in massage and bath blends for arthritis, gout, rheumatism, and sciatica. It increases the flow of urine, helping to ease the symptoms of cystitis and urethritis.

As a compress or fomentation, celery seed oil relieves cramps and spasm in the uterus, encourages and regulates menstrual flow, and increases the production of breast milk.

Celery seed used as a massage oil over the abdomen aids digestion, relieves cramps and spasms in the intestines, and will help with flatulence and indigestion.

Caution: *Avoid using during pregnancy.*

Arctium lappa

Asteraceae
Burdock
Also known as lappa and beggar's buttons

A traditional medicinal herb, burdock is an imposing biennial that grows up to 5 ft (1.5 m) or more, with large, dull green, bitter tasting leaves. The globular flowers are covered with stiff, hooked burrs that cling to clothing, and are a well-known source of burrs matted in dogs' hair.

Uses: HERB

Burdock root is one of the classic herbs used to produce a beneficial change in bodily functions, especially when combined with yellow dock root and red clover flowers, taken either as a tea or a tincture (40–60 drops) three times daily. It is used for a wide range of inflammatory conditions including boils and sores.

The herb is widely recommended for use both internally and externally for the relief of dry, scaly skin conditions such as eczema and psoriasis. It is also useful for treating acne. Use in ointments for skin eruptions, minor burns, and wounds.

Seed extracts have been shown to reduce blood glucose.

The fresh roots and leaf stalks can be used as a vegetable in salads and stir-fries.

Caution: It is recommended that dosage should be small to begin with, as burdock may provoke a symptomatic crisis in severely toxic conditions. Increase the dosage cautiously. If you are taking insulin or an oral medication to reduce blood glucose, it is possible that burdock will increase its effect.

Growing and harvesting

Burdock is normally collected in the wild. If you grow it in your garden, you'll find it readily self-seeds. Lift the mucilaginous roots in the fall, and dry for making decoctions, teas, tinctures, and ointments.

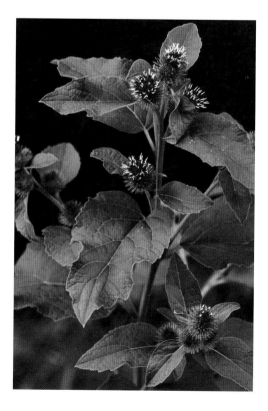

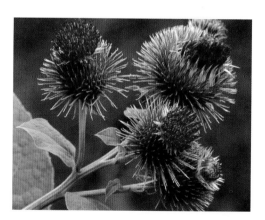

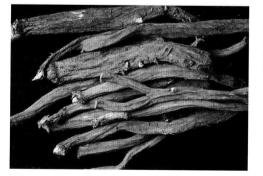

All parts of burdock are of use in natural medicine. The dried root is a traditional source of ointments and tinctures while the stems and leaves can be eaten.

Amoracia rusticana

Brassicaceae
Horseradish
Also known as spoonwart, red cole, mountain radish

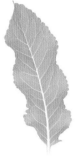

Horseradish is a hardy perennial growing to 2–3 ft (60–90 cm) with a large, fleshy, and very pungent, branched taproot, and large (up to 20 in/50 cm), toothed leaves.

Uses: HERB

Grated, fresh horseradish (on its own or as a sauce with vinegar or cream) complements beef to perfection, and goes well with egg and vegetable dishes, sauces, vegetable juices, and dressings. Keep in mind that a little goes a long way. Try the fresh young leaves in salads and sandwiches. This is not a pot herb—heat destroys the volatile oils that produce the eye-smarting pungency.

If you are stoic, clear sinus congestion by chewing and swallowing one teaspoon of freshly grated root. Neat.

A horseradish poultice can ease the pain of arthritis, rheumatism, and muscular aches and pains.

When taken internally as a diuretic, to stimulate the stomach secretions, and for respiratory and urinary infections, use strictly in accordance to recipe dosage directions—too much can cause vomiting.

Caution: *Not to be used by people with depressed thyroid function or stomach ulcers.*

Growing and harvesting

Grow horseradish from root division, but beware—the root is very invasive, and the plant will take over the garden if allowed. It grows best in sun, is dormant in winter, likes moderate water, and it is resistant to frost. Plant near apple or apricot trees, and potatoes. Pick leaves in spring and use fresh. Lift roots in the fall and use in poultices and cooking.

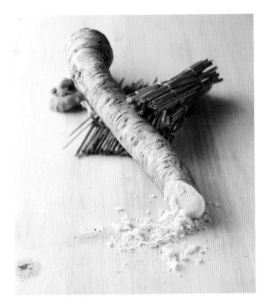

Strong, pungent, and irresistible, horseradish is cultivated world-wide for culinary and medicinal uses. Even the Japanese wasabi is a form of horseradish. The root is the most popular but for those desiring a kick to their salads, try the leaves fresh.

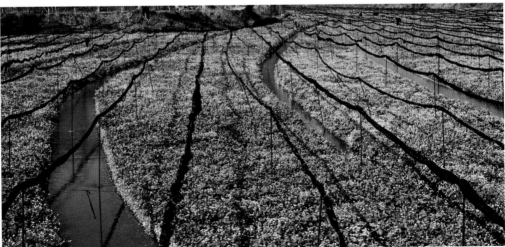

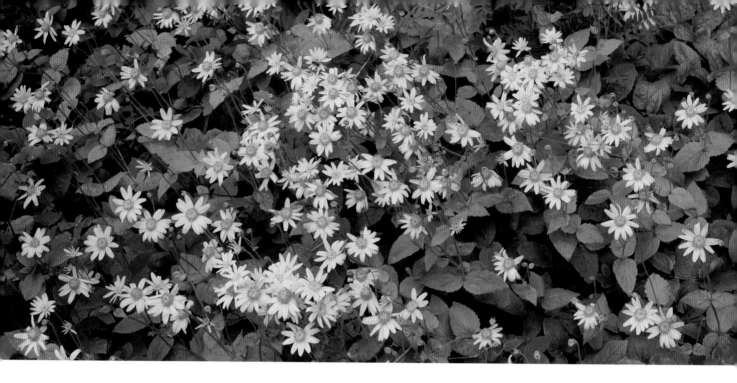

Arnica montana

Asteraceae
Arnica
Also known as leopard's bane, mountain arnica, wolfsblane

Arnica is a perennial plant with slightly hairy, single, or lightly branched stems that reach a height of 2 ft (60 cm). Each plant has numerous large, yellow, daisy-like flower heads.

Pure essential arnica oil contains a high percentage of toxic constituents, and is not for home use. Arnica essential oil can be bought as 2 percent essential oil in 98 percent jojoba oil or other carrier oil. This is safe to use on unbroken skin.

Arnica infused oil or ointment is a valuable addition to the family first aid box. The infused oil is one of the best remedies for sprains, strains, and bruises, but remember it should never be applied to broken skin or open wounds.

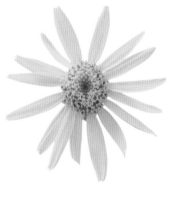

Uses: HERB, INFUSED OIL
Used externally as an ointment, infused oil, or tincture on unbroken skin, arnica promotes the healing of bruises, and relieves the pain of arthritis, and stiffened, cramped and sore muscles and joints. It can also be used in blends to relieve rheumatism and other inflammatory conditions. Used as massage oil it will help to reduce pain and swelling. It can also be used to great effect in the treatment of repetition strain injury.

Caution: For external use only. Extended use may cause allergic dermatitis.

Growing and harvesting
Arnica can be very slow to germinate, taking 25 days to two years! Sow seeds in sandy soil in full sun with moderate water. Pick flowers in spring, and dry on racks in a sheltered, airy place for use in infusions, tinctures, and creams.

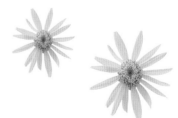

Artemisia absinthium

Asteraceae
Wormwood
Also known as old woman, green ginger, absinthe, sage brush

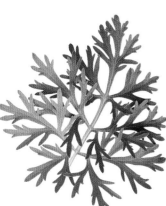

Wormwood, a bushy perennial growing to about 3 ft (1 m), has a silvery appearance as the stems and leaves are covered in fine, whitish hairs. It has been referred to as a "cure-all," and has been used in a wide range of conditions, as it works in a truly holistic way to stimulate the entire digestive system. It is notable for the large number of powerful ingredients it contains, making it a single-handed pharmacy of bitters.

Like most herbs, care is always needed, and there are far more pleasant-tasting herbs that can replace wormwood for the beginner in herbalism. Dandelion leaf and root, for example, are good substitutes.

Consult with a health-care professional knowledgeable in herbal medicine before taking wormwood internally. It can be used with discretion for short periods (2–4 weeks maximum), and no more than two cups of tea a day. The tea should be taken before meals in half-cup doses, or 20 drops of tincture in water.

"While Worm-wood hath seed, get a handful of twaine, To save against March, to make flea to refrain: When chamber is sweep'd, and Wormwood is strewne, No flea, for his life, dare abide to be known. What savour is better. If Physic be true, For place infected than Wormwood or Rue? It is a comfort for heart and the brain, And therefore to have it, it is not in vain."
—THOMAS TUSSER: *FIVE HUNDRED POINTS OF GOOD HUSBANDRY,* 1573

Uses: HERB

Fomentations using this herb can be used externally to ease the pain of irritations, bruises, and sprains or strains. I include it in ointments for its antiseptic and pain-easing properties.

The spicy fragrance of wormwood repels moths, silverfish, and other indoor insects.

It is an excellent outdoor insect repellent when leaves are sprinkled among plants in the garden.

Wormwood makes a good garden border that also discourages dogs and cats from entering your garden.

Caution: Do not use wormwood oil as it is highly toxic. Use only in amounts recommended. Avoid excessive or longer term (over four weeks) use. Not to be used during pregnancy. Do not use for children, the frail, or the elderly.

Growing and harvesting

Wormwood grows to about 3 ft (1 m) tall, with silky, grayish white leaves and stems. It requires little attention or water. Gather the leaves in the spring just as the plant is beginning to flower, prune at this time also or the plant becomes straggly. It dies back in the fall to rest over the winter.

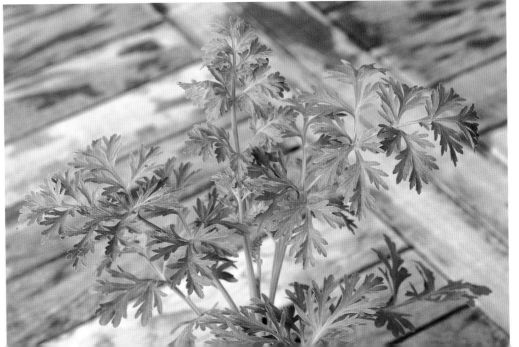

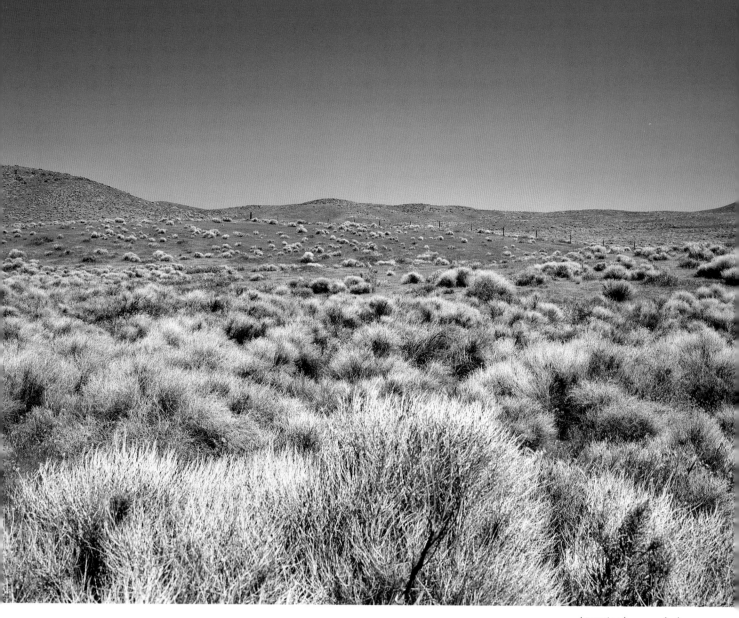

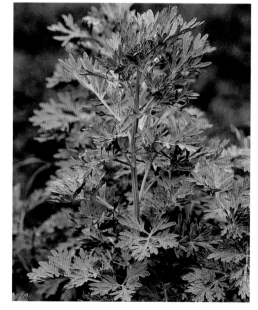

Artemesia arborescens, also known as wormwood or sage brush.

Wormwood (bitters) stimulates the appetite, promotes the flow of juices from the pancreas, duodenum, and liver, increases the flow of bile, helps the liver with its detoxification, and regulates the secretion of insulin. Other plants classified as "bitters" include rue, gentian root, dandelion, golden seal, mugwort, yarrow, southernwood, blessed thistle, and hops.

Wormwood can be used as a tea to stimulate digestion.

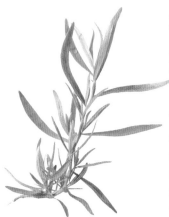

Artemisia dracunculus

Asteraceae
Tarragon
Also known as little dragon, estragon,
French tarragon

Tarragon is a bushy, semi-hardy perennial
that has a rather sprawling habit. It grows
to 1–3 ft (30–90 cm) and has long, narrow,
dark green leaves, and small, insignificant
flowers. Don't let yourself be fobbed off
with Russian tarragon—it is very inferior in
flavor. Always select French tarragon.

In the kitchen, tarragon is best with
delicate foods such as seafood, poultry, eggs,
cheeses, and vegetables. It is also excellent in
salads, dressings, vinegars, and can be used as
a garnish.

Tarragon contains the oil eugenol, which
is also the major constituent of anesthetic
clove oil, making it useful for temporary
relief of pain such as toothache.

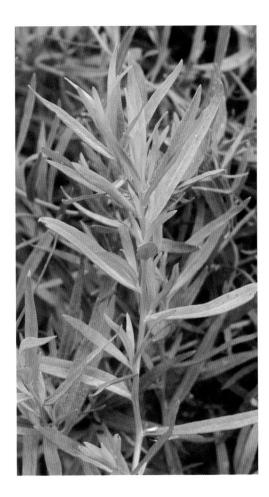

Uses: HERB
Use the leaves as a tea to act as a diuretic,
to stimulate menstrual flow, and to soothe
the stomach.

Growing and harvesting
Grow the herb from root division in a sunny
spot with moderate water. It is dormant in
winter but resistant to frost. True French
tarragon grows steadily from seed, but
packets of seed seldom mention variety. So
beware—it is much better to beg or buy a
piece of root from an established plant. After
two or three years the plant begins to lose
much of its distinctive flavor. Strike new
plants from pieces of root. Harvest leaves as
the flower buds appear until late in the fall.
Dry in bunches or on racks in a warm airy
place and strip leaves to store.

With its vague licorice
flavor, French tarragon
is an essential in any herb
garden. Ground, it makes
a wonderful tea.

Astragalus membranaceous

Papilionaceae
Astragalus
Also known as Huan-Qi, yellow vetch, milk vetch, yellow emperor

Astragalus is a sprawling, perennial legume with spikes of yellow, pea-like flowers followed by pendulous pods in the fall. It grows to about 16–24 in (40–60 cm).

In Chinese medicine the root of this herb (often combined with ginseng) has been used for thousands of years for its tonic properties to strengthen the immune system, and it is still an important ingredient in many traditional Chinese and East Indian medicines.

Uses: HERB

Astragalus is most useful when used as an immuno-stimulant for people suffering from chronic conditions (as opposed to echinacea, which is a short-term immune booster). The four-year-old root is the part used. It is best purchased as an extract and taken according to the directions given. The typical adult dosage is three cups of tea, 30 drops of tincture, or 500 mg capsules every three hours, when symptoms are most acute, reduced to twice a day as improvement is seen, and then to once a day as a maintenance dose.

Astragalus is used to treat complaints such as chronic fatigue, glandular fever, Ross River fever, and other persistent viral infections.

It can also be used in remedies to fight bacteria and inflammation.

Astragalus has hepatic and diuretic properties.

Caution: Do not use while inflammation is present.

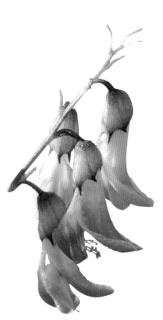

Growing and harvesting

Propagate from roots or from seeds that need to be scratched (scarified) before planting by rubbing briefly between two pieces of fine sandpaper. The seeds should be planted in the early spring in a good seed-raising mix or in small peat pots. A full-sun location is recommended, and it likes deep, sandy, well-drained soil that is somewhat alkaline. The roots should be harvested in the fourth year. Pulverize the root (finely but not to a powder) and use as a tea, to make a tincture, or to fill empty gelatine capsules.

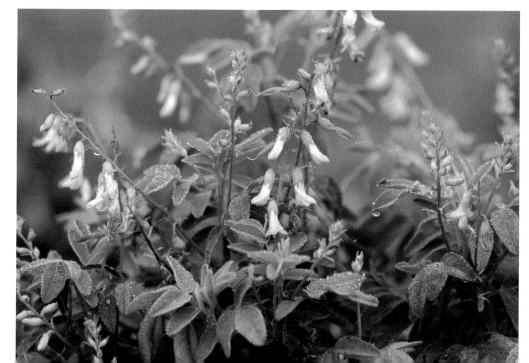

Bacopa monnieri

Scrophulariaceae
Brahmi

Brahmi is an Indian Ayurvedic herb that's also frequently used in Japanese traditional medicine—primarily as a nerve tonic, to treat insomnia and nervous tension. In the folklore of Indian medicine, it was a popular memory booster given to infants to improve memory power, intelligence, and mental health. The name comes from Brahma, the creator god of the Hindu pantheon of deities.

Brahmi is a hardy, perennial ground cover growing to 6 in (15 cm) in height, with small, oval-shaped leaves that form in pairs along the stems. Tubular, white flowers bearing five petals (with a faint tinge of blue on the outside of the petals) grow in the leaf forks, and can blossom for many months of the year. It is sometimes confused with gotu kola (*Centella asiatica*). Although they have similar applications they are very different looking herbs.

Uses: HERB

A bitter plant, the leaves and stems of brahmi can be used as a tea, tincture, or decoction, and may be sweetened with honey. It's used in salads, soups, and as a cooked vegetable in India and Asia, where bitter flavors are more widely accepted.

Brahmi is one of the main revitalising herbs for the nerves and the brain cells. It is said to increase intelligence, improve short- and long-term memory, and delay the onset of senility and ageing. It has a calming effect on the nerves, and is reputed to increase sex drive.

Brahmi can be used for inflammatory conditions including arthritis, rheumatism, and backache, and chronic skin diseases such as eczema and psoriasis. It is useful also to treat bronchitis, chronic coughs, asthma, and hoarseness.

Growing and harvesting

This tropical or semi-tropical plant won't tolerate frost, so in cold climates it needs to be grown in a pot, and moved to a warm, sheltered spot in winter. Although it is considered a bog plant it will grow in pots or in the garden, in sun or shade. Water well in dry weather as the roots are fairly shallow—remember it is a bog plant. Propagate by seed or root division. Pick when growth is at its strongest. Best collected and used fresh as needed, but it can be carefully dried.

Although originally an Indian herb, brahmi is an essential ingredient in Japanese medicine. Its tea is said to improve sex drive!

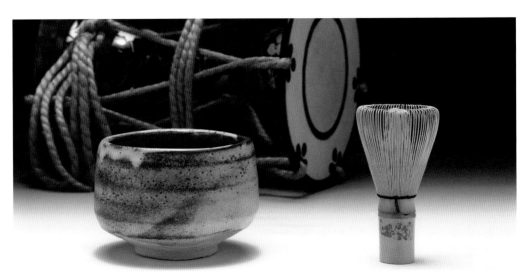

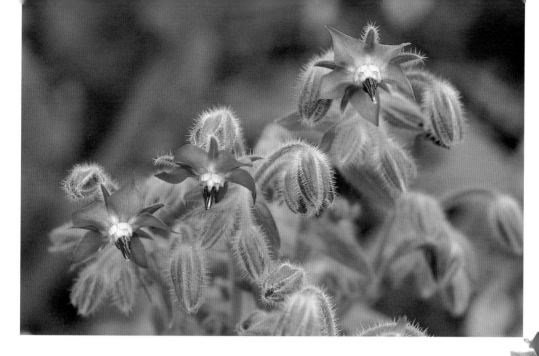

Borago officinalis

Boraginaceae
Borage
Also known as burrage, starflower

Borage was once known as the "herb of courage," and its dainty blue flowers were embroidered by ladies on the jerkins of knights about to embark upon crusades. The flower is exquisite—bright blue and star-like, with very prominent black anthers growing from its center. Borage is an annual, growing to about 1–3 ft (30 cm–1 m). The multiple branched, hollow stems, and the large, gray-green, oval, pointed leaves are hairy. The flowers hang down, so to see them at their best, plant borage on a bank or wall where you can look up to them.

Uses: HERB
The flowers and leaves are reputed to cool any liquid in which they are steeped. Whether or not this is true, the flowers look lovely floating in a jug of lemonade, and they bring a delicate cucumber flavor to the drink. Add flowers to hot vegetable dishes, soups, and stewed fruit. Cold, they enhance salads, fruit salads, drinks, and dressings, and they can also be crystallized.

Borage is recommended for the entire digestive system. The leaves and flowers are used for their softening and lubricating properties internally and externally, and for their ability to cool the body down. Three cups of the tea, or 40–60 drops of the tincture daily, is the recommended dose.

The herb may be used to reduce fever, to ease and soothe coughs, sore throats and colds, and to restore vitality during convalescence. Use also as a wash for sores and ulcers, and the tea as a gargle for sores in the mouth and throat.

Borage is a good companion to strawberries, deters Japanese beetles and tomato hornworms, and brings bees into the garden.

Caution: The hairs on the leaves and stems can cause throat and stomach irritation or contact dermatitis on some sensitive skins. Strain carefully if used internally.

Growing and harvesting
Borage is an easily grown annual that self-seeds so readily that, unless kept under control, can take over the whole garden. It likes plenty of space in a sunny location and moderate water. Gather leaves in spring, and use fresh or dried in infusions.

Gerard says: "put into wine make men and women glad and merry, driving away all sadnesse, dulnesse and melancholy, as Dioscorides and Pliny affirme. Syrrup made of the floures of Borrage comforteth the heart, purgeth melancholy, and quieteth the phrenticke or lunaticke person."
——JOHN GERARD,
THE HERBALL OR
GENERALL HISTORIE
OF PLANTES

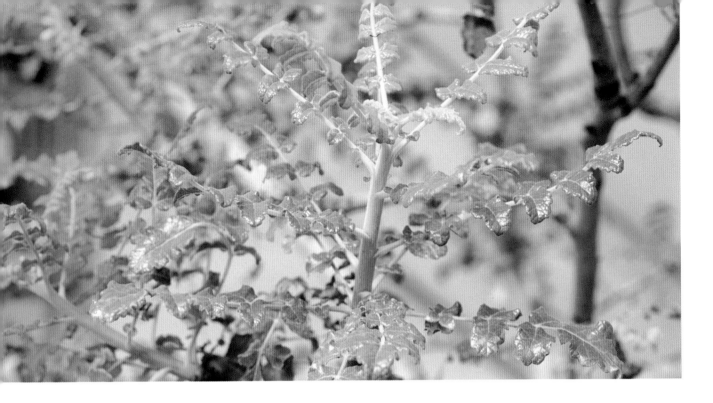

Boswellia sacra

syn. *B. carteri*

Burseraceae
Frankincense
Also known as mastic tree, olibanum

This ancient essential oil comes from a small, resinous, evergreen tree, native to the tropical regions of Arabia and Africa. Damaged bark (originally natural cracks, but now cut deliberately) exudes a resin from which the essential oil is distilled. It has a perfume that is spicy, woody, and sweet, and blends well with basil, citrus, cypress, lavender, patchouli, pine, and sandalwood.

The essential oil is used for incense, in perfumery, soap making, and cosmetics as a fixture and fragrance.

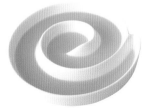

Uses: ESSENTIAL OIL

Frankincense helps to destroy infection-causing bacteria, and contracts and tones tissue. A gentle "balancer" for oily skin, it helps to regenerate ageing skin, keeps wrinkles at bay, and possibly smooths out some existing ones! It is a good cleanser for boils, wounds, and ulcers.

This oil is particularly valuable for congestive lung problems as it helps to loosen and remove mucus from the lungs, and is a pulmonary antiseptic. Used in chest massage, it slows down the breathing which is helpful during attacks of asthma. Use also as an inhalation or massage oil to ease coughs, chronic bronchitis, laryngitis, and shortness of breath.

Frankincense tones and strengthens the uterus particularly during labor. It regulates heavy menstrual flow.

It helps to expel gas from the intestines, and generally aids digestion. Its diuretic and antiseptic properties help with urinary tract and genital infection such as cystitis, urethritis, and leucorrhea.

Caution: Patch test—may cause irritation on sensitive skin.

Calendula officinalis

Asteraceae
Calendula
Also known as marigold, pot marigold

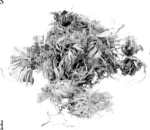

Calendula's bright flowers range in color from yellow to vivid orange. Its alternate, slightly hairy, pale green, toothed leaves are very widely spaced, and it grows to a height of about 18 in (45 cm). Be careful not to confuse this bushy, aromatic annual with African (Aztec American) marigold (*Tagetes erecta*) or French marigold (*T. patula*).

This is the herb to take with you as an ointment or tincture in your car or on trips. It's a fine healer for burns, cuts, or lacerations, helping to promote rapid healing without infection and with minimal scarring. Some people believe that the hybridized calendula is less effective than the traditional, single variety, but I believe them both to be equally effective.

Uses: HERB, INFUSED OIL
The leaves and flowers are used in poultices, washes, compresses, and fomentations, as an astringent and an antiseptic, helping to reduce bleeding, and heal wounds. It is a good treatment for sore nipples, ulcers, sprains, and varicose veins.

Made as a very strong tea and used as a spray or local application, it helps to reduce inflammation and pain from stings, as well as from measles and chickenpox spots.

Tincture of calendula is a most important addition to a first-aid box and very simple to make.

An infused oil made from the petals has powerful skin-healing properties. This makes it useful as the main oil in creams and ointment for cracked skin, burns, eczema, inflammations, rashes, work-rough hands, nappy rash, grazes, and wounds. It is an excellent treatment for sore nipples—use the oil alone rather than a cream. It also helps to fade old scars, and can be used in the treatment of ulcers and varicose veins.

The flower petals will add color and flavor to rice, salads, sandwiches, curd (cottage) cheese, and fruit dishes, and may also be crystallized.

Calendula will repel eelworm, and is a good companion to beans, lettuce, potatoes, roses, and tomatoes.

Growing and harvesting
Calendula is a readily self-seeding annual. Plant seeds in spring (or fall) direct into the garden in a sunny, well-drained spot with moderate water. Pick the flower heads daily to encourage more growth. Use flowers, fresh or dried, in infusions, tinctures, to make infused oil, and in your cooking.

Be sure that you are using true calendula [marigold] as there is often confusion with African [Aztec American] marigold [*Tagetes erecta*] or French marigold [*T. patula*]. These plants don't have the same properties and aren't suitable for therapeutic use. African or French marigolds are a little similar in appearance and are used as companion plants but are never used medicinally or in cooking.

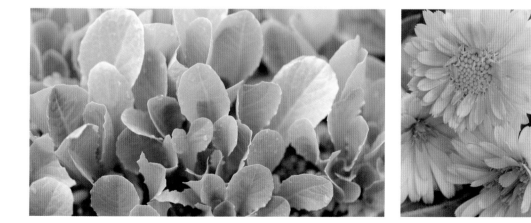

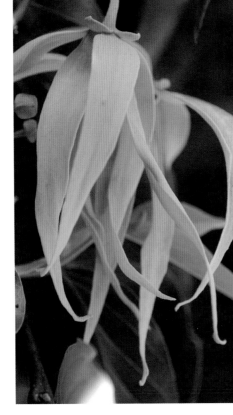

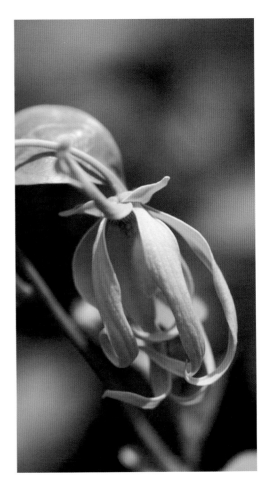

Cananga odorata

Annonaceae
Ylang-ylang
Also known as ilang-ilang and Macassar oil tree

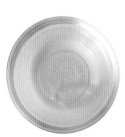

The Malay name means "flower of flowers," or maybe the name is derived from "along-ilang" for the way in which the flowers hang.

Ylang-ylang is prized for its fragrant pink, mauve, and yellow flowers. And it's from these flowers (particularly the yellow ones) that the essential oil is steam-distilled.

Ylang-ylang blends well with bergamot, jasmine, lemon, neroli, rose, rosewood, and sandalwood, but one needs to be aware that this oil can be overwhelmingly sweet (to the point of nausea) unless blended with the sharper citrus oils. This oil can create a calming environment in which to tackle unpleasant jobs or issues.

Affordable, ylang-ylang is often used as a substitute for expensive jasmine essential oil as its properties and perfume are similar. It is one of the most used fragrances and fixatives in perfumes, colognes, cosmetics, and soaps.

Uses: ESSENTIAL OIL
Ylang-ylang has a sebum-balancing effect, making it useful for all skin types, and is used in oils and tonics to encourage hair growth and shine.

It has a balancing effect on hormones, making it useful to treat menopausal and menstrual problems.

It exerts a deeply tranquilizing and strengthening effect on the nervous system. If used quickly as the situation arises, it will lower raised blood pressure, slow rapid breathing or palpitations that are due to shock, anger, or fright. Obviously, if these symptoms are not due to sudden trauma, or if they don't respond quickly, then a health professional needs to be consulted.

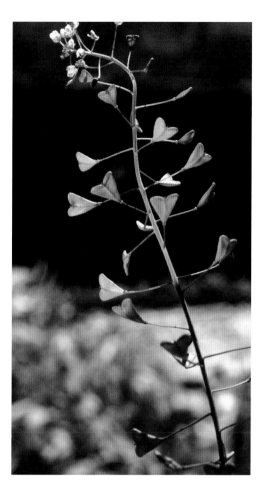

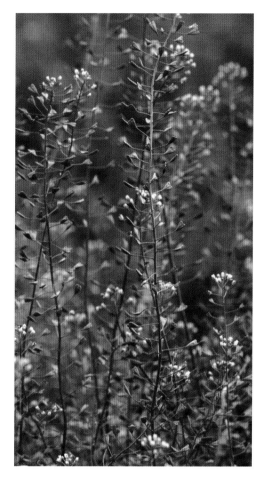

Capsella bursa-pastoris

Brassicaceae
Shepherd's purse
Also known as shepherd's bag,
lady's purse, Chinese cress, nazuna,
pickpocket, toywort

This invaluable annual is often viewed as
a weed. The main leaves, which are green,
rough, and divided like a feather, form a
rosette from which the erect stem rises to
tiny white flowers. You can add the leaves
to salads or cook as a vegetable. The small
flat, heart-shaped pods (like old-fashioned
purses) are the best way to identify this
plant which reaches 1–16 in (3–40 cm) high.

Uses: HERB
Use the whole plant for its stimulant,
antiseptic, and wound-healing properties.
The tincture may be used to help to control
internal hemorrhage, and 30 drops of
tincture in one tablespoon (15 ml) of water
might even save your life in an emergency.

Caution: Not to be used during pregnancy or by
anyone with a history of kidney stones.

Growing and harvesting
Give the shepherd's purse a special place
in a "wild" area of your garden. Grow
it from seed in a sunny place with
moderate water, or gather it from the
wild if you don't want to be invaded.

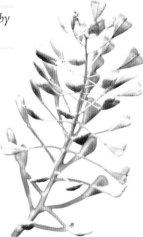

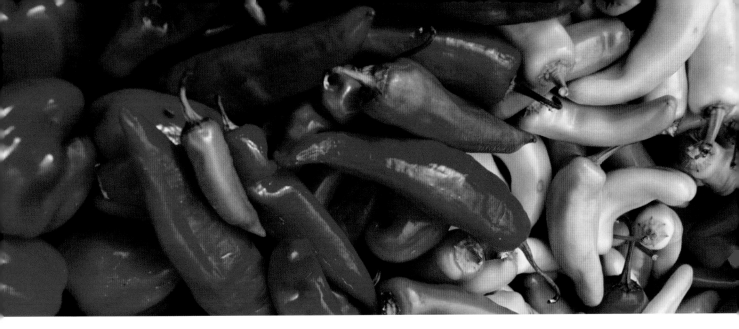

Capsicum frutescens

syn. *C. minimum*

Solanaceae
Cayenne
Also known as capsicum, hot pepper, bird pepper, chili pepper, red pepper, spur pepper, Tabasco pepper

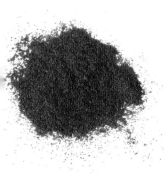

HANDLING CHILIES
The name "capsicum" is derived from the Greek "kapto," meaning "I bite." Remember this when handling fresh chilies, as the oil can create severe burns or blisters, specifically if you touch your eyes with the juice on your hands. Wear rubber gloves to prepare large quantities, or use a fork to hold the chili if just cutting one or two.

The chili plant grows to 2–3 ft (60-90 cm), has shiny, bright green leaves, and small, drooping, white flowers. The pungent slender, green fruit ripens to the familiar red. Spike meals with a little cayenne. It makes savory dishes, sauces, dressings, and juices sparkle, and is good to have on the table for those who "like it hot." Don't overdo it. Overuse can damage the digestive tract. Well-known as an ingredient in Tabasco sauce and Creole cooking, cayenne is also the catalyst that strengthens the remedy in herbal combinations in addition to adding its own valuable properties.

Uses: HERB

Use a cayenne tincture of 6–15 drops three times daily. Make a tea by pouring one cup (250 ml) boiling water over $1/_2$ teaspoon of cayenne powder. A teaspoon of this tea can be mixed with water and drunk three to four times daily.

Include the powder or tincture in recipes for colds, fevers, and sinus.

Cayenne increases heart action without raising blood pressure, and improves circulation to cold hands and feet. Two drops of cayenne tincture under the tongue will help to revive someone in shock.

A few drops of the tincture, or a pinch of the powder in water, will ease stomach pains and cramps, cysts, cystitis, neuralgia, and sore throats. Make a gargle with 10 drops of Tabasco sauce in a glass of warm water.

Five to ten drops of cayenne tincture diluted in four tablespoons (60 ml) of water can be used internally to treat frostbite and hypothermia. It warms hands and feet and the whole body by dilating the blood vessels.

Dab a little cayenne powder or tincture on cuts that are bleeding profusely to help the blood coagulate.

Use cayenne tincture in liniment to ease the pain of arthritis, rheumatism, fibromyalgia, and lumbago.

Growing and harvesting

Grow from seed or seedlings in full sun away from frosts in well-drained, rich soil. To obtain the best fruit, grow as an annual. Pick ripe fruits as required and use fresh or dried.

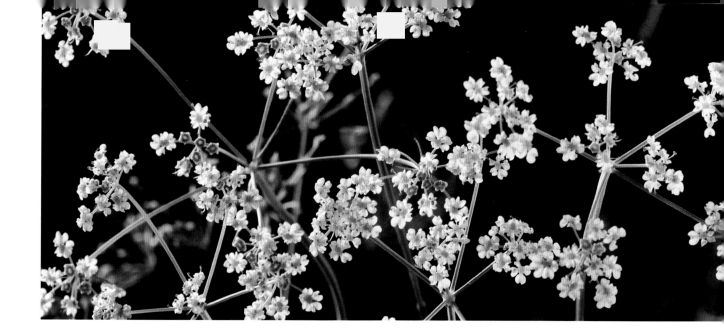

Carum carvi

Apiaceae
Caraway
Also known as caraway seed

Biennial caraway grows to 2–3 ft (60–90 cm), has a furrowed, hollow stem, finely-cut, feathery leaves, and flat-topped clusters of white flowers in summer. The crescent-shaped, dark brown, aromatic seeds have five distinct ridges.

Uses: HERB

Make a tea with the seeds to use as a digestive to soothe gripe and wind, and as an expectorant.

A combination of enteric-coated peppermint oil and caraway can reduce the pain of irritable bowel syndrome.

Caraway combined with anise and fennel can effectively deal with windy matters, especially in children.

Add caraway seeds to vegetable or fruit dishes.

In the garden caraway repels aphids, flies, and fruit moths; indoors it deals with mosquitoes.

Growing and harvesting

Grow caraway from seed in a sunny place direct in the garden. Gather the leaves and roots fresh to use as a vegetable. Cut the flower heads in the fall and spread out to dry in a warm, airy room. When dry, the seeds will fall from the shriveled flower heads.

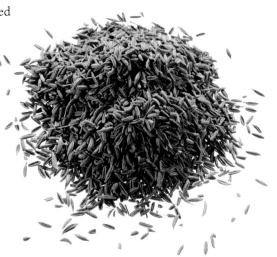

Faith, hope and caraway seeds. Records show that caraway has been used for more than 5,000 years, and legend would have us believe that caraway seeds made into a potion and fed to straying husbands made them become faithful. Some pigeon fanciers use the seed in the mash of homing pigeons, so maybe there is some truth in the old legend!

Cedrus atlantica

Pinaceae
Atlas cedar

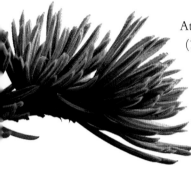

Atlas cedar is a majestic, tall 50–80 ft (15–25 m) tree that grows in the Atlas mountains in North Africa. It's highly prized for its insect-repellent, scented wood that is used for making chests for storing precious items. In ancient Egypt, cedarwood oil was used for embalming bodies, and the sarcophagi were also made from the wood. Double insurance?

Cedarwood essential oil, steam-distilled from the leaves and sawdust, has a warm, sweet, and woody perfume. It kills bacteria, deals with fungal infections, is insecticidal, and mildly astringent. It blends well with benzoin, bergamot, cypress, frankincense, juniper, lavender, lemon, and rosemary.

Uses: ESSENTIAL OIL

Add to oil blends, steams, and masks to treat acne, eczema, dermatitis, fungal infections, ulcers, and psoriasis. It is a useful treatment for oily skin, and a lovely oil to use in aftershaves and other preparations for men who appreciate its "masculine" perfume. Nice for personal insect-repellent blends too.

Include in massage and bath blends for easing arthritis, and chronic rheumatism. It is well-known for its ability to treat urinary tract infections as it is a strong antiseptic, and also increases the flow of urine.

A powerful bronchial tract antiseptic and decongestant, it helps to loosen and remove mucus during attacks of bronchitis, coughs, colds, influenza, and other congestive conditions.

Cedarwood soothes the overexcitable and relieves mental strain, and gently helps those suffering insomnia.

Caution: Not to be used during pregnancy. Patch test first—may irritate sensitive skin. Do not confuse with white cedar.

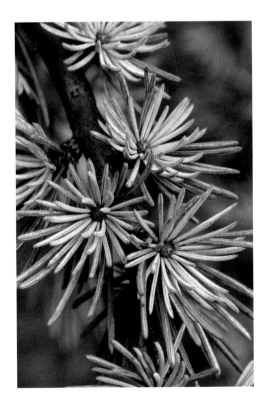

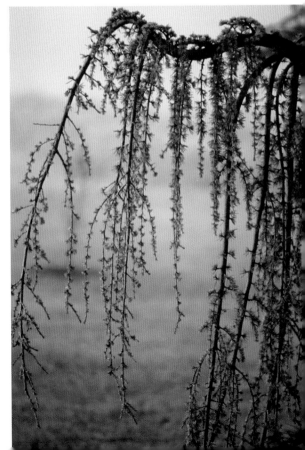

Centella asiatica

Apiaceae
Gotu kola
Also known as Indian pennywort, marsh penny, water pennywort

Gotu kola is gaining quite a reputation for itself. A humble perennial that thrives in and around water, it has a creeping habit that can become invasive if not checked. Its fan-shaped, bright green leaves are about the size of an old British penny—hence the common names. Don't let the "kola" concern you. It's not to be confused with kola nut (*Cola nitida*), an active ingredient that contains caffeine, and used in the manufacture of Coca Cola.

Uses: HERB

Gotu kola is called "food for the brain" and is one of the best herbs for improving mental clarity and concentration. In recent years it has become popular as a nerve tonic to ease anxiety, promote relaxation, and to enhance memory. Its calming properties make it well-suited for dealing with insomnia.

It is used as a tonic to speed wound healing, purify the blood, promote healthy skin, treat skin inflammations, and as a mild diuretic.

Three to four leaves a day eaten in sandwiches or salads have been shown to help people who are inactive or confined to bed due to illness.

Caution: Not to be used during pregnancy or while breastfeeding. Not recommended for children.

Growing and harvesting

If you live in a tropical area, sow seeds in spring. Harvest the whole plant or leaves once mature.

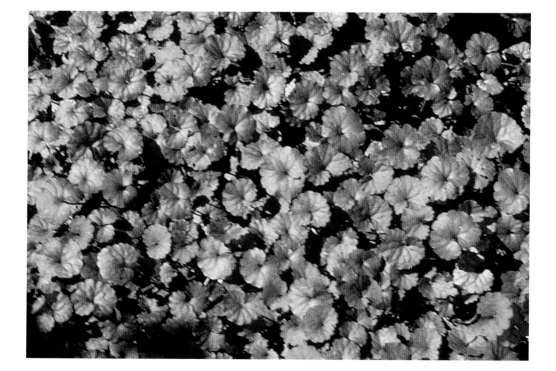

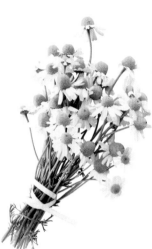

Chamaemelum nobile

syn. *Anthemis nobilis*

Asteraceae
Chamomile

Chamaemelum
comes from the
Greek meaning
"earth apple,"
and the perfume
of chamomile
is refreshing,
pleasant, and
remarkably apple-
like. All varieties
of chamomile
have this sweet
"apple" scent.

*Anthemis
tinctoria* [dyer's
chamomile]
is a perennial
that grows as a
compact, bushy
plant to about
3 ft [90 cm]. The
bright, golden-
yellow flowers
make this a
valuable dye plant.

Chamaemelum nobile (Roman chamomile)
is a low-growing, spreading perennial with
aromatic leaves and tiny, white, daisy-like
flowers. Thickly planted as a lawn, it will
withstand a certain amount of traffic but
needs regular mowing (blades set high) to
keep it lush.

Matricaria recutita (German or wild
chamomile) is a rather wispy annual. The
leaves are very narrow. The flowers are daisy-
like with white petals and yellow centers.
It is also used for herbal remedies.

The use of chamomile for healing
dates back to antiquity. It is probably the
most widely drunk herbal tea, enjoyed
for its pleasant flavor and soothing action.
Chamomile's healing powers can be
attributed to a complex blend of substances
contained in the heads of the flowers, which
when distilled, yield a medicinal oil.

Chamomile essential oil blends well with
geranium, lavender, patchouli, and rose, and is
widely used in pharmaceutical preparations,
the perfume industry, and food products. The
chamomiles are very similar, and the essential
oil distilled from the flowers of both varieties
contains chamazulene, a powerful anti-
inflammatory agent.

Uses: HERB, ESSENTIAL OIL
Chamomile is a popular remedy for
digestive upsets. It will help with colic,
colitis, indigestion, an upset stomach and
irritable bowel syndrome, and heartburn
caused by stress.

For the nervous system it can relieve
headaches, depression, and insomnia.

For the skin it is an excellent
antibacterial and anti-inflammatory,
useful to help treat eczema, urticaria,
and dermatitis.

Chamomile is also an aid in the
treatment of urinary tract infections,
and menstrual and menopausal problems.
Furthermore, the natural antihistamine
properties of chamomile can ease the
miseries of hay fever and allergic reactions.

Babies suffering from colic may be given
teaspoon doses of weak chamomile tea to
ease pain and calm fretfulness.

To lighten fair hair, make a paste of
mashed flowers, massage through the hair,
cover with a shower cap and leave for
an hour or two before rinsing out. This
treatment will need to be repeated every
time you wash your hair for the blonding
effect to become noticeable.

The oil softens and soothes tight, dry,
and itchy skin. In baths, creams, or lotions,
the anti-allergenic properties of chamomile
oil will benefit those who suffer from
allergic skin reactions such as dermatitis,
hives, and eczema. It prevents or destroys
fungal infections, kills bacteria, reduces
inflammation, promotes the formation of
scar tissue, and is widely used to treat skin
complaints such as acne, allergies, burns,
blisters and cold sores, dermatitis, eczema,
inflammations, insect bites, cuts, and boils.

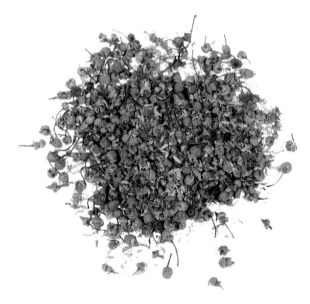

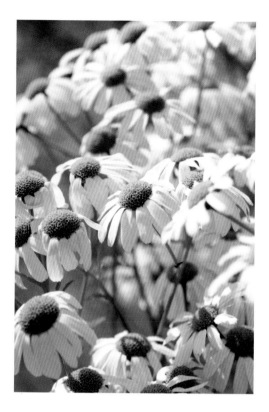

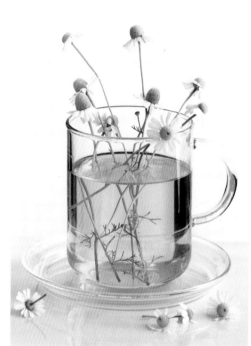

Nothing is more soothing than a cup of warm chamomile tea at the end of a stressful day.

Chamomile eases pain and is useful in fomentations, baths, and massage blends to treat the discomfort of arthritis, rheumatism, inflamed joints, sprains, strains, neuralgia, toothache, headaches, and migraine. It seems to be particularly beneficial in combination with other oils for massage, and bath treatments for lower back pain.

Chamomile increases the flow of urine, stimulates bile production and aids digestion, stimulates and strengthens the liver, and tones the digestive system. When used in baths, massage, or fomentations, it will help to treat flatulence, diarrhea, gastritis, colitis, cystitis, peptic ulcers, nausea, and other stomach complaints.

Chamomile is a popular oil for treating problems connected with the reproductive system as it encourages and regulates menstrual flow, and regulates irregular painful periods. The calming effect helps to reduce irritability felt during menopause and PMS.

The classic and popular bedtime anti-insomnia drink is chamomile tea, and the same effect can be achieved by using the oil in a pre-bedtime bath, shower, or massage, and also in an air spray in the bedroom. It sooths the overexcitable, relieves mental strains and stress, depression, and insomnia.

When used as directed, this is a safe and gentle oil for babies and children. It eases colic, the pain of teething, and soothes restlessness and "miseries."

Cautions: Patch test—may cause irritation on sensitive skin. Not to be used during the first four months of pregnancy.

Growing and harvesting
Chamomile thrives in a sunny, well-drained position. Sow seed in spring in well-drained soil and cut flowers in summer for using fresh, or dried for herb teas and infusions.

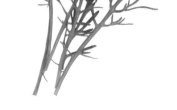

Citrus aurantiifolia

Rutaceae
Lime

The essential oil can be expressed from the peel of unripe fruit and from whole ripe fruit. See caution. The perfume is fresh, sweet, and lemony, and blends well with angelica, bergamot, citronella, clary sage, geranium, lavender, palmarosa, rose, rosemary, and ylang-ylang. Lime oil needs to be used fresh as older oil can develop carcinogenic properties.

Uses: ESSENTIAL OIL

Although limes have a stronger flavor and are more acidic than lemons, the essential oil has a similar fragrance, the same properties, and can be used in just the same way. Use no more than three drops in a bath or one percent in blends.

In skin care products such as body lotions and creams, lime helps contract and tone tissues.

In healing ointments, it is useful in removing warts, and it soothes and prevents infection of insect bites and stings. It helps to stop external bleeding such as that from nosebleeds, wounds, and after tooth extraction.

With its antibacterial and fever-lowering action, it is an extremely valuable oil in the treatment of sore throats, bronchitis, coughs, throat infections, colds, and influenza. Use as a gargle, an inhalation, as a room spray, or in a massage oil.

Caution: Patch test—may cause irritation on sensitive skins. If using an oil expressed from peel, do not use on skin exposed to sunlight. The safest lime oil to use is that which is distilled from the peel and although phototoxic it is not sensitizing.

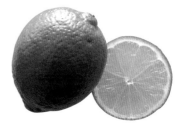

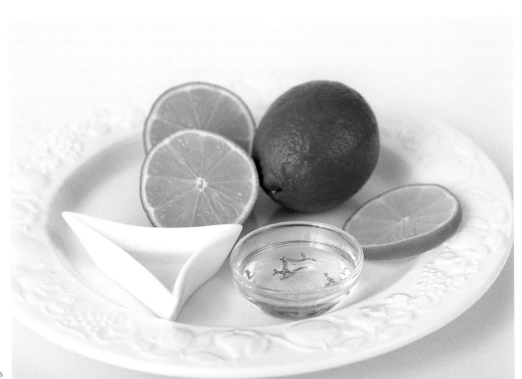

Citrus aurantium

Rutaceae
Seville orange
Also known as bitter orange

Petitgrain

Petitgrain essential oil is extracted from the leaves and twigs of the Seville orange tree. The perfume is sweet with sharper under-notes of citrus, and blends well with benzoin, bergamot, clary sage, geranium, lavender, neroli, and palmarosa.

Uses: ESSENTIAL OIL

It can be used as a less expensive substitute for neroli as it has similar qualities, but the perfume is not as subtle, and the therapeutic properties not as profound.

Petitgrain is an antiseptic tonic and sebum regulator for oily skin and hair, particularly for oily dandruff. It is lovely to use in baths or added to antiperspirant/deodorant preparations. It is useful in perfume blends to add a fresh note and to act as a middle note moderator, balancing top and base notes.

Its properties have a mildly stimulating effect on the immune system, lifting the spirits, easing nervous indigestion and flatulence, aiding convalescence, and soothing anger and panic.

Neroli
Also known as orange blossom

Neroli essential oil is extracted from the flowers of the Seville orange tree. The sweet perfume blends well with other oils. Neroli is a very expensive oil, and substituting with equal parts of mandarin and petitgrain oils will give almost the same therapeutic effect. But there is no substitute for neroli if you are making a special perfume.

Uses: ESSENTIAL OIL

Neroli is an excellent skin-care oil. It has a reputation for regenerating skin cells and maintaining or restoring elasticity, particularly in mature, prematurely aged, or sensitive skin. It helps to prevent wrinkles, remove scars, stretch marks, and lessen thread veins.

When used as a massage oil, neroli relieves cramps and spasms, and helps to expel gas from the intestines. It will ease diarrhea and indigestion that are related to shock or nerves. It also relieves cramps and spasms in the uterus.

It is a very tranquilizing oil, used for relieving long-term anxiety, calming nerves, and soothing the spirit, and easing the turbulent emotions that often accompany PMS and menopause.

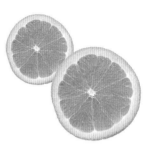

Neroli's exquisite scent isn't immediately apparent in undiluted oil, but when added to a carrier oil or other base the true aroma appears. It is then that you realize why this oil is an ingredient in the best and most expensive perfumes and eau de colognes in the world.

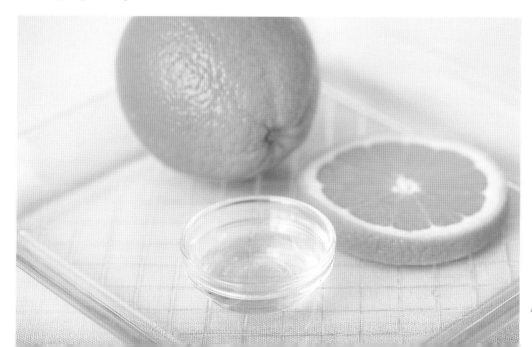

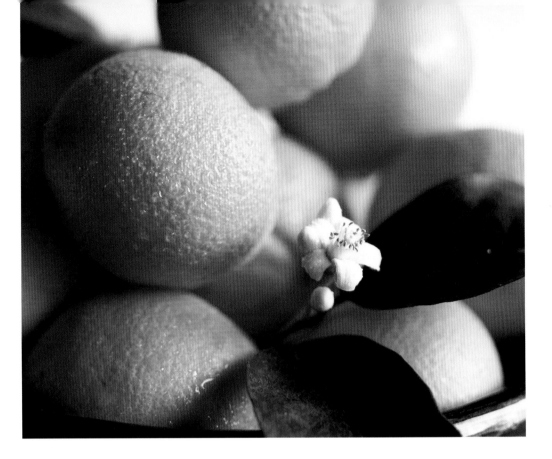

Citrus bergamia
syn. *C. aurantium* var. *bergamia*

Rutaceae
Bergamot orange

Oil of bergamot is expressed from the skin of the fruit just before it ripens. With its unique citrus and floral aromas, it blends well with cypress, geranium, lavender, lemon, neroli, palmarosa, patchouli, and ylang-ylang. The oil is useful as a fixative in cosmetic preparations and perfumes, and is an important ingredient in eau de cologne.

Uses: ESSENTIAL OIL
Used at 0.5–1 percent in a carrier oil, bergamot eases skin irritations, and softens cracked and dry skin. It is an excellent oil for treating many skin complaints. It eases pain, is antifungal, aids in wound healing, and helps to clear skin infections. It is said it will inhibit the virus responsible for cold sores if one drop is dabbed on the site immediately after the first warning tingle is felt.

Added to deodorant blends, it reduces body odor, and is also a very good personal insect repellent.

Bergamot's properties help increase the flow of urine, and act as an antiseptic and disinfectant making it useful in remedies to treat the infection and inflammation that characterize cystitis and urethritis.

Used in inhalations and chest rubs, it can ease the symptoms of bronchitis, coughs, chills, colds, and laryngitis.

It is a useful oil to use in air sprays, oil burners, and bath and massage blends to treat tension and anxiety.

Caution: *Patch test—may cause irritation on sensitive skin. Avoid using on skin that will be exposed to sunlight.*

Citrus limon

Rutaceae
Lemon

Lemons are an amazing and versatile fruit with a deliciously clean, sharp, fresh fragrance. Rich in vitamin C, lemons have abundant culinary, medicinal, and cosmetic uses in and around the home. The essential oil, which is expressed from the rind of the lemon, is used widely by the food and perfume industry. It blends well with benzoin, chamomile, eucalyptus, frankincense, grapefruit, lavender, orange, rosemary, sandalwood, and ylang-ylang.

Uses: HERB, ESSENTIAL OIL

A drink made from a whole pulped lemon—peel, pith, and juice—is particularly beneficial if you have a cold threatening or have a fever. Make it fresh—it becomes bitter on standing.

Lemon juice on its own is used to treat rheumatism, and to reduce the size of kidney stones and gallstones. Juice held in the mouth will stop the bleeding from gums and sockets.

Cosmetically, lemon juice is used diluted as an astringent for oily skin and as a bleach for discolored skin. It is also used as a rinse to balance oily hair or to highlight fair hair.

All creams and lotions containing 0.5–1 percent lemon oil may help to smooth skin and contract and tone tissue, and because of the mild bleaching action, can be used to treat oily, dull skin. It is successful in removing warts, and soothes and prevents infection when used on insect bites and stings.

Lemon is valuable oil in the treatment of sore throats, bronchitis, coughs, throat infections, colds, and influenza. It eases indigestion, expels gas from the intestines, and purifies the blood.

Caution: Avoid using on skin that will be exposed to sunlight. Patch test—may cause irritation on sensitive skin.

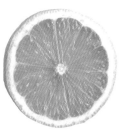

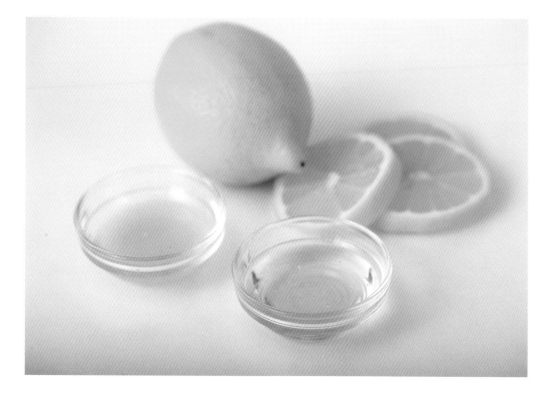

Citrus × paradisi

Rutaceae
Grapefruit

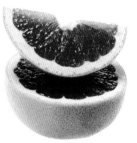

Mandarin and tangerine are not the same. The names mandarin and tangerine are often used to describe the same oil, but they are in fact different cultivars within the same species, and the oils have slightly different properties.

The best essential oil is expressed from the peel of fresh, ripe grapefruit; the distilled oil is inferior. It has a fresh, sweet, citrus aroma and blends well with basil, bergamot, cedarwood, chamomile, frankincense, geranium, palmarosa, rosewood, and ylang-ylang.

Unlike the other citrus oils, grapefruit is not a photosensitizer and may be used as a substitute for them in skin-care preparations if the skin is to be exposed to sunlight. However, grapefruit oil oxidizes quickly, so only buy in very small amounts and use within a short time.

Uses: ESSENTIAL OIL

Grapefruit oil contracts and tones tissues, and is useful in blends for oily skin and acne.

It eases muscle stiffness, soreness, and fatigue, and is a useful oil for a bath or shower blend, to relieve travel fatigue and jet lag.

Grapefruit's properties balance and tone the digestive system, and have a cleansing effect on the kidneys, liver and gall bladder, and the lymphatic system.

Citrus reticulata

Rutaceae
Mandarin orange

Mandarin oil is expressed from the peel of the ripe fruit. An inferior oil is steam-distilled from leaves and twigs. Mandarin is a safe, delicate oil to use in baths and massage oils for children, the elderly and during pregnancy, and as a terrific "pick-me-up" for those recovering from illness. The perfume is intense—a deliciously sweet, citrus-floral that blends well with basil, bergamot, black pepper, chamomile, grapefruit, lavender, lemon, lime, neroli, orange, palmarosa, petitgrain, and rose.

Uses: ESSENTIAL OIL

A lovely oil to use in blends to prevent or treat stretch marks and scars, and also for ageing and mature skin.

One of the main applications is when included in a massage oil for use over the stomach where it will act as a digestive tonic. Used in this way, it is particularly good for babies suffering from the "miseries" and pain of colic, as the digestive properties will relieve the cramps, and the sedative action will calm the fretfulness.

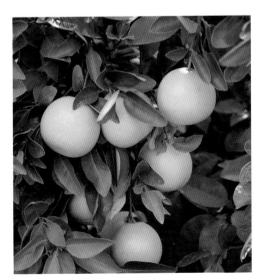

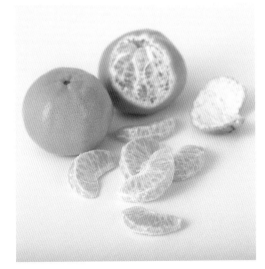

Citrus sinensis

Rutaceae
Orange
Also known as sweet orange

Glowing and sunny, fresh oranges and orange juice are rich in vitamin C and among the most popular fruits and juices. The essential oil is expressed from the orange peel. The perfume is happy and "citrussy," and blends well with angelica, benzoin, cinnamon, cypress, frankincense, lavender, neroli, nutmeg, petitgrain, rose, and rosewood. It is widely used as a fragrance in soaps, cosmetics, colognes, and perfumes, and also as a flavoring component in liqueurs, soft drinks, and food.

Orange oil will oxidize. Buy in small amounts and use within three to four months.

Uses: ESSENTIAL OIL
Orange oil is a good skin tonic for all skin types. It stimulates and brightens oily skin but is also useful for dry and normal skin. In blends with other oils, it is useful to treat fungal infections, and to kill bacteria.

Used in massage oil and applied over the stomach and abdomen, it has a toning effect on the digestive system and relieves wind, cramps and spasms in the intestines, settles a nervous stomach, and eases indigestion.

Orange oil's properties act to increase energy, boost the immune system, and reduce fever during cold and influenza.

Use only four drops dissolved in vegetable oil to baths to prevent irritation.

Caution: Patch test—may cause irritation on sensitive skin.

Cnicus benedictus

Asteraceae
Blessed thistle
Also known as holy thistle

Blessed thistle has a long history as a digestive and general tonic—it was a popular cure-all in the Middle Ages. It is usually found growing (to around 16 in/40 cm) along the wayside or in wasteland. The leaves are long, slender, sharply-toothed, and spiny, making it a very unfriendly plant to collect. The creamy yellow flowers are surrounded by a calyx that is just as spiny as the leaves.

Uses: HERB
The leaves, flowers, and seeds are all used as both a tea and a tincture. Take either three cups of tea or 20–40 drops of tincture in two tablespoons of water daily.

As with all bitters, it has a stimulant effect on the digestive tract, increasing the flow of gastric juices. This may make it useful for the physical treatment of anorexia. It is also an astringent, making it useful as a treatment for diarrhea, especially when combined with meadowsweet.

Caution: Not to be used during pregnancy. Excessive use can cause vomiting. This herb is subject to legal restrictions in some countries.

Growing and harvesting
It will grow in poor soil, needs little water, and likes the sun. Harvest leaves, flowers, and seeds in summer, and dry for later use.

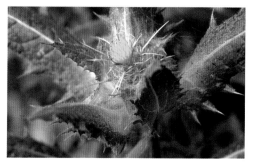

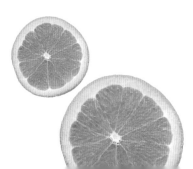

Commiphora myrrha

Burseraceae
Myrrh

Myrrh was widely used in ancient times throughout the Middle East, especially in Egypt where it was valued for its rejuvenating properties, and as an ingredient in the embalming process. Today the oil is obtained by steam distillation from the crude myrrh oleoresin that exudes from the trunk of the tree. The perfume is smoky, musky, slightly acrid and blends well with benzoin, frankincense, galbanum, lavender, patchouli, and sandalwood.

Uses: ESSENTIAL OIL, TINCTURE

The cooling action of myrrh reduces inflammation, and helps to heal boils, ulcers, weeping eczema, and infected wounds. The antifungal properties are helpful when treating athlete's foot.

Add a few drops of myrrh oil to skin-care blends for mature or prematurely ageing skin, chapped skin on lips, hands, and rough cracked skin on heels.

The tincture and oil are used commercially in toothpastes and mouthwashes as myrrh is possibly the best remedy to heal mouth ulcers, gum infections, gingivitis, and sore throats. The best way of using myrrh in the mouth is either to buy tincture of myrrh from the pharmacy or health-food store, or to make a three percent essence by dissolving 40 drops of myrrh oil into three tablespoons of high proof vodka or brandy. The essence or tincture may be dabbed neat into mouth ulcers, or one teaspoon added to one tablespoon water as a mouth rinse or gargle.

A powerful treatment for respiratory infections where the cleansing and drying properties help kill infection, and loosen and remove mucus during attacks of asthma, bronchitis, coughs, and colds.

Used in massage oil or fomentations for the abdomen, myrrh acts as a tonic and strengthener to the digestive system, easing diarrhea, indigestion, and flatulence. Add to ointments or carrier oil for treating hemorrhoids.

The antifungal action can be employed successfully to treat thrush, leucorrhea, and pruritus.

Caution: *Not to be used during pregnancy.*

Often purchased dry, myrhh has a cooling effect while the oil is indispensable in the treatment of mouth ulcers.

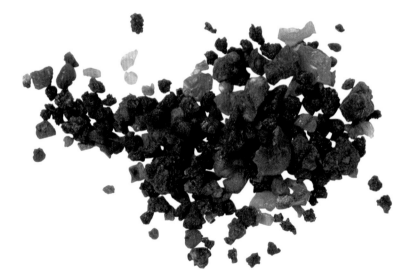

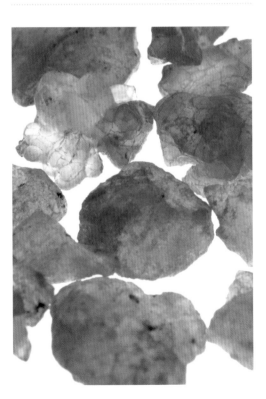

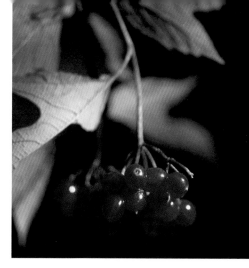

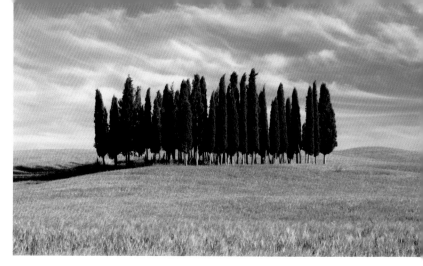

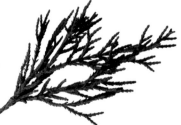

Reminiscent of the past, groves of cypress cover the landscape of central Italy.

Crataegus laevigata
syn. *C. oxyancantha*

Rosaceae
Hawthorn
Also known as may, quickset

Hawthorn, an attractive bush growing to about 23 ft (7 m) with sharp thorns, small white flowers, and bright red berries, is steeped in myth and tradition. *Crataegus laevigata* and *C. monogyna* are used interchangeably for medicinal purposes. Hawthorn has long been used as a heart tonic—both in natural therapies and clinical medicine.

Uses: HERB
Taken as capsules, tea, tincture, or extract, hawthorn is a safe herb that can be used long-term. It is the most widely used herb for cardiovascular problems including mild forms of angina and blood pressure. But remember, such conditions need to be monitored by a qualified practitioner.

Growing and harvesting
Plant hawthorn in well-drained soil in full sun or part shade. Water regularly. Harvest flowering sprigs in spring and dry for infusions, decoctions, tinctures, and teas. Collect ripe fruits late in summer or fall, and dry for tinctures.

Cupressus sempervirens

Cupressaceae
Cypress

Cypress, one of the safest and most gentle oils you can use, is distilled from the leaves, twigs, and needles. The clean, woody perfume blends well with juniper, lavender, pine, rosemary, and sandalwood.

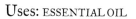

Uses: ESSENTIAL OIL
Use cypress as a tonic and sebum balancer for oily skin. It tones tissue and helps to reduce the appearance of broken capillaries. Include in aftershaves for its astringent action and woody perfume. It's a good wound oil as it stops or reduces external bleeding. Cold compresses can soothe and reduce hemorrhoids and varicose veins.

Add it to blends for deodorants and insect repellents, or use in a mouthwash.

Use in fomentations, baths, and massage blends to help relieve painful cramps and spasms, regulate the menstrual cycle, reduce heavy blood loss, and the symptoms of menopause. Its circulatory properties increase energy, warm cold hands and feet, and ease muscle cramps and rheumatism.

A cypress inhalation and chest rub can help reduce the spasms of asthma, coughs, bronchitis, and whooping cough.

Curcuma longa
syn. *C. domestica*

Zingerabaceae
Turmeric

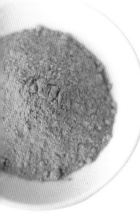

Pungent turmeric is a tropical perennial growing from underground rhizomes (the part used) to reach a height of about 3 ft (90 cm). It has long, oval-shaped leaves, and bears yellow flowers on a long stem.

We tend to think of this plant as a spicy seasoning but it is much more than this. Certainly, it is a prime component of curry powders, and is used for its color and flavor in many types of food in various cuisines. But it can also be used as a digestive aid, and a remedy for jaundice and other liver ailments.

Ground turmeric not only adds scrumptious flavor to curries but its wonderful color gives any rice dish a traditional Eastern look.

Uses: HERB

Turmeric can be effective easing the pain of acute inflammation although somewhat less so for chronic inflammation. Use an infused oil of turmeric as a massage oil in the treatment of sprains, cramps, bruises, and muscle pain.

Topical applications of the dried, powdered root are used to promote the healing of wounds and skin conditions.

Turmeric is a useful expectorant. When taken as a tea, it may help to treat bronchitis, colds and coughs, flatulence, and diarrhea.

Recent studies are showing that it may have a role to play in lowering blood cholesterol levels.

In cosmetics, turmeric is mainly used as a dye in lipsticks, skin foundations, and hair tints.

Caution: *Large amounts or long-term use of turmeric may cause heartburn or other gastric disturbances. Because of the biliary secretion properties of turmeric, it should not be taken by anyone with a biliary tract obstruction. Take with food, as it may upset the stomach. Not recommended for people taking blood-thinning medication.*

Growing and harvesting

Although a tropical plant, it can be grown in temperate areas in a warm, sunny spot in well-drained soil. Water and fertilize regularly. Propagate by rhizome division in fall. Lift rhizomes when the lower leaves turn yellow, and steam or boil before drying and grinding for use in teas, decoctions, poultices, and powders. Or use it to make an infused oil.

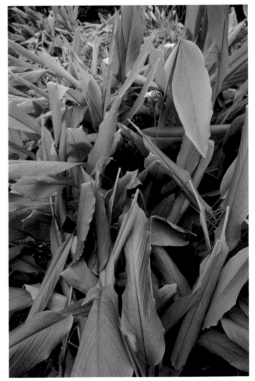

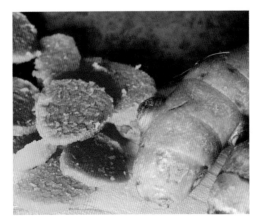

Turmeric roots have a thin dry skin and knobby appearance.

Cymbopogon citratus

Poaceae
Lemon grass

A semi-hardy perennial, lemon grass grows in clumps to about 5 ft (1.5 m) in height. The leaves grow from the base and are pale green and reed-like. The fleshy white base of the stems of lemon grass is widely used in Southeast Asian cookery, especially curries and satay sauces. The leaves themselves are tough and virtually inedible. However, it is from these leaves with their strong fresh lemony fragrance when crushed or bruised that the essential oil is distilled. Lemon grass oil blends well with cedarwood, geranium, jasmine, lavender, neroli, palmarosa, rosemary, and tea tree.

Uses: HERB, ESSENTIAL OIL

Lemon grass is a good herb for refreshing and cooling drinks. Use the leaves and white parts at the bottom of the stems in teas.

Use three drops only in a bath and no more than one percent in blends.

It is a refreshing, cleansing, and stimulating tonic to the skin. A good oil to include in blends to treat athlete's foot (or any fungal condition) where the deodorant and antifungal properties are of help. Use also in deodorants.

A good insect repellent, it protects animals and humans from fleas, lice, and ticks.

Added to shampoos, it gives shine to hair.

Lemon grass kills bacteria, fungal infections, and also has very powerful antiseptic and tonic properties.

It cools and reduces fever, and strengthens all bodily systems, making it a useful oil in the prevention and treatment of infectious diseases and during convalescence.

It stimulates the circulation, and helps to ease muscular pains and aching feet.

Caution: Not to be used during pregnancy. Not suitable for babies or toddlers. Patch test—may cause irritation on sensitive skin.

Growing and harvesting

Propagate lemon grass by root division or from seed, in well-drained soil in a sunny spot. Water regularly. This plant doesn't like its feet to be either cold or dry and will not tolerate frost. It is dormant in winter and may be slow to recover in spring. In a warm climate it grows a flowering stem, but it is unlikely to flower in cooler areas. Cut and use fresh in your cooking or fresh or dried for infusions or teas.

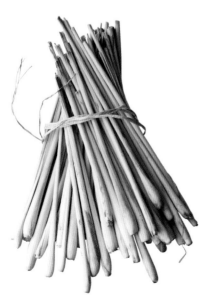

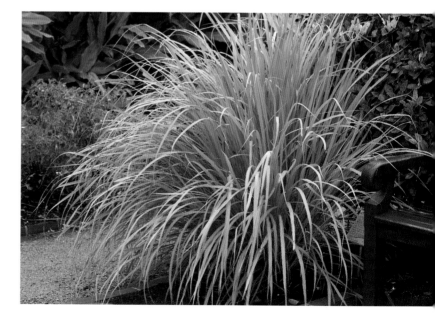

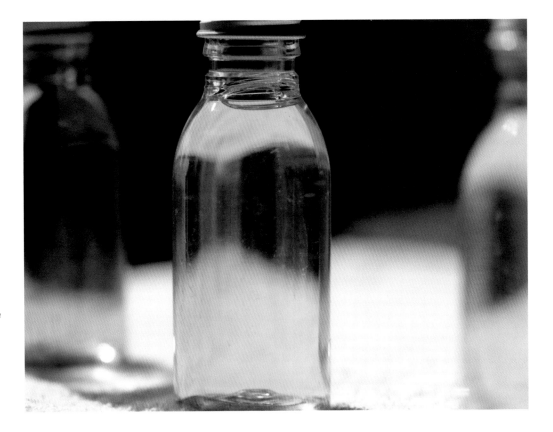

Palmarosa essential oil not only helps treat eczema and other skin conditions but it also emits a delectable floral scent.

Cymbopogon is a genus of some 50 species of grasses including a number with aromatic foliage that are of considerable economic importance for their oils, including lemon grass [*C. citratus*], citronella [*C. nardius*], and palmarosa [*C. martini*]

Cymbopogon martini

Poaceae
Palmarosa

Palmarosa essential oil is steam- or water-distilled from the whole plant. It is also widely used in making soap because, unlike other oils, it retains its sweet, rose-like, floral perfume that blends well with bergamot, citronella, geranium, cedar, jasmine, lavender, organe, petitgrain, sandalwood, and ylang-ylang.

Uses: ESSENTIAL OIL
One of the most valuable skin oils, palmarosa restores and maintains the correct water balance, and moisturizes, stimulates cell growth, and regulates the production of sebum. If used regularly, it will help to smooth and tone wrinkles and crepey skin.

Its antibacterial action makes it useful in skin-care products for acne, dermatitis, eczema, scars, sores, and skin infections.

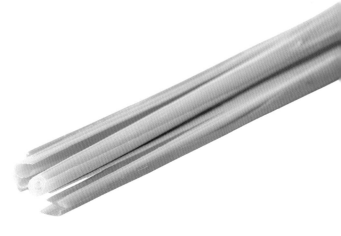

Cymbopogon nardus

Poaceae
Citronella

The essential oil is distilled from all parts of the plant and has a clean, powerful, and distinctive lemony perfume that blends well with bergamot, eucalyptus, geranium, lavender, neroli, peppermint, petitgrain, and ylang-ylang.

Uses: ESSENTIAL OIL

Citronella is mainly used in air sprays and body rubs as an insect repellent (particularly good against mosquitoes) for both humans and animals. It can be used in deodorant blends but should be added cautiously as the scent is quite overpowering.

Citronella encourages perspiration, increases energy and quickens the function of glands making it quite useful in bath and massage blends to treat colds, influenza, and other infections.

Caution: *Not to be used during pregnancy.*

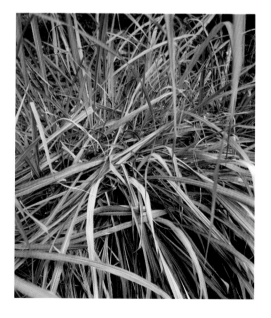

Daucus corota

Apiaceae
Carrot

The essential oil is distilled mainly from the seed of the wild carrot but oil is contained in the whole plant. The perfume is dry, warm, and sweet, and has the characteristic smell of carrots. It blends well with bergamot, cedarwood, geranium, juniper, lavender, lemon, lemon verbena, lime, melissa, neroli, orange, petitgrain, and rosemary.

Uses: ESSENTIAL OIL

Rich, golden, carrot seed oil (used discreetly) is wonderful for skin—it contracts and tones tissues, kills bacteria, and adds elasticity (especially with prematurely ageing skin), and it may remove or fade "age spots" and scars.

It is exceptionally healing, and may be included in small amounts in blends for dermatitis, anal or vaginal itching, eczema, ulcers, boils, and psoriasis.

Carrot seed oil helps to rid the body of toxins, so it is useful added in small amounts to bath and massage blends for treating arthritis, gout, and rheumatism.

It acts as a powerful tonic for the digestive system particularly the liver and gall bladder, aiding digestion, and helping to expel gas from the intestines. It is currently being used in the treatment of some cancers and jaundice.

Because of its regulating effect on hormone production it may be employed in blends for all menstrual problems, PMS, and menopause.

Echinacea angustifolia

syn. *Rudbeckia purpurea*

Asteraceae
Echinacea
Also known as purple cone flower,
rudbeckia

The name of this fascinating plant comes from the Greek word "echinos," meaning "hedgehog," and when you see and feel the prickly scales of the flower's rounded center you will appreciate the naming.

Echinacea is a remarkable herb, being non-toxic and having few side effects. It was widely used by Native Americans for a variety of conditions including the treatment of wounds. The root is medicinally the most commonly used part of all varieties, although the whole plant may be used, especially in ointments.

Echinacea angustifolia and *E. purpurea* are strong and handsome plants with dark green leaves and daisy-like flowers that bloom for several months, making them an attractive addition to a perennial border. *E. purpurea* grows to approximately 4 ft (1.2 m), with wide leaves, large pink-purple flowers that droop and a high, central, blackish cone. *E. angustifolia* is shorter, has narrow leaves and the flower petals are purple and more upright.

Uses: HERB

Take as a tincture, extract, or in capsules. Between 40-60 drops of the tincture taken three times daily in water is to be preferred. Echinacea is now being used as a premier immuno-stimulant remedy for building resistance to, and lessening the effects and duration of colds and influenza, and upper respiratory infections.

It is recommended for acute conditions temporarily affecting the immune system. For chronic, deep-seated illnesses it is recommended to begin a course of treatment with astragalus (see *Astragalus*), and then to follow up with echinacea.

In addition to taking echinacea internally, use the tincture externally on cuts, sores, and skin problems such as psoriasis, eczema, and acne. This herb is useful in ointments and extracts for the treatment of wounds, minor burns, cuts, and mouth sores. It also encourages cell regeneration.

Growing and harvesting

Grow from seed or root cuttings in fertile soil in a sunny position in the garden or deep pots (not seed trays). Once planted it doesn't like to be disturbed. It prefers not to be too wet and is winter dormant. If the position is wet, the roots might rot over winter and the plant will not regenerate in spring. Lift rhizomes in the fall and dry for use in decoctions, infusions, extracts, ointments, capsules, and tinctures.

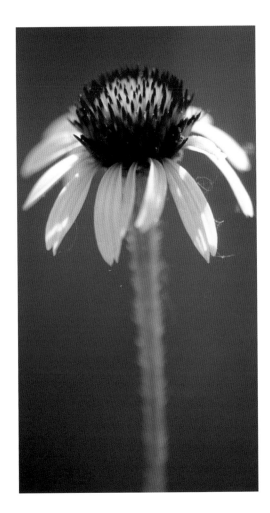

Elettaria cardamomum

Zingiberaceae
Cardamom

Cardamom has been used in cooking, medicine, perfume, and incense for more than 3,000 years. The essential oil is steam-distilled from the seeds. The perfume is warm, spicy, and blends with other spice oils, frankincense, geranium, juniper, orange, and rosewood. It is related to ginger and they have several properties in common particularly that of being able to warm and tone the system.

Uses: ESSENTIAL OIL
The main use for cardamom oil is for its tonic and digestive action. When used in baths, massages, or fomentations, it will stimulate appetite, ease colic, flatulence, indigestion, nausea, and the griping pains of diarrhea. It may also help to treat bad breath due to poor digestion.

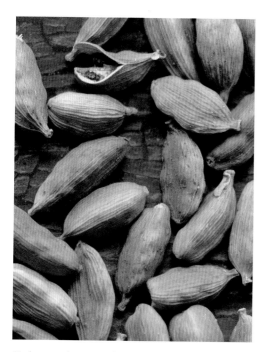

Cardomom pods are ground to make the powder used in curries, while the distilled oil is perfect for massage.

Eleutherococcus senticosus
syn. *Acanthopanax senticosis*

Araliaceae
Siberian ginseng

Siberian ginseng is a distant cousin of the true ginsengs. This deciduous shrub is also a larger plant than *Panax ginseng* with a height of 8–22 ft (2.5–7 m). The roots and root bark have long been used in Chinese medicine especially for rheumatic complaints. It has apparently been used by cosmonauts and Olympic athletes to reduce stress, and as a general tonic.

Uses: HERB
Siberian ginseng is a pungent, bitter-sweet, warming herb. It's more useful for maintaining good health rather than treating poor health. It acts as a tonic for people who are run-down, or feeling weak and lacking in energy. It helps to reduce high blood pressure, reduces physical and mental stress, and improves stamina and resistance to stress.

Caution: Not be taken in large doses or for prolonged use (more than six weeks at a time).

Growing and harvesting
Siberian ginseng grows from seed in rich, moist soil. Harvest rootstock in fall and dry for use in extracts, decoctions, and infusions.

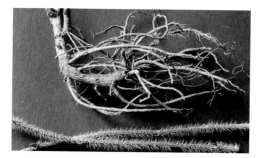

The tangled, hairy roots and bark of ginseng are the base of a stress-relieving tonic.

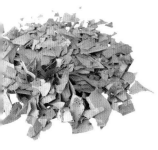

Eucalyptus globulus

Myrtaceae
Eucalyptus
Also known as Tasmanian blue gum,
blue gum

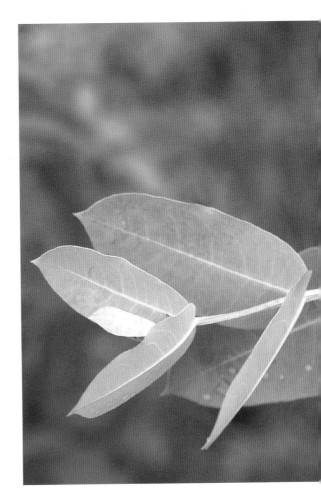

The handsome Tasmanian blue gum was the
first eucalypt to be introduced to Europe and
North America. This impressive tree can grow
to over 150 ft (50 m). Eucalyptus essential oil,
one of the most powerful natural antiseptic
oils, is distilled principally from its fresh
leaves and twigs, and has a clean, camphoric,
and cleansing perfume that blends well with
lavender, rosemary, and pine.

The oils of other varieties are used too,
notably *Eucalyptus citriodora* (lemon-scented
gum) and *E. dives* (Australian peppermint or
broad-leaved peppermint).

Use eucalyptus oil with care. If a recipe
says one drop, then that's all that's required!
Two drops will not be better.

Uses: ESSENTIAL OIL

Eucalyptus oil is used in the treatment of
burns, blisters, cuts, wounds, and sores, as
it prevents bacterial growth, inhibits the
growth of viruses in the damaged tissue,
and eases pain.

It is one of the best oils to use in blends
to kill head lice, ease the itch of insect bites,
and act as an insect repellent.

It is used in low concentrations in
creams for cold sores, and for genital herpes.

Added to baths and massage oils
or creams, it will ease the pain of sore
muscles, aches and pains, rheumatism, and
rheumatoid arthritis.

Eucalyptus has long been respected for
its ability to lower temperature, and help the
respiratory tract by loosening and removing
mucus during attacks of bronchitis, coughs,
and influenza, sinusitis, and throat infections.
Added to a foot bath it is a prime remedy
during feverish attacks.

Used in an air spray, its antibacterial and
antiviral properties will help to prevent the
spread of epidemics and diseases including
chickenpox, mumps, or measles. Its antiviral
and antibacterial action will deter further
growth of the bacteria and viruses. At the
same time it will also have the effect of
giving some protection to other members of
the family.

A fomentation containing eucalyptus
will increase the flow of urine, and this
combined with its other properties will help
to ease cystitis and urethritis.

Another useful and interesting property
of eucalyptus oil is that it removes many
stains and grease marks from clothes.

It's definitely a brain cleanser—
crystallizing the mind like a breath of fresh
air and aiding concentration.

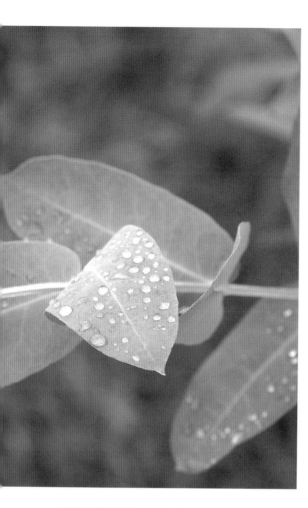

Filipendula ulmaria

Rosaceae
Meadowsweet
Also known as queen of the meadow

A striking, clump-forming perennial growing to a height of 2–4 ft (60 cm–1.2 m), meadowsweet bears large, dense heads of small, sweet-smelling, creamy white flowers on stiff reddish stems. The plant contains salicylates that act to ease pain in a similar way to aspirin.

Uses: HERB

Meadowsweet used as an infusion, decoction, extract, or tincture generally has alterant action, healing, soothing and relieving pain.

It is an excellent herb for using in remedies for easing heartburn, acidity, and disturbed digestion.

An anti-inflammatory, it can ease the pain of rheumatism, arthritis, and aching muscles and joints.

Meadowsweet is also helpful in reducing fevers, and helps in the treatment of urinary tract infections.

Growing and harvesting

Meadowsweet grows easily from seed or root cuttings in a sunny spot with moderate water. Harvest and dry plants as flowering begins. Gather flowers separately for infusions if you wish.

Caution: *Not to be used if you have high blood pressure, suffer from epilepsy, have an inflammatory disease of the gastrointestinal and bile ducts, or a severe disease of the liver. Do not store near homeopathic remedies or use in conjunction with them.*

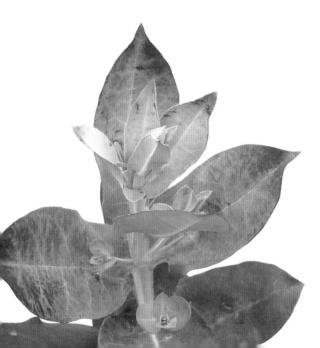

Foeniculum vulgare

Apiaceae
Fennel

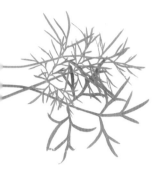

Fennel is a tall and handsome perennial, graceful and feathery. The stems are strong, tubular, and bright green and grow to a height of about 6 ft (2 m). The leaves grow from sheaths that surround the stem; they are feathery and similar to dill, but much larger. The flower heads are flat umbels of bright yellow florets blooming from late spring onwards. The seeds are slightly curved and grayish green in color, becoming brown when dried. The leaves, seeds, and roots of the plant are all useful.

The variety used in aromatherapy is sweet fennel (*Foeniculum vulgare* var. *dulce*) as it is less sensitizing. The seeds are crushed and distilled to produce an essential oil with a perfume similar to aniseed that blends well with frankincense, geranium, lavender, rosemary, and rose.

Uses: HERB, ESSENTIAL OIL

Fennel is best known for its tonic, antispasmodic, and cleansing action on the digestive system. It acts as a liver cleanser and eases digestive problems, such as indigestion, constipation, cramps and spasms, colic, nausea, flatulence, and hiccoughs. It is also useful as a tea for people who have difficulty with fat absorption. To make the tea put a teaspoon of the seeds in a tea pot and leave to "steep," strain, and pour.

It is similar to aniseed in its calming effect on bronchitis and coughs, and its licorice-like flavor helps to disguise bitter cough remedies and other unpleasant-tasting preparations.

Fennel works well on the reproductive system where its estrogen-like and antispasmodic properties are helpful in relieving cramps and spasms in the uterus, scanty and irregular menstrual flow, PMS, and water retention. It stimulates the adrenal glands to produce estrogen after the ovaries have stopped working and, in so doing, helps to correct menopausal irregularities due to fluctuating hormones. The hormone activity also increases the production of milk in nursing mothers.

Externally, the essential oil or infused oil eases muscular and rheumatic pains. The tea may be used as an eyewash or compress to treat conjunctivitis, tired and sore eyes, and inflammation of the eyelids.

Fennel is a cleansing tonic for oily skin, and has a reputation for retarding the appearance of wrinkles.

Caution: Avoid using on skin that will be exposed to sunlight. Not to be used during pregnancy or if you suffer from epilepsy. Do not use in blends for children.

Growing and harvesting

Plant seeds or seedlings in a sunny and sheltered (remember it's tall) part of the garden in rich, well-drained soil. Water regularly. Keep away from dill or cilantro (coriander) to reduce the chances of cross pollination. Cut back the old growth in winter months. Pick young stems; leaves can be picked when you need them, and collect and dry the seeds for use.

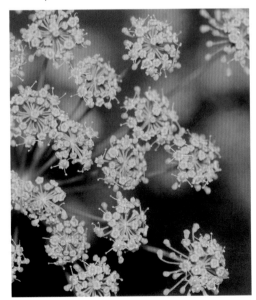

Ginkgo biloba

Ginkoaceae
Ginkgo
Also known as maidenhair tree

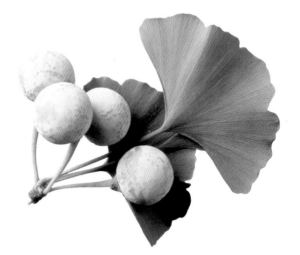

Deciduous ginkgo grows to 130 ft (40 m) and is a beautiful, stately tree with fan-shaped leaves. While it's possible to grow this tree, be aware that it takes a long time for it to become big enough to use and by then it may be too big for the average garden.

Uses: HERB

Ginkgo has become a very popular remedy and is used for a variety of conditions associated with ageing including memory loss and poor circulation. Extracts of ginkgo leaves have antioxidant effects and also increase blood circulation, thus helping to ease cold hands and feet, pain in the hands, legs, or lower back, and eyesight problems that are caused by poor capillary function. It has been used clinically for tinnitus (ringing in the ears).

Health professionals commonly use ginkgo in the treatment of early-stage Alzheimer's disease.

Caution: Ginkgo is generally well tolerated, but it can increase the risk of bleeding if used in combination with blood-thinning medications such as warfarin.

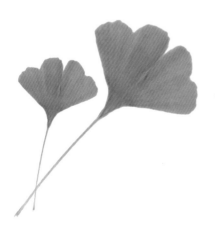

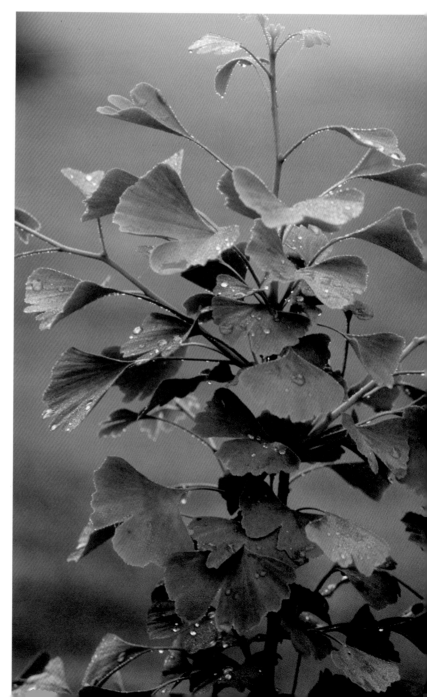

Glycyrrhiza glabra

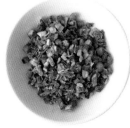

Fabaceae
Licorice
Also known as licorice root, sweet licorice

It is worth growing this plant, as it is a large and handsome addition to the garden while you are waiting for the roots to mature. It is a perennial, initially slow growing then spreading rapidly outwards and up to 5 ft (1.5 m) tall. Small, dark green, graceful leaves stand up by day and droop by night. Mauve, pale blue, or yellowish flowers grow from the axils. The roots are made up of two parts. One is long, brown, cylindrical and many-branched, while the other comprises horizontal rhizomes which run just below the ground and throw up shoots, causing the plant to spread over a large area. Both parts of the root are used.

Many people prefer to buy licorice root from the health-food store rather than grow it, as it takes four years for the plant to be ready to harvest. Even then it has to be dried and ground into a powder or chopped. The other form in which it is used (and which I prefer) is as an extract, which cannot easily be made at home. It is available from pharmacies or health-food stores.

Licorice is an invaluable herb and one of the most widely used medicinal plants for which it's not easy to find an alternative. As well as having healing properties, it makes putrid-tasting herbs more acceptable to the palate, in tinctures, teas, and decoctions. This is of particular importance when treating children, as they are very resistant to unfamiliar tastes but will accept licorice readily.

Uses: HERB
It has wide applications in tinctures, teas, and decoctions in treating respiratory tract infections, coughs, mucous congestion, lung congestion, and viral infections.

Licorice itself makes a delicious tea that may be served hot or cold.

Caution: *Not to be used during pregnancy. Not for prolonged use except under supervision by a qualified health practitioner. Do not use if you have hypertension, cardiovascular disease, kidney or liver disorders, or diabetes. Avoid excessive doses; use only in amounts recommended. Eat more potassium-rich foods (such as bananas and dried apricots) while using licorice.*

Growing and harvesting
It can be grown from seeds, suckers, or root division, but be careful to control it, as it is invasive. It likes moderate water and a sunny position, and will resist frost.

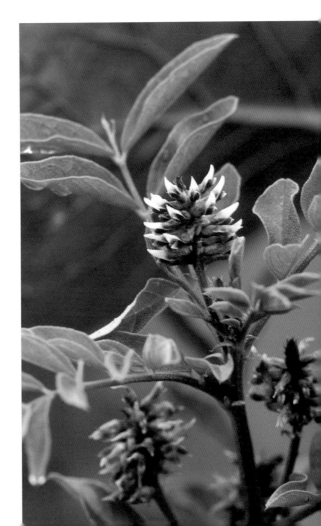

Harpagophytum procumbens

Pedaliaceae
Devil's claw
Also known as grapple plant, arthritis tea

Devil's claw, a native of southern Africa and the island of Madagascar, has thorny fruit that catch in animal fur. The roots or tubers are used.

Uses: HERB

The main use of devil's claw is in the treatment of rheumatic pain and joint problems, mainly arthritis and lumbago. It needs to be taken continuously as a tea or tincture three times a day for up to four weeks before noticeable pain relief is felt. It can be combined with other herbs like meadowsweet, angelica, celery seed, or nettles. The normal dosage is one teaspoon of dried root as a decoction made with one cup water taken three times a day (drink one cup of tea three times daily) or 20–40 drops of the tincture taken three times daily in water.

Caution: Not to be used during pregnancy. Not to be used if you have cardiovascular problems, a gastric or duodenal ulcer, or if you are taking blood-thinning medications such as warfarin.

Growing and harvesting
Grows easily from seed sewn in sandy soil in a warm climate. Lift tubers in winter and dry for later use.

Helichrysum italicum
syn. *H. angustifolium*

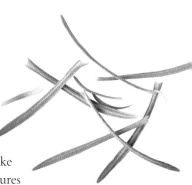

Asteraceae
Immortelle
Also known as everlasting flower, curry plant

Immortelle has strongly aromatic daisy-like flowers that become dry as the plant matures but retain their color and perfume. There are many varieties of helichrysum but only *H. italicum* is used for making the essential oil. Steam-distilled from fresh flowers, it has a honey-sweet perfume that blends well with chamomile, clary sage, frankincense, lavender, geranium, clove, and citrus oils.

Uses: ESSENTIAL OIL
Immortelle is ideal to use in blends for acne, allergic reactions such as hives, dermatitis, eczema, inflammations, psoriasis, and wounds. It promotes cell growth making it valuable in skin-care preparations.

Blended with lavender and mandarin, it makes a safe, sweetly perfumed oil for massaging babies and children where it can help to treat asthma, bronchitis, coughs, and ease the distressing "whoop" of whooping cough.

Use in baths and massage oils for rheumatism, muscular aches and pains, sprains, and strains.

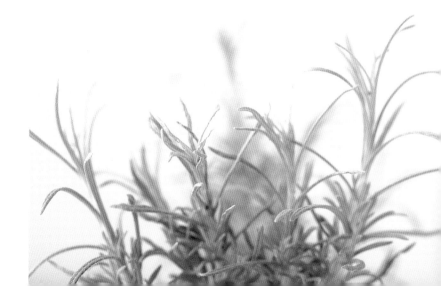

Hydrastis canadensis

Ranunculaceae
Goldenseal
Also known as orangeroot and yellowroot

This North American herb was used for a variety of medicinal purposes by the Native Americans, became a popular "cure-all" home remedy with the new settlers especially for its wound-healing properties, and is now recognized and respected the world over. Goldenseal grows in humid shady woodlands with rich soil and deep humus. It has been collected to the point of near extinction, and was listed as an endangered species in 1997. It is now being commercially cultivated to meet demand. The rhizome is the part used.

Uses: HERB

Combine goldenseal with echinacea as a tea or tincture for cold and influenza symptoms, coughs, and sore throats. Take 15 drops of tincture in water, or one cup of tea three times daily. Children and the elderly should take smaller doses.

As a diluted, well-strained infusion, goldenseal is a valuable herb for using as a wash to treat skin diseases, wounds, and sore inflamed eyes, and as a mouthwash for gum disease. It is also an effective wash or douche for yeast infections.

The ointment will help to heal hemorrhoids, herpes, impetigo, psoriasis, eczema, athlete's foot, scabies, and ringworm.

Sprinkle the finely powdered root directly onto open wounds to disinfect and promote scab formation.

Taken internally, goldenseal aids digestion.

It is useful in the treatment of menstrual disorders, urinary infections, rheumatic and muscular pain, and as an antispasmodic.

Caution: Avoid excessive or prolonged use. Not to be used during pregnancy or given to children under the age of two.

Growing and harvesting

Goldenseal is not really for the home garden as germination is unreliable, and it will be several years until plants will be large enough to harvest. Sow seeds in rich, well-drained soil in a shady position in the garden, or propagate by rhizome division. Lift rhizomes in the fall, and dry for using in decoctions, teas, tinctures, powders, ointments, and capsules.

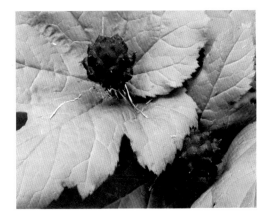

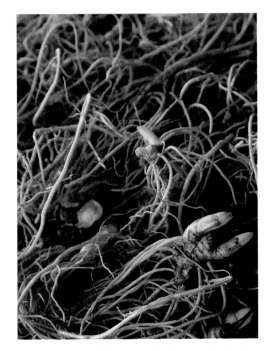

The common names of orangeroot and yellowroot aptly describe the knotted rhizomes that are used to make teas or tinctures.

Hypericum perforatum

Clusiaceae, formerly Guttiferae
St John's wort
Also known as common St John's wort, perforate St John's wort

St John's wort is a sprawling perennial herb growing to 2–3 ft (60–90 cm), with dark green leaves and bright yellow flowers that appear to have dots on the petals when held up to the light. These "dots" are glands holding little droplets of oil which, when the flowers are steeped to make an infused oil, release themselves resulting in a glowing, ruby-red liquid. The infused oil, also known as hypericum-infused oil, is available in most good health-food stores but if you can find the plant in flower, you can make this oil yourself.

Uses: HERB, INFUSED OIL

Taken in infusion, tincture, or tablet form, St John's wort is an excellent herb to allay anxiety, relieve general stress, and deal with mild to moderate depression. As well as having a calming and tranquilizing effect, it also appears to strengthen the immune system, and improve mental clarity. It is a useful herb for insomniacs.

Massage muscles and joints with the infused oil to ease the pain of sprains, fibromyalgia, rheumatism, neuralgia, sciatica, and other muscle pain.

Use the ointment or infused oil for inflammations, wounds, burns, bruises, skin ulcers, shingles, and varicose veins.

Caution: Consult a health professional before taking St John's wort if you are on any medication. Do not rely on it as a treatment for severe depression. Might decrease the effectiveness of oral contraceptives. May cause photosensitivity—avoid exposure to direct sunlight when using.

Growing and harvesting

This herb isn't fussy where it grows, although it does prefer a little shade. Be careful where you plant it, as it is very invasive. In fact in some parts, it's declared a noxious weed. Harvest as flowering begins, and use fresh or dried in infusions, tinctures, tablets, ointments, or to make an infused oil.

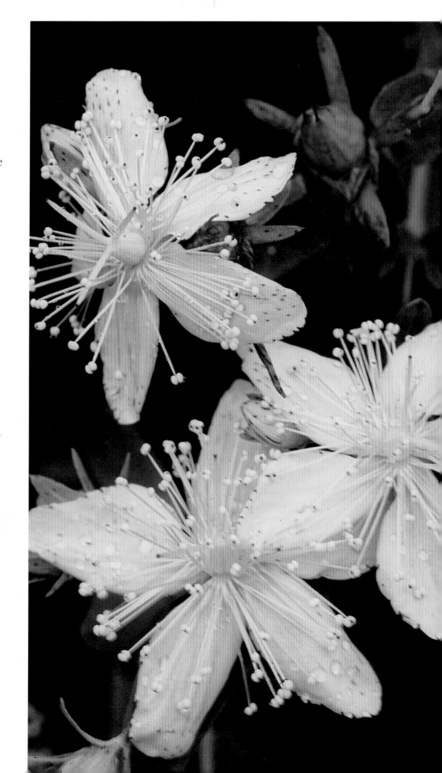

Hyssopus officinalis

Lamiaceae
Hyssop

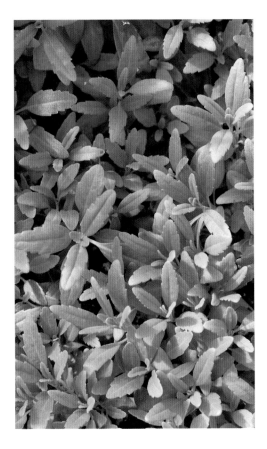

Hyssop is bushy perennial herb that can grow to 2 ft (60 cm) or more. It has woody stems and narrow dark leaves, which have a sweet scent when bruised, and are sometimes added to salads, or to legumes (pulses) or meats during cooking. Its pink, blue, or white flowers are very popular with butterflies and bees.

The essential oil is distilled from the leaves and flowers. The perfume is difficult to describe—it's a combination of camphor and spice, and blends well with citrus, geranium, lavender, rosemary, and sage.

This is a questionable oil to use as the pinocamphene and thujone content makes it fairly toxic. I prefer to use fresh or dried hyssop only, as there are safer essential oils that perform the same functions.

Uses: HERB, ESSENTIAL OIL

The use of hyssop leaves for respiratory infections has been recorded from Greek and Roman times to today.

Hyssop taken as a weak tea or well-diluted tincture three times daily is particularly valuable for children suffering from influenza, bronchitis, and coughs, and may be mixed to advantage with elder flowers and peppermint.

It is a general insect repellent and works well in sprays.

Grow near cabbages or grapes but away from radishes.

Use hyssop essential oil only in conjunction with other oils, and not exceeding 0.5 percent of total essential oil content.

Hyssop oil used in ointments is quite useful for bruises, cuts, eczema, and wound healing.

Use as a massage oil to reduce fever, and help to relieve congestion.

Mixed with other digestive herbs and taken as a tea, hyssop aids digestion—helping to expel gas from the intestines, and easing mild constipation. It is beneficial for menstrual problems, encourages and regulates menstrual flow, and increases the flow or urine.

Caution: The essential oil is not to be used during pregnancy. Avoid if you suffer from epilepsy or high blood pressure. Use only recommended doses.

Growing and harvesting

Grow hyssop from seeds or cuttings in a sunny, well-drained position in the garden. It is frost hardy. Remember, it's bushy, so you will need to cut it back to maintain shape. Pick leaves and flowers as the buds open, and used fresh or dried in infusions, extracts, tinctures, and teas.

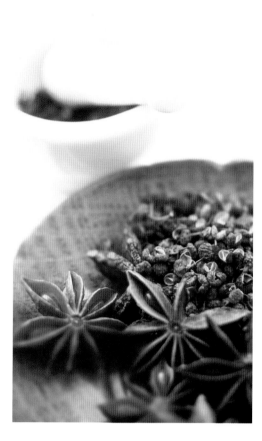

flavoring food and drinks. It has been widely used in Europe since the sixteenth century as a flavoring agent for liqueurs.

Uses: ESSENTIAL OIL

Add to inhalations and massage blends at 0.5 percent (2 drops in 4 teaspoons/20 ml carrier oil) to treat respiratory complaints where there is a mucus problem such as during bronchitis, sinusitis, and colds.

It is helpful for dispelling flatulence, and easing the digestive pains and colic. It eases constipation by encouraging a stronger action of the bowel.

It has a warming effect that could help with pain such as rheumatism and lumbago—complaints that are aggravated by the cold.

Caution: *Not to be used over the whole body. Not to be used in high concentrations or for prolonged periods.*

Illicium verum

Illiciaceae
Star anise
Also known as badian

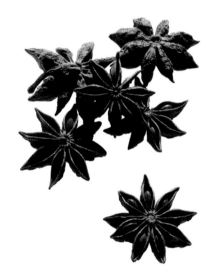

Star anise essential oil is extracted by steam distillation from the fresh, green, star-shaped fruits of *Illicium verum*. The oil has a licorice-like aroma, and blends well with other spice oils, lavender, pine, orange, and rosewood.

Although the perfume and properties of star anise and anise/aniseed (*Pimpinella anisum*) are almost the same, the two oils aren't related, and star anise is a much safer oil to use. However, it needs to be treated with great care, and shouldn't be used for a total body massage

Star anise is used in pharmaceuticals to mask the taste of less pleasant tasting ingredients, and by the food industry for

Jasminum officinale

Oleaceae
Jasmine
Also known as common jasmine, jessamine

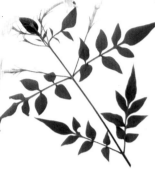

Jasmine is synonymous with sweet and heady fragrance. Its essential oil, sometimes called the "king of the oils," is one of the most expensive as the extraction process is a lengthy business—only the flowers are used and they have to be picked at night when the perfume is most intense. It is one of the most important oils in high-quality perfumery work.

Jasmine's sensual and relaxing perfume blends well with most other oils, especially rose and citrus oils. Substituting ylang-ylang will give almost the same effect in recipes and blends.

Jasmine flowers alone in a bowl are enough to evoke the romance of a summer evening.

Uses: ESSENTIAL OIL

Jasmine softens and smooths dry irritated skin, and balances the production of sebum thus making it useful in skin-care preparations for most skin types. It eases dermatitis and is said to encourage a glorious head of hair when used in shampoos and hair tonics.

Used in massage oils and fomentations, jasmine strengthens and tones the uterus, particularly after childbirth (do not use until labor has started), and relieves cramps and muscular spasms of the uterus during painful periods.

Jasmine can be sniffed straight from the bottle to great effect when the heart is beating rapidly and there is breathlessness due to shock or anxiety. It will also help to reduce high blood pressure.

The scent of jasmine is best known for its ability to stimulate our responses, and to create and increase sexual desire. It is one of the most important oils for helping to ease depression.

Caution: *Avoid during pregnancy. Overuse can cause headaches or nausea. Unsuitable for the very young.*

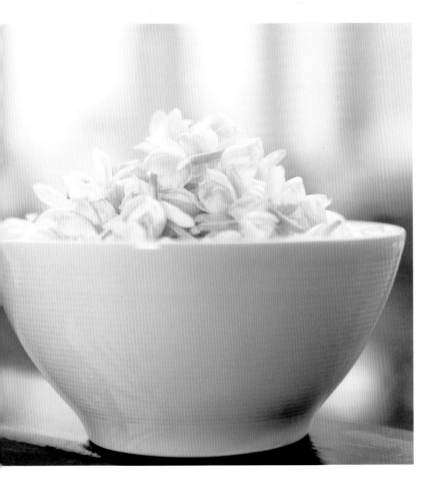

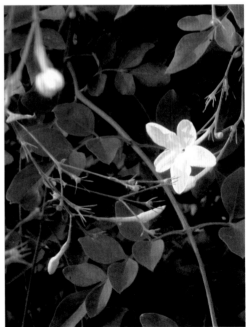

Juniperus communis

Cupressaceae
Juniper
Also known as common juniper

The best essential oil is steam-distilled from the ripe berries; an inferior oil is produced using the berries, needles, and twigs. The aroma is sharp and stimulating, and blends well with citrus oils, cypress, lavender, and pine. The berries, which take a couple of years to ripen, are also used to flavor gin!

Users of this oil should be aware that due to its powerful detoxifying action it might produce a "healing crisis," and the condition may appear to worsen before it begins to improve.

Uses: ESSENTIAL OIL

Juniper's perfume and properties make it ideal to use in air sprays and oil burners to purify air in sick rooms.

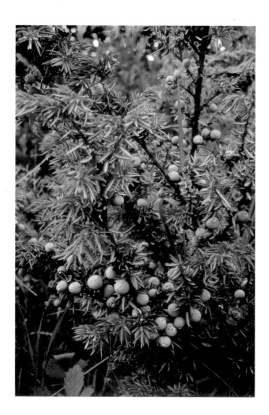

Used in baths, massages, or fomentations, it can increase the flow of urine in fluid retention, enlarged prostrate gland (only after medical opinion has been sought), and kidney stones. It also acts as an antiseptic for relieving cystitis and urethritis.

Juniper is one of the most useful oils to include at one percent in creams, lotions, and hair products for clearing oily skin and scalp. The detoxifying action is indicated for treating the possible causes of acne, dermatitis, psoriasis, and eczema.

It is useful to include in personal insect repellent blends for humans (and dogs), where it may be used to deter ticks and fleas.

It can be added (no more than one percent) to cream, gel, or oil for external application to hemorrhoids.

It is a very important tonic and powerful detoxifier for such conditions as food poisoning, an excess of rich food or alcohol, gout, and rheumatism.

Its ability to increase perspiration and reduce temperature make it suitable for baths and massage oils to treat feverish conditions such as colds, influenza, and infectious diseases.

It produces localized redness and warmth when applied to the skin, which eases muscular pain. Juniper works well on the reproductive system where it relieves cramps and spasms in the uterus, and encourages and regulates menstrual flow.

This vital oil will dispel the anxiety, nervous tension, and stress created by leading a busy, people-filled life.

Caution: Not to be used during pregnancy nor if suffering from kidney disease. Do not use for a prolonged period (more than six weeks).

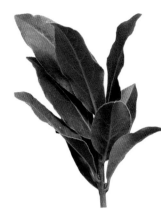

Laurus nobilis

Lauraceae
Bay laurel
Also known as sweet bay

A tall stately tree, bay laurel has shiny, dark green leaves and is often grown in tubs as an ornamental shrub. The leaves, which are spicily fragrant, are used in cooking or kept in dried foods as a deterrent to weevils. Leaves were once woven into wreaths by the ancient Greeks and Romans to crown their victors. The highly perfumed flowers come in creamy yellow clusters and are loved by bees. In warmer climates the bay tree can grow to a height of about 50 ft (15 m), but in cold regions it is much smaller, looking more like a big shrub. Bay trees can be grown in large pots and are often used for topiary work.

The oil is steam-distilled from the leaves and twigs, and has a spicy almost medicinal aroma that blends with clary sage, cedarwood, citrus, cypress, eucalyptus, ginger, lavender, marjoram, rosemary, and all spice oils. Commercially, it is used in many products ranging from detergents to cosmetics, and perfumes, and also in processed foods.

Uses: HERB, ESSENTIAL OIL

Fresh bay leaves are quite bitter so it's preferable to use dried leaves in cooking. It is a very strongly flavored herb, and is best when added in small amounts (one to two leaves to a dish for four people) to soups, sauces, and stews.

The leaves dry well and are useful insect repellent if fastened inside the lids of storage containers for grainy foods such as rice or barley. Placed on bookshelves they will help to deter silverfish.

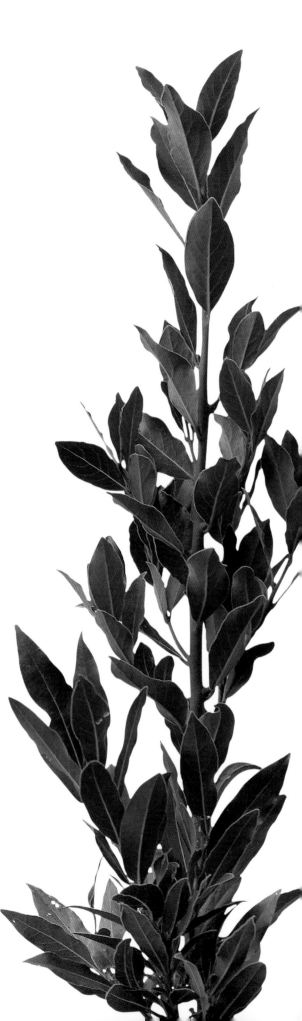

As with other spicy oils, bay helps the digestive system where it has a tonic effect on the liver and gall bladder. It can be used in small amounts (2–3 drops in $2^{1}/_{4}$ tablespoons/40 ml of vegetable oil) to massage the abdomen, and ease the discomfort of indigestion, flatulence, and loss of appetite.

A mild immune system booster and with the capability of encouraging sweating, it can be included in blends for inhalations and massage to treat fever, infectious diseases, and bronchitis.

Caution: *Not to be used during pregnancy. Use only on small areas of the body. Unsuitable for using in baths as it may cause skin irritation.*

Growing and harvesting

Grow this tree from cuttings (there's a high failure rate germinating seeds), which will strike more readily if given bottom heat. It likes a sunny spot with good quality, well-drained soil. It's quite hardy, but a slow grower, and susceptible to white scale. Pick mature leaves year round to use fresh or dry in bunches in a warm airy place. Dried leaves lose their flavor if kept for more than a year or so.

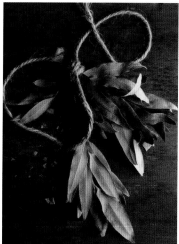

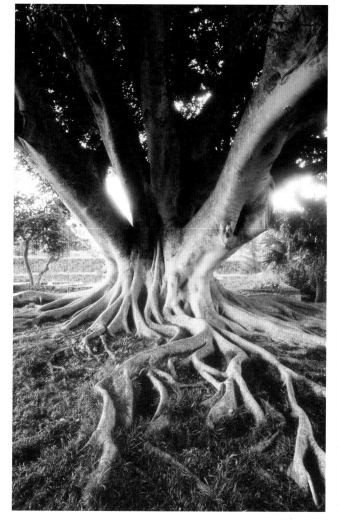

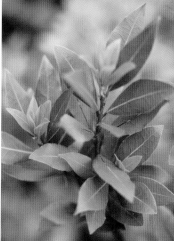

Lavandula angustifolia
syn. *L. officinalis*, *L. spica* in part, *L. vera* in part

Lamiaceae
Lavender
Also known as English lavender

Today this is probably the best-known and loved of herbs. The flowers are used in potpourris, sachets, and sleep pillows for their calming fragrance. In addition to being a favorite, lavender is also one of the most versatile herbs, being used for perfume, healing, as a household cleanser, a culinary ingredient, and a disinfectant.

In the kitchen, the flowers can be used to flavor sugar and jams. Crystallized lavender flowers make an attractive decoration on desserts. Not many herbs can lay claim to such a variety of uses.

There are about 25 species of lavender—aromatic evergreen perennials and shrubs. *Lavandula angustifolia* (formerly *L. vera*) is most commonly cultivated for its precious oil. Growing to 24–28 in (60–70 cm, it has grayish green, narrow, pointed leaves that are covered with soft, downy hairs. Tiny mauve flowers are borne in clusters or whorls at the top of long spikes.

Other varieties include *Lavandula dentata* (fringed lavender), which grows into quite a large shrub, and is useful for hedging, provided it's regularly pruned after flowering to prevent it from becoming bare and woody at the base.

Lavandula allardii (Mitcham lavender or giant lavender) has all the benefits of other lavenders in one plant and is my preferred lavender. It can grow up to 4–5 ft (1.2–1.5 m) high and 3 ft (90 cm) wide, with long flower heads on tall spikes. Its scent alone makes it worth growing and using in the home.

With its "balancing" qualities, lavender has to be the most used essential oil, and probably the one with the longest list of applications. If you can afford only one essential oil, choose lavender—it is safe, versatile, and gentle, and may be used undiluted over small areas. It is steam-distilled from the flowers and the powdery aromatic leaves.

For perfumery choose English lavender for its softer, sweeter scent. The perfume is comfortably familiar, fresh, clean, floral, and soft, and it blends well with most other oils. Spike lavender (*L. latifolia*) is very similar but its refreshing, penetrating perfume is clearer and stronger. It blends well with bergamot, citrus oils, eucalyptus, geranium, jasmine, lavender, and rosemary. For medicinal purposes spike lavender seems to have a more profound effect.

Uses: HERB, ESSENTIAL OIL

Flowers and leaves can be sipped in tea to calm stress and ease stress headaches. The tea, made triple strength, also makes a soothing and refreshing addition to the bath, or when patted over the body after a shower. The tea is also effective as a douche to treat thrush, and other vaginal infections.

Lavender is one of the most valuable oils for skin care and skin conditions as it stimulates the growth of new cells, kills bacteria, is antibiotic, antiviral, prevents scarring, and eases pain. Use it to treat abscesses, acne, athlete's foot, boils, bruises,

The name is derived from the Latin verb *lavare*, meaning "to wash," and lavender was widely used by the Romans for laundry and bathing.

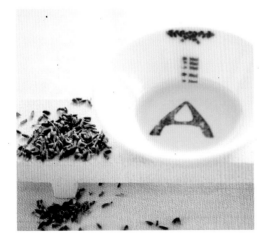

Lavender flowers and oil—the cure-all for almost anything.

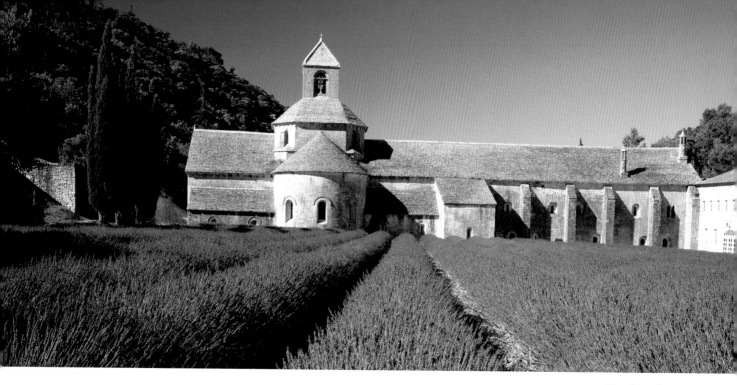

inflammations, dermatitis, eczema, insect bites, stings, psoriasis, scabies, sunburn, burns and scalds (minor), sores, spots, ringworm, and wounds. Include it in deodorants as it reduces body odor.

Lavender is renowned for its effective relief of the pain and inflammation caused by arthritis, lumbago, muscular aches and pains, rheumatism, sciatica, and muscular pain arising from tension. The best way of using lavender oil for these problems is in a synergistic massage or bath blend with other oils where it will strengthen their properties.

The antiseptic, antiviral, and antibiotic properties combined with the ability to loosen and expel mucus make it an ideal oil to use as an inhalation and chest rub for bronchitis, coughs, colds, laryngitis, mucus, and throat infections.

Used in baths, massages, or fomentations, it eases problems with the digestive system, respiratory and urinary systems, relieves cramps and spasms in the intestines and uterus, and stimulates bile production. It helps to expel gas from the intestines, and encourages and regulates menstrual flow.

It is a good companion to silver beet. It repels beetles, mosquitoes, sandflies, and flies, and is a good indoor insect repellent.

Caution: *Not to be used during the first four months of pregnancy—longer if there is a history of miscarriage.*

Growing and harvesting

Grow it from seed, seedlings or stem cuttings in a sunny spot in the garden (or in a pot) in well-drained soil. It really doesn't like damp or shady places. Prune after flowering. Harvest stems on a dry day before the heat of the sun has drawn out the volatile essences. Hang in bunches or spread on racks to dry in a warm, airy place. Use fresh or dried in infusions, teas, tinctures.

Magnificient Senanque Abbey in Provence in the south of France forms a backdrop for the ripe lavender fields that dominate the landscape in summer.

TIP REMEMBER THAT IN AN EMERGENCY, LAVENDER FIXES ALMOST ANYTHING

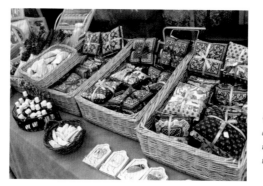

Open-air herb and food markets can be found any day of the week in the villages and towns that dot the French countryside.

Leptospermum scoparium

Mytaceae
Manuka
Also known as New Zealand tea tree

Manuka is an evergreen shrub or small tree growing to 26 ft (8 m). Its brown bark sits loosely on the trunk and branches. It has tiny white flowers, which generally bloom in spring and summer. The prickly, narrow leaves have a sharp perfume when crushed, and are used to produce a lovely and powerful essential oil. I use it in preference to tea tree as I much prefer the smell. The perfume is sweet and soft, and blends well with cinnamon, clary sage, clove, cypress, eucalyptus, geranium, ginger, lavender, lemon, lemon grass, mandarin, marjoram, rosemary, and thyme. Unfortunately, unless you live in New Zealand, this essential oil is quite expensive compared with tea tree.

Uses: ESSENTIAL OIL

It may be used undiluted on small areas of skin or in a carrier oil to treat abscesses, ringworm, corns, mouth ulcers, blisters, warts, and cold sores.

Add to baths and foot baths to treat athlete's foot, wounds, sunburn, burns, and scalds (minor). Use as a mouthwash or gargle to treat bad breath, gingivitis, and tonsillitis.

The antihistamine action of manuka is useful for treating insect bites and stings, and allergic reactions such as hives.

Diaper rash can be avoided or healed if you add 0.5 percent manuka oil to the cream used on your baby's bottom.

Manuka oil has the capacity for loosening and removing mucus and this, combined with its other properties, makes it a valuable remedy to use in baths, massage oil, and inhalations to treat bronchitis, catarrh, colds, influenza, fevers, coughs, sinusitis, tuberculosis, and whooping cough.

When used in an oil burner or air spray, it will help to prevent the spread of infectious diseases.

It can be used to treat urinary tract infections such as urethritis and cystitis, vaginal trichomonas, candida, thrush, herpes, and vaginitis.

LEMON TEA TREE CAN BE USED INSTEAD OF CITRONELLA

Lemon tea tree (*Leptospermum petersonii* syn. *L. citratum*) is an evergreen shrub growing to 13 ft (4 m) tall, with flaky bark, lemon-scented, narrow, dark green leaves, and five-petaled, scented, white flowers from early spring to early summer. The oil is distilled from the leaves. The perfume has a delightfully fresh and rosy tone, and blends well with cedarwood, lemon grass, and patchouli.

Uses: essential oil

- Possibly the best known use of lemon tea tree is as an insect repellent where its fresh scent is to be much preferred to that of the previously popular citronella. Use in combination with cedarwood, lemon grass, and patchouli as an anchor.
- May be included in any product where an antimicrobial action is needed. Useful as an ingredient in deodorant products.
- Lemon tea tree has been also shown to be active against *Aspergillus niger*, *Candida albicans*, *Pseudomonas aeruginosa*, and *Staphylococcus aureus*.

Litsea cubeba

Lauraceae
Mountain pepper
Also known as may chang, exotic verbena, tropical verbena

This is a small tropical tree native to China, and other regions in East Asia, that has scented flowers and foliage, and small berries shaped like peppers. The essential oil is produced by steam distillation from the fruits, and has an intense lemon perfume similar to that of lemon grass. The oil blends well with basil, geranium, jasmine, lavender, lemon grass, neroli, orange, petitgrain, rose, rosemary, rosewood, and ylang-ylang.

Uses: ESSENTIAL OIL

Use it in lotion and cream blends to treat acne, dermatitis, spots, greasy skin, and in deodorants where it will help to control perspiration.

It has digestive properties, and could be added to fomentations or massage blends to ease digestion and flatulence.

Caution: Patch test—may cause irritation on sensitive skin.

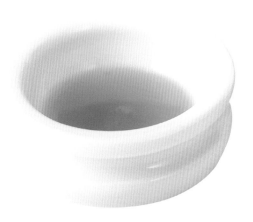

Mountain pepper essential oil blended with orange, rosemary, and a drop of patchouli.

Medicago sativa

Papilionaceae
Alfalfa
Also known as lucerne

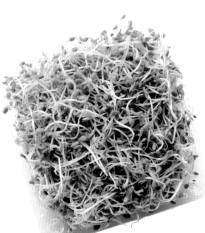

Alfalfa is a perennial herb that grows to 12–32 in (30–80 cm), with blue-violet flowers that appear during the summer months. Unless you have a lot of land it's not practical to grow this plant, or other plants such as red clover, mung beans, lentils, and fenugreek. These are better to sprout—they take up less space that way.

Uses: HERB

This is a most nutritious plant for humans and animals—a valuable supplement to our diet. Fresh alfalfa sprouts are delicious in sandwiches and salads, and leaves and flowers may be taken as a tea three times daily.

Use for easing indigestion, stimulating appetite, and as a tonic for conditions relating to the kidneys and the reproductive system. It cleanses toxins from the body and helps to control bleeding. It can be used as a poultice for boils and insect bites.

Caution: Avoid alfalfa if you have auto-immune problems or are taking blood-thinning medication. Not to be used during pregnancy, while breastfeeding, or for young children.

Growing and harvesting

Alfalfa is grown easily from seed sown in spring or fall. Cut plants before flowering and dry for infusions. New leaves can be used fresh.

Sprouting seeds

Sprouting seeds and grains is a way of growing fresh greens, even if you live in a one-room apartment. Sprouts are full of vitamins and minerals. They taste good and are cheap, easy, and fun to grow.

It's always a temptation to sprout too much seed when you first begin. As a guide to quantities, remember that a quarter of a cup of seeds becomes two cups of sprouts, and its better to maintain a steady supply of fresh sprouts than to have bowlfuls of sprouts losing goodness in the refrigerator.

CONTAINERS FOR SPROUTING

All sorts of containers can be used for sprouting. Look around and you will find many things that can be used: colanders, sink strainers, sieves, or one of the ideas following:

Unglazed flowerpot saucers

These are inexpensive, easily available, aesthetically pleasing to have around the kitchen, and they work well. Different sizes allow you to grow different-sized sprouts. You will need two of each size at any one time.

Wash and soak the containers in water to prepare them before starting the sprouting. Sprinkle the soaked and strained seeds evenly in the bottom of one saucer, and invert the other saucer to cover it. Stand these saucers in a dish of water—the water will be absorbed through the unglazed terracotta. Keep near the stove or in a kitchen cupboard. Another good place is on top of the refrigerator towards the back, where the heat escapes. Top up the dish of water as needed. When the plants are as tall as you want, take the top saucer off, leaving the bottom one standing in the container of water, and put near a window for a day or so. The sprouts will grow a little more during this time and develop their green leaves. Store in a cool, dark place, or in the refrigerator.

Plastic containers

Square or round $^{1}/_{2}$ gallon (2 liter) plastic containers such as those for ice cream, make excellent sprouting trays. They don't look pretty, but they don't cost anything, and are very efficient. To prepare them punch a lot of holes in the bottom with a skewer.

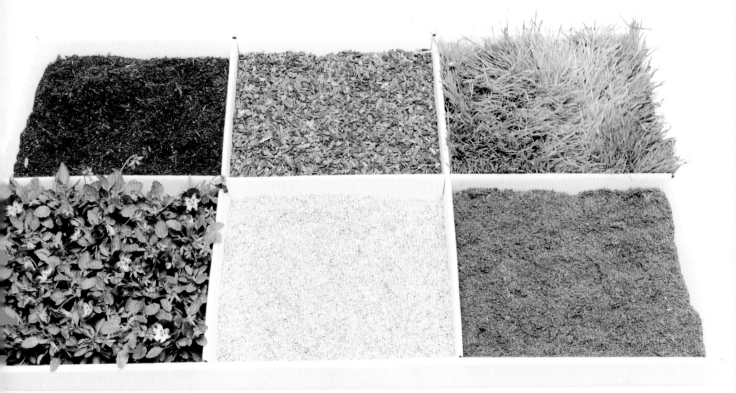

Growing your own herbs from seed is a rewarding experience and can be done in almost any container found around the home.

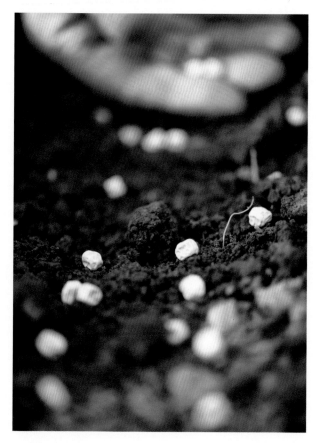

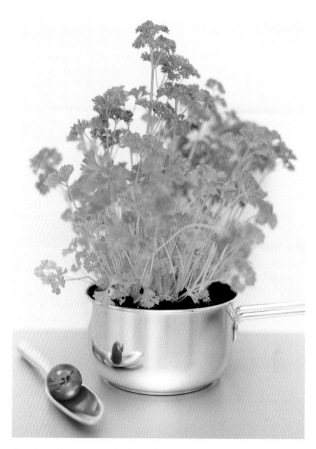

Seeds from larger herb varieties and vegetables can be planted straight in the ground.

Growing herbs can be a work of art when planted in a stylish kitchen container.

I use these containers for big seeds like mung beans, lentils, and fenugreek, but you can make them suitable for small seeds by laying blotting paper, cheesecloth, or nylon fly netting in the base.

Spread the soaked and strained seeds evenly over the bottom of the container, and put the lid on. Twice a day stand the container in enough water to come up through the holes and just cover the seeds, then lift it out and let it drain. Treat the sprouts in the same way as described for flowerpot saucers.

Glass jars

Any sized glass jar can be used. You will need some sort of cover (not a lid) for the jar. This must allow air to circulate among the sprouts, otherwise they will rot. A piece of coarse cheesecloth, net curtain, or old pantihose will do, with an elastic band to hold the cover on. Keep in mind the eventual size of the plants, for it becomes difficult to rinse them properly if they are too closely packed.

Keep the jar on its side and grow the sprouts in the same way as described previously, rinsing them daily. To keep out as much light as possible, cover all but the mouth of the jar with a folded cloth, or place in a cupboard.

HOW TO SPROUT SEEDS

First, remove any debris or broken seeds before you begin sprouting. If these bits are left in, they may rot and spoil the whole batch.

Rinse the seeds and soak in warm water overnight. Drain and pour the drained water on indoor plants, or use it for stock in cooking. Put the seeds in your chosen container, and keep them moist (not wet), in dark and warm conditions. They need rinsing each day or they will begin to either rot or dry out.

When alfalfa and red clover sprouts are about $3/_4$ in (2 cm) high, and the little leaves appear (after three to five days), they can be exposed to sunlight for a time until the leaves turn green. Mung beans, lentils, and fenugreek can be eaten as soon as the roots are $1/_4$ in (7 mm) long. Don't leave them too long or they will become bitter. When ready, take them out of the sprouting container, rinse well, and put them in a covered dish in the refrigerator or other very cool place. Try to use within four to five days (rinsing each day to gain the maximum goodness).

Melaleuca alternifolia

Myrtaceae
Tea tree

There is no doubt about it, tea tree (also called ti tree) is tops when it comes to healing oils. Ranking as the number two antiseptic oil (after thyme), it is reputed to be 100 times stronger than carbolic acid, and safer to use than thyme. Tea tree is closely related to cajuput (*M. leucadendra*) and niaouli (*M. viridiflora*) oils but is more powerful than both.

The distilled essential oil is widely used in household and personal toiletries, and cleansers, as well as in natural remedies. The perfume is resinous and slightly musty, and blends well with cinnamon, clary sage, clover, cypress, eucalyptus, geranium, ginger, lavender, lemon, lemon grass, mandarin, marjoram, rosemary, and thyme.

Uses: ESSENTIAL OIL

Tea tree oil is a "first aid in a bottle" treatment for abscesses, acne, athlete's foot, blisters, boils, burns and scalds (minor), rashes, gingivitis, mouth ulcers, insect bites, diaper rash, ringworm, and infected wounds.

One drop of undiluted tea tree oil applied to a cold sore will often prevent it from getting worse. Corns and verrucas can also be treated in this way (using the oil directly on the corn or verruca and covering with a plaster) but will take a little longer to heal. Pimples also will often respond to the one-drop treatment.

It is one of the most important oils to use in gargles, baths, massage blends, air sprays, and oil burners to treat respiratory tract infections such as bronchitis, catarrh, colds, coughs, influenza, fevers, sinusitis, tonsillitis, tuberculosis, and whooping cough. Add it to air sprays and oil burners to prevent infectious diseases from spreading.

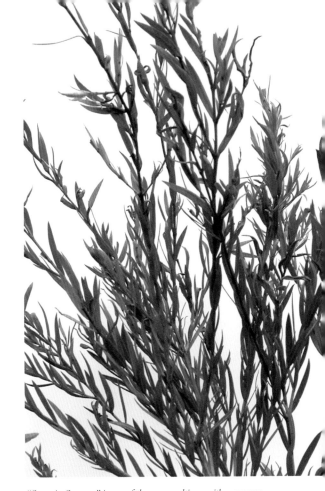

"Snow in Summer" is one of the many cultivars with a common name of tea tree.

It is one of the few oils that I recommend for use in douches and other genital treatments for vaginal trichomonas, candida, thrush, pruritus (itching of the anus and genital area), and genital herpes.

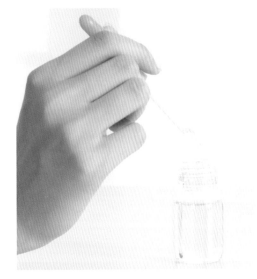

One drop of undiluted tea tree oil is a great acne treatment.

Melaleuca leucadendra

Myrtaceae
Cajuput
Also known as weeping paperbark,
weeping tea tree

Cajuput, a tall, vigorous, robust tree also called the weeping paperbark, is related to eucalyptus, clove, myrtle, tea tree, and niaouli. Along with these oils cajuput has the ability to successfully combat and prevent infection. The oil is extracted by steam distillation from the buds, leaves, and twigs. The perfume is similar to eucalyptus but sweeter. Cajuput blends well with angelica, bergamot, clove, geranium, lavender, niaouli, nutmeg, rosewood, and thyme. It is used in pharmaceutical preparations as an antiseptic, and thanks to this property it is also used in manufacturing soaps, detergents, and cosmetics.

Uses: ESSENTIAL OIL

Cajuput oil is useful for treating insect bites, acne, psoriasis, and spots. It is also a very valuable insecticide.

Its similarity to tea tree means that it can be used in many of the same situations, but it is particularly useful in massage oils for easing rheumatic pains, arthritis, muscular aches and pains, and rheumatism. It also relieves cramps and spasms in the intestines and uterus.

It is a fine respiratory tract treatment for helping to loosen and remove mucus, increase perspiration, and cool and reduce fever. Asthma, bronchitis, sinusitis, sore throat, feverish colds, laryngitis, and viral infections will all respond to treatments with cajuput oil—including baths, massage and inhalation (not for asthma sufferers), and air sprays.

Its antiseptic properties also help in the treatment of cystitis and urethritis, and it can be used as a mild painkiller for easing toothache.

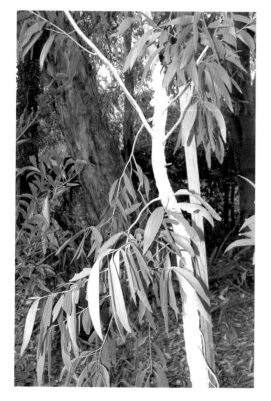

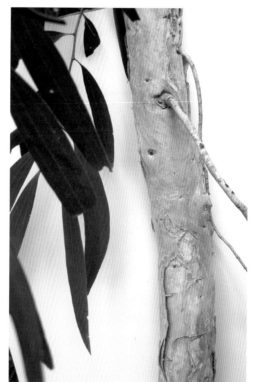

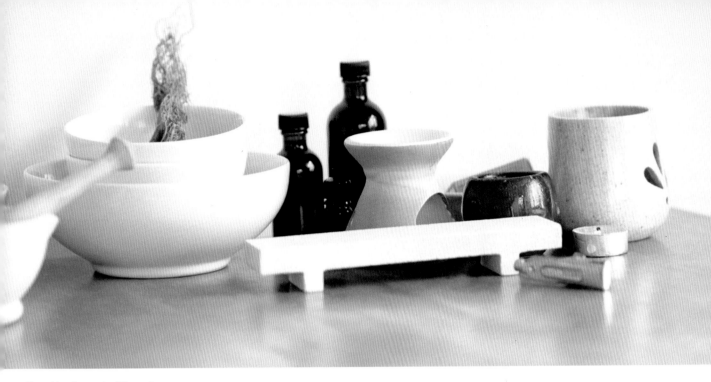

Essential tools to make full use of all the properties of niaouli.

Melaleuca viridiflora

Mytaceae
Niaouli
Also known as broad-leafed paperbark

Niaouli essential oil is extracted by steam distillation from the leaves and young twigs of the broad-leafed paperbark tree. Its natural antiseptic qualities make it ideal for the medicine cabinet. The perfume is strong, camphor-like and clean, and blends well with juniper, lavender, lemon, lemon grass, lime, oregano, pine, peppermint, and rosemary.

Although niaouli and cajuput oils are closely related, niaouli is a better choice for using on the skin as it is less likely to irritate. It is used in commercial preparations such as gargles, toothpastes, and breath fresheners.

Uses: ESSENTIAL OIL

Acne, boils, cuts and minor burns, grazes, insect bites, sores, spots, and wounds will all be helped to heal by the application of the diluted oil. It eases pain and kills bacteria.

Used in a mouthwash, it will help to sweeten bad breath caused by gum disease or bad teeth (obviously in this case a visit to a dentist is also recommended).

Included in a bath or massage blend, niaouli will help ease muscular aches and pains, rheumatism, poor circulation, and neuralgia.

Inhalations will loosen and remove mucus and, as it also cools and reduces fever, it may be used to treat bronchitis, coughs, colds, sinusitis, laryngitis, influenza, and whooping cough.

Melissa officinalis

Lamiaceae
Lemon balm
Also known as melissa, balm, honey plant, bee balm

This perennial herb grows to 12–32 in (30–80 cm). With its sweet, soft, and lemony smelling flowers, leaves and abundant nectar, lemon balm brings bees to the garden. Lemon balm has been used to flavor many well-known alcoholic drinks such as Chartreuse and Benedictine.

The oil is extracted by steam distillation from the leaves and flowering tops. As there is so little oil in these parts of the plant, melissa is very expensive to extract. A blend of lemon and petitgrain gives an approximation of its properties and scent. Melissa blends well with basil, chamomile, frankincense, geranium, ginger, lavender, rosemary, and ylang-ylang.

Uses: HERB [LEMON BALM], ESSENTIAL OIL [MELISSA]
Lemon balm is a gently tranquilizing herb. The leaves and shoots are best used fresh or frozen as a tea or tincture, which is suitable for treating anxiety, depression, heart flutters, stomach nerves, and high blood pressure. It also eases nausea, colic, and flatulence.

Give hot teas to treat influenza, colds, fevers, mumps, and headaches.

This is an excellent herb for young children, as the action is effective but gentle, and the taste is softly lemony and delicious.

Skin allergies respond well so use to treat acne, eczema, and bee stings—useful also as an insect repellent, and in general garden insect sprays.

As an oil, use only three drops of melissa in a bath, and no more than one percent in any blends.

Melissa oil will relieve cramps and spasms, cool and reduce fevers, and calm the heart, slowing palpitations, lowering blood pressure, and easing headaches and migraine.

It is one of the best oils for treating allergies both of the skin (allergic skin reactions) and the respiratory system, where it can be used to relieve hay fever and asthma.

Caution: Not to be used during pregnancy. Patch test could cause irritation.

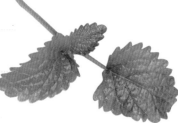

Growing and harvesting
Grow lemon balm from seed, cuttings or root division, and plant in full sun or a semi-shaded place. It doesn't like having roots in cold and wet, and may die right back in winter. Harvest as flowering begins, and use fresh or dried in infusions, extracts, ointments, and tinctures.

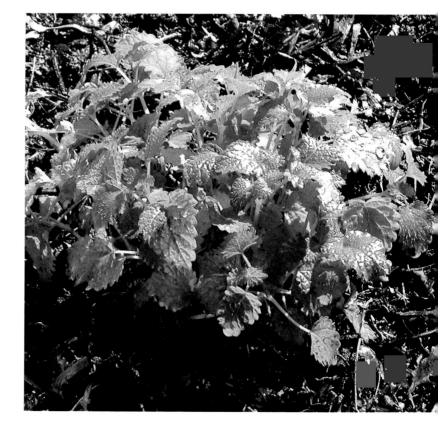

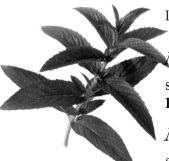

Mentha *species*

Lamiaceae

Mentha × *piperita*
syn. *M. nigricans*
Peppermint

M. spicata
syn. *M. crispa, M. viridis*
Spearmint

M. pulegium
Pennyroyal

Refreshing **peppermint** has a variety of uses. It is one of the most popular of the herbal teas, and the leaves add a delicious tang to cool drinks. In fact, its clean refreshing flavor and therapeutic qualities ensure that it is widely used in the food and pharmaceutical industries. The most important chemical element is menthol from which the well-known menthol crystals are formed. The refreshing, cooling, and warming oil is extracted from the leaves by steam distillation. The perfume is highly penetrating and minty and blends well with benzoin, eucalyptus, lavender, marjoram, lemon, rosemary and other mints. Peppermint and lavender oil have an affinity for each other and work in a complementary and synergistic way. Peppermint oil is one of my most loved and most used oils.

Spearmint stands out from the crowd in the culinary department. In the kitchen, spearmint leaves go well with fish, lamb, vegetables, and stewed fruit dishes, especially when added late in the cooking. Use them in salads and fruit salads, drinks (float a few sprigs in a jug of lemonade for a wonderfully refreshing summer drink), dressings, vinegars, and as a garnish, fresh or crystallized.

Pennyroyal is best known as the flea herb. It makes a great ground cover in a damp, shady spot and although you can snip a few leaves and add to soup or salads, keep in mind it's not to everyone's taste.

Uses: HERB, ESSENTIAL OIL

A tea or tincture made with peppermint leaves will help ease indigestion, wind, and gripe problems, reducing colic and cramps. Use spearmint in preference to peppermint for easing indigestion and colic in children and during pregnancy, as the action is gentler. Peppermint and spearmint will also help to ease diarrhea by soothing the lining and muscles of the colon.

For indigestion after a meal, mix one drop only of peppermint oil with a little honey in a glass, fill the glass right up with warm water (at least 1 cup/250 ml), stir, and sip the contents at once. The "burping" that follows is almost immediate and most satisfactory. The same treatment can be used to ease nausea or vomiting caused by food or travel sickness.

Use pennyroyal leaves as a tea for its soothing sedative and perspiration-

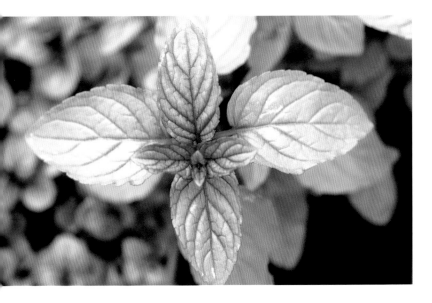

Mentha *"Chocolate" is a seductive addition to the mint family with its subtle flavor combination of dark chocolate and refreshing mint.*

promoting qualities, and to relieve gripe. It is also suitable to stimulate menstrual flow.

Peppermint and spearmint promote perspiration and cooling when treating fevers, headaches, and migraines. When combined with elder flower and yarrow, a tea of these mints makes a first-rate treatment for influenza.

If you feel you are about to catch a cold, try a hot bath containing three drops only of peppermint oil, three drops marjoram oil, and four drops lavender oil, dissolved in one teaspoon of vegetable oil. Sip a cup of peppermint, yarrow, and elder flower while you bathe. If a feverish cold has already struck, peppermint or spearmint oil will help to loosen mucus and reduce the fever.

The cooling and pain-relieving action of both oils is immensely soothing to hot, tired, and aching feet and legs. One percent of the oil can be used in a spray or gel to apply to the legs and feet. It shouldn't be rubbed in but allowed to dry naturally on the skin.

Treat headaches, mental fatigue, nervous stress, shock, palpitations, vertigo, dizziness, and fainting attacks by applying cold compresses made with peppermint or spearmint oil to the forehead. Alternatively, smell the oil directly from the bottle or use in an oil burner or air spray.

Rub dried, powdered pennyroyal into your pet's coat to deter fleas.

Peppermint oil deters insects and rodents—they detest its odor.

Growing mint in the garden will repel caterpillars and cabbage moth. For this reason it is a good companion to cabbages.

Caution: Not to be used during pregnancy. Use oils in small quantities—0.5 percent is plenty in a blend. Do not use in conjunction with homeopathic remedies and store separately.

Growing and harvesting

Grow mints (including some of the other delicious varieties such as chocolate and apple mint) from seed, root division, or runners, in semi-shade in rich, moist soil or indoors in a pot with lots of water. Take care to control them in the garden as they are invasive and can take over. Cut back to ground level in winter. To harvest, cut leafy stems just before they flower and hang in bunches in a warm, airy spot to dry. Use fresh or dried in cooking and herbal preparations.

WHICH MINT IS THAT?

Peppermint has dark green leaves, purple-tinted stems and lilac flowers. With a creeping rootstock, it grows to about 1–3 ft (30–90 cm).

Spearmint stems are square, with bright green, short-stemmed, pointed leaves with irregularly serrated edges. Pale lilac flowers appear in whorls at the top of the stem.

Pennyroyal has pale purple flowers that grow in clusters and small, bright green leaves that are quite unlike others of the mint family. It grows to about 16 in (40 cm) cm tall.

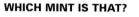

These aromatic perennials with their vigorous creeping rootstock have a place in every garden. With all varieties, especially if you grow more than one, it's essential to pick off the flower heads as they bloom. If you neglect to do this they will cross-pollinate each other and the plants will become not-so-useful "bastard" mints, lacking any distinct flavor or perfume.

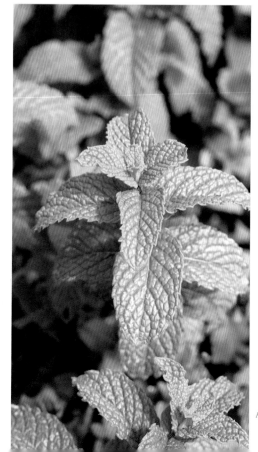

Mentha × piperita

Monarda didyma

Lamiaceae
Bergamot
Also known as bee balm, Oswego tea

The *Monarda* genus was named in honor of Spanish physician Nicolas Bautista Monardes [1508–88] whose *Joyfull News Out of the Newe Founde Worlde* was the first book to describe tobacco, coca, passion vine, guava, and sarsparilla. Monardes imported medicinal plants and established a botanical garden in Seville for the study of New World plants. He never visited the Americas.

There are twelve species in the *Monarda* genus, but it is *M. didyma* that is grown most frequently. It makes a beautiful and useful addition to the herb garden.

Bergamot is a most attractive, spreading perennial that grows to about 2 ft (60 cm). The stem is square, stiff, and hairy, with opposite, rough, serrated, grayish green leaves. Pale green, leafy bracts support scarlet flower heads at the end of the stem. The whole plant has a delicious fragrance and is loved by bees.

The Oswego Indians of North America are said to have used this plant as a medicinal tea to treat colds, respiratory tract ailments, skin complaints, and inflammation. During the Boston Tea Party in America, when British tea was boycotted, bergamot tea was drunk as a substitute.

There is a common misconception that the oil of this herb is used to flavor Earl Grey tea—this is not so. In fact, the flavor comes from the oil expressed from the rind of a small, orange-like fruit, *Citrus bergamia*.

Uses: HERB

The flowers and leaves are used as a stimulant and for relief of gripe and wind.

The very young leaves and petals of bergamot combine well with salads and fruit dishes and may also be crystallized or used as a garnish. Both the leaves and the petals may be dried and used in potpourri.

Growing and harvesting

Grow from seed or root division and plant in a sunny position in the garden in rich, moist soil. Cut leaves before flowering or harvest plants when flowering and use fresh or dried in infusions.

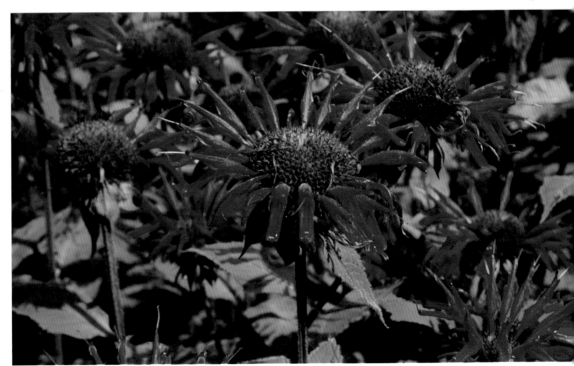

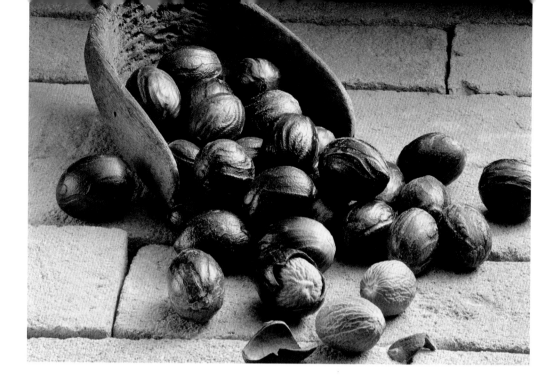

Myristica fragrans

Myristicaceae
Nutmeg

The fruit of the nutmeg tree has many culinary and medicinal uses. The dried kernel is grated and used to flavor sweet and savory dishes, especially those with milk or cheese. (I can't image rice pudding without a thick sprinkling of nutmeg baked into the skin on the top!) Its outer "jacket" is harvested for mace. The perfume is sweet-spicy and blends well with black pepper, clary sage, cypress, frankincense, geranium, lemon, lime, orange, patchouli, petitgrain, and rosemary. It is widely used by the pharmaceutical industry in analgesic and tonic preparations and also as a flavoring in many commercially prepared foods.

Uses: ESSENTIAL OIL

Nutmeg is beneficial to the hair when added to hair tonics and shampoos.

The most powerful use of nutmeg oil is its toning action on the digestive system where it will help to control vomiting and nausea, relieve cramps and spasms in the intestines, help to expel gas from the intestines, and ease indigestion, diarrhea, vomiting, nausea, and poor indigestion. It stimulates the appetite and helps to digest fatty foods.

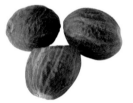

A massage blend containing the warming and pain-relieving nutmeg oil will be very soothing and comforting for muscular aches and pains, arthritis, gout, poor circulation, and rheumatism. It can also be used in a bath to ease these problems, but only use three drops (no more!) dissolved in a little vegetable oil or it may irritate the skin. A hot fomentation, again only using three drops of the oil, will help the pain of neuralgia.

Nutmeg is a natural hormone, imitating estrogen, and it also acts as a tonic to the reproductive system. Used as a massage or fomentation blend it encourages and regulates menstrual flow, reduces spasms and cramps of the uterus, and regulates scanty menstrual flow.

Caution: Do not use in large doses or for prolonged periods of time. Use one percent only in blends and three drops only in inhalations, fomentations, compresses, and baths.

Myrtus communis

Myrtaceae
Myrtle

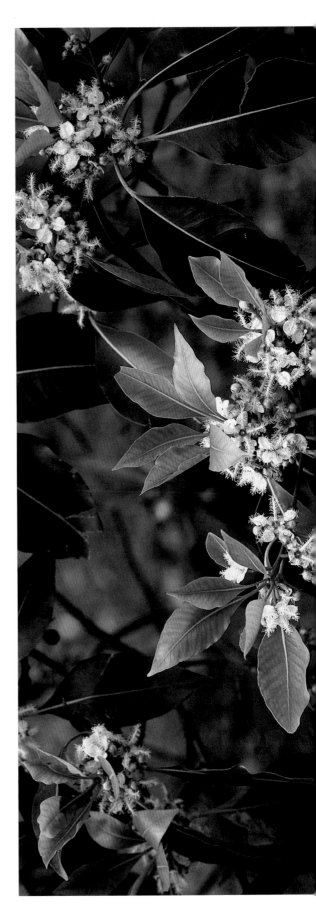

Myrtle comes from the same family of plants that includes cloves, allspice, and eucalyptus. Native to southern Europe and northern Africa, myrtle has been cultivated for many years and these days it is mainly grown for its essential oil.

This evergreen shrub has dark green leaves which have sweet, spicy, and aromatic fragrance when crushed or bruised. During late spring and summer it is covered in creamy white, scented flowers that are followed by blue-purple berries in the fall. The essential oil is steam-distilled mainly from the leaves and twigs. The oil has a clear herbaceous perfume and blends well with bergamot, clary sage, hyssop, lavender, lemon, lime, rosemary, spice oils, thyme, and tea tree.

Myrtle has long been associated with romance—it was sacred to Aphrodite, the goddess of love, and a favorite flower for using in wedding wreaths and bouquets.

Uses: ESSENTIAL OIL

A gentle oil, it is particularly effective for respiratory problems and suitable for the very young and the elderly. It helps to loosen and remove mucus and this, combined with the antiseptic properties, helps to treat asthma, bronchitis, catarrh, colds, and coughs.

It also helps to prevent infectious diseases, making it a good choice to use in blends for air sprays and burners when there are epidemics.

Myrtle helps to destroy infection-causing bacteria and contracts and tones tissue, so can be used in blends to treat acne, bruises, hemorrhoids, oily skin, and psoriasis. The antiseptic action will be found useful for clearing cystitis and urethritis.

Nepeta cataria

Lamiaceae
Catnep
Also known as catnip, catrup, field balm

Even the most docile, aged, and dignified cat goes quietly silly when it smells bruised catnep. Very superior cats may be seen lying on their backs, flapping their paws in the air in ecstasy as they roll on the newly transplanted small herb, usually destroying it in the process.

Catnep is a perennial, medium-sized, shrubby plant growing to 1–5 ft (30 cm–1.5 m) in height. The branching stems are square, erect, and hairy, with gray-green, ovate, toothed leaves. The whole plant is covered in a fine, soft, whitish down, particularly the underside of the leaves. The flowers, whitish with lilac spots, grow in whorls on spikes from midsummer through to winter.

Uses: HERB

Throughout history the leaves and flowering tops of this herb have been used to produce a sedative effect, and an infused oil is particularly useful in baths, and for massages for children suffering from measles, chickenpox, whooping cough, colic, fevers, hives, insomnia, and hyperactivity.

This is one of the best herbs for children if used as directed. Catnep tea is also ideal to calm restless children. Give one to two cups a day (in $\frac{1}{2}$ cup doses), sweetened with honey, to soothe and aid recovery from any of the complaints listed above. Children often prefer to drink this tea cold.

Catnep is useful for reducing fevers, as it raises body heat and thus induces sweating. It also settles the stomach, and is useful in treating headaches related to digestive problems.

A tincture makes a good friction rub for rheumatic and arthritic joints.

Caution: In large or strong doses this plant can induce vomiting.

Growing and harvesting

Grow catnep from seeds, cuttings, root division, mounding, or layering. It likes a sunny spot with moderate water and will tolerate frost. The plant self-sows so readily that you rarely need to transplant it. Harvest and use fresh, or hang in bunches or spread out in a warm, airy place to dry.

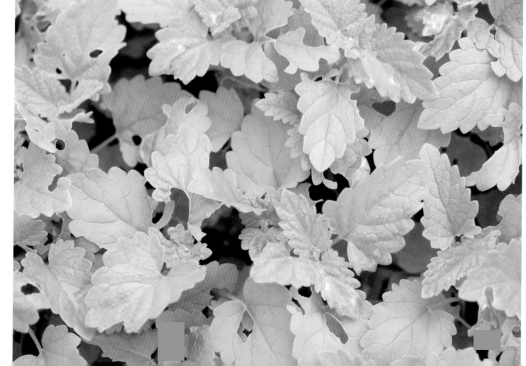

Ocimum basilicum

Lamiaceae
Basil
Also known as sweet basil

Basil is an annual and grows to about 12–24 in (30–60 cm) with opposite, smooth green leaves and white or pale lilac flowers, occurring in whorls at the base of the leaves. To prolong the life of the plant the flower buds should be picked off regularly before they fully open. The scent of the leaves when bruised is very strong and clove-like. The leaves are the part used, both medicinally and for cooking, and are at their best before the plant flowers.

Basil is one of the most popular herbs for use in the kitchen. A tomato salad is nothing without the accompaniment of fresh, sweet, spicy, shredded basil leaves. The leaves can also be used in moderate quantities with other salads and vegetables. It livens up cheese dishes, soups, stews, sauces, salads, dressings, sandwiches, and some fruit dishes and who amongst us can resist a plate of pasta with pesto? In hot dishes its best added towards the end of cooking or the flavor is lost and the herb can become bitter.

The flowering tops and leaves are distilled to produce the oil, which blends well with bergamot, geranium, and hyssop. The Latin name for basil is derived from the Greek for a king and, like a king, this powerful oil needs to be treated with a little respect—two drops in $2\frac{1}{2}$ tablespoons (40 ml) of a blend will be enough.

Uses: HERB, ESSENTIAL OIL
Basil is a useful herb for complaints of the stomach and digestive organs. Sip a cup of basil tea after meals to ease the symptoms of constipation, gastric catarrh, stomach cramps, enteritis, indigestion, vomiting, and to increase appetite. It will relieve nausea, even that induced by chemotherapy, and helps to soothe the spasms of whooping cough.

Basil oil is an appetite stimulant and, used as an inhalation or massage oil, it tones the digestive system, aiding digestion and helping to expel gas from the intestines. It also eases hiccups, heartburn, nausea, and gastroenteritis.

Basil is an excellent oil for the brain, stimulating the intellect, clearing the mind and aiding concentration. Simply sniffing the oil directly from the bottle or used in an oil burner, it is useful for easing headaches and migraine. It lifts depression, eases hysteria, insomnia, and anxiety, and provides endurance and stamina.

Basil oil is a popular choice for blends to treat respiratory problems such as bronchitis, colds, and influenza, where it helps to loosen and remove mucus and reduce fever. Incorporate it with other oils in blends for inhalations, massages, and baths. Furthermore, it is reputed to improve blood circulation and ease fevers, colds, influenza, coughs, and sinusitis.

The oil has estrogen-like properties that may help to relieve cramps in the uterus and intestines, encourage menstrual flow, and increase production of breast milk. Used in a compress and applied to the breasts it can reduce engorgement but must only be used at 0.5 percent.

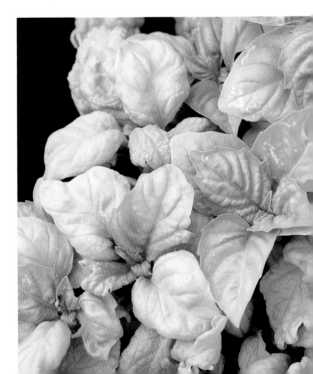

The tonic and antiseptic properties of basil oil are helpful for treating skin problems like acne and abrasions, and it's worth including in blends to ease insect bites and stings, and to repel insects.

Included in blends with lavender, marjoram, and black pepper, basil makes an excellent massage and bath oil for overworked muscles and muscular aches and pains.

It is a very good hair tonic when blended with oils such as rosemary, lavender, and jojoba.

A sprig of basil in the wardrobe will keep moths and other insects at bay. It has a reputation for repelling flies, but when I tested this out by putting a pot of basil on my patio, the flies used it to rest on!

It's a good companion to apricot trees, asparagus, grapes, and tomatoes (it improves the growth and flavor of both the tomatoes and the basil), and repels aphids, flies, fruit moths, and also mosquitoes. Basil dislikes rue intensely.

Caution: *Never use basil oil internally. Use only 0.5 percent in blends used externally. Avoid using basil oil during pregnancy.*

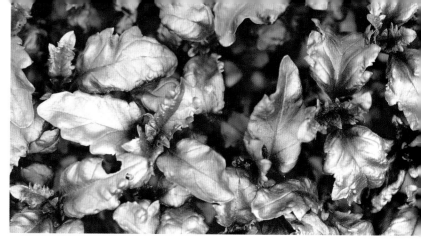

Growing and harvesting

Plant seeds or seedlings in a sunny, well-drained spot in the garden and pick leaves before flowering begins to use fresh or freeze. Basil doesn't dry well, in fact it tastes like dry grass. I freeze some of the leaves whole in zip-top plastic bags, others I grind to a paste with olive oil (sometimes I add garlic, ginger, etc.). Or I make basil ice cubes—I grind to a paste, add water and freeze in ice-cube trays. Each cube equals approximately one tablespoon and can be dropped into dishes towards the end of cooking time—excellent for adding flavor to stir-fries.

Basil is grown in many varieties, such as Ocimum basilicum *"Purple Ruffles."*

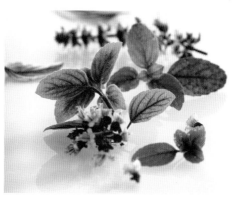

Another variety Ocimum basilicum *"Africa Blue."*

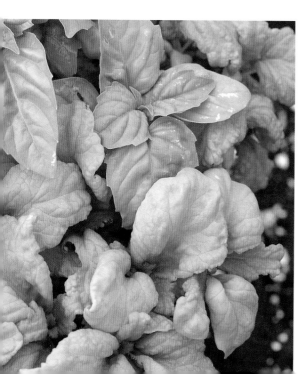

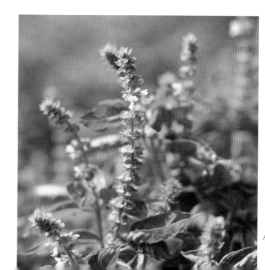

Origanum marjorana
syn. *O. hortensis*

Lamiaceae
Marjoram
Also known as sweet marjoram, knotted marjoram, joy of the mountains

Oregano and marjoram are among the few herbs that retain their pungent and distinctive odor after drying. The flowers of oregano also carry the perfume, to an even greater extent than the leaves. This is rare in the herb world and it means that the plant can be gathered while in full bloom, and both leaves and flowers dried.

Marjoram is a very aromatic herb long used for both cooking and herbal medicine. It is a perennial but you may like to treat it as an annual, as it tends to become straggly and woody. Growing to about 2 ft (60 cm) in the right position, it has, small, grayish green, rounded leaves, and flowers like clusters of little knots. The leaves are used fresh or dried in many Mediterranean dishes and give them their distinctive flavor. The perfume is gently pungent and warm, and blends well with bergamot, black pepper, cedarwood, chamomile, clary sage, cypress, eucalyptus, juniper, lavender, mandarin, nutmeg, patchouli, peppermint, petitgrain, rosemary, and tea tree.

Its intense perfume made it a favorite for "strewing" in medieval days. This powerful scent has a modern-day application as a "smelling salt" to restore the faint or dizzy. Just holding a few crushed sprigs under the patient's nose can restore him or her.

Marjoram has a similar flavor to oregano but is less pungent. The leaves, used discreetly, add flavor to meat, vegetable, seafood, bean, cheese, and tomato dishes.

Uses: HERB, ESSENTIAL OIL

The whole herb is used in teas and tinctures for its tonic powers, and to stimulate menstrual flow.

Marjoram is a warming and relaxing oil. It helps to loosen and remove mucus, and increases perspiration, making it useful in air sprays, inhalations, baths, and massage oils, to ease respiratory complaints and fevers such as asthma, bronchitis, coughs, colds, influenza, and sinusitis.

Marjoram dilates arteries and small blood vessels making it an ideal massage oil to treat arthritis, lumbago, sprains, bruises, rheumatism, and joint and muscle pain. The same property will help with chilblains, fainting, headache, migraine, and high blood pressure.

As with several other culinary herbs, marjoram is an excellent toner of the digestive system, and may be used in baths, fomentations, and massage oils to treat intestinal cramps, flatulence, diarrhea, indigestion, and constipation. Menstrual cramping, scantiness, and irregularity can also be eased by laying a marjoram fomentation over the lower abdomen.

Combined with lavender in a bath or massage oil before bedtime, it calms the nervous system and makes it a good remedy for insomnia (particularly if the sleeplessness is cause by stress), hyperactivity, or PMS.

It will repel ants and is a good companion to cucumber.

Caution: Not to be used during pregnancy. Overuse can dull the senses and cause drowsiness. Avoid if you suffer from very low blood pressure.

Growing and harvesting
Plants seeds or seedlings, or grow from cuttings in a sunny position in the garden in well-drained soil. Cut out the old wood at the end of winter before the spring growth, and replace plants when they get too woody. Cut the long stems and flower heads, and use fresh, or hang to dry in a warm, airy place.

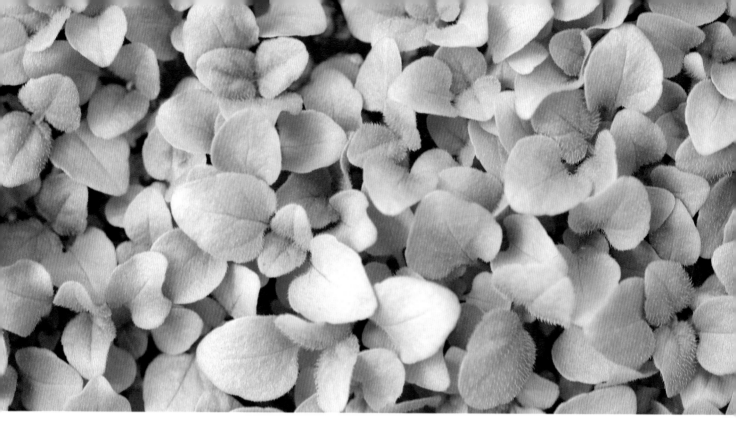

Origanum vulgare

Lamiaceae
Oregano
Also known as wild marjoram, mountain mint

A perennial plant with a creeping rootstock, oregano has purple-tinged, woody stems, and usually grows up to 12 in (30 cm) in height. It has small, bright to dark green, rough-textured leaves. The white or pale purple flowers grow in terminal clusters.

In the kitchen, oregano leaves and flowers (fresh or dried), add flavor to cooked meat, fish, vegetable, and egg dishes, as well as soups and stews. Add towards the end of cooking. Use more sparingly to enhance salads, dressings, and vinegars.

Uses: HERB
Oregano is an excellent herb for those who suffer from poor digestion. In this way it may also be helpful in teas and tinctures in easing headaches caused by digestive problems.

It repels bacteria and ants, and is good near cabbage or cucumber.

Growing and harvesting
As for marjoram, page 130.

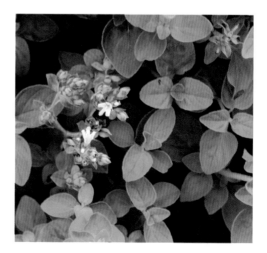

Panax *species*

Ariliaceae

Panax ginseng
Ginseng

P. quinquefolius
American ginseng

The perennial ginsengs with their carrot-shaped, aromatic rootstock are native to Korea (*Panax ginseng*) and North America (*P. quinquefolius*). Both varieties, however, are chemically almost indistinguishable. Be aware that ginseng is difficult to grow from seed and it is also hard to mimic the natural habitat. Add to this the fact that the roots need to be several years old before they are mature enough to use, and you will see that it's probably best to buy your ginseng extract from the health-food store.

They are considered by some to be a panacea for all aliments, but in fact ginseng isn't recommended for inflammatory diseases.

Uses: HERB

It is used as a tonic, an aphrodisiac, a stress reliever, to improve stamina, regulate blood pressure, and to enhance immunity and resistance to infection.

Growing and harvesting

Somewhat difficult to cultivate but best done from ripe seed kept very damp, even in moss. Plants are six to seven years old before roots can be lifted and used fresh or dried in decoctions or extracts. The flowers can be harvested in spring and summer for similar uses.

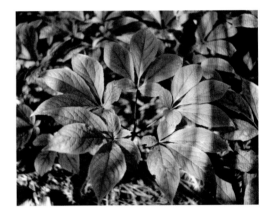

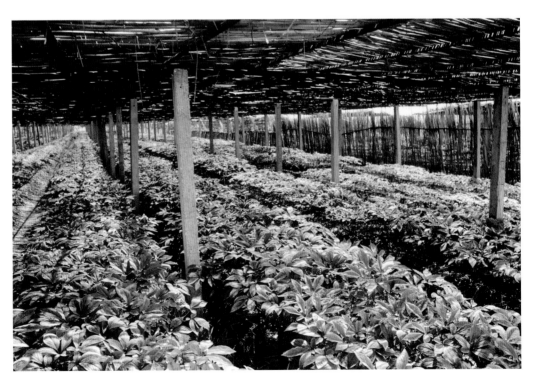

Ginseng is farmed commercially in Asia.

Pelargonium *species*

Geraniaceae
Geranium

Pelargonium graveolens
Rose geranium

P. odoratissimum
Apple geranium

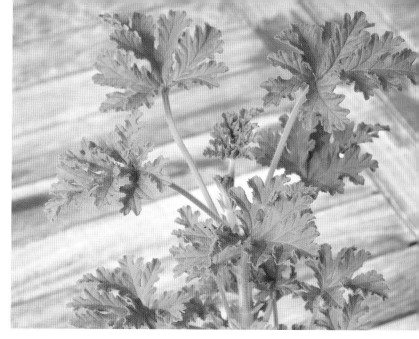

Pelargonium graveolens

Fragrant pelargoniums (commonly called geraniums) are succulent, soft-wooded herbs that have long been cultivated for their intensely aromatic foliage. Rose geranium leaves are used to make a tea, and to flavor cakes, jellies, sauces, and even vinegars. A rose geranium sorbet is a delicious dessert to finish a meal. Lay whole leaves under cakes where they will release their subtle flavoring. Toss the delicate flowers into salads.

Geranium essential oil is distilled from two species—either from the leaves, flowers and stems of the rose geranium (*Pelargonium graveolens*) or (rarely) from the apple geranium (*P. odoratissium*). Geranium essential oil, with its heady, languorous, and relaxing aroma, is much used in the perfume industry. It blends well with most other oils and harmonizes and balances other scents.

Uses: ESSENTIAL OIL
Geranium encourages speedy healing, can help to stop bleeding, and is an antiseptic, which makes it a valuable oil to use as a diluted wash for wounds and cuts. Use it also to treat acne, bruises, burns and scalds (minor), dermatitis, eczema, ulcers, and hemorrhoids.

Head lice and ringworm also respond to this oil.

It is a good essential oil for making skin-care products for all skin types as it balances sebum production (the fatty secretion in the sebaceous glands that helps to keep skin supple) and stimulates both dry and oily, sluggish skin.

Geranium eases pain by numbing nerves, so use in gargles and mouthwashes for sore throat, tonsillitis, and mouth infections (remember to spit the gargle out). It also exerts a tonic and diuretic action on the urinary system and the liver that helps to rid the body of toxins.

Sometimes it is called the "woman's oil" because of its regulatory action on the hormones secreted by the adrenal cortex. This property makes geranium an appropriate and valuable remedy used in baths and massage for problems caused by a fluctuating hormone balance. These include engorged breasts, menopausal problems, and PMS.

Caution: Patch test—may cause irritation on sensitive skin.

Growing and harvesting
Pelargoniums like well-drained, neutral to alkaline soil in a sunny position in the garden. Grow from softwood cuttings and cut plants back in the early spring to encourage new growth. In the right spot they will grow to 3–5 ft (90 cm–1.5 m). Pick leaves as required for use in infusions, and in cooking or dry to add to potpourri.

Petroselinum crispum

Apiaceae
Parsley

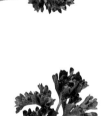

Parsley is a clump-forming biennial with bright green foliage, deeply divided, curling leaves and a flower stem, which appears in the second year with tiny, white and green flowers. Parsley ensures well-digested food, sweet breath, and a good supply of minerals, and vitamins. It is one the most popular culinary herbs, and can be added to almost every savory dish, hot or cold, including dressings and vegetable juices.

The Greeks believed it came from the blood of heroes and this led to the notion that it could be used medicinally. Of the many types of parsley available, *Petroselinum crispum* is the most widely used medicinally. A good digestive aid, parsley stimulates the appetite, helps to digest food (eat the parsley that decorates your food in restaurants), and eases nausea and wind. It is used in some pharmaceutical preparations for digestive remedies. It is also used by the perfume industry.

The essential oil is steam-distilled from the leaves, root, and (mainly) from the seed. The perfume is warm, spicy, and blends well with clary sage, lavender, lime, marjoram, oregano, rosemary, and tea tree.

Uses: HERB, ESSENTIAL OIL

The plant may be drunk as a tea, its diuretic action ridding the body of excess water. Massage blends and fomentations made with no more than 0.5 percent parsley oil increase the flow of urine and reduce water retention during menstruation, or in other conditions where oedema is a problem, such as swollen ankles and PMS. The increased flow of urine and parsley's antiseptic action can also be used to treat cystitis and urethritis. It must not however be used when there is kidney disease or inflammation, or during pregnancy, as it stimulates muscle contractions in the uterus. Contraindicated also when periods are painful as it could cause cramping.

A tea from the leaves is used to treat late menstruation.

Strain weak tea through coffee filter paper and use as an eyewash to treat conjunctivitis and styes.

Extract the juice and add it to pineapple juice as a drink to relieve the pain of arthritis.

Parsley helps to shrink small blood vessels, and can be used in ointments and lotions to treat hemorrhoids, bruising, and thread veins.

Taken as a tea, parsley relieves cramps and spasms, expels gas in the intestines, and eases colic, indigestion, and nausea.

Parsley grows best when planted near asparagus, roses, and tomatoes.

Caution: *Use 0.5 percent parsley oil only in blends. Not to be used during pregnancy or painful menstruation. Not to be used by people with inflammatory kidney disease.*

Growing and harvesting

Grow it from seed or seedlings in a frost-free sunny place or partial shade in well-drained soil with moderate water. To prolong the life of the plant, cut the stems right back regularly or it will go to seed and die. Pick leaves before flowering and use fresh, frozen, or hang in bunches in a warm, airy place to dry. The leaves, root, and seeds can all be used.

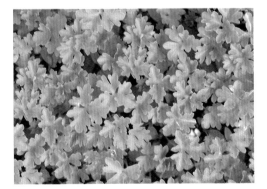

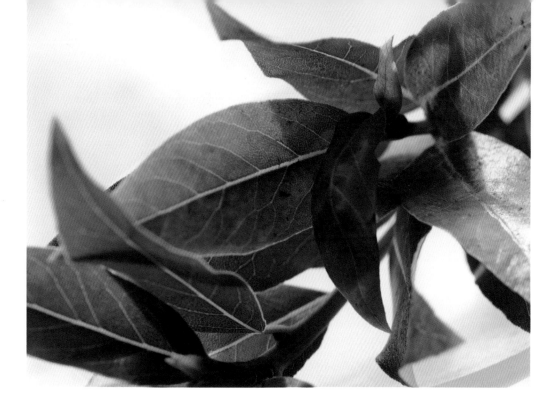

Pimenta racemosa
syn. *P. acris*

Myrtaceae
West Indian bay
Also known as bay rum tree

The leaves of the tropical evergreen West Indian bay tree are distilled with rum to produce the famous "Bay Rum" hair tonic that was reputedly tonic and fragrant—lessening grease and stimulating hair growth. West Indian bay essential oil is still used extensively in commercial soaps, perfumes, aftershaves, and hair preparations. The aroma of this oil is fresh and balsamic, blending well with citrus and spice oils, lavender, geranium, rosemary, and ylang-ylang.

Uses: ESSENTIAL OIL
The main use of West Indian Bay essential oil is still in hair preparations as a scalp stimulant to restore the appearance of lank and greasy hair, to encourage growth, and to help to treat dandruff.

It has been suggested that it could be useful for treating muscular pain and problems, but as it is moderately toxic I feel that there are safer and more effective oils that can be used.

Caution: Use 0.5 percent only in hair preparations.

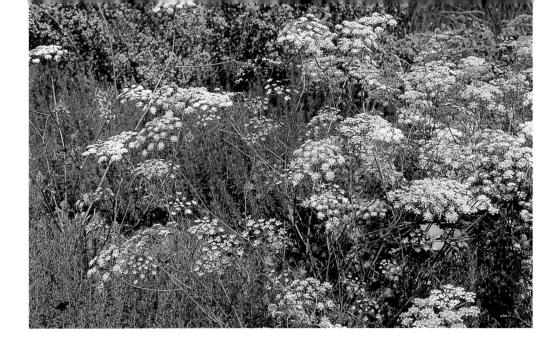

Pimpinella anisum

Apiaceae
Anise
Also known as aniseed

A dainty annual of very similar appearance to caraway, anise grows to about 20 in (50 cm) high. The stem is ribbed, with kidney-shaped lower leaves, and feathery leaflets of bright green above. Clumps of creamy white flowers are followed by gray-green, aromatic seeds with a licorice-like flavor. These seeds are the part normally used.

In the kitchen, use sparing amounts of the crushed or whole seed and the leaves to flavor cabbage, carrots, salads, tomato and vegetable juices, as well as biscuits, stewed fruits, and liqueurs. Anise is the main flavoring in Pernod, anisette, and ouzo.

Uses: HERB

Aromatic anise can be used to disguise unpleasant-tasting herbs, and may be used as an antiseptic expectorant to ease the symptoms of whooping cough, and to treat griping pain and wind. A tea made from equal parts of anise, caraway, and fennel makes an excellent intestinal purifier, and if sipped before a meal it promotes digestion and improves appetite.

Anise alleviates cramps and nausea, coughs, colds, and bad breath, and a few crushed seeds infused in a glass of hot milk and drunk before bedtime will help you fall asleep easily.

Anise acts as a good insect repellent for most plants, and is especially good as a companion to asparagus, beans, broccoli, Brussels sprouts, cabbage, carrots, cauliflower, celery, cucumber, lettuce, parsnips, radishes, silverbeet, strawberries, tomatoes, and zucchini (courgette).

Growing and harvesting

Grow the plant from seed in a sunny spot in well-drained soil with a moderate amount of water. Be aware that the seeds won't ripen unless grown in a warm climate. Harvest seeds as they ripen and use dried for tinctures, or dry for culinary use, whole or ground.

Pinus sylvestris

Pinaceae
Pine
Also known as Scots pine

The Scots pine is the only pine indigenous to the United Kingdom, and is also the most common one found growing throughout Europe. Pine essential oil is steam-distilled from the needles, twigs, and cones. Its refreshing, clean perfume makes pine one of the most "commercial" of the oils, and its aroma is in demand for products ranging from perfumes to household disinfectants, detergents, and insecticides. Pine oil blends well with cedarwood, clary sage, eucalyptus, rosemary, and tea tree.

Uses: ESSENTIAL OIL
Pine oil is one of the best oils to use in ointments and washes to treat scabies, cuts, head lice, and sores.

Pine is a strong pulmonary antiseptic, and has a particularly powerful effect on the respiratory system where, when used in baths, massage oil, or inhalations and air sprays, it kills bacteria, helps to loosen and remove mucus, increases perspiration, and acts as a restorative. It can be used to great advantage in the treatment of bronchitis, catarrh, coughs, sinusitis, sore throat, colds, and influenza.

It's a warming and soothing treatment for tired sore muscles when used in baths and massage oils. Sufferers from arthritis, rheumatism, muscular aches and pains, poor circulation, gout, fatigue, and nervous exhaustion will all benefit from a mentally and physically restorative pine bath.

Pine fomentations or sitz baths will ease the symptoms of cystitis, urethritis, and other urinary infections.

Caution: Note that the oil from dwarf Swiss mountain pine (P. mugo var. pumilo) is hazardous and must never be used.

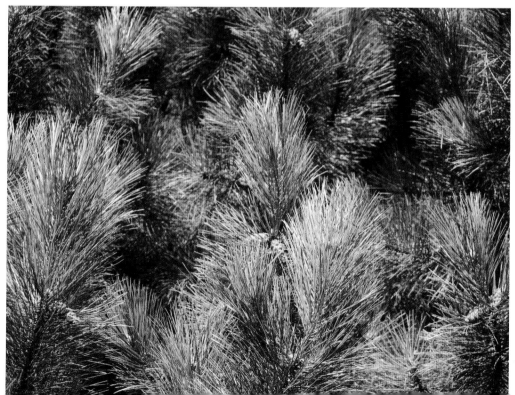

Piper nigrum

Piperaceae
Pepper
Also known as black pepper

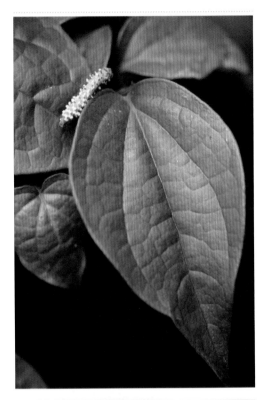

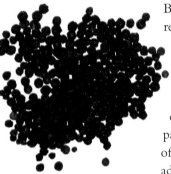

Black pepper is a climbing vine that can reach to 12 ft (4 m) if left unpruned. The dried black fruit is ground as a spice for cooking and for steam distillation as an oil. The perfume is warm, spicy, and familiar, and blends with basil, bergamot, cypress, frankincense, geranium, citrus oils, palmarosa, sandalwood, and ylang-ylang. It is often used in tiny amounts in perfumery to add a warm, deep, and spicy note.

Uses: ESSENTIAL OIL

Black pepper oil is one of the important oils for treating muscular problems. It dilates blood vessels, and produces localized redness and warmth when applied to the skin, relieving aching, tired muscles. Used in a massage oil prior to sport (particularly for runners, dancers, etc.), it can reduce the strain on muscles by increasing the blood flow to the area. It may be used in small amounts in bath and massage blends to ease arthritis, rheumatism, muscular aches and pains, sprains, strains, poor muscle tone, muscular stiffness, neuralgia, chilblains, and poor circulation. It eases pain by numbing nerves, and kills bacteria.

It tones and stimulates the nervous, circulatory and digestive systems, aiding digestion, relieving cramps, wind and spasms in the intestines and uterus, and eases colic, constipation, diarrhea, and nausea. It reputedly counteracts the effects of poison.

Use black pepper oil in small amounts (three drops only) in baths to increase perspiration and to cool and reduce fever during chills, colds, and influenza. It strengthens the immune system, and helps to prevent viral infections.

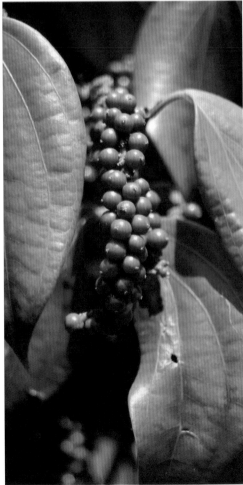

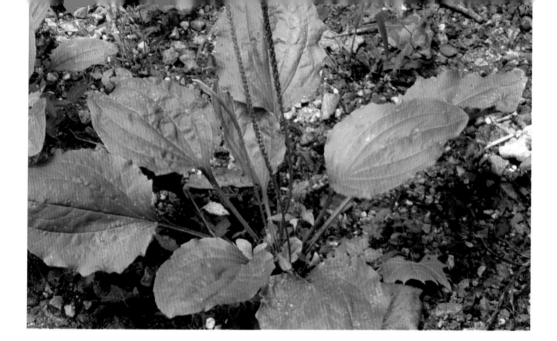

Plantago *species*

Plantaginaceae
Plantain
Also known as common plantain, broad leaf plantain, greater plantain, lance leaf plantain, rat-tail plantain, ribwort, white man's foot

Plantain grows everywhere "white man has trodden," hence "white man's foot." Like the nettle, plantain is treated as a pest by those who are unaware of its worth. Make a place for it in your garden and learn to appreciate its virtue.

Broad leaf plantain (*Plantago major*) is a perennial weed with a radial rosette of wide, ribbed, grayish green, hairy leaves which can grow to 16 in (40 cm). The flower stalk is erect, with grayish green, inconspicuous flowers. It's also known as common plantain, rat-tail plantain, and greater plantain.

Narrow leaf plantain or ribwort (*P. lanceolata*) has bright-green, pointed and ribbed leaves, and a grooved flower stalk topped with a flower head having slim, white filaments tipped with greenish yellow anthers, forming a halo around the base of the head.

The seeds of *P. psyllium* (flea seed, fleawort, Spanish psyllium) can be sprinkled over cereals, or similar, to treat constipation, and are used in many over-the-counter products sold for this purpose. The tiny seeds have a gelatinous coating, which swells on contact with moisture, and increases movement within the bowel. It should always be taken with plenty of liquid.

Uses: HERB

Drink plantain tea or syrup to treat bronchitis, catarrh, coughs, colds, and all respiratory problems.

Use the leaves and seeds in ointments, poultices, and washes for the herb's astringent, analgesic, emollient, and cleansing qualities. Plantain encourages healing and eases the pain of problems such as insect bites and stings, cuts, scratches, wounds, boils and ringworm, and to reduce black eyes and swellings, swollen glands, varicose veins, and cysts. Use to stem the bleeding of hemorrhoids and sores.

Growing and harvesting

Grow plantain from seed in a sunny position in well-drained soil with moderate water or, if you don't want it invading your garden, find it in an unpolluted area in the wild. It self sows easily. Cut plants during the growing season, and use fresh or dried for infusions, extracts, and tinctures.

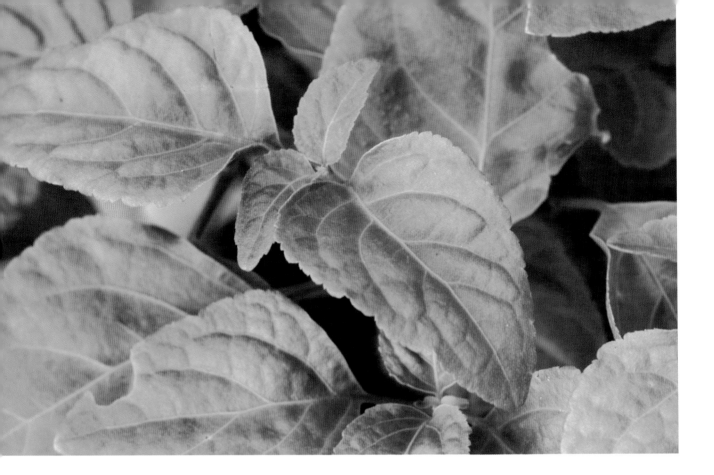

In India, sprigs of patchouli leaves and flowers are laid between clothes and linen to protect them against insects.

Pogostemon cablin

syn. *P. patchouli*

Lamiaceae
Patchouli

The patchouli plants of tropical East and Southeast Asia are renowned for their aromatic oils. *Pogostemon cablin* is widely used in perfumery or to provide a sensuous, earthy "bottom" note. The essential oil is steam-distilled from the leaves. Its earthy aroma is reputed to balance the emotions but that rather depends on whether or not you can tolerate the smell.

Unlike many essential oils, the hot, heavy, oriental perfume improves with age and, if used in very discreet amounts, it blends well with most other scents, and is one of the best perfume fixatives. The quality of this oil can be likened to harvest time—rich, fruitful, and abundant. It can rekindle desires in relationships, which have become jaded through familiarity.

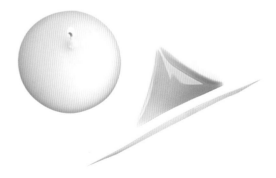

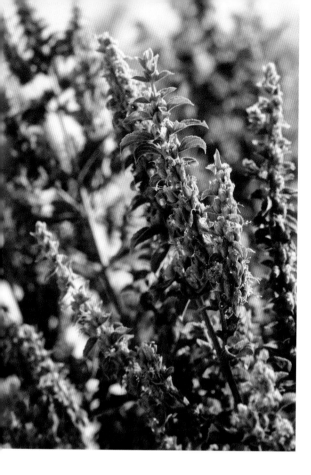

Ravensara aromatica
syn. *Agathophyllum aromaticum*

Lauraceae
Ravensara

Ravensara is an aromatic, evergreen tree growing to around 65 ft (20 m), native to the humid eastern rainforests of Madagascar. The leaves, bark, and nut are all fragrant. The anise-flavored bark is used in making a local rum. The essential oil is steam-distilled from the leaves and is almost colorless, with an aroma similar to that of rosemary and lavender. A relatively recent addition to the aromatherapy medicine chest, deliciously scented ravensara is as safe to use as lavender and well worth the hunt to find it. It blends with lavender, manuka, pine, rosemary, tea tree, and thyme. It's the oil to "get you going" when you feel down.

Many people find the smell unpleasant but if a small amount is included in a blend, the powerful aroma is somewhat neutralized.

Uses: ESSENTIAL OIL
Patchouli oil reduces inflammation, kills bacteria, and prevents or destroys fungal infections. It is also a cell regenerator. This impressive list of properties makes it a valuable oil for use in skin-care blends, ointments, creams, and lotions for treating skin problems, including acne, athlete's foot, cracked and chapped skin, dermatitis, eczema (weeping), fungal infections, and insect bites.

It increases the flow of urine making it useful when used in baths or fomentations over the abdomen for fluid retention, and is possibly helpful for cystitis and urethritis.

Uses: ESSENTIAL OIL
Make good use of the immuno-stimulant and virus-inhibiting properties of ravensara to protect the body during epidemics of influenza, or other virus infections. Use it in a bath, followed by a massage containing the oil. Protect the family by using it in an air spray and inhalation. Use it in this way for treating respiratory tract infections such as bronchitis, catarrh, sinusitis, colds, and coughs.

As it is powerfully antiviral it can be used for cold sores, genital herpes, and shingles, where it can be blended with oils such as lavender or chamomile in healing ointments to ease pain. Used in air sprays, it will help to prevent the spread of diseases such as chickenpox and measles.

Arthritis, rheumatism, sore joints, and sore, tense muscles will all benefit from the muscle-relaxant pain relief that is offered by this oil when used in baths, fomentations, or massage oils.

Rosa *species*

Rosaceae

Rosa centifolia
Cabbage rose

R. damascena
Damask rose

R. gallica
French rose

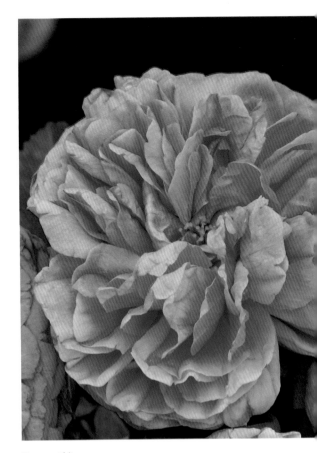

Rosa centifolia

The rose, for so long, has been prized for its beauty and perfume that it is hard to imagine in centuries past it was more highly regarded for its gentle medicinal qualities. "Rose juice" seems to have been something of a cure-all for every imaginable ailment in medieval Europe. It has long been a symbol of love and purity, and rose petals are still strewn in the path of the bride and groom.

Although it is thought to be the first plant from which essential oil was distilled, the main method of extraction is by effleurage, a labor-intensive (expensive) method that needs huge amounts of petals to yield a small amount of oil known as an "absolute." The perfume is sweet, sensual, and romantic, and blends with almost all other oils. Sensual but never sensuous, rose encourages us to be loving, caring, and compassionate to ourselves, and to others. Warmly relaxing and gentle, this oil calms us, reducing stress and tension.

Rosewater is a by-product of the steam distillation process.

Uses: ESSENTIAL OIL

Rose oil is good for all skin types especially dry and sensitive skin. It soothes inflammation, and constricts capillaries making it useful for those suffering from thread veins. It can be used to treat eczema and herpes.

It's considered to be a "woman's oil," partly because of its perfume, but largely because of its affinity with the female reproductive system. When used as a massage oil, it tones the uterus, encourages and regulates menstrual flow, eases problems such as menstrual irregularity, excessive menstrual loss, cramps and spasms in the intestines and uterus, and leucorrhea.

Damask rose

Government and Virtues. – It is under the dominion of Venus. Botanists describe a vast number of roses, but this, and the common red rose, and the dog rose, or hip, are the only kinds regarded in medicine.

"There is a syrup made from the flowers of the damask rose, by infusing them twenty-four hours in boiling water, then straining off the liquor adding twice the weight of refined sugar to it. This syrup is an excellent purge for children and grown people of a costive habit; a small quantity taken every night will keep the bowels regular. There is a conserve made of the unripe flowers, which has the same properties as the syrup; there is likewise a conserve made of the fruit of the wild or dog rose, which is very pleasant, and of considerable efficacy for common colds and coughs. The flowers of the common red rose, dried, are given in infusions, and sometimes in powder, against the overflowings of the menses, spitting of blood and other hemorrhages. There is likewise an excellent tincture made from them, by pouring a pint of boiling oil on an ounce of the dried petals, and adding fifteen drops of oil of vitriol, and three or four drams of the finest sugar in powder, after which they may be stirred together, and left to cool. This tincture, when strained, is of a beautiful red colour. It may be taken to the amount of three or four spoonfuls, twice or three times a day, for strengthening the stomach and preventing vomiting. It is a powerful and pleasant remedy in immoderate discharges of the menses, and all other fluxes and hemmorhages. The damask rose, on account of its fragrance, belongs to the cephaltics; but the next virtue it possesses, consists of its cathartic quality. After the water, which is a good cordial, is drawn off in a hot still, the remaining liquor, strained, will make a very good purging syrup from two drams to two ounces. An infusion made of half a dram to two drams of the dried leaves, answers the same purpose."

– Nicholas Culpeper, *Culpeper's Complete Herball* (Originally published in 1652, Reprinted, W. Foulsham & Co., Ltd., London, n.d.)

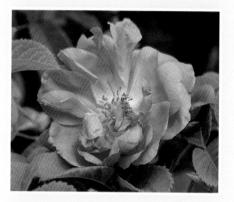

Rosa *"Trigintipetala" (syn. "Kazanlik") is a* Rosa damascena *cultivar that is grown commercially in south-eastern Europe for the famous "attar of roses."*

Despite it's seemingly "female only" uses, it also has a reputation for increasing the production of semen.

Rose oil tones the digestive system, stimulates and strengthens the liver, stimulates the secretion of bile, and relieves liver congestion making it useful in blends inhaled from the bottle, or massaged over the stomach and abdomen as a digestive, and to ease nausea and vomiting. It has a tonic action on the heart, eases palpitations, and stimulates circulation.

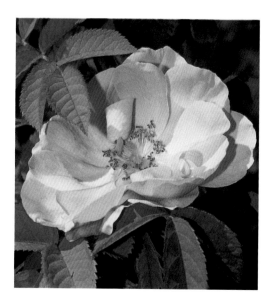

Rosa gallica

Rosmarinus officinalis

Lamiaceae
Rosemary
Also known as compass plant, komero, polar plant

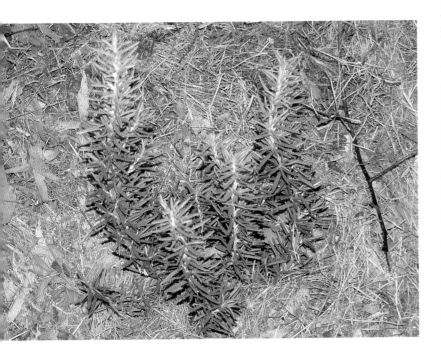

One of the best-known and loved herbs, versatile rosemary is a member of the mint family, and has been grown through the centuries for culinary, medicinal, and decorative uses. It is renowned for the fragrance of its foliage, and has a long history as the herb of remembrance, and is used to improve brainpower and failing memory.

This bushy, evergreen shrub thrives in a Mediterranean-style climate, and in the right conditions grows to around 5 ft (1.5 m). Its long narrow, shiny, leathery leaves are deep green on top, and pale, almost silvery gray, underneath. The flowers are small, pale to dark blue, and the whole plant is very aromatic if bruised, as the leaves are rich in volatile oils.

In the kitchen, fresh chopped rosemary leaves or sprigs are added to meat dishes (especially lamb or chicken), and to flavor baked potatoes, and other root vegetables. It makes a delicious addition to sauces, soups like minestrone, and stews. The leaves can also be added to biscuits, salads and fruit salads, pickles, vegetable juices, punches and liqueurs, and for making fragrant vinegars and infused oils.

The best essential oil is distilled from the flowering tips and leaves, but sometimes the whole plant is used, resulting in a much inferior oil. The perfume is sharp and penetrating, and blends well with basil, bergamot, cedarwood, all citrus oils, lavender, and peppermint.

Uses: HERB, ESSENTIAL OIL

Taken as tea, rosemary seems to relieve headaches in the same way that aspirin does, but without irritating the stomach. It can also soothe an upset digestive system where there is flatulence and poor liver function.

Rosemary leaves and flowers are added to ointment blends to fight bacterial and fungal infections, heal cuts, sores, stings, and bites.

A strong astringent, rosemary oil is useful to help contract and tone skin that is loose and sagging. It kills bacteria, and prevents or destroys fungal infections, making it a good oil to treat acne, dermatitis, eczema, athlete's foot, and scabies.

It's an excellent hair and scalp treatment, which is why it's a good idea to include rosemary in shampoo, rinses, and hair tonic, where it will control dandruff, greasy hair, and oily scalp. It is also used in treatments for head lice.

Use rosemary in baths and massage oils to ease the pain of aching muscles, arthritis, bruises, neuralgia, gout, rheumatism, and sports injuries such as sprains and strains.

Restorative rosemary tea sipped in $\frac{1}{4}$ cup amounts four times a day for one week is a good tonic, and helps ease digestive problems such as colitis, indigestion, flatulence, and cramps and spasms in the intestines.

"As for rosemary, I let it run all over my garden walls, not only because my bees love it but because it is the herb sacred to remembrance, and to friendship, whence a sprig of it hath a dumb language."

SIR THOMAS MORE
[1478–1535]

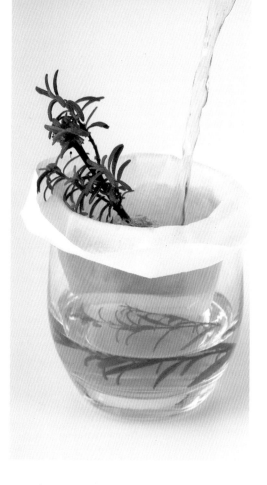

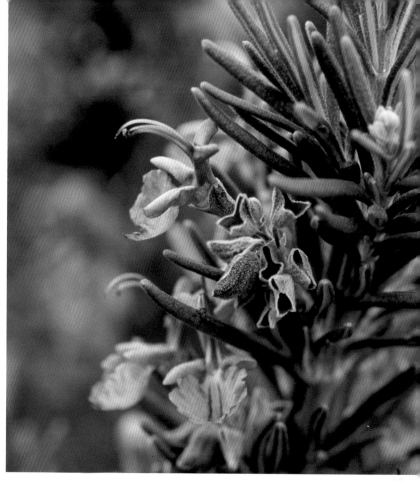

Left: *Rosemary tea is useful in relieving congestion.*

It has a reputation for having a tonic effect on the lungs, which is useful when treating asthma, bronchitis, colds, coughs, and whooping cough—sip ¼ cup rosemary tea four times a day for one week.

As an aromatic, rosemary is used in potpourri for scenting clothing or linen, and deterring moths. The stripped stems can be burned on a barbeque or in the fireplace.

Caution: *A word of caution—drink no more than one cup of rosemary tea daily for no longer than one week. Not to be used during pregnancy. Avoid if you suffer from epilepsy.*

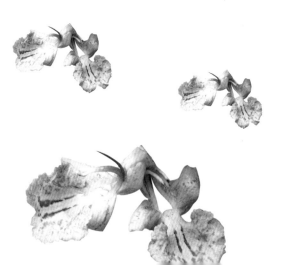

Growing and harvesting

Rosemary is usually propagated from tip cuttings and layering—seeds can be hard to germinate. Choose a sunny, well-drained location in the garden, and plant in early spring or fall in light, sandy, or alkaline soil. Regular trimming encourages growth, and pruning after flowering will prevent the plant from becoming woody and straggly.

When harvesting or picking to use fresh, resist the impulse to "strip" off the leaves with a downward action as this will tend to remove some of the outer stem bark too. The leaves also exude a sticky resin if stripped from the branches this way. To pick, hold the bottom of the stem in one hand and pluck the leaves off with an upward motion. Cut the branches before flowering, and hang them in bunches in a shady, airy place with a cloth or paper spread underneath or spread out on wire racks. Remove the crisp-dry leaves from the stems, crumble them into small pieces, and store in airtight, labelled containers away from the light.

"The distilled water of the flowres of Rosemary being drunke at morning and evening first and last, taketh away the stench of the mouth and breath, and maketh it very sweet..."

— GERARD

Rubus *species*

Rosaceae

Rubus fruticosus
Blackberry

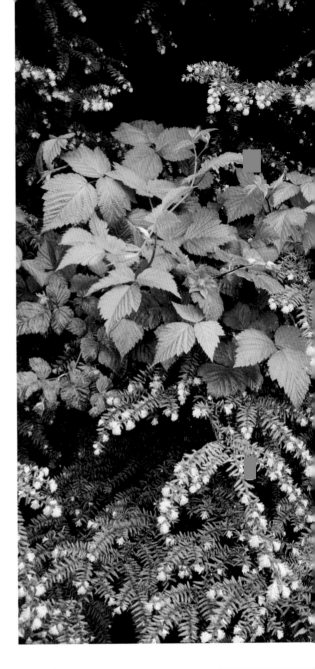

Blackberry is a trailing, semi-evergreen, prickly perennial growing to around 12 ft (4 m). The slender branches feature sharp prickles, and the leaves are finely hairy with three to five leaflets. The white, five-petaled flowers appear from mid-summer to fall, followed by the juicy black fruit that can be picked to make delicious pies, wine, brandy, and cordial. But all parts of the plant are useful (leaves, stem, and roots), and have a well-known and documented history as herbal remedies.

Uses: HERB

Blackberry tea is most easily made with the leaves and/or fruit, and is an astringent remedy for diarrhea and dysentery.

A tea is also useful when applied externally as a lotion, and may be of help in the treatment of psoriasis, and other scaly conditions of the skin.

Caution: It is not advisable to take blackberry preparations for more than a week at a time.

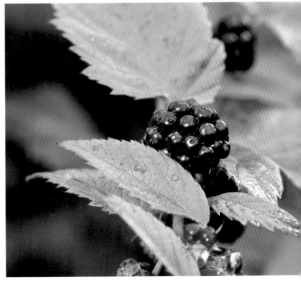

R. idaeus
Raspberry
Also known as red raspberry, hindleberry, wild raspberry

Raspberry is known as the king of the berries. This deciduous shrub with bristly canes grows to about 3–6 ft (1–2 m). The leaves are feather-shaped, with three to seven notched lobes, green above, whitish green and hairy beneath. The loose, greenish white flowers turn to strongly scented and delicious, red fruits that ripen during the summer months and look like jewels set among the leaves. The mouth-watering fruit can be served plain or in fruit salads, puréed, or to make a delicious pouring sauce for sponge and other plain puddings.

Uses: HERB
The best known property of this herb is to strengthen the tissue of the uterus in preparation for labor, where it will assist contractions. Drink tea made of the leaves increasingly during the last three months of pregnancy, starting with two cups a day, and increasing to four cups. Sip the tea during labor to decrease the risk of hemorrhage.

The astringent properties of raspberry are valuable when the leaves and fruit are used as a gargle for mouth and throat infections (such as mouth ulcers, bleeding gums, and inflammations).

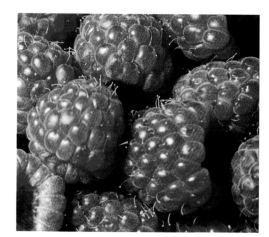

Growing and harvesting
These bramble plants can be grown from seed, cuttings or tip layering (blackberry). They like moist, well-drained soil in a sunny position, or partial shade. They tend to be invasive so need to be controlled in your garden. Pick leaves before flowering, and dry for making infusions, and liquid extracts. Harvest fruit when ripe, and use fresh or dry for making decoctions.

Blackberry is subject to control restrictions in some countries, particularly parts of Australia, where it infests an estimated 22 million acres (8.8 million hectares) of land, and has been known to completely invade grazing properties, waterways, and even abandoned buildings. If tempted to pick blackberries from the wayside, be aware that wild blackberries may have been subjected to poisonous sprays.

Berried treasure

Blackberries and raspberries are a good source of vitamin C and fiber, and also supply essential minerals such as iron, calcium, magnesium, and phosphorus. Blackberries are also a source of vitamin E. They are rich in anthocyanins—the purple and red pigments in these berries function as antioxidants, minimizing the damage to cell membranes that occurs with ageing.

Berries are best eaten as soon as possible after purchase. If you need to keep them for a day or two, here's how to minimize mold. Take them out of the punnet, and store in the refrigerator on a couple of layers of paper towel, and cover loosely with plastic wrap. Don't rinse them until you are about to eat them or use them in your cooking.

SERVING SUGGESTIONS
- Combine one cup of blackberries or raspberries (or a combination) with a little powdered (caster) sugar to taste, and a tablespoon of balsamic vinegar. Let the flavors develop then serve.
- Purée berries for coulis, salsas, sauces, sorbets, and ice creams.
- Top your breakfast cereal or porridge with berries.

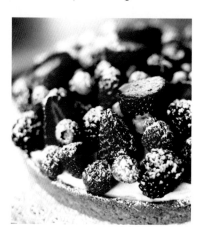

Rumex crispus

Polygonaceae
Yellow dock
Also known as curled dock

Yellow dock is a cousin of French sorrel. It is a hardy, perennial plant growing to 1–5 ft (30 cm–1.5 m) in height with light green, lance-shaped leaves and pale green flowers borne on spikes in summer. The root (which is the important part of the plant) grows very deep. It has a rusty brown, quite thick bark and whitish flesh.

Uses: HERB
Yellow dock gently encourages the bowels. It is an excellent herb to use in combination with dandelion and burdock in tinctures and teas taken three times daily. In this way it has a cleansing action that will help to treat chronic skin complaints such as eczema and psoriasis.

Caution: Not recommended for use if there is a history of kidney stones.

Growing and harvesting
Plant seeds in moist, well-drained soil in a sunny position in the garden or partial shade. Be aware that once it's there, it's hard to get rid of. Because dock is very difficult to eradicate, it's unpopular with gardeners and is subject to weed control restrictions in certain parts. If you don't want the plant to spread, it's best to cut the flowerheads off as they appear. Lift roots in the fall for use in decoctions, extracts, and tinctures.

Ruta graveolens

Rutaceae
Rue
Also known as herb of grace, herby grass, herb of repentance

Rue is perennial shrub with a yellow or yellow-green flowers, and blue-green leaves with a pungent smell. The plant rarely grows to more than 24 in (60 cm) high. It was once used extensively as a healing herb, but research has shown that many of the active ingredients are toxic and certainly not suitable for use by anyone other than a trained clinical herbalist.

Uses: HERB
The main uses for rue are to be found in the garden, where it is a most effective insect repellent, especially for ants, flies, snails, and slugs.

Caution: Internal use can cause poisoning. Contact may cause dermatitis. Not to be used during pregnancy, or by people taking blood-thinning medication.

Growing and harvesting
Grow rue from seed or cuttings in a sunny place in well-drained soil. Plant it well away from cabbages.

Judges were, until quite recently, given sprigs, or "tussie-mussies" (small bouquets) of rue. It was believed that the perfume would protect them from the jail fever being carried by the prisoners.

Rue seems to have been one of the main herbs used to try and protect against the plague. It was one of the ingredients in the "Vinegar of the Four Thieves," used by a band of criminals who robbed the bodies and homes of the dead during the plague. The vinegar was used as a wash to protect the thieves from catching the disease.

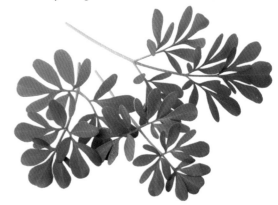

Salix alba

Salicaceae
White willow

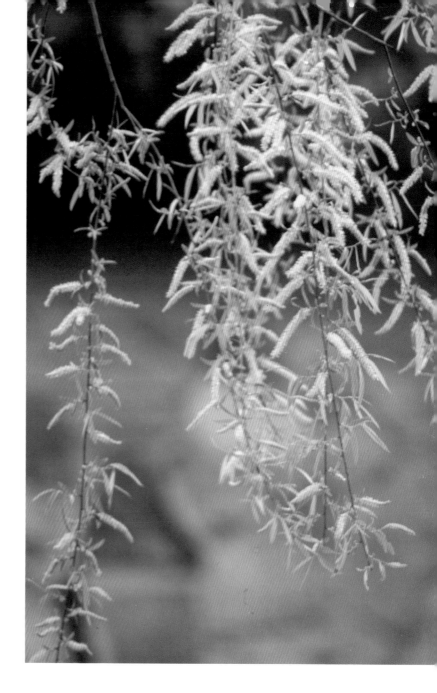

The graceful willow tree, with its silvery white foliage, is a common sight along riverbanks and damp meadows. White willow bark is often called "herbal aspirin." Its active ingredient is salicin, the forerunner of aspirin (aspirin is a trade name which stands for acetylsalicylic acid). White willow is the species most often used medicinally, but other salicin-rich species, including crack willow (*Salix fragilis*), purple willow (*Salix purpurea*), and violet willow (*Salix daphnoides*), are also sold as willow bark.

Uses: HERB

A decoction is prepared from one teaspoon of dried bark simmered in one cup (250 ml) of water in a covered pan for 10 minutes. Three to five cups of this decoction may be drunk each day. The tincture is also used, commonly in the amount of 20–40 drops, three times a day.

Analgesic, anti-inflammatory, and astringent properties relieve inflammation and swelling, and improve mobility in painful joints, making it an extremely effective herb for treating joint, hip, and back pain. Willow bark is also used to manage high fevers, and may help ease tension headaches and migraines.

Willow bark taken as a decoction or tincture (as described above), assists during menopause by reducing sweating during hot flashes and night sweats.

The bark eases internal and external bleeding; it can also be used as a gargle to ease sore throats, laryngitis, and tonsillitis.

A decoction or diluted tincture is used to wash wounds, burns, and sores.

Caution: Long-term use of willow is not advisable, as it may cause some of the same problems that aspirin does. However, willow is considered to be much safer than aspirin.

Salvia officinalis

Lamiaceae
Sage
Also known as garden sage,
common sage

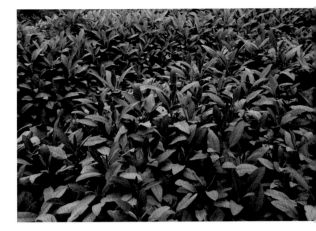

There are several hundred species of sage,
most of which are ornamental, but a few
are useful to herbalists. Garden or common
sage (*Salvia officinalis*), the most widely used
medicinally, is a hardy perennial growing
to about 12 in (30 cm) high with velvety,
grayish green leaves and purple-grey flowers.
Sage leaves are particularly good in savory
dishes and can be used with vegetables,
poultry, soups, stews, stuffings, cottage
cheeses, and dressings. This is a very strongly
flavored herb so use with a little discretion.

Uses: HERB

Sage is the classic remedy for mouth and
throat problems such as ulcers, sore tongue,
laryngitis, and tonsillitis. Use as a gargle,
mouthwash or, for convenience and pain
relief, freeze a very strong sage tea in ice
cube trays and break a cube into chips to
suck for relief from mouth ulcers.

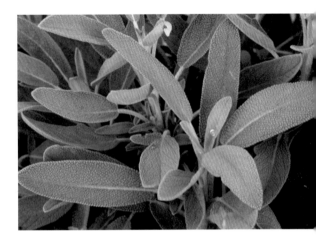

Use the leaves in washes, ointments, and
fomentations for their anti-inflammatory
and astringent qualities to treat abscesses,
sores, ulcers, wounds, and varicose veins.
When drunk as an infusion, sage reduces
"night sweats" and excessive perspiration.

In the garden, sage repels cabbage moth,
carrot fly, snails, and slugs. Grow it near
cabbages, carrots, or strawberries.

Caution: *Not for prolonged use. Not to be used
during pregnancy.*

Growing and harvesting

Grow it from seed, seedlings, or cuttings in
a sunny spot in well-drained soil. Pick leaves
and use fresh or hang in bunches in a warm,
airy place, and dry for using in infusions,
extracts, tinctures, washes, ointments, and
also fomentations.

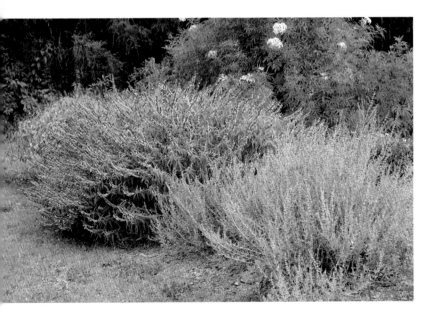

Salvia sclarea

Lamiaceae
Clary sage
Also known as cleareye, muscatel sage

Clary sage with its greenish white spikes tinged with purple flowers is a native of southern Europe. It's a natural antidepressant and the essential oil is distilled from the whole herb. It is also one of the most powerful relaxants in the essential oil pharmacy and is used in preference to other varieties of sage as its toxicity levels are much lower. Its perfume is intoxicating— sweet, floral, and fixative, blending very well with cedarwood, geranium, juniper, lavender, and sandalwood.

Uses: ESSENTIAL OIL

Clay sage's antiseptic and sebum-regulating action is useful in the treatment of acne, boils, and inflammation of the skin. It has a reputation for combating hair loss and dandruff. Use the oil in blends for care of mature, dry skin, and also as a deodorant.

Clary sage is a soothing and powerful muscle-relaxing oil that will help to ease muscular aches and pains, whooping cough, and asthma attacks, when used as a massage oil. Its tonic and hormonal properties help to regulate and encourage labor (but should not be used until after labor has begun). It can tone, strengthen, and relieve cramps and spasms in the uterus, ease period pain, encourage and regulate menstrual flow, and help with pre-menstrual problems.

Clary sage may be used in compresses and massage and bath blends to help tone the digestive system, aid digestion, expel gas from the intestines, and treat colic, cramp, and flatulence.

The warming and spasm-relieving properties can be employed in fomentations and/or gentle massages when dealing with colic and stomach or intestinal cramps. It may also be used to reduce sweating.

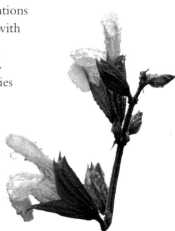

Its tonic and antidepressant properties in baths and massage oils are useful when people are recovering from illnesses, feeling weak and depressed. It calms and reduces stress.

Caution: Use in small amounts only. Large amounts may cause a severe headache and poisoning. Not to be used during pregnancy. Avoid using when drinking alcohol.

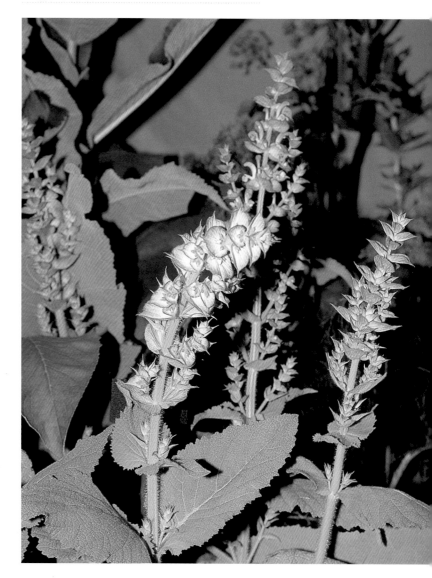

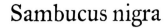

Sambucus nigra

Caprifoliaceae
Elder
Also known as common elder, black elder, European elder, German elder

The elder, long regarded as the medicine chest of country people, is a small, deciduous tree with a dense, spreading habit that grows to about 20 ft (6 m). The rough gray-brown stems bear large leaves and large, creamy white heads of small, sweet-smelling flowers. Flowers are by drooping bunches of purple berries that contain more vitamin C than any other herb except rosehip.

For centuries people have found a use for each and every part of the elder—leaf, bark, wood or branch, flower, and fruit. The flowers and berries are the most widely used part, medicinally and in the kitchen, where they are used in making tea, cordials, wines, jams, jellies, chutneys, fruit tarts, ice cream, and fritters—simply dip the flower heads in a light batter, deep fry them and sprinkle with powdered (caster) sugar.

The flowers are the parts to use to make elder flower infused oil. I make and keep a good supply of this infused oil for blending with calendula infused oil to make moisture lotions and creams. The resulting blend is softening, anti-inflammatory, healing, and good for all skin types.

Uses: HERB, INFUSED OIL
When drunk in a tea, the flowers act as a febrifuge (an agent for reducing fever), and diaphoretic (an agent for promoting perspiration), to improve feverish conditions such as colds and influenza, particularly when combined with peppermint and yarrow. The flowers are also decongestant and helpful in any catarrhal conditions of the upper respiratory tract. They may also be used as a mouthwash and gargle for mouth and throat inflammations and infections.

Elder leaves can be very purgative and I restrict their use to external treatments—ointments, compresses, fomentations, and poultices for bruises, sprains, and wounds.

I use elder flowers in almost every healing cream and skin preparation that I make.

Elderberry juice is a wonderful cleanser and tonic for the reproductive and glandular system, and appears to be useful in all rheumatic complaints. The juice needs to be brought to the boil and cooled before drinking or the action may be purgative.

The plant repels aphids and caterpillars.

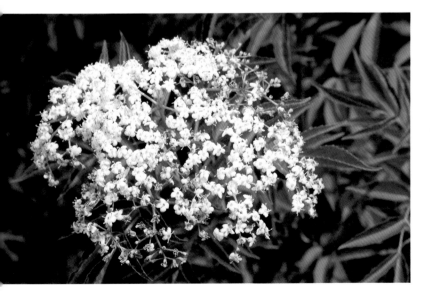

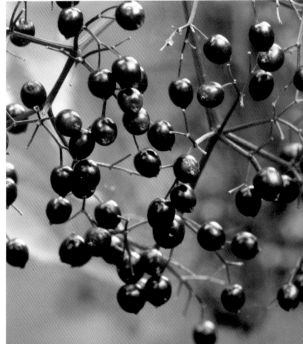

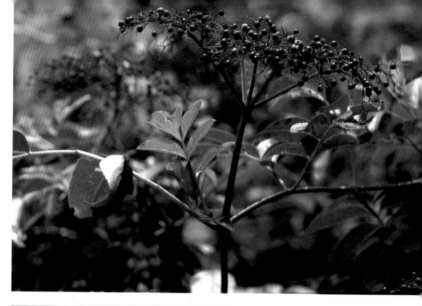

Growing and harvesting

Grow it from cuttings in rich, moist soil in a sunny position in the garden with partial shade. It is frost resistant and prefers a cool climate to fruit properly. Elder trees are not only hardy, they are hard to eradicate and have a spreading habit, so be aware before you plant that this tree is likely to outlast you. Cut back hard in winter. Collect and dry flower heads when fully open for infusions, extracts, ointments, and tinctures.

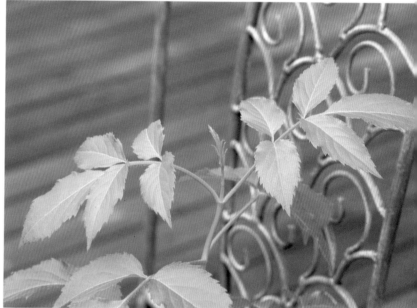

ELDER FLOWER SPARKLING WINE

A delicious non-alcoholic elder flower wine that is easy to make, quick to mature and delicious to drink.

$5^1/_2$ oz (150 g) sugar

3 cups (750 ml) hot water (hot enough to dissolve the sugar but not to evaporate the essential oil in the skin of the lemon)

2 lemons

4 large elder flower heads

$^1/_4$ cup (60 ml) white wine vinegar

$1^1/_2$ gallons (6 liters) water

- Add the sugar to the hot water in a large stainless steel pot, stir to dissolve well.
- Thinly peel the yellow rind from the lemons in narrow strips (no white pith please!), juice the lemons and add the juice and rind to the syrup.
- Add the remaining ingredients, stir, cover and leave for four days.
- Strain into sterilized, screw-top bottles, and leave for six days or until effervescing (don't leave for too long or the bottles may burst).
- Serve chilled.

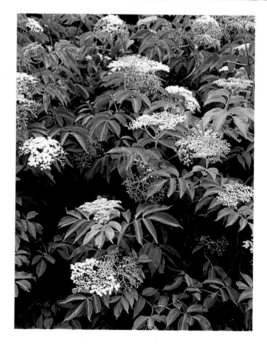

Santalum album

Santalaceae
Sandalwood
Also known as Indian sandalwood, white sandalwood

Sandalwood is a small, semi-parasitic tree that feeds through suckers attached to the roots of other trees. The oil is steam-distilled from the heartwood of trees at least 25 years old. Renowned for its spiritual and uplifting qualities, sandalwood incense and oil was (and still is) used in temples, and to aid and deepen meditation.

"If I had a palace made of pearls, inlaid with jewels, scented with musk, saffron and sandalwood, a sheer delight to behold—seeing this, I might go astray and forget You, and Your Name would not enter into my mind."
SRI GURU GRANTH SAHIB

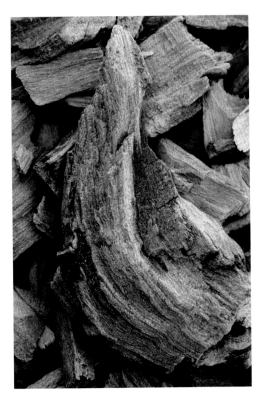

Today, that distinctive mysterious, spicy aroma is used as a fixative and fragrance in the manufacture of perfumes, cosmetics and toiletries, such as soaps and aftershaves. It blends well with most other essential oils but especially benzoin, rose, neroli, and petitgrain. The essential oil worth using is that from Indian sandalwood—the oil from Western Australian sandalwood (*Santalum spicatum*) is definitely inferior.

Uses: ESSENTIAL OIL
A lovely moisturizing oil to use in blends for all skin types but it is particularly beneficial on dry, thin, ageing skin, and cracked chapped skin. A good oil to include in aftershave preparations as it prevents inflammation, moisturizes the skin, and has an aroma that is very acceptable to men. Use in compresses or creams to heal dry eczema, acne, and to cool inflammations.

Sandalwood is a pulmonary antiseptic and also helps to loosen and remove mucus. Use it in inhalations, and chest and throat rubs, where it will ease chronic bronchitis, mucus, dry, irritating cough, and sore throat.

It acts as a urinary system cleanser as it increases the flow of urine and is antiseptic; it can be used in fomentations and massage to ease cystitis and urethritis.

Sandalwood oil is recognized as one of the few true aphrodisiacs and can help to promote sexuality in those who suffer from impotence and frigidity.

Caution: Sandalwood has a very penetrating and long-lasting perfume—use in very small amounts in blends.

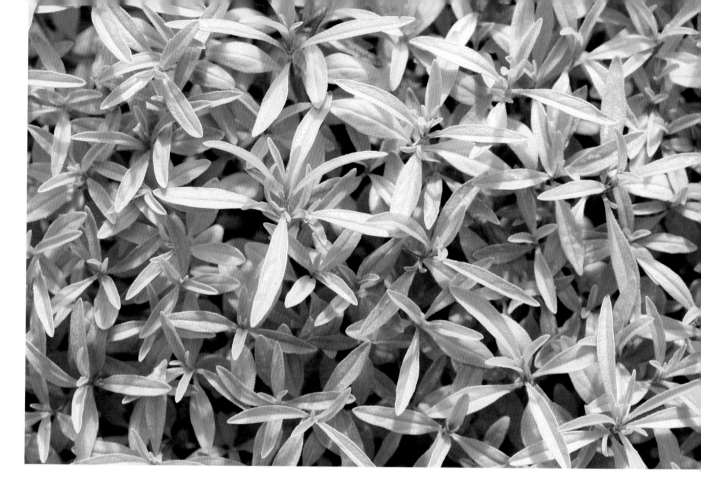

Satureja *species*

Lamiaceae

Satureja hortensis
Summer savory

S. montana
Winter savory

Summer savory (*Satureja hortensis*) is a bushy annual that grows to about 12–24 in (30–60 cm) high with opposite, straight, dark green leaves and pinkish mauve flowers in clusters. Winter savory (*S. montana*) is much smaller and a perennial. The plant is branched and woody, with dark green, glossy leaves, and lots of creamy white flowers from midsummer until the end of fall.

In the kitchen, use savory to flavor delicate dishes, or add to salads. Winter savory is reputed to reduce the flatulence factor with legumes.

Uses: HERB

Use the leaves of both summer and winter savory fresh or dried in infusions to soothe the stomach or gripe pains.

Savory repels beetles and grows well with beans.

Growing and harvesting

Grow from seed or (winter variety) cuttings, mounding, or layering in a sunny, well-drained spot. Harvest leaves during the growing season as required, to use fresh or dried.

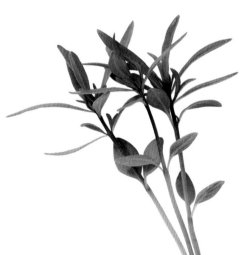

Scutellaria laterifolia

Lamiaceae
Skullcap
Also known as mad dog skullcap, Virginian skullcap

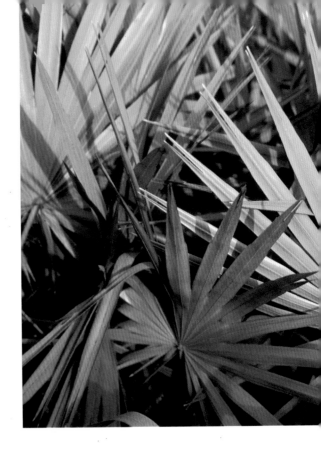

This is a small and fairly inconspicuous perennial plant native to North America, rarely growing taller than 12 in (30 cm). The leaves are thin and finely toothed at the edges and are one of the most valuable nervines in the herbal pharmacy. The plant's name refers to the helmet-shaped calyx on the outer whorl of the plant's tiny blue (occasionally white or pink) flowers. In the nineteenth century it was used to treat rabies—hence the common name, mad dog skullcap.

Uses: HERB

Soothing, astringent skullcap acts as a tonic for the nervous system and especially for nervous and convulsive disorders. Use the leaves in the form of a tea or tincture to treat nervous tension or exhaustion, mild depression, insomnia, excitability, PMS, irritability, and restlessness. To make a tea, add one teaspoon of the finely chopped dried herb to one cup of boiling water. Cover and steep for 10 minutes. Drink one cup three times a day, or 40–60 drops of tincture in water three times a day. The tea also reduces symptoms in those suffering from chronic hepatitis, improving liver function.

Caution: It is not advisable to increase the dose recommended above as it can result in dizziness and mental confusion. Not to be used during pregnancy.

Growing and harvesting

Plant seeds or cuttings (or propagate by division) in well-drained soil in a sunny position or partial shade. Cut leaves as required for using fresh or dried in infusions.

Serenoa repens

syn. *S. serrulata*

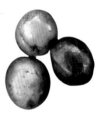

Arecaceae
Saw palmetto

Saw palmetto is a hardy palm growing to around 2–9 ft (60 cm–2.7 m), native to the south-eastern United States and the West Indies. Its fragrant, white flowers produce dark purple, edible berries in the fall, which are wild harvested (mainly in Florida) for their medicinal properties.

Clinical studies have shown that the extract of saw palmetto berries is a safe and effective remedy for the symptoms of an enlarged prostate gland (benign prostatic hypertrophy or BPH), increasing urine flow and reducing the frequency of night-time urination.

Uses: HERB

Take as recommended as an over-the-counter extract. The primary use of this plant is to strengthen and tone the

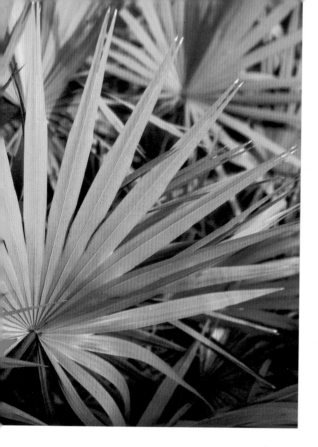

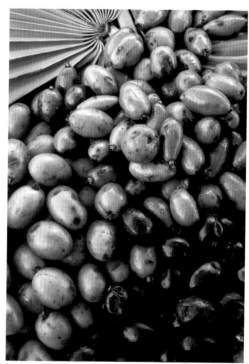

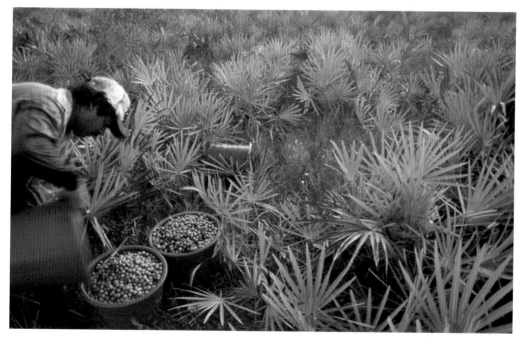

The edible berries of the saw palmetto are harvested in the fall.

male reproductive system. It is an anti-inflammatory, and also acts as a boost to the male sex hormones. It is also useful to deal with urinary tract infections, and problems of the gastrointestinal system.

Caution: *Saw palmetto should only be used for BPH after proper diagnosis by a physician.*

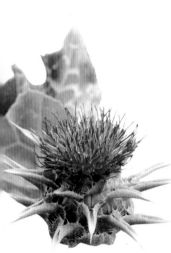

Silybum marianum

syn. *Carduus marianus*

Asteraceae
Milk thistle
Also known as blessed thistle

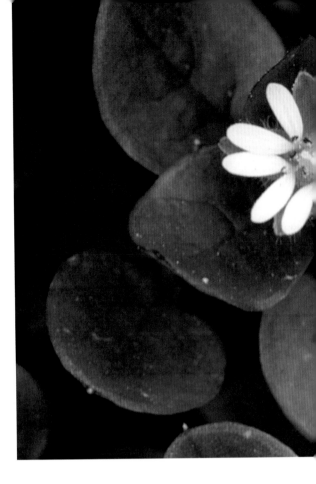

This prickly annual or biennial grows to 4–5 ft (1.2–1.5 m). It has spiny green leaves and bears an attractive flower head, topped with a purple, thistle-like tuft. The leaves can be eaten as a vegetable, raw or cooked. All parts of the plant are of interest. They contain an active compound known as silymarin, which works in a number of ways to restore liver health. Milk thistle extract, in pills, capsules, tincture, or infusion, improves liver function, protects against liver damage, and stimulates the growth of new liver cells. It has also been used to reduce the side-effects of chemotherapy.

Uses: HERB
Take a cup of milk thistle tea made by infusing one teaspoon of the seeds for 10–15 minutes in boiling water or 40 drops of tincture in water three times daily to treat food intolerances and skin conditions caused by poor liver function.

Growing and harvesting
Grow seeds in well-drained soil in a sunny position and collect ripe seeds for use in infusions and tinctures. It is subject to weed control regulations in some countries.

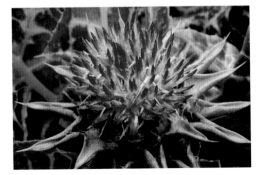

WHY IS IT CALLED CHICKWEED?
People noticed that chickweed provided birds and other wild life with much needed fresh greens. John Gerard commented in *The Herball* [1633 edition]: "Little birds in cadges [especially Linnets] are refreshed with the lesser Chickweed when they loath their meat [lose their appetite]; whereupon it was called of some *Passerina.*"

Stellaria media

Caryophyllaceae
Chickweed
Also known as starweed

Chickweed is an annual with long, sprawling branches that trail on the ground, pale green, ovate leaves, and small, white, star-shaped flowers. Usually despised as an obnoxious weed by the keen gardener, this lovely and valuable little plant is found in gardens and wastelands throughout the temperate regions of the world. Culpeper calls it "a fine, soft, pleasing herb."

Make the most of its cleansing and alterative properties in the kitchen by adding torn leaves to salads, cooking leaves and stems as a vegetable, or juicing leaves and stems with other vegetables as a tonic.

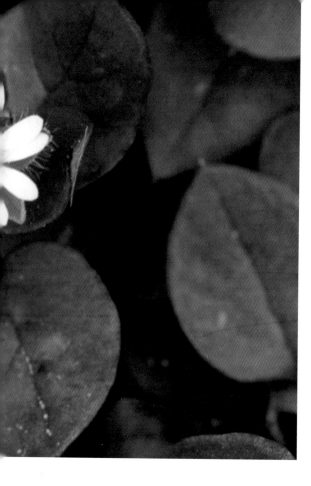

Styrax benzoin

Styracaceae
Benzoin
Also known as gum Benjamin

Benzoin oil is prepared from the crude resin that exudes from the trunk of a tall, evergreen tree native to Indonesia. To harvest the resin, deep incisions are made in the trunk of the tree, from which the grayish colored sap exudes. This hardens into a resinous lump and is then collected. It is an ingredient in the world famous friar's balsam.

Benzoin is not true essential oil as the resin is then dissolved in alcohol. It blends well with spice oils, bergamot, cypress, juniper, lavender, myrrh, petitgrain, and sandalwood.

I use it when making ointments, creams, and lotions for both its healing and preservative action, and also in perfumes for its fixative properties.

Uses: HERB

The whole plant can be used both internally and externally—as a compress, fomentation, ointment, tincture, or tea. There is no finer remedy for soothing and healing inflammation, ulcers, eczema, psoriasis, and other itchy and/or inflamed skin conditions.

Taken as a tincture or tea, it has a reputation as a remedy for easing the pain of rheumatism. Infuse the leaves and stems and drink one cup three times daily or take 40 drops of tincture in two tablespoons of water three times daily.

Growing and harvesting

Grow seeds in moist soil in a sunny position or partial shade. Or simply allow it to grow freely in your garden wherever it chooses. It doesn't become troublesome, as it's very easy to pull up by the roots when ready to harvest. Use the leaves, stems, and roots, fresh or dry, for infusions, tinctures, ointments, and extracts.

Uses: ESSENTIAL OIL

Benzoin oil helps to destroy bacterial and fungal infections of the skin and reduces inflammation. It is useful in blends for ointments, creams, and lotions to heal skin irritations and ease itching, and excellent when added to creams to soothe and soften cracked and dry skin. It contracts and tones tissue, stops external bleeding, helps to heal wounds, and reduces body odor.

Benzoin is a warming oil and this, combined with its tonic and mucus-loosening properties, gives it a very old reputation for helping with respiratory problems such as asthma, bronchitis, coughs, chills, colds, and laryngitis when used in inhalations or chest rubs.

It is helpful for arthritis, poor circulation, and rheumatism when used in massage oils. In fomentations it may be a good remedy for problems such as cystitis and infected urinary tract.

WHY IS IT CALLED BENZOIN?
In the fourteenth century, the Arabs who traded this "incense of Java" [it was a useful substitute for frankincense], called it "luban jawi" which over time became "benjawi," "benjamin," and then "benzoin."

Symphytum officinale

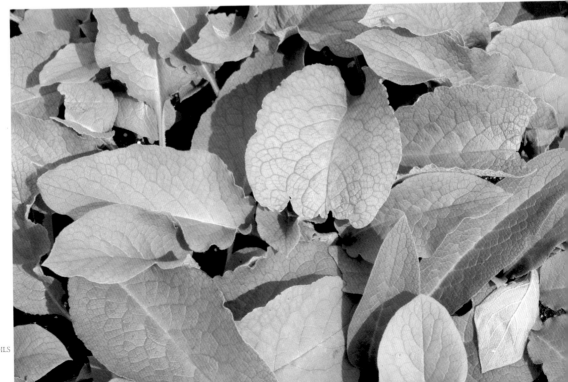

Boraginaceae
Comfrey
Also known as knitbone, knitback, bruisewort, gum plant

Prickly comfrey is a leafy, spreading perennial, dormant in winter and growing as tall as 4 ft (1.2 m) under good conditions—it thrives in soft, wet ground in fields, meadows, or valleys. The fleshy rootstock is blackish on the outside, white and fleshy inside, and oozes a thick, sticky juice when cut. The hairy leaves are green, long, and oval-shaped, growing very large at the base of the plant and decreasing in size further up the stem. Comfrey blooms in summer with clusters of pale pink, pale yellow, or pale mauve, softly drooping, bell-shaped flowers. In medieval times, comfrey was used topically to mend fractured bones—hence knitbone and boneset.

Uses: HERB, INFUSED OIL

The roots and leaves of comfrey are used externally when the skin is unbroken in compresses, fomentations, ointments, and poultices, for their anti-inflammatory, softening, lubricating, and wound-healing properties. They treat boils, bruises, fractures, sore breasts, eczema, ulcers and tropical ulcers, minor burns, aching joints, sprains, and swellings, including arthritis and bunions.

An infused oil made from roots and leaves is an essential in the medicine chest. Comfrey infused oil is impressive in its healing powers for clean wounds, ulcers, strains, muscular injuries, and fractures. It may also be used to good effect on dry eczema, itchy skin, and rough skin.

Caution: Comfrey is for external use only. Do not use on abraded skin; nor on unbroken skin long term. Not for use during pregnancy.

Growing and harvesting

Grow comfrey from root division in a sunny place or partial shade, and remember it likes moist soil. Keep it under control or it can take over the garden. Comfrey is one of the few plants that will tolerate fresh manure. Pick leaves as required and lift roots to use dried for decoctions, extracts, and ointments.

Syzygium aromaticum

syn. *Eugenia caryophyllata*

Myrtaceae
Clove
Also known as nelkin, ting-hiang

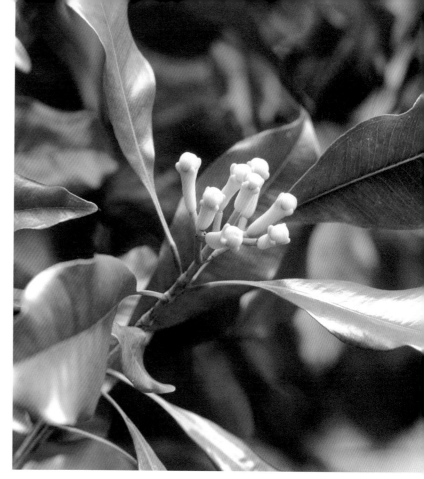

The aromatic cloves you use in cooking are the unexpanded dried flower bud from a tropical evergreen tree, native to a handful of tiny islands in eastern Indonesia—the Moluccas. Clove trees don't start producing until they are about six to eight years old and even then they usually only deliver a bumper crop every four years or so. When the flower buds are full size, the clove clusters are hand picked. The buds are then removed from the flower stems by twisting the cluster against the palm of the hand and spread out on woven mats to dry in the sun. This is when the flavor develops thanks to the enzymatic reaction that forms eugenol—a volatile oil that may remind you of the dentist's chair. Now and again, you will see a flutter of yellow amongst the darkening cloves, when a bud has burst into flower just at picking time. The essential oil, steam-distilled from the flower buds, has a pungent and spicy aroma. Clove essential oil is often used in toothpastes and other dental preparations, germicides, perfumes and mouthwashes, and in commercial foods and drinks.

Cloves combine endurance and strength with assertiveness and determination. Why choose the rest when you can have the best? Clove reaches deep into the recesses of the mind to stimulate memory.

Uses: ESSENTIAL OIL

A very good oil to include in blends for compresses, fomentations, and baths for treating infectious sores, leg ulcers, acne, athlete's foot, bruises, and burns. It is also a good insect repellent.

Cloves and their oil are well known for their power to ease toothache by numbing the nerve and causing loss of sensation. This pain-numbing property may also used as a mouthwash to ease mouth ulcers, and to relieve the pain of neuralgia, arthritis, and rheumatism in massage blends.

Clove oil's other claim to fame is from the benefits it bestows on the digestive system. Used in compresses, fomentations, baths, massages, and mouthwashes, it tones the digestive system, relieves cramps and spasms in the intestines, helps to control vomiting and nausea, expels gas from the intestines, aids digestion, and sweetens bad breath that is due to fermentation in the stomach.

It has the power to increase energy and quicken the function of the glands, and is often included in chest massage blends to relieve asthma and bronchitis.

Caution: Never use neat or in a high concentration in skin preparations.

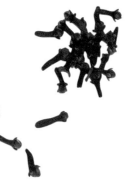

Cloves were one of the major spices, along with nutmeg, right in the middle of that ruthless business popularly known as "the spice trade" when a handful of cloves was worth a handful of silver and more.

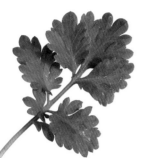

Tanacetum parthenium

syn. *Chrysanthemum parthenium,*
Matricaria parthenium

Asteraceae
Feverfew
Also known as featherfew, featherfoil,
flirtwort

A traditional cottage herb, feverfew seems to have been used as a whole pharmacy on its own. Gerard and Culpeper back in the 1600s were both fans. Gerard, for instance, says: "very good for them that are giddie in the head." Culpeper says that: "Venus commands this herb, and has commended it to succour her sisters [women], to be a general strengthener of their wombs..." He goes on to agree with Gerard saying: "It is very effectual for all pains in the head..."

Feverfew has had many names over the centuries, which means that it was well known and used. The name "feverfew" seems to come from "febrifuge," which describes the herb's capacity to reduce fever. The plant is a hardy perennial growing to 18–24 in (45–60 cm) tall, with light green, feathery leaves and tiny, sunny, daisy-like flowers with yellow centers, white rays, and toothed edges. Use the flowers in floral arrangements, especially traditional posies, as they will last well indoors. Remember to replace the water every two days or so.

Uses: HERB

Use the whole herb as a tea sipped after a meal for its digestive qualities. It soothes indigestion, gripe, and wind.

Feverfew is an anti-inflammatory and also dilates veins, so has been found to be useful when three or four leaves are chewed to relieve migraine headaches if they are of the type that is relieved by heat. **Note the caution.** This property also helps to ease arthritic inflammation. A cold extract has a tonic effect.

Use in teas, taken three times daily where menstrual flow is sluggish and after childbirth to hasten cleansing and toning of the uterus. Feverfew has a reputation for reducing the symptoms of vertigo.

Feverfew teas can be used cosmetically to help fade freckles and age spots.

To repel insects, a tincture made from feverfew and rubbed on the skin will keep away gnats, mosquitoes, and other pests, and also has the power to relieve the pain and swelling caused by the bites.

Caution: Not to be used by anyone taking blood-thinning medication or during pregnancy. Excessive use can cause vomiting and diarrhea. In rare cases chewing the leaf can cause mouth ulcers.

Growing and harvesting

Feverfew is not a fussy grower, tolerating some shade, most soils, and dry (but not wet) conditions. Plant seeds in a sunny position with moderate water. It can also be propagated by dividing established plants into fairly large pieces in spring, or from cuttings taken from young shoots with a heel attached, planted out in the fall. Set plants 12 in (30 cm) apart. It will resist frost and repel insects, but take care—once established it tends to wander over the whole garden and pop up between pavers if not controlled. Pick leaves as required, or harvest after flowering, and use fresh or dry for making infusions, extracts, powders, and tinctures.

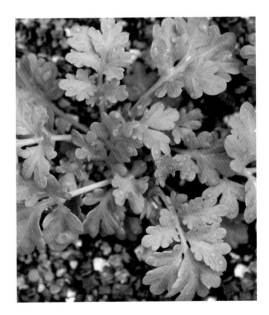

Tanacetum vulgare
syn. *Chrysanthemum vulgare*

Asteraceae
Tansy
Also known as buttons, bachelor's buttons, stinking willy

Tansy is a hardy perennial that spreads from runners. It is almost as invasive as the mint family. The rootstock sends up an erect, grooved, leafy stem that grows to a height of about 3 ft (90 cm) with fern-like, dark green leaves and attractive yellow clusters of button-like flowers developing in the fall.

One of the most interesting uses for tansy in the past was as an embalming agent and meat preservative.

Uses: HERB
Use the whole herb externally in massage oils and ointments to treat inflammations, cuts, sprains, and varicose veins.

It repels ants, aphids, beetles, cabbage moths, and cutworms, and acts as a general insecticide indoors.

It is a useful herb for those with pets, grown around kennels, or dried and rubbed into the fur of dogs to help keep flea populations under control.

It is a good companion to apple, peach, and apricot trees, and cabbage, cauliflower, grapes, as well as raspberries and roses.

Caution: For external use only. Not to be used during pregnancy.

Growing and harvesting
Grow tansy from root division in a sunny spot with moderate water. Pick leaves as required, or harvest after flowering and use fresh or dry for making infusions, extracts, powders, and tinctures

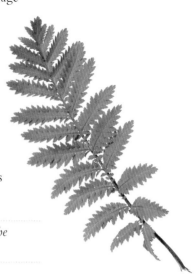

These members of the daisy family are all rich in insecticidal compounds. The pyrethrum that's used commercially in sprays to control flies and other insect pests is derived from *T. cinerariifolium*, a cousin of feverfew and tansy.

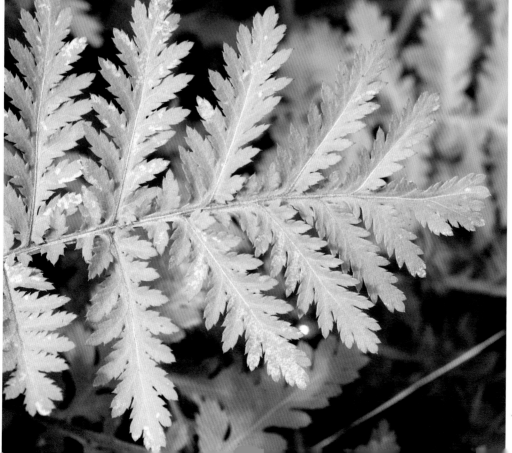

Taraxacum officinale

Asteraceae
Dandelion

Often viewed as a weed (especially by people trying to remove it from a lawn), it is a powerhouse of goodness—right up there with broccoli and spinach. Perennial dandelion has a thick, juicy root (which can be used for making "coffee"), and pale green leaves that rise directly out of the root. Many plants look like dandelion. One of the distinguishing features is the single, smooth, pale green (sometimes tinged with mauve) flower stem that also rises from the root. It is hollow and ends in a single flower head with a collection of gold petals that turn into a white, downy, "puffball" head of seeds. When snapped, the stem exudes a white "milk" (latex).

The very young leaves are a delicious and healthy addition to salads, sandwiches, and vegetable juices (older ones become very bitter). Moderate quantities of petals also make a nice addition to salads. The flowers can be used for making a wine.

The fall and winter roots are the sweetest and this is the best time to harvest them. Scrub them clean, chop into small pieces and roast in the oven until brittle and dark brown, but not burned. They may then be ground and used as a coffee-like drink.

Uses: HERB

When drunk as a tea two or three times daily, the leaves are a safe and powerful diuretic; they are a source of the vital potassium that is normally stripped from the body by other diuretics. Loss of potassium can intensify cardiovascular problems.

When drunk as a decoction two or three times daily, the roots gently stimulate the liver and gall bladder.

The roots and leaves are used for their anti-inflammatory cleansing properties. Dandelion helps to relieve joint inflammation when taken as a tea or decoction.

The latex that oozes from the cut flower stem is traditionally the best way of getting rid of warts. The latex should be applied several times a day to the wart only and not to the surrounding skin, where it can cause irritation.

Caution: Do not use dandelion if you have an obstruction of the bowel or the bile duct.

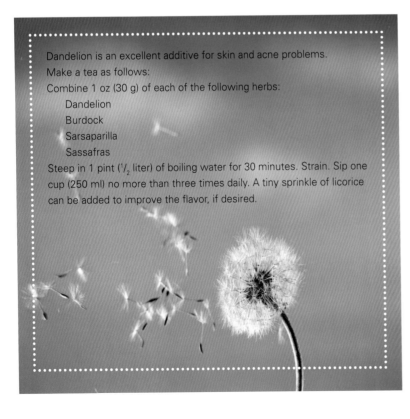

Dandelion is an excellent additive for skin and acne problems.
Make a tea as follows:
Combine 1 oz (30 g) of each of the following herbs:
Dandelion
Burdock
Sarsaparilla
Sassafras
Steep in 1 pint (1/2 liter) of boiling water for 30 minutes. Strain. Sip one cup (250 ml) no more than three times daily. A tiny sprinkle of licorice can be added to improve the flavor, if desired.

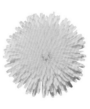

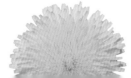

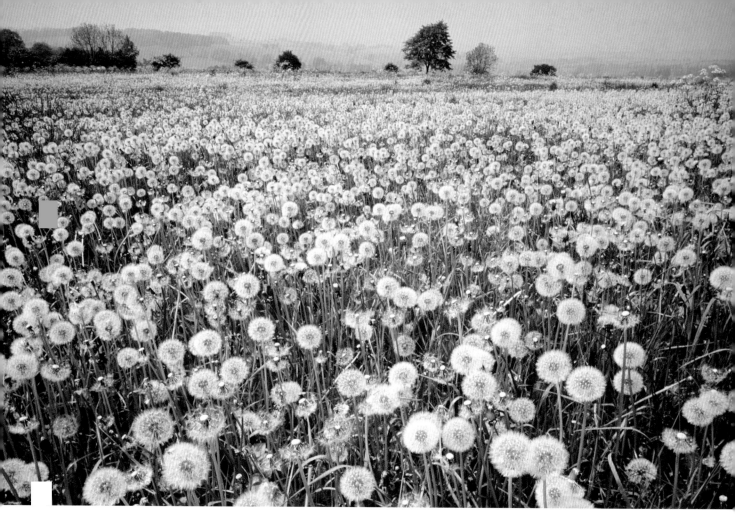

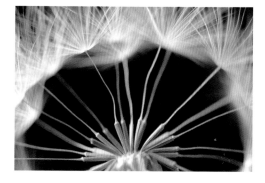

A field of dandelions ready to explode their seeds across the English landscape.

Growing and harvesting

Grow from seed in full sun with little water if you wish to cultivate it, but be careful—it can take over the garden. If you do grow it, a wise precaution is to deadhead plants to prevent seeding. But it's not usually too difficult to find wild stocks if you want to use this herb. Don't however, collect from places that are near road traffic fumes or plants which may have been sprayed. Pick leaves in late spring and use fresh or dry for making decoctions, extracts, infusions, and tinctures. Lift the roots and dry for decoctions, extracts, infusions, and tinctures.

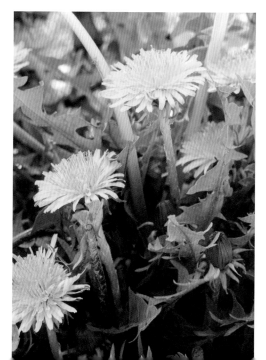

Thymus vulgaris

Lamiaceae
Thyme
Also known as common thyme,
garden thyme

There are between 300 and 400 varieties of
thyme. All have slight differences in aroma
and appearance, and they are often used
as sturdy ground covers in cottage
gardens. Garden thyme is a small,
bushy perennial with hard, branching
stems growing to about 10 in (25 cm)
high. The leaves are very small and
grayish green in color. Light purple flowers
are borne from late spring onwards.

Lemon thyme (*Thymus × citriodorus*) is
very similar to garden thyme but slightly
smaller, with brighter, yellowish green foliage
and a slightly darker mauve flower. It's not as
strong medicinally, but is a wonderful culinary
herb well worth growing.

Aromatic thyme, a perennial herb with
culinary, medicinal, and cosmetic uses, has
long been associated with strength and well-
being. It is a powerful antiseptic herb. It is
also antispasmodic and astringent.

In the kitchen, the leaves of the various
culinary thymes can be used to flavor most
meat and vegetable dishes, seafood, eggs,
and cheese. Thyme also makes excellent
vinegars. If you find the flavor of zucchinis
(courgettes) bland, try sautéing them
in a little butter with lemon thyme and
basil. The final flavor is very reminiscent
of mushrooms!

Thyme is a powerful essential oil doubly
distilled from the flowers in order to remove
some of the more irritant properties.
Chemotype "linalol" thyme oil or lemon
thyme contains few of the toxic phenols and
is safer to use, particularly for the skin, and
in blends for children. Thyme's perfume is
warmly, sweetly pungent, and blends well
with bergamot, cedarwood, chamomile,
juniper, lemon, mandarin, niaouli, petitgrain,
and rosemary.

Uses: HERB, ESSENTIAL OIL, INFUSED OIL
Thyme is a powerful healer for all types of
skin infections and is suitable for treating
abscesses, acne, boils and carbuncles, bruises,
burns and scalds (minor), cold sores,
dermatitis, eczema, and insect bites. Use
thyme leaves as a tea, or in ointment and
infused oils, to treat cuts, sores, wounds,
and ulcers. Thyme essential oil used in skin-
care preparations must always be well diluted
as it can sting and cause irritation. Thyme
oil can be used as a scalp cleanser and hair
tonic and in shampoos to treat dandruff and
hair loss.

Thyme leaves, taken as a tea, aid
digestion, easing griping pains and acting as
a tonic. In massage and bath blends, thyme
oil acts as an intestinal antiseptic aiding
digestion, relieving cramps and spasms in
the intestines, and easing flatulence and
gastric infections.

Thyme is also an expectorant. A tea plus
an inhalation will be effective to treat the
catarrhal congestion and distressing spasms
of bronchitis, croups, asthma, and whooping
cough. Use as a gargle to treat laryngitis,

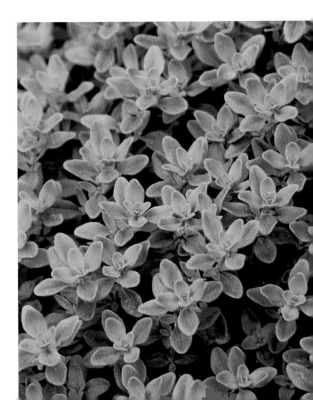

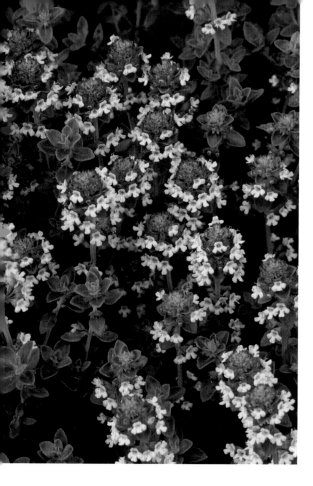

Thyme oil increases the flow of urine and this, combined with the antiseptic action, makes it useful in abdominal fomentations to treat cystitis and urethritis. Use three drops only dissolved in one tablespoon full-cream milk. The diuretic action helps to remove uric acid, making it useful in blends for easing arthritis, gout, rheumatism, and sciatica.

Thyme oil is the reviver, having a stimulant action on the immune system, and a strengthening and tonic action on the circulation. It encourages and regulates menstrual flow when used in a massage oil over the abdomen.

Thyme is useful in treating insomnia, headaches, nervous debility and stress—it seems to give courage and strengthen the nervous system. Sip a cup of tea four times daily for three weeks only.

Thyme repels cabbage moth, black fly, and some bacteria, and is a good companion to Brussels sprouts, broccoli, and cauliflower

Caution: Not to be used during pregnancy. Avoid using if you have high blood pressure.

Thyme is very powerful—use only 0.5–1 percent of the oil in blends. Never use it neat. Take no more than one teaspoon (about 1–4 g) of dried leaf daily. Not to be taken for more than three weeks at a time, as thyme can be toxic in large quantities.

tonsillitis, and sore throats. In chest rubs, or used in an oil burner, it will ease the symptoms of asthma. Use in massage blends or add three drops to an inhalation to treat bronchitis, catarrh, chills, coughs, colds, croup, sinusitis, whooping cough, and many other chest complaints.

Growing and harvesting

Grow thyme in a sunny spot from seed, root division, mounding, or layering. It requires moderate water. Once it is established, garden thyme will grow better and have more flavor in slightly dryer conditions. It is a great survivor—frost resistant and spreading in habit. Cut bushes back after flowering and renew every couple of years. Harvest leafy branches just before flowering and dry for making infusions, decoctions, tinctures, ointments, and extracts.

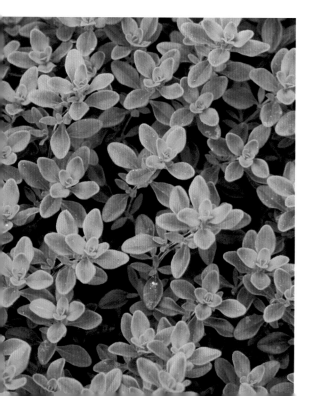

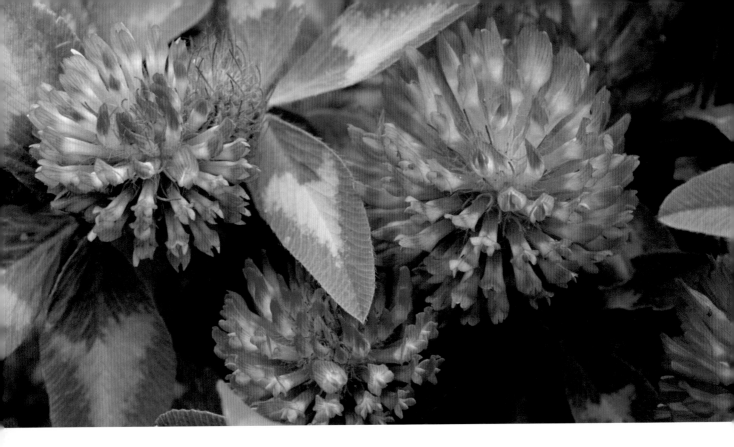

Trifolium pratense

Papilionaceae
Red clover
Also known as purple clover, trefoil

Red clover is a perennial with 12–24 in (30–60 cm) stalks rising from a short rootstock. The bright green, three-lobed leaves are sometimes finely toothed on the leaflets. The flowers grow in dense, globular heads and vary considerably in color from deep red to white.

This is a well-known fodder and soil-improvement plant—a nitrogen fixer used by farmers in many countries. Lots of space is needed to grow a reasonable quantity of red clover, so it is often sprouted in the same way as alfalfa. Red clover sprouts are a vitamin-rich tonic. Add them late in the cooking of cheese, egg, rice, and vegetable dishes, and in soups and stews. They are also good in leafy salads, sandwiches with curd (cottage) cheese, and as a garnish. They are an excellent food supplement for children, particularly if they are troubled with skin conditions.

Uses: HERB
Use the flowers in salads or the sprouted whole herb for its powerful alterant, anti-inflammatory, cleansing, diuretic, and expectorant qualities.

Red clover is particularly useful taken as sprouts or tea three times daily in the treatment of skin complaints, such as psoriasis and childhood eczema. Used the same way, it also encourages the loosening and expelling of phlegm in coughs, bronchitis, and is particularly effective for whooping cough.

This herb stimulates liver and gall bladder function, and can be taken as sprouts or a tea three times daily for constipation, rheumatism, and gout.

Growing and harvesting
Grow it from seed in a sunny place in well-drained soil. Harvest flower heads and leaves and dry for making infusions, extracts, ointments, and tinctures.

Trigonella foenum-graecum

Papiloniaceae
Fenugreek

Fenugreek is a small, somewhat delicate annual from the pea family (hence the sickle-shaped pods), growing to a height of 2 ft (60 cm) with slender, smooth stems. The aromatic, light green leaves have a grassy sweetness and can be used as a vegetable (add a few to a spinach frittata). It has pale yellow flowers. The dried seeds have a rather sharp, appetizing taste and are used, sparingly (too much spoils the flavor), in spice mixtures, curries, and North African casseroles. An extract from the seeds is also used by the food industry to make artificial maple syrup.

The small golden brown seeds are delicious sprouted, but need frequent rinsing, as they can become sticky as the mucilage is released. Use them in salads and sandwiches with a light oil and lemon dressing.

Uses: HERB

It is an excellent herb to use during convalescence as a tea from the crushed seeds; it stimulates the appetite and aids a digestive system that may be weak. The tea is also useful as a decongestant for treating lung infections such as bronchitis and pneumonia, or as a gargle for sore throats.

Fenugreek is one of the best teas for producing perspiration and as such is equally helpful in reducing fever. The tea made from the crushed seeds tastes a little like a broth.

Like fennel, fenugreek is a useful tea for those people who may have difficulty with fat absorption. It may also be effective for treating teenage acne. The tea may be applied topically where it can have a slow but beneficial effect.

The phytoestrogens in fenugreek are good for the treatment of many menstrual disturbances from premenstrual syndrome to menopause. Fenugreek is also used to promote the production of breast milk.

Growing and harvesting

Grow from seed in a sunny, well-drained position in the garden. Pick leaves as required to use fresh or dried in infusions or as a vegetable; harvest seeds and dry for decoctions, teas, and tinctures.

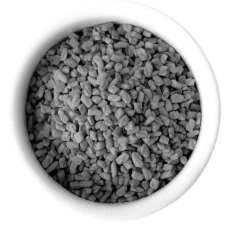

Tropaeolum majus

Tropaeolaceae
Nasturtium
Also known as garden nasturtium,
Indian cress

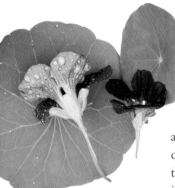

Nasturtium is an annual, self-seeding, creeping and climbing plant with large, round, pale green leaves and bright, showy, trumpet-shaped flowers ranging from pale yellow to dark red. It is a lovely and useful herb to grow in your garden, but can become a pest by growing so rampantly that it suffocates and chokes any plants in its path—remember it can cover a bank or fence within weeks of planting. Overcome this problem by pinching off the tips of all shoots when the plants are as large as you desire, or buy seeds of the new "non-running" cultivars.

Nasturtium belongs to the same family as watercress and has the same peppery "bite." Use the leaves in cheese and egg dishes. Try the flowers in soups and stewed fruits, or use them to make flavored vinegar. The leaves and flowers can also be added to curd (cottage) cheese, salads, sandwiches, and used as garnishes.

The ripe seeds can be roasted and ground as a seasoning. The unripe seeds can be pickled and used in place of capers. Simply soak the seeds in a brine made from one heaped tablespoon of salt dissolved in $1^1/_2$ cups (375 ml) water—the water should just cover the seeds, so pour off any excess. Change the brine every day for three days. Drain and rinse the seeds well and place in a clean jar. Add enough white wine vinegar or cider vinegar (whichever you prefer) just to cover the seeds. Leave for five to six weeks before using.

Uses: HERB

The nasturtium is a tonic herb with anti-infective and expectorant properties. Include the leaves, flowers, and seeds in your diet as often as possible.

It repels beetles and aphids, and is good to plant near apple trees, broccoli, Brussel sprouts, cabbage, cauliflowers, cucumber, grapes, kohlrabi, and zucchini (courgette).

Growing and harvesting

Grow it from seed in a sunny, frost-free place with moderate water. Pick leaves and flowers, and use fresh as vegetables for salads and soups.

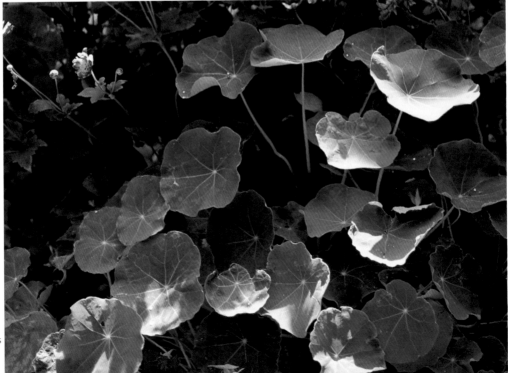

Uncaria tomentosa

Rubiaceae
Cat's claw
Also known as una de gato,
"champion cat"

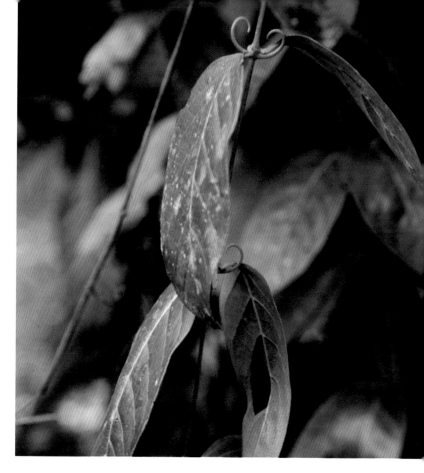

This large, woody, climbing vine (liana),
native to the tropical rainforests of Peru,
is currently causing quite a stir. Although
scientific research has just recently begun to
explore cat's claw's many healing properties,
it has apparently been used by the Ashaninka
Indians in Peru for hundreds of years as
a contraceptive and abortifacient, and for
treating intestinal disorders, rheumatism,
and inflammation. The name comes from
the small thorns at the base of the leaves
(rather like a cat's claw), that let the vine
climb over trees reaching heights of up
to 100 ft (30 m).

I think that it is possible, as with many
newly discovered herbs, that the benefits of
cat's claw are somewhat exaggerated. But
the fact remains that this herb seems to be
an impressive healer. Time alone will tell.

Uses: HERB

Cat's claw is becoming firmly entrenched as
an exceptional immune response stimulator
and appears to be proving useful in the
treatment of many different complaints,
including aids and cancer, as it seems to
alleviate many of the side-effects of the
medications and therapies used, including
radiation. Extracts are used for a variety
of conditions including gastrointestinal,
menstrual disorders, arthritis and
rheumatism, chronic inflammatory disorders,
and allergic conditions.

Make a tea using one teaspoon of
powdered bark in one cup of boiling
water, simmered (covered) for 10–15
minutes. Take three cups daily. Alternatively,
$^1/_4$–$^1/_2$ teaspoon (1–2 ml) of tincture can be
taken up to twice daily.

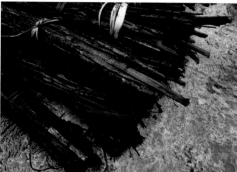

*Cat's claw roots and vines bundled
ready for drying.*

Caution: *Contraindicated in auto-immune
illness, multiple sclerosis, and tuberculosis. Avoid
combining this herb with hormonal drugs, insulin,
or vaccines. Not suitable for use while pregnant
or breastfeeding, or for children under the age of
three. Not for use by those who have received
organ transplants.*

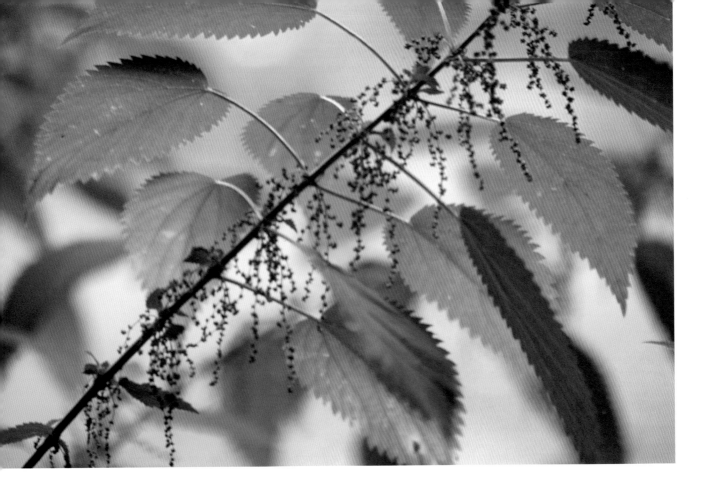

Urtica dioica

Urticaceae
Nettle
Also known as stinging nettle

There are two types of nettle. An annual (*Urtica urens*) with a delicate, pale green, opposite leaf and shallow root system, rarely growing taller than 8–12 in (20–30 cm) high. The other is a perennial (*U. dioica*) with a much coarser, darker leaf, and a creeping rootstock, commonly found growing along the wayside or in hedgerows. The leaves of both are hairy, deeply serrated, and pointed. The whole plant is covered in sharp, stinging points that cause irritation and local swelling. Stinging nettles, wrote Culpeper "need no description, they may be found by feeling, in the darkest night." (*The English Physitian Enlarged*, or the *Herball*, 1653). In the United Kingdom it's common to find dock growing near nettle patches. A crushed dock leaf rubbed onto

the stings brings instant relief just as the traditional rhyme describes: "Nettle in, dock out. Dock rub nettle out!"

To most people this is a despised weed, yet it is one of our most valuable herbs. If you can't find it growing wild it deserves a place of honor in your garden. Perhaps you have a spot behind the shed or in a corner where it can grow and multiply without stinging anyone?

Nettles are mineral-rich to eat and lose their sting when cooked. Only use the young leaves of young nettles in your cooking, for vegetable dishes, stews, and soups, as the older leaves become very bitter and coarse. Not to be eaten raw.

Nettles were once used to make a cloth very similar to linen. Scottish poet Thomas Campbell wrote: "In Scotland, I have eaten nettles, I have slept in nettle sheets, and I have dined off a nettle tablecloth. The young and tender nettle is an excellent potherb. The stalks of the old nettle are as good as flax for making cloth. I have heard my mother say that she thought nettle cloth more durable than any other species of linen."

Uses: HERB

The whole herb is used (suitably processed), as an alterant and tonic to support and nourish the body. Used externally, it acts as an astringent and can stop bleeding, cleanse, and heal wounds. Taken as a tea or tincture, it can help in the treatment of poor peripheral circulation and anemia. It also promotes milk production in nursing mothers and can be used internally to stay bleeding, such as uterine hemorrhage.

Nettle is useful to fight urinary tract infections. Drinking nettle leaf tea has become popular in Germany for treating bladder infections and other inflammations of the lower urinary tract.

The herb taken as a tea or tincture, may help minimize hay fever discomforts, supplying compounds that inhibit the release of histamine, the inflammatory substance triggered by seasonal allergens.

Nettle root appears to be particularly useful for men with benign prostatic hyperplasia (BPH), a condition in which the prostrate gland gradually enlarges, slowly narrowing the urethra that drains urine from the bladder and ultimately causing urination difficulties.

It is a specific for treating infantile eczema, especially in combination with chickweed. The two herbs may be mixed together, given as a tea, and used externally as a wash.

The whole plant makes a first-rate treatment for hair, and its uses extend even to the making of fine linen.

Use it in a general spray for the health of your garden.

Growing and harvesting

Nettle can be grown from seed. It likes little water and a sunny spot, but it will tend to invade the garden and should be contained. Always wear gloves and long sleeves when handling nettles. Collect from the wild if you can find unpolluted nettles, or harvest fresh from the garden and use for infusions, tinctures, ointments, and powders.

Nettles growing in the Wasatch Mountains in Utah, USA.

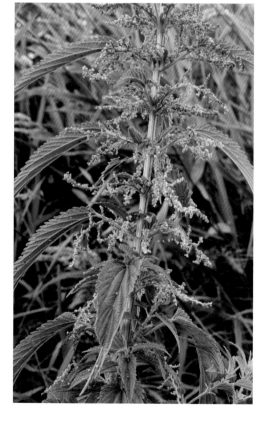

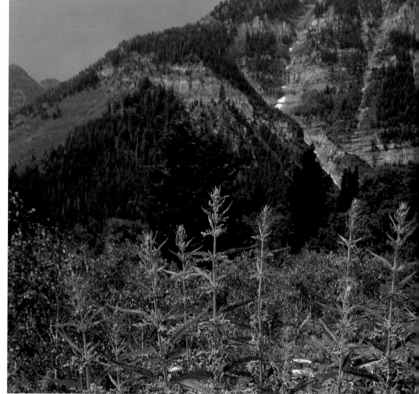

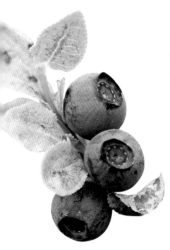

Vaccinium myrtillus

Ericaceae
Bilberry
Also known as huckleberry,
whortleberry

The bilberry comes from the same family that gives us cranberries and blueberries. It is a deciduous shrub with angular green stems that grow from a creeping rootstock to a height of 12–18 in (30–45 cm). Its shiny, dark green leaves turn yellow then red in the fall. Reddish pink or red and white flowers appear in late spring, followed by blue-black (may be red in some areas), five-seeded berries which resemble currants. They are usually gathered wild.

The leaves and berries of the bilberry have been used medicinally since at least the sixteenth century and probably long before that. We now know that they are rich in antioxidants thanks to the blue pigment they contain (called anthocyanins).

Like blueberries and cranberries, they are popular for eating fresh, or using in pancakes and smoothies, muffins, jams, as a snack, and in many other dishes and desserts.

Bilberry is used as a leather dye to produce brown and yellow colours, and when combined with other chemicals it produces shades of red, blue-purple, green, and blue for wool, cotton, and linen materials.

Uses: HERB

The berries are effective in the treatment of many eye disorders such as chronic glaucoma, tired, sore eyes, and inflamed eyes. Bilberry is a well-known folk remedy for poor vision, especially for people who suffer from "night blindness." In fact, bilberry jam (along with carrots), was give to Royal Air Force pilots who flew night-time missions during World War II.

Bilberry berries are used also for treating sinusitis, and kidney and bladder problems.

The leaf is effective as a remedy for diarrhea when brewed as a tea. The fruit can be used to ease indigestion and colitis.

The fresh berry juice makes an excellent gargle for sore throats, or as a mouthwash for inflamed gums.

There is evidence that bilberries help to prevent blood clots.

Externally, use a tea of the leaves as a wash for skin problems, sores, wounds, ulcers, and burns.

Caution: Be very careful to obtain a definite identification before using this herb. There are many very different herbs that have the same common name.

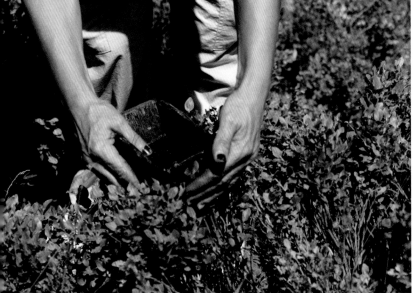

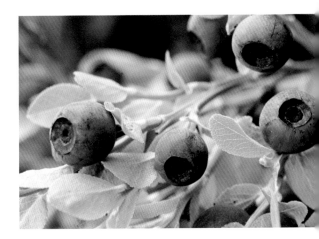

Valeriana officinalis

Valerinaceae
Valerian
Also known as setwall, all-heal, amantilla, fragrant valerian

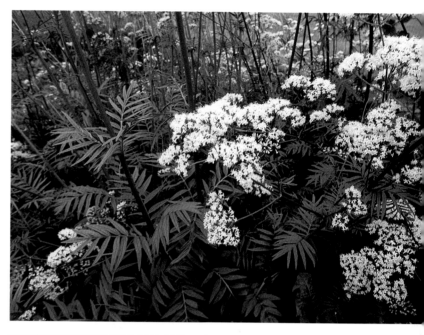

Valerian is a clump-forming, hardy perennial with one hollow, furrowed stem rising to a height of about 5 ft (1.5 m), usually in the second year of growth. The large leaves are pale green, opposite and serrated, and the stem divides to form flower stems with clusters of small pink flowers at the tip.

The flowers of this plant smell bad and the root, after drying, even worse. But it is this evil-smelling root that contains constituents that provide us with one of nature's finest nervines. Valerian is best used in compounds or capsules, as it's easier to disguise the taste in this way.

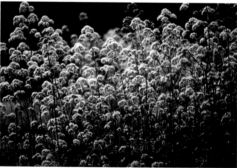

Caution: Valerian can cause headaches, depression, and palpitations if overused. Take in recommended doses only. A few individuals may experience nightmares after taking valerian.

Uses: HERB

Taken internally as a tea or tincture, valerian is pain- and anxiety-relieving, calming, and antispasmodic. Use for stress, insomnia, nervous tension, and migraine. It is also beneficial for premenstrual syndrome, stress, headaches, and tension. Valerian decreases muscle spasms, so use for stomach and menstrual cramps, irritable bowel syndrome, and nervous indigestion.

Valerian taken as a tea or tincture is an effective, safe and pleasant way to induce sleep. Unlike prescription medication, it doesn't interfere with the natural sleep process. It isn't habit forming and, in recommended doses, doesn't produce a heavy-head side-effect the next day.

It has been found to be a very useful herb in the treatment and calming of hyperactive children.

The leaf may also be included in ointments and massage oils, as it is analgesic, and also hastens the healing of wounds.

Growing and harvesting

Grow it from root division in a well-drained spot with moderate water. It is happy in sun or shade. It resists frost but is dormant in winter. Encourage rhizome growth by snipping the flowers and lift the root at the end of the second year of growth after the leaves have died off. Use fresh or dried for decoctions, teas or tinctures, ointments, or massage oils.

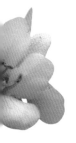

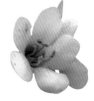

Verbascum thapsus

Scrophulariaceae
Mullein
Also known as Aaron's rod, great
mullein, lady's foxglove, blanket herb,
flannel plant

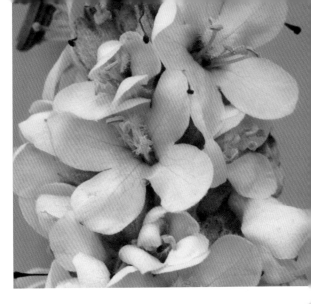

Mullein is a tall, handsome, biennial growing
up to 6 ft (2 m) in good conditions, with
huge, wooly, gray-green base leaves. The tall,
straight stem grows in the second year and
may be simple or branched. The flowers are
bright yellow and heavily clustered on the
top of the stem. In medieval days tall flower
stalks of mullein would be dried, dipped
in melted tallow, and lit, to carry through
the streets as torches, lighting the way for
processions and parades.

If you can find wild mullein in a clean,
unpolluted area, its medicinal properties are
reported to be more powerful than those of
the cultivated variety.

Uses: HERB

Today mullein is regarded as a valuable
respiratory remedy. Use the leaves and
flowers as infused oil to massage on the
chest if suffering bronchitis or other
bronchial problems, or as an antispasmodic
and analgesic to ease pain and spasms.

Drink a tea of leaves and/or flowers for
the herb's decongestant, demulcent, cleansing,
and expectorant properties when there is
painful, hard, and unproductive coughing.

Apply mullein fomentations or
compresses to treat arthritis, bronchitis,
bursitis, cysts, swollen glands, inflammation,
neuralgia, sore nipples, and sore throats.

The yellow flowers and olive oil make a
very valuable infused oil for the treatment
of simple earache. Prolonged or more severe
earache needs urgent professional treatment.

The infused oil can be used for painful
and inflamed conditions such as wounds
and hemorrhoids. An ointment, poultice, or

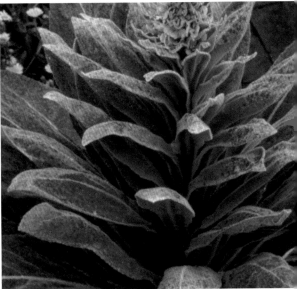

fomentation made from the leaves makes a
pain-soothing treatment for hemorrhoids,
ulcers, and tumors.

Caution: Teas made from mullein must be
carefully strained through coffee filter paper to trap
the fine hairs of the plant, which can cause severe
irritation or choking.

Growing and harvesting

Grow mullein from seed in a sunny, well-
drained position with moderate water. It
self-sows freely, so you may end up with
more mullein than you can handle. Harvest
leaves and flowers in summer, use fresh or
dried for teas, tinctures, making infused oil,
ointments, compresses, and fomentations.

Viburnum opulus

Caprifoliaceae
Crampbark
Also known as snowball tree,
guelder rose

Few people who have a beautiful snowball
tree in the garden realize what a valuable
herb it is. This large, spreading, deciduous
bush grows to around 15 ft (5 m) tall. The
tiny white flowers cluster together to form
large semi-circular "snow" balls in summer
followed by black berries.

Uses: HERB
Taken as a tea or tincture, this astringent
herb relaxes muscle spasm, aiding both
muscular and ovarian or uterine cramps,
which may make it helpful with threatened
miscarriage. It helps to control excessive
menstrual or menopausal bleeding, and has
been shown to relieve asthma, convulsions,
treat palpitations, and rheumatism.

Place two teaspoons of the finely
chopped dried bark in a small saucepan,
add one cup of water, cover and simmer
for 10 minutes. Strain, bring back to one
cup (250 ml) of liquid with hot water and
sweeten with honey. One cup should be
drunk three times a day. (The full amount
for one or two days can be made at once
and stored in the refrigerator). Alternatively,
one teaspoon (5 ml) of the tincture may be
taken in three times a day.

Caution: The uncooked berries are poisonous
*even when eaten in small quantities. Not
recommended for use by anyone who has ulcers.*

Growing and harvesting
Plant your tree in well-drained soil in sun
or partial shade. The bark is stripped and
dried for making decoctions, infusions,
and tinctures.

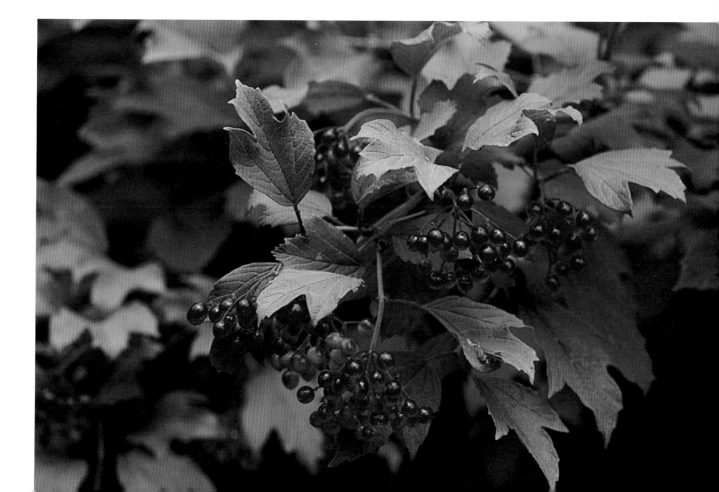

Viola odorata

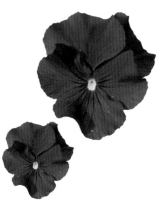

Violaceae
Violet
Also known as sweet violet, garden violet

This little perennial plant must surely be known to everyone, with its heart-shaped leaves, and sweet-scented flowers ranging in color from pink through to deep purple. In the kitchen, violets can be added to salads, or can be crystallized to make beautiful decorations on cakes and desserts.

Uses: HERB

A good vulnerary, anti-inflammatory, and antiseptic herb, the whole plant can be used in ointments to heal sores and ulcers, and to reduce inflammation.

Internally, when taken as a tea or tincture it will promote perspiration and act as an expectorant for catarrh and bronchial complaints, and as a diuretic.

Growing and harvesting

Propagation is by runners and unless the plant is regularly divided it will produce very few flowers. It likes a shady spot with moderate water and will resist frost. Collect plants and dry for making decoctions, or use the flowers fresh in salads.

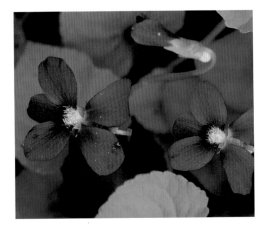

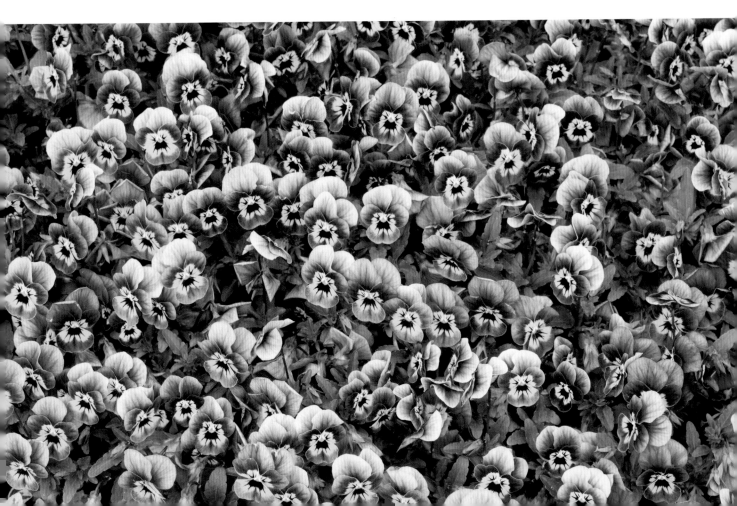

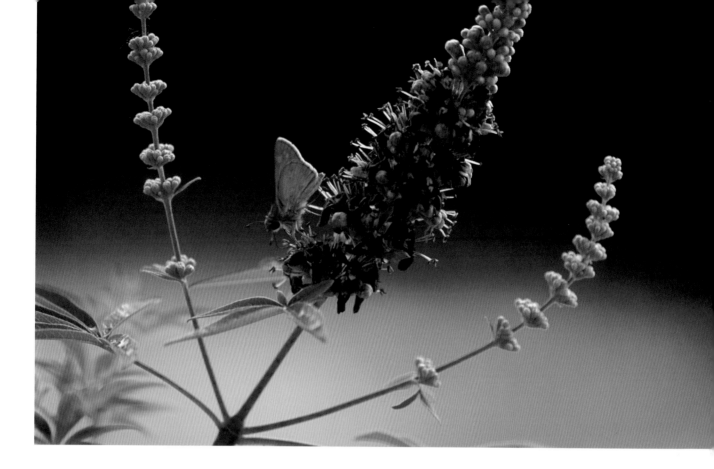

Vitex agnus-castus

Lamiaceae/Verbenaceae
Vitex
Also known as chaste tree, the woman's
herb, monk's pepper

This is a summer-flowering, deciduous
shrub growing in tropical and subtropical
areas to 25 ft (8 m) with aromatic leaves,
tubular, lilac-colored flowers, followed by
red-black fruits. The dried fruit, which has a
pepper-like aroma and flavor, is considered
to be one of the major herbs for women.

Many problems that are linked to the
menstrual cycle, such as migraine and acne
have been eased by the use of vitex. Women
who are having difficulty conceiving due to
hormonal imbalance may find the balancing
action of vitex helpful.

Uses: HERB
Used as a tea, it appears to regulate
hormones, balancing progesterone and
estrogen production, as well as inhibiting
male androgens. It increases breast milk
production in nursing mothers and can be
taken as a decoction or a tincture.

Use this herb to treat menstrual
irregularities ranging from premenstrual
syndrome as well as heavy, absent, or
irregular periods.

Other conditions where this herb may
be useful are in the treatment of fibrocystic
breast disease and menopausal symptoms.

This is not a fast-acting herb and may be
taken safely for periods of several months.

*Caution: Vitex is not recommended during
pregnancy, but if taken in the weeks after
giving birth it will encourage the production
of breast milk.*

Zingiber officinalis

Zingerberaceae
Ginger
Also known as African ginger,
race ginger

Ginger is a perennial plant with a thick, fibrous, knotted rhizome that is highly aromatic. The simple, red-tinged stem grows to about 5 ft (1.5 m) high. The long, narrow leaves grow from sheaths on the stem. Yellowish white flowers grow on spikes coming straight from the rhizome.

Ginger (fresh or dried and powdered) has been used in cooking and medicine since ancient times. In the kitchen, ginger can be used moderately with beef, chicken, seafood, and vegetables, especially in spicy dishes like curries and Indonesian dishes. It's a nice addition to cooked and fresh fruit. It's also good in baking, and small amounts can be tossed through salads, or used in drinks and liqueurs. The fresh root may be sliced and stored in either vinegar or dry sherry.

The essential oil is distilled from the root and produces perfume that is rich and spicy, blending well with lavender, lemon, oregano, and petitgrain.

Uses: HERB, ESSENTIAL OIL

Ginger tones the digestive system and stimulates the production of gastric juices. It increases appetite, aids digestion, and relieves cramps and spasms in the intestine and uterus. It will help ease diarrhea, colic, and flatulence. It calms a queasy stomach such as morning sickness, and is the best remedy for travel sickness when taken in powder or capsule form an hour before setting off, and sniffing the oil every half hour during the journey.

The pain-relieving and warming properties of ginger make it a good choice in blends to treat arthritis, rheumatism, muscular aches and pains, poor circulation, sprains, and strains. It should be used no more than 1–1.5 percent in fomentations, massage creams, and massage oils.

Catarrh, chills, colds, coughs, fever, influenza, sinusitis, and sore throats are

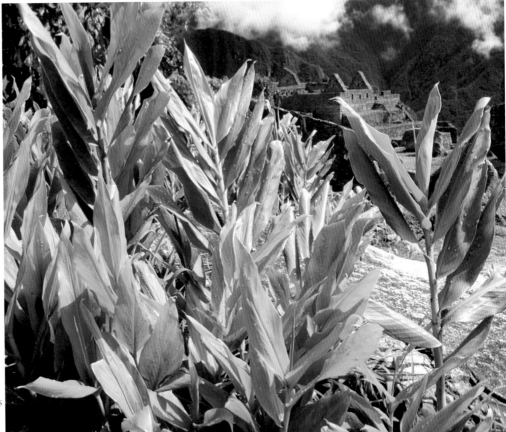

all helped by ginger. It reduces fever by increasing sweating.

The fresh, pressed juice is useful for applying to minor burns, boils, sprains, and infected hangnails where it heals, disinfects, and alleviates pain.

Taken as a tea and used in cooking, the stimulant properties improve circulation and help to prevent or alleviate cramps and chilblains.

Caution: Patch test—may cause irritation on sensitive skin.

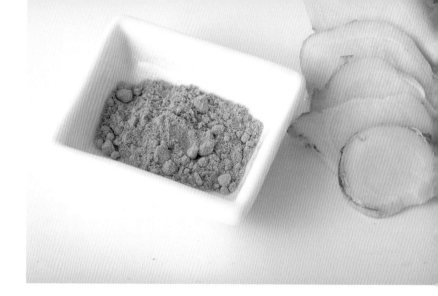

Growing and harvesting

This is a tropical plant and is propagated by root division. It may do well in the subtropics or temperate areas if in a very sheltered sunny spot, or if you have a heated greenhouse or conservatory. It likes full sun and moderate water. The root (the part used) needs to be twelve months old before using.

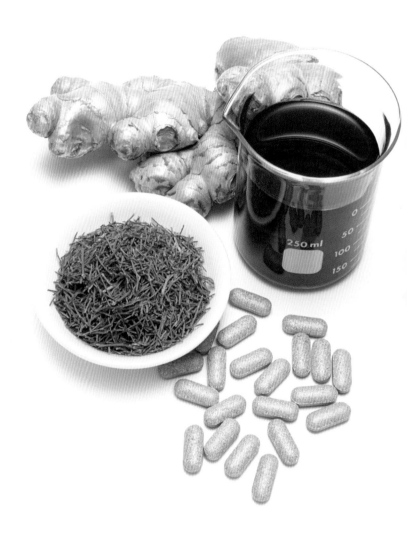

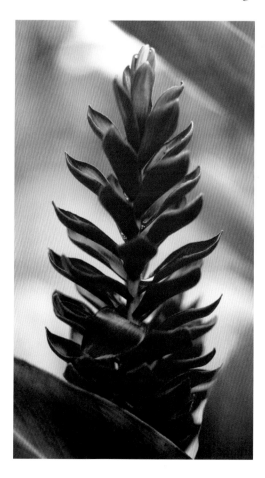

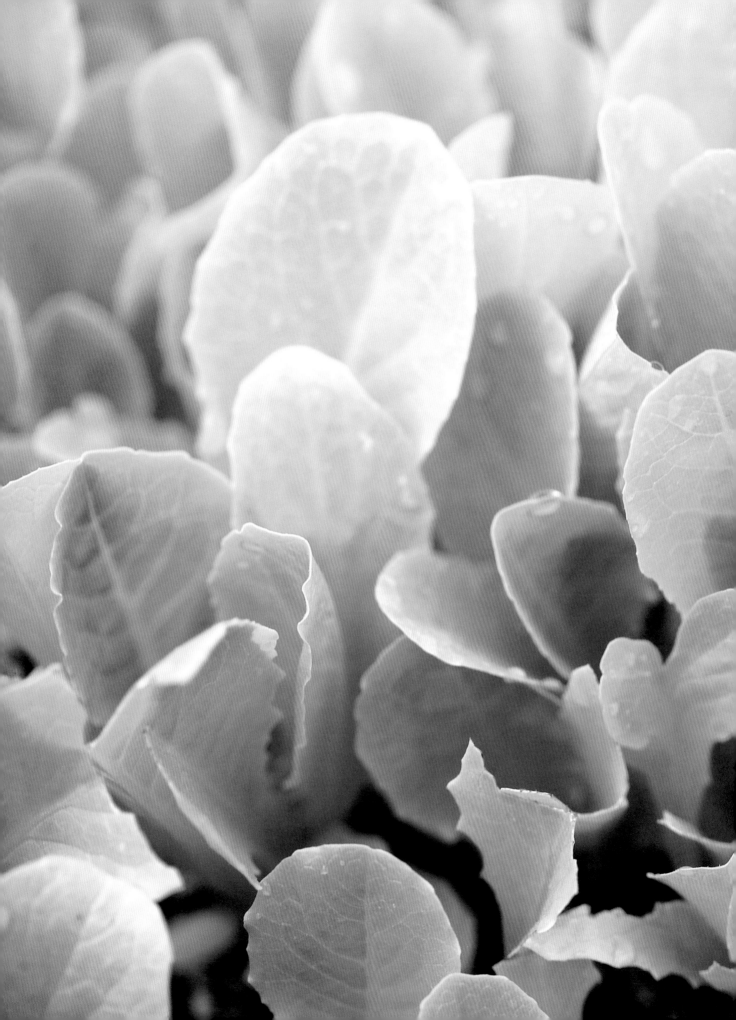

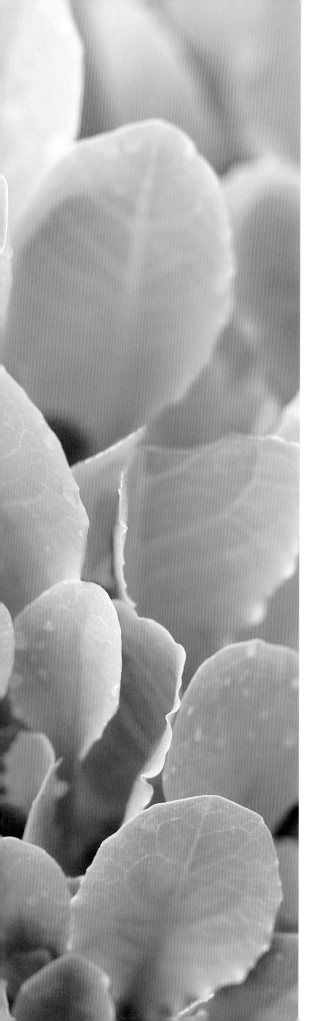
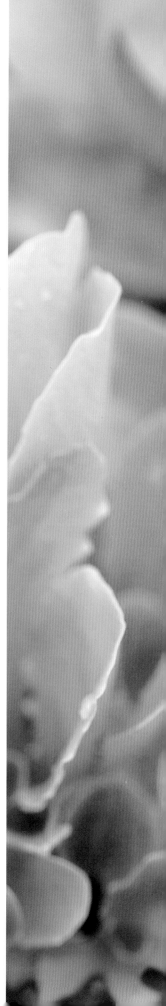

A–Z FIXED OILS

Oils are often the mainstay of the skin-care items we make. It's important to choose the right oil for the job and the right oil for the skin type. This A–Z Fixed Oils directory will help you determine which oils will suit your purpose and pocket best—be aware that many oils are very expensive and that there may be a cheaper one that will fit your criteria just as well.

COLD-PRESSED OR NON-COLD-PRESSED?

I like to use cold-pressed for all recipes that require little heating, such as emulsions and salves. I feel that the cold-pressed oils retain more of the vitamins and oxidize less quickly.

I use non-cold-pressed oil for soap making, as I'm sure that any benefits such as vitamin content are totally destroyed by saponification. The essential fatty acids remain the same during the process of soap making and these are what we look for in soap.

High oleic oils

These oils are produced from a special breeding program that makes the seed rich in oleic fatty acid. Since oleic is less subject to oxidation than the linoleic acid, these oils are more stable.

It is claimed that these oils retain the benefits of the original oil for food and cosmetic applications, but I haven't ever

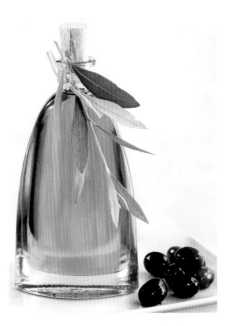

used them because I try to avoid anything that is genetically modified. The choice however is yours, as oils like sunflower and other very unstable oils become more stable and possibly more moisturizing once they become high oleic oils.

Storing oils

If you live in a climate that gets very hot in summer you will need to refrigerate your oils to keep them in peak condition for longer. We occasionally get temperatures over 105°F (40°C) where I live, so all my oils are refrigerated. This has another benefit in that light is an enemy of oils and it's dark in the fridge.

Keep your oil bottles as full as possible as air is another factor in deterioration. It's worth decanting oil into a smaller bottle when necessary—particularly if it's an expensive oil.

You can extend the life of all oils by adding one percent vitamin E d-alpha-tocopherol. As an alternative you can use rosemary oil extract, but it has the disadvantage of odor—it smells a little strange. It is also more expensive than vitamin E.

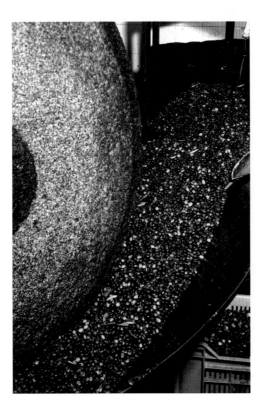

Olive harvest being crushed in a stone press in Tuscany, Italy.

Almond oil, sweet

Prunis dulcis

This is a fine, emollient, non-drying, fixed oil expressed from the kernel of the sweet almond. Odorless, it is used for conditioning and softening the skin and it is great for dry, itchy skin. It is used in massage oils, lotions, balms, soaps, and even the most simple of moisturizers.

* May be used as 100 percent of the base oil to use in creams and lotions formulated for dry, normal, and combination skins.
* For massage oils, use 50 percent of almond oil and 50 percent of a lighter oil such as grape seed, fractionated coconut, rice bran, sunflower, or apricot kernel oil.
* Stable for six months to one year.

Almond oil, bitter

Prunis amygdalus var. *amara*

The delicious scent of this oil, which is expressed from the kernel of the bitter almond, makes it a popular addition to perfumes and soaps. Although bitter almonds may yield from six to eight percent prussic acid (hydrogen cyanide) this oil is safe to use, as by law the prussic acid is removed in the extraction process.

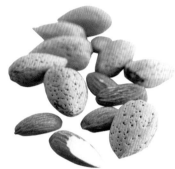

* Stable for six months to one year.

Clockwise from top: *Whole sweet almonds; ground sweet almonds; sweet almond oil.*

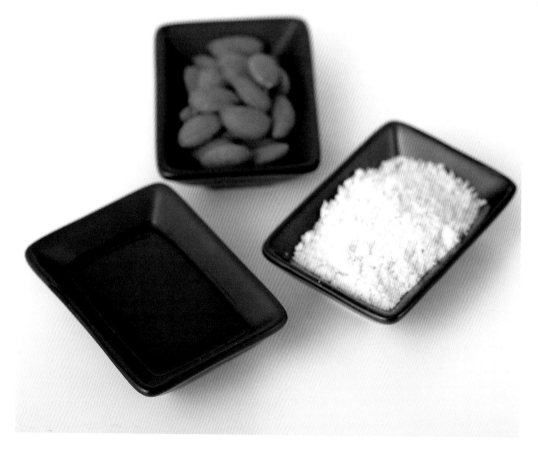

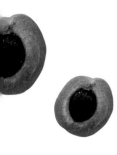

Apricot kernel oil

Prunus armeniaca

This is a pale golden oil obtained from the kernel of the apricot seed. It is a light, rich oil, especially good for mature, dry, or sensitive skin. Use in creams and lotions. This oil is lovely used alone for removing makeup and softening delicate skin around the eye. A skin-conditioning agent, it is emollient, non-greasy, and ideal for dry, tired, and mature skins. This oil is reputed to rejuvenate and repair skin cells due to the high vitamin A and B content.

* May be used as 100 percent of the base oil in recipes.
* Stable for six months to one year.

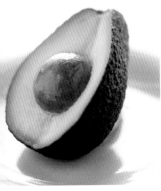

Avocado oil

Persea americana syn. *Persea gratissima*

This is a beautiful, thick, heavy, green, semi-drying oil extracted from the flesh of the avocado. Rich in nutrients including vitamin E, fatty acids, and the youth mineral potassium, this highly therapeutic oil is said to have healing and regenerating properties. Avocado is reputed to be beneficial in reducing age spots, healing scars, and moisturizing the upper layers of the skin. It is rich, nourishing, and invaluable in moisture creams and lotions, particularly for sensitive and sunburnt skins. Studies have shown that treatment with avocado oil significantly increases the water soluble collagen content in the dermis, which affects the age of the skin. The vitamin E content helps to preserve other oils in blends.

* Because of its thick consistency its best to use no more than 5–10 percent in massage and face oils.
* Stable for up to one year.

According to Mrs Carl F. Leyel in her book *Herbal Delights:* "Avocado Pear oil...used as a cosmetic, has greater powers of penetration than any other vegetable oil...it conveys vitamins and nourishment to the glands that lie beneath the skin."

Borage oil

Borago officinalis

Reputed to rejuvenate skin cells due to the high gamma linoleic acid (GLA) content, borage oil also has the highest known content of essential unsaturated fatty acids. These are great skin conditioners. They regulate the hydration of the skin and are humectants.

* Use no more than 10 percent in massage and face oils. Evening primrose also contains a high GLA and may be substituted.
* Stable for three to six months.

Canola oil

Brassica napus

This light, non-drying oil has properties similar to olive oil. It is excellent in soaps, massage oils, and in creams and lotions for dry and normal skins. Use it in massage oil blends. It's not an oil that I use (I prefer rice bran or grape seed oils) and you won't find canola oil in recipes in this book.

* May be used as 100 percent of the base oils in preparations.
* Stable for six months to one year.

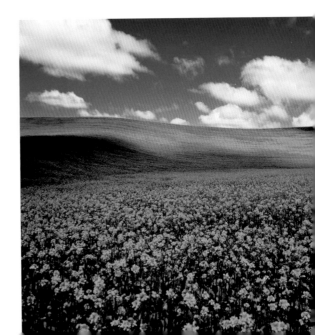

Castor oil

Ricinus communis

This rich, non-drying oil is pressed from the seeds of the castor oil plant. The seeds themselves are very poisonous. The oil is rich in fatty acids and lubricating to the skin. It is useful in combination with other oils in soap making. It is an invaluable oil for use in hair conditioners, in hot packs on sore muscles, or to draw splinters that are deeply embedded in the flesh. It creates a moisture barrier and is richly emollient if included in small quantities in night creams, lip salves, and soaps.

* Stable for up to one year or more.

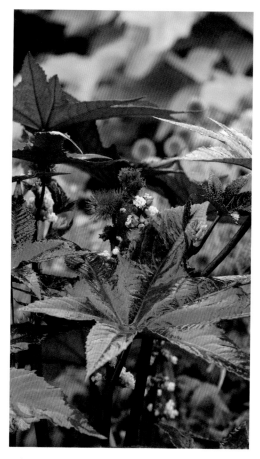

A handsome plant, Ricinus communis *is also grown as an ornamental in Europe.*

Sulfated castor oil

Also known as turkey red oil, it is made by adding sulphuric acid to castor oil—hence sulfated castor oil. The resulting oil is water-soluble and useful for making dispersible bath oils.

* Stable for up to one year or more.

MINERAL/PARAFFIN OIL

Not good for anyone and certainly not for babies! Cosmetic companies who make baby products, cleansers, moisture creams, and lotions use it extensively because it's cheap, hypoallergenic and is completely inert, which gives it indefinite shelf life. If used alone it remains on the surface of the skin but once incorporated in an emulsion it is absorbed into the skin in the same way as other oils. The only advantage that this oil has for the home user is that it doesn't go rancid. Many books on natural cosmetics state that mineral oil leaches the vitamins from the skin—this is not strictly accurate. All oils used both internally and externally will collect fat soluble vitamins (A, D, E, K) as they travel through the body, but natural oils are then absorbed through the intestines, hence the vitamins aren't lost. Mineral oil isn't absorbed into the intestinal wall and the oil is excreted, along with the vitamins.

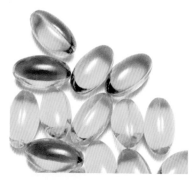

Coconut oil

Cocos nucifera

Coconut oil is a semi-solid, saturated fat extracted from the white meat of the coconut. It is a wonderful lubricant and moisturizer for delicate eye and throat areas. If used very discreetly it conditions and gives a glossy shine to hair. It's sometimes possible to buy saponified coconut oil to make shampoos and bath foams.

* If refrigerated it remains solid but liquefies easily when at room temperature.
* Stable for up to a year.

The many forms of the versatile coconut (clockwise from top): fresh meat; coconut sugar (whole and grated); virgin coconut oil; whole coconut oil; and coconut milk (in the glass).

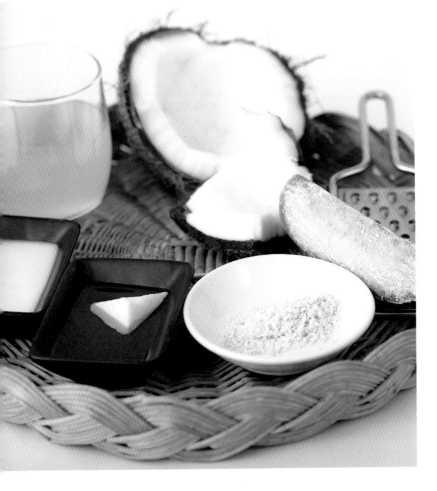

Fractionated coconut oil

Whole coconut oil is semi-solid at room temperature, fractionated is liquid. Fractionated coconut oil is a clear, light-textured oil, which is odorless and tasteless. It is completely soluble with essential oils. It can be used as base oil for aromatherapy and massage therapy as it penetrates the skin well. It is non-staining and washes off massage table sheets and towels easily, which makes it popular with massage therapists. It's ideal for perfume makers who don't want to use alcohol as a carrier because it's so light it will spray through a pump sprayer with ease. It leaves your skin feeling silky smooth without that greasy feeling. If blended with other oils it will help to extend the shelf life of the final product.

* It has an indefinite shelf life.

Virgin coconut oil

Virgin coconut oil is cold-pressed from the fresh meat of the coconut and then run through a centrifuge to remove all remaining insoluble proteins and milks until only a pure, high-quality coconut oil is left. This oil still retains the delicious scent of coconut, making it a perfect way to scent your lotions and lip balms.

* Stable for up to one year.

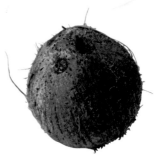

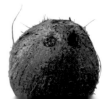

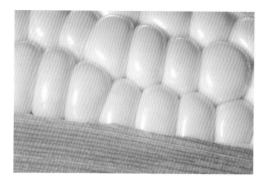

Corn oil

Zea mays

Corn oil is a good cosmetic and soap oil, but Jeanne Rose in *The Herbal Body Book* comments, "I cannot recommend its use since a large percentage of the pesticides and fungicides that are employed in this country [USA] are used on corn." I haven't been able to establish if the situation is the same in other countries, so it becomes a case of buyer beware. Corn oil goes rancid more quickly than most other oils, so store carefully.
* Stable for six months to one year.

Evening primrose oil

Oenothera biennis

Expressed from the seeds of evening primrose, a tall, weedy herb with yellow flowers, evening primrose oil contains 10 percent gamma-linolenic acid. It is a very nourishing, emollient, soothing, healing oil when added to creams and massage blends to help heal acne, dermatitis, eczema, psoriasis, and other inflammatory skin conditions. It also repairs damaged skin, keeps skin healthy, and helps repair sun-damaged and mature skin. It removes tangles and repairs damaged hair while providing a non-greasy shine. Evening primrose is full of vitamins and minerals—best for dry skins.
* Use 10 percent in massage oils or blends.
* Stable for three to six months only.

Flax seed oil

Linum usitatissimum

Flaxseed oil is pressed from the seeds of the flax plant. It has a high concentration of omega-3 essential fatty acids. It is useful for treating eczema, psoriasis, burns, and inflammatory skin conditions.
* It is super polyunsaturated so is very unstable and must be refrigerated.
* Unstable (less than three months).

Grape seed oil

Vitis vinifera

As the name suggests, this oil is pressed from grape seeds. It's one of the lightest of all oils, a fine, semi-drying, polyunsaturated oil, which makes it suitable for most skins except for the very oily. It is widely used in hypoallergenic natural products because it does not often cause allergic reactions in the highly allergic. It is very good basic carrier oil, as it is light, clear, and has no smell.
* Stable for three to six months only.

Vineyards near Stellenbosch, South Africa. Grape seed oil is a byproduct of wine grapes.

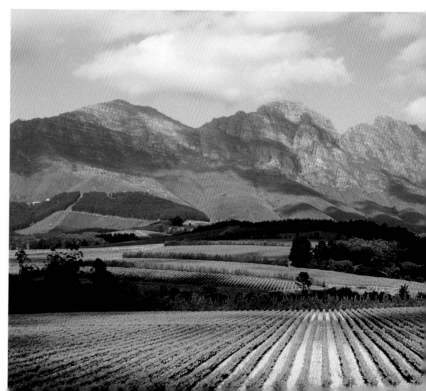

Hazelnut oil

Corylus avellana

This fine, yellow oil is pressed from the kernel of the hazelnut and is good for all skin types. Easily absorbed by the skin, this oil's phospholipid content gives a better and longer lasting moisturizing potential to cosmetic emulsions.

* If you are feeling reckless and want to make a superlative cream or oil, 100 percent hazelnut oil may be used but as this oil is becoming increasingly difficult to buy you may want to use it more sparingly.
* Unstable (less than three months).

Whole hazelnuts can be pressed to produce hazelnut oil.

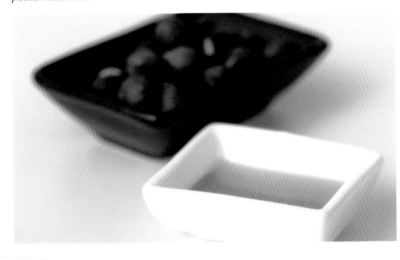

Hemp seed oil

Cannabis sativa

Hemp contains proteins and high-quality fat. It is wonderful oil for dry or mature skin since it is an emollient and said to help stimulate cell growth. Natural hemp seed oil is dark green and has a nutty, rich scent. It can help to make the skin feel softer and smoother, reducing roughness, cracking, and irritation, and it just may slow down the fine wrinkles of ageing.

* Stable for three to six months only.

A flower head of Cannabis sativa. These later produce seeds, a source of a high-quality oil; but such heads are also dried and smoked for their hallucinogenic drug content.

Jojoba oil

Simmondsia chinensis

Technically not an oil, this is a yellow wax pressed from the bean of a desert plant. It is similar to the skin's own sebum. It contains a substance, similar to collagen, which gives skin a silky smooth feel. Jojoba oil penetrates deeply to increase skin softness and reduce superficial lines and wrinkles for several hours after use. It seems that the reason jojoba works so well is that the skin accepts it as sebum and allows it to penetrate. Useful for acne, eczema, hair conditioner, inflamed skin, and psoriasis. Refined jojoba has been deodorized and bleached, but there is no need for this as the cold-pressed, natural, golden jojoba has no discernible scent and adds a lovely golden tint to toiletries.

Macadamia oil

Macadamia integrifolia

This oil has an unsurpassed reputation of being able to penetrate skin, replenishing oils lost during the day. Suitable for all skin types and excellent as part of a massage blend, it is a lovely light oil.

* Use as 100 percent of oils in a formula.
* Stable for six months to one year.

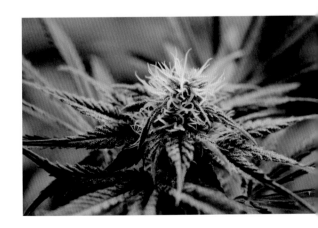

Meadowfoam seed oil

Limnanthes alba

Meadowfoam oil is pressed from the seed of *Limnanthes alba*. The oil is stable, resistant to oxidation, and is lovely to use in cosmetics and body-care products. It is non-greasy and rapidly absorbed, leaving the skin soft, smooth, and silky. It moisturizes the skin in ways few other oils do. In shampoos and soaps it helps add shine and moisture to hair and scalp. Research suggests that this oil may increase the shelf life of less stable oils.

* Stable for one year.

Neem oil

Azadirachta indica syn. *Melia azadirachta*

The oil is pressed from the kernels of the seeds of the neem tree and sometimes extracted by other methods. Neem is one of the important detoxicants in Ayurvedic medicine. It is used widely in India as an antibacterial, antiviral, antifungal, antiseptic, antiparasitic agent in toiletries, soap, toothpaste, and skin/hair care products. In toothpaste it helps relieve swollen and bleeding gums and kill the bacteria that cause gingivitis. And if that's not enough, neem oil can be sprayed on plants to keep insects from devouring the leaves. Neem powder can be used in a foot bath powder to kill fungus and bacteria. Mixed with clay, it makes a great facial for those with acne and other skin problems. Add to liquid soap base for an antibacterial hand soap. Use in insect-repellent lotion bars to keep the bugs away. Use in pet soaps to kill and repel fleas and to treat hot spots.

* Stable for up to one year.

Olive oil

Olea europaea

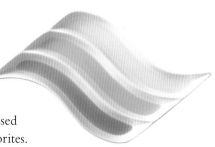

This is a rich, non-drying oil expressed from ripe olives. It is one of my favorites. I use extra virgin through to extra light depending on the end product. Olive oil is too rich for oily skins but is excellent for massage oils, creams, soaps, and lotions for dry and normal skins. It is a lovely oil to use on the skin of babies. There are three grades of olive oil that are suitable for toiletry making.

Virgin: Green in color, with a strong scent and taste, it is cold-pressed and the most expensive and usually reserved for cooking. When used in soap, it makes a very hard bar. And it may give a green tinge to your soap.

Light: This has a golden coloring with little odor. Soap made with light olive tends to be a hard, long-lasting bar, with no discernible olive scent or color.

Pomace: Oil is removed from the ground flesh and seeds of olives through solvent extraction. It is then deodorized, bleached, and colored. I personally don't like pomace and would recommend that its use be confined to soap, at only 20 percent or less of the total oils.

* Stable for up to one year.

Palm oil and palm kernel oil

Elaeis guineensis

These are hard, white oils generally used in soap making. They help boost the lather of the bar much like coconut oil and also add hardness to the bar, making it long lasting. They have similar properties to coconut oil.

* Usually limited to 20 percent of the total oils as it may be drying to the skin.
* Stable for a year or more.

From top: *Light extra virgin olive oil, cold pressed exra virgin olive oil, heat pressed olive oil.*

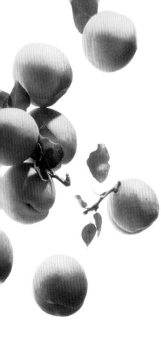

Peach kernel oil

Prunus persica

This is a light, rich oil especially good for mature, dry, or sensitive skin. Use it in creams and lotions. It is lovely used alone for removing makeup and softening delicate skin around the eye. A skin-conditioning oil, which is emollient, non-greasy and ideal for dry, tired, and mature skins, it also contains minerals and vitamins. It is reputed to rejuvenate and repair skin cells due to the high vitamin content.

* May be used as 100 percent of the base oils.
* Stable for six months to one year.

Peanut oil

Arachis hypogaea

A pale yellow, non-drying, and conditioning oil with a faint, pleasant, nutty odor and bland, nutty taste, it is good for dry and normal skins and may be used in the same way as olive oil. Having said this I must add that I have completely discontinued using peanut oil as even a drop can be fatal to those who suffer from an allergy to peanuts. It is also susceptible to fungus.

* Stable for six months to one year.

Rice bran oil

Oryza sativa

Rice bran oil is produced from the bran of the rice kernel. It is rich in vitamin E complex, squalene and a unique antioxidant known as gamma-oryzano. This antioxidant property gives the oil a very good shelf life compared to other vegetable oils. Gamma-oryzanol is also considered effective in absorbing ultraviolet light making it useful in sunscreen formulations. It is very emollient oil and penetrates the skin quickly. Use especially for dry, sensitive, mature skins in lotions and creams, and to add body and shine to hair.

* Use at 0.5–7.0 percent in lotions and creams.
* Stable for up to one year.

Rosehip oil

Rosa canina

Pressed from the seed and flesh of the wild or dog rose, rosehip oil is reputed to renew skin cells and lessen scarring. Richly moisturizing, it may possibly retard fine wrinkles. Rosehip oil is often used in products made for stretch marks, burns, scars, and mature dry skin. This oil is a rich source of omega-3 and omega-6 fatty acids and is high in gamma linoleic acid (GLA) and vitamin C. It is to be avoided if you have oily skin.

* Add no more than one percent of total oils but may be applied neat to scars.
* Unstable (less than three months).

Sesame oil

Sesamum indicum

A semi-drying oil expressed from ripe, unroasted sesame seeds, sesame oil contains natural antioxidants, vitamins, minerals, proteins, lecithin, and amino acids. It is useful in all moisturizing creams and lotions. Sesame oil absorbs ultraviolet rays from the sun so it may be used in sun-tanning preparations but shouldn't be relied upon for protection from UV rays.
* Stable for six months to one year.

Soybean oil

Glycine max

This is an unsaturated, drying oil expressed from the soybean. Most of the lecithin used in cosmetics is derived from soybeans. Soybean oil may be used in small amounts in cleansing creams, moisturizers, and massage and bath oils.
* Stable for three to six months.

Sunflower oil

Helianthus annuus

This is a semi-drying oil that may be used even by those with oily skin. It is rich in both vitamins A and E. Sunflower oil is very high in essential fatty acids and helps to moisturize, regenerate, and condition the skin. Can be used as the main oil or in a blend. Good for mature, sensitive, dry, and damaged skin. Excellent on throats and around the eyes where there are few oil glands and the skin is very thin.
* Stable for three to six months.

Vegetable oil

This is a broad term to cover a mixture of oils. The oils are usually chosen for their cost or availability at any given time. It's not possible to ascertain the percentages of each oil in the blend.

Natural vitamin E [d-alpha tocopherol]

This is one of the most impressive natural fat-soluble antioxidants in use, particularly when combined with vitamin C and vitamin A. It is excellent for helping to fade scars.
* May be used at one percent to help to prevent oxidation of oils.
* Frequent allergen.
* Stable for up to one year.

Wheatgerm oil

Triticum vulgare

This is a richly nourishing, fine, healing oil pressed from the golden inner germ of wheat. The vitamin E content makes it useful for most skins, especially dry, prematurely aged skin, or for skin troubles such as eczema or psoriasis. It is good in anti-stretch mark blends. It helps to make the skin feel softer and smoother, reducing roughness, cracking, and irritation and may possibly retard fine wrinkles. It also helps to preserve other oils. This oil is very emollient but needs to be blended with other oils as it has an extremely sticky texture.
* Ten percent is a valuable addition to creams and lotions, massage oils, and soaps.
* Stable for up to one year.

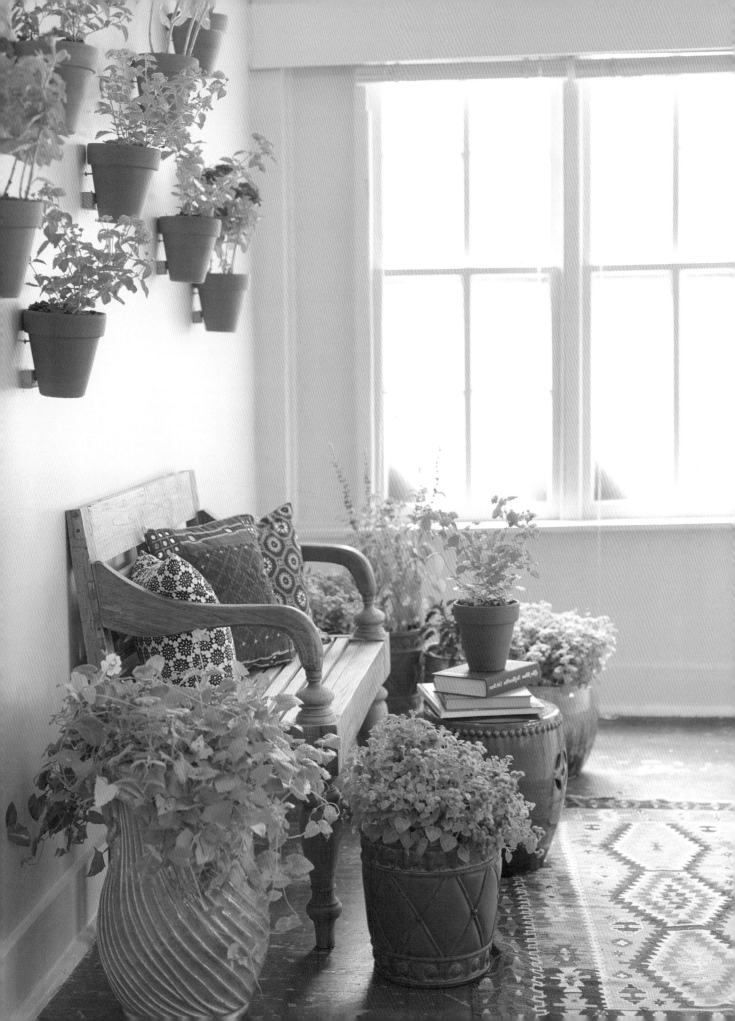

Growing herbs

I feel that the herbs that are most beneficial for us are those that we have grown in our own garden or that we have collected from the wild. There is a powerful "energy exchange" that happens when you plant a seed and watch it grow to maturity, then gather it, and make healing and beautifying preparations, or delicious food. You know every stage of the life of this plant and will have an understanding of the many ways in which it will be of benefit to you.

If you have never grown herbs before, you are about to experience a very joyful time as you watch the plants grow, gather them, and create your own herbal products for your home, family, and friends. You will also see the benefits to your garden as the herbs give their minerals to the soil and their essential oils to the air.

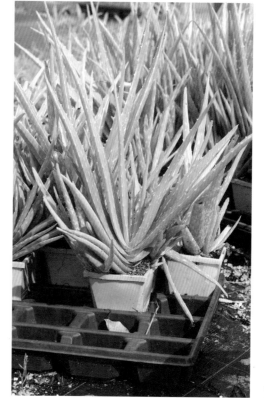

Aloe vera will grow quite large in a small pot. These plants are commercially grown, awaiting shipment.

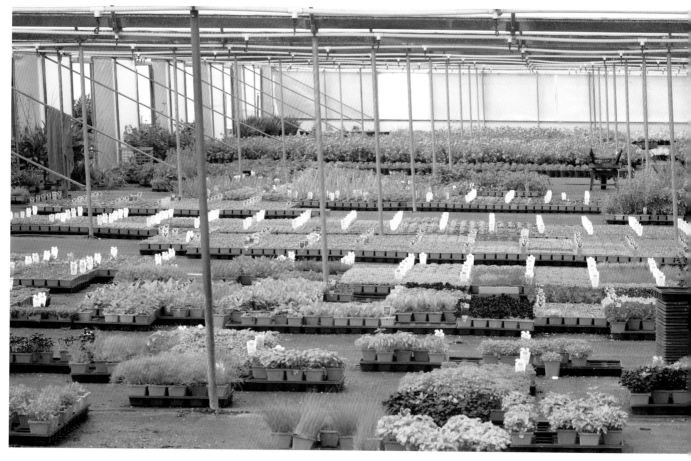

Herbs are raised from seed by commercial growers and nurtured in a controlled environment.

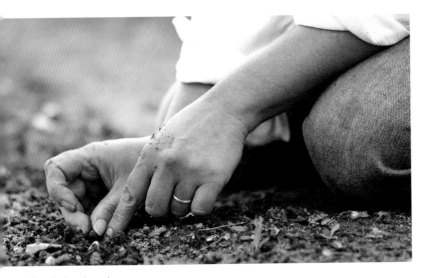

Some herb seeds can be sown directly into the ground where they are to grow.

Opposite: Lavender is cultivated commercially in many parts of the world and harvested by machine.

Creating your herb garden

Many people think that a garden is made up of a herb patch, some flower beds, and the vegetable plot. In the gardens I have had over the years, a border may be woolly yarrow, parsley, or some other low-growing herb, and silver beet grows cheek by jowl with roses and borage—a great color combination. Tomatoes, capsicums, and other vegetables share very happily with the herbs and flowers. The only precaution you need to take is to make sure the vegetables get the extra space and food they always need.

It has been said that wild herbs are more potent than herbs grown in a garden, and this may well be true, but these days there is also a risk that they are more contaminated. In this section you will find many ways to ensure that your garden plants are full of vigor and goodness. You will discover how to grow your herbs, how to harvest, dry and store them, and how to use them as companion plants and insect repellents.

If you wish to begin with only a few plants, choose those which appear most often throughout the book. In this way, you will begin with a selection that has wide applications.

If you have very little space, select small herbs that will suit you. For instance, if you have a pocket-sized garden you will not be able to grow angelica, bay, or elder. Perhaps you can find a few friends who also want to grow herbs and divide the cost and growing space between you. You will benefit in lots of ways—expense, space, and the sharing of an interest.

The A–Z section on herbs provides information on the general growing conditions needed by individual herbs. Plants will, as a general rule, adapt to different soils and different amounts of sunlight; they will often tolerate some shade, even if they are specific as "full sun" plants.

The amount of water needed is the one condition that herbs seem least willing to change. Too much water on sage or lavender for example, will cause them to die very quickly. If you deprive angelica or the mints of water, their growth will be very stunted and they may even die. Try to arrange your garden so that plants that like plenty of water live together, and the ones that enjoy drier conditions are in their own area.

From now on, be very careful of well-wishers who offer to do some weeding for you. It's more likely you will find your precious dandelions, shepherd's purse, and plantain in a dying pile and your friend very happy at having done such a good job. You will develop a whole new attitude towards "weeds" when you realize that they are all valuable, though not necessarily in the position they have chosen to grow. Give them their own place and watch them flourish.

If you really have to remove some of them, carry a bucket to put them in. Cover the plant material with water, fasten down with a lid and forget about it for three to four weeks. When you take the lid off the bucket it will really stink, but the liquid is fantastic liquid fertilizer. Dilute it until it looks like weak tea and pour it over plants or over the compost heap. In this way you will have shown respect for the "weeds" which, after all, are just plants that are growing in a place where we arrogant humans don't want them.

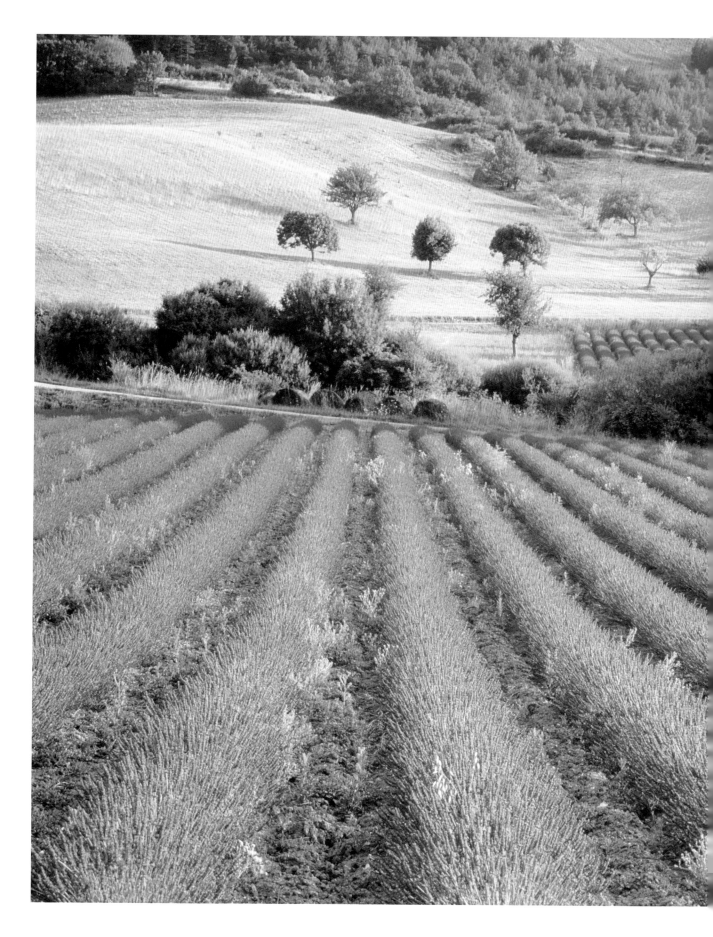

GLOSSARY OF GARDENING TERMS

This is a very short list of terms, sufficient for the scope of this book. If you want to know more, consult one of the many good books on organic gardening that are now available.

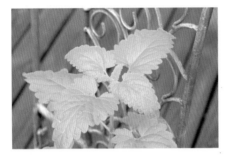

ACID

Soil, water, and so on, with a pH level below 7.0, indicating the absence of lime.

A simple soil test can be done at home using litmus paper (available from many pharmacies). Put a teaspoon of soil in a non-metal dish, cover with water and, when the sediment has settled, dip the litmus paper into the water. If the paper turns red then the soil is acid, if blue it is alkaline. If you'd like a more accurate test you can buy a special testing kit, available from gardening stores.

For a home-grown acid test, collect two jarfuls of violet blossoms, fill them with boiling water to the top, then seal and steep overnight. Divide the contents of one of the jars into two containers. Add lemon juice to one. It will turn purple/red; this is your acid indicator. Add baking soda to the other jar. It will turn green/yellow; this is your base indicator. Pour the contents of the "neutral" jar into as many jars as you have soil samples to test. Match the colors in these to the two indicators.

The application of good compost balances most soils. However, if you have azaleas or other acid-loving plants in your garden, you must remember to mulch them with pine needles, sawdust or other acidic materials.

ALKALINE

Soil, water and so on with a pH above 7.0. See Acid.

ANNUAL

A plant which completes a whole life cycle in one year.

BIENNIAL

A plant which fruits in its second year then dies.

DAMPING OFF

A condition in which a seedling rots at the base where it touches the soil. "Damping off" is usually a fungal problem.

DRILL

A channel made in the soil to sow seed, usually twice as deep as the circumference of the seed.

HUMUS

Decomposed organic matter.

MULCH

Material that is laid around plant to protect the roots, conserve moisture, or deter the growth of unwanted plants. Examples of mulch materials are straw, seaweed, rotted sawdust, grass clippings, newspaper, and rocks.

PERENNIAL

A plant that lives for more than two years.

SLAKED LIME

Otherwise known as hydrate of lime or quicklime. This is lime which has been treated with water, making it less caustic and more readily available to the soil. It is used to treat clay soils.

VERMICULITE

A water-absorbing substance made from mica. It is very useful for mixing with soil in pots, and as a medium for growing seeds and cuttings, as it helps to hold water and air in the soil.

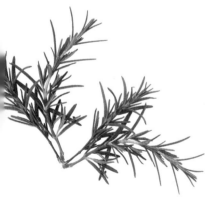

Garden equipment

Buy the best tools you can afford. They will work more efficiently and last longer. A basic selection of garden equipment should include:

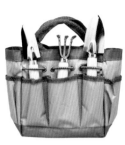

Fork
Spade
Shovel
Plastic grass rake
Secateurs
Trowel
Hand fork
Wheelbarrow
Selection of stakes
Watering can
Plastic garbage bins (for compost, liquid sprays, and fertilizers)

Craft/pop sticks for marking rows of seeds
Spray bottles
Soft twine for tying up plants
Garden sieve
Garden hoses
Gardening gloves
Plastic pots
Small jars for storing seeds
Large jar for storing dried herbs
Cheesecloth bags for drying seed heads
Old fly screen from a window for drying herbs
Sharp garden knife and scissors
Black plastic
Fine-tip waterproof markers
Selection of trays for seed sowing

A "tool belt" is useful to keep tools handy.

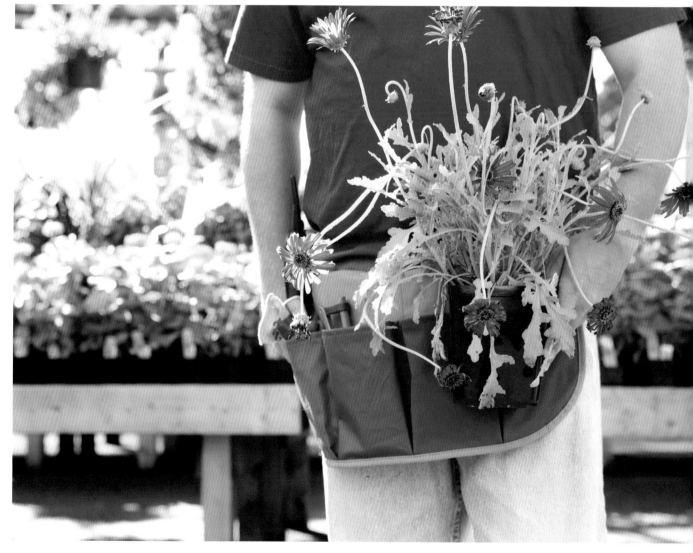

Some suggestions for garden planning

Herbs loved by bees and butterflies

Plant these throughout your vegetable garden, under fruit trees, or anywhere that you want good pollination to take place.

Anise	Bergamot
Catnep	Lavender
Basil	Borage
Dandelion	Lemon balm
Mallow	Mints
Sage	Valerian
Marjoram	Rosemary
Thyme	Yarrow

Gray or silver herbs

Catnep	Sage
Lavenders	Southernwood
Rue	Wormwoods

White flowers

Anise	Catnep
Feverfew	Winter savory
Basil	Chamomile
Lemon balm	Caraway
Elder	Marjoram
Yarrow	

Blue, mauve, or purple flowers

Borage	Hyssop
Rosemary	Catnep
Lavender	Thymes
Chives	Pennyroyal
Violet	

Red/pink flowers

Bergamot	Cilantro (coriander)
Valerian	Clover
Mallow	Yarrow
Comfrey	Summer savory

Aromatic herbs

Angelica	Catnep
Lavender	Mints
Tansy	Basil
Chamomile	Lemon balm
Rosemary	Thymes
Bergamot	Cilantro (coriander)
Marjoram	Southernwood
Wormwood	

Yellow/orange flowers

Aloe	Dill
Calendula	Nasturtium
Tansy	Dandelion
Rue	

Flowers for salads

Bergamot	Dandelion
Nasturtium	Borage
Elder	Rosemary
Calendula	Fennel
Violet	

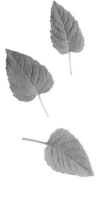
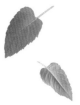

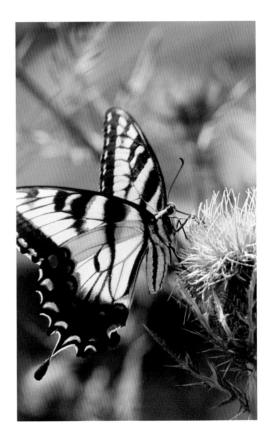

Flowers produce sweet nectar to attract pollinators like butterflies.

GROWING HERBS INDOORS

It's possible to grow some herbs indoors in pots. The soil used is most important, as it needs to retain plenty of moisture but also to drain well. I use half-and-half compost and sandy loam. A bought potting mix could replace the sandy loam. Choose your potting mix carefully, as some brands are much better than others. If you have a good nursery nearby, take the advice of the staff and then only buy a small bag, to try it out. If I have to rely on a commercial potting mix I add a few handfuls of natural compost or slow-release fertilizer to the bag.

Herbs grown indoors never seem to get as big or strong as those grown in the garden. Let's face it, there's no such thing as an indoor plant. There are only plants which will tolerate being indoors or which need to be wintered indoors because they are not in their native habitat. With all this in mind, it is worth giving it a try. The prime requirements are good light (but not burning heat through glass), fresh air without a draft, and not much artificial heat. Try to give the herbs a day every now and again in a sheltered place out of doors.

The best place for herbs indoors is a warm, well-lit spot near a window.

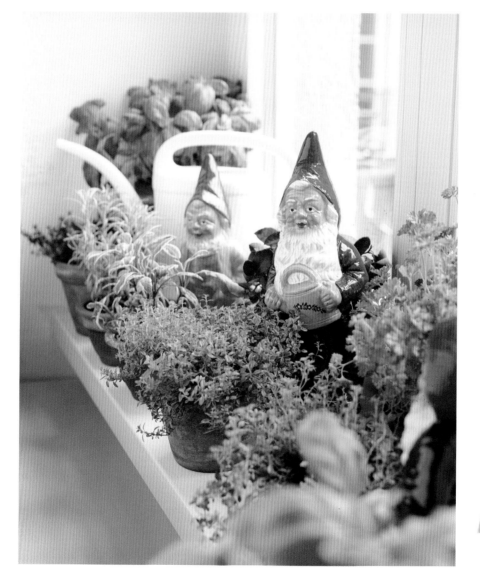

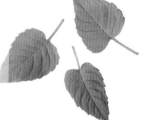

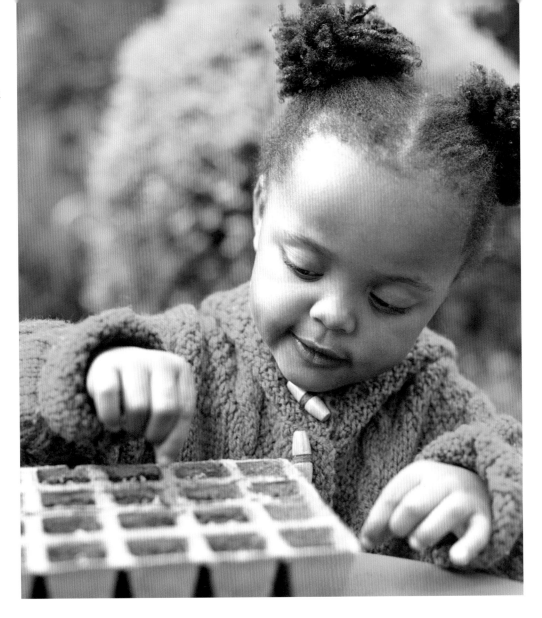

Children are fascinated by the process of growing plants from seed.

Propagating your own herbs

It's infinitely gratifying, quite easy, and much less expensive to propagate your own herbs. There are a few simple rules to observe, but you have the pleasure of knowing that you have raised new plants and known their entire history.

Propagating herbs from seeds

Seeds can be planted in containers and then transplanted, or sown directly in the garden where you want them to grow. The decision depends on several factors, such as the size of the seed, the difficulty of transplanting, and the weather conditions.

Assuming you are going to use trays, which is the safest way to be sure of raising a crop, you will need a bag of good quality seed-raising mix, or some sieved compost, and some seed trays. Cardboard egg cartons make good seed trays, as you can cut the carton when the plant is $^1/_2$–1 in (1–2 cm) tall and plant each portion, complete with its little seedling, without disturbing the roots. The carton will rot, adding humus to the soil. Other favorites of mine are large, square plastic ice-cream containers. I cut these down to a suitable height and punch holes in the bottom with a skewer.

Fill your container with seed-raising mix and firm the surface to within $^1/_2$ in (1 cm) of the top, then water it down with Chamomile Spray (see recipe page 224) and make drills (channels) in which to sow the seed. (If you are using cardboard egg cartons, the drills aren't necessary.) Sprinkle the seed as thinly as possible and cover with very finely sieved soil to about twice the thickness of the seed. If possible, place the whole tray in water when needed rather than watering from above, as there is less chance of disturbing the seed. Occasionally, give a spray of chamomile tea to prevent "damping off."

The seed will need a good light to germinate, but mustn't be left in full sun. A shadehouse or similar is ideal. The surface of the soil should never be allowed to dry out completely, but neither should it be sodden, otherwise the seeds or seedlings will rot. If you like you can cover the seed tray with a sheet of plastic or glass, removing it for an hour early morning and evening. This helps to prevent drying out and keeps the seeds warmer. The plastic or glass should be removed as soon as the plants show through the surface of the soil.

The seedlings should be thinned out as soon as possible. Do this by nipping off surplus plants at surface level (choose the weaker ones, where possible) until there are no plants touching each other.

Transplant seedlings when they are about 1 in (2.5 cm) high, being very careful not to damage the delicate roots as you take them from the soil. I use a tool like a delicate, two-pronged fork, but a wooden craft stick or ice-cream stick is fine. Water the hole before planting the seedling, and then again after planting. Gently firm the soil around the plant and finish with a dose of one of the garden sprays, such as Chamomile or General Spray (page 224), to ensure a good start.

Propagating herbs from cuttings

The advantage of growing a plant from a cutting is that you will get a clone. The best time of day to take cuttings is in the early morning, before the sun has made the plant soft and limp. Winter is the best time of year to start cuttings of deciduous plants, and late spring for non-deciduous plants.

Sandy soil, river sand, or vermiculite may be used to strike the cuttings. If you have problems striking your cuttings, you can buy a hormone powder (rooting powder) that can assist and hasten the growth of roots. Simply dip the fresh cutting into the powder, shake off the excess and plant as usual.

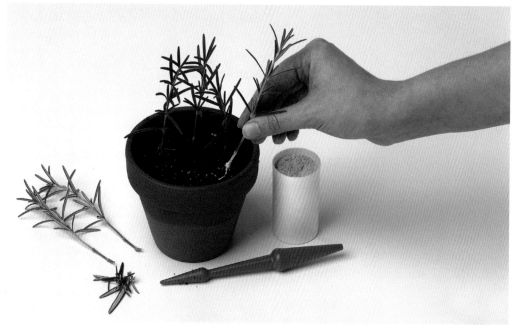

Dip cuttings in rooting hormone before planting to encourage a successful "strike."

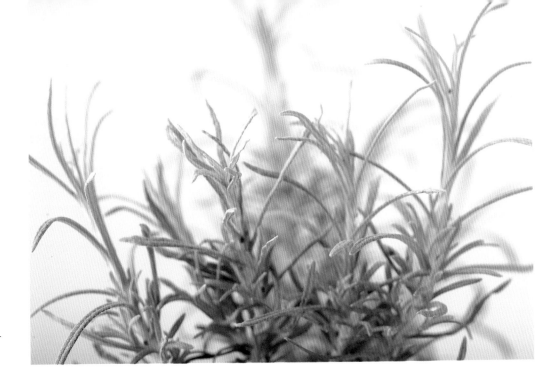

Helichrysum italicum, *the curry plant, has beautiful silver-gray foliage.*

The best cuttings are "heels." These are small branches, pulled off gently downward or cut with a sharp knife from the main stem of the parent plant. The next best are sprigs of about 4 in (10 cm) long, where there is a node (growing point). Trim the top leaves at half their length and strip the remaining leaves off the stem. Using a stick, make holes in the potting mixture, put the cuttings in the holes and firm well, leaving about 2 in (5 cm) showing.

You can put a lot of cuttings in each pot—in fact, they seem to prefer this to being alone. When the pot is full, water it, place in a plastic bag in which you have punched two or three air holes and seal the top of the bag (or place a plastic bag over the top of the pot and fasten with an elastic band). This stops the cuttings from drying out. Leave the pot in a semi-shaded position for three to four weeks, when the new plants should be ready to plant out. Open or remove the plastic bag every three to four days to give the plants some fresh air and the prevent molds from developing. Plant in the same way as seedlings, keeping the roots cool and moist.

I live on sandy soil and often put cuttings straight in the ground, where they are to grow. I cover them with a plastic bag with some holes in it, weigh the edges down with stones or rocks and leave the bag on until I see some new top growth. I then take the bag off for about an hour, three times a week, to give a good airing to the plant.

Propagating herbs by root division

The best time for this method of propagation is spring, when the new growth is just beginning to appear. It is not only desirable but necessary to divide perennials as it gives them a new lease of life and prevents clumps from becoming too big and straggly.

This is a really easy way to grow new plants, each one having its own piece of root. Trim the tops and roots back equally to avoid stressing the new plant. Replant as quickly as possible and water in very well. If for some reason you can't plant immediately, be sure to cover the roots with a wet sack or cloth or prevent them from drying out.

Some plants, particularly comfrey and horseradish, can be propagated by chopping their roots into several parts (ensuring that each part has an "eye"). These separate pieces of root will each grow into a plant.

Propagating herbs by mounding

Some plants may be very easily propagated by mounding. The best time to do this is in fall. The plant is mounded over with soil and then shaken lightly to enable the soil to get right down among the branches. About 5–6 in (12.5–15 cm) of the top of the plant must be left exposed. Leave the plant over winter, topping up with soil if needed. In spring, lift the whole plant and, with secateurs, cut away all the newly rooted cuttings.

Mounding is a good system to use to rejuvenate plants that have become leggy and bare at the base. Thyme, lavender, small rosemaries, and winter savory are some of the plants that benefit from being treated in this way.

Propagating herbs by layering

This is similar to mounding, but only single stems are treated.

Pegs are needed to hold the stem or branches on the ground, and all but the tip is covered with soil. After a few weeks the soil may be removed and the rooted stem cut away from the main plant. The pegs may be pieces of wire about 4 in (10 cm) long and bent into a "U" shape.

In small gardens or terraces a "herb table" means you can enjoy the look and the taste of fresh herbs.

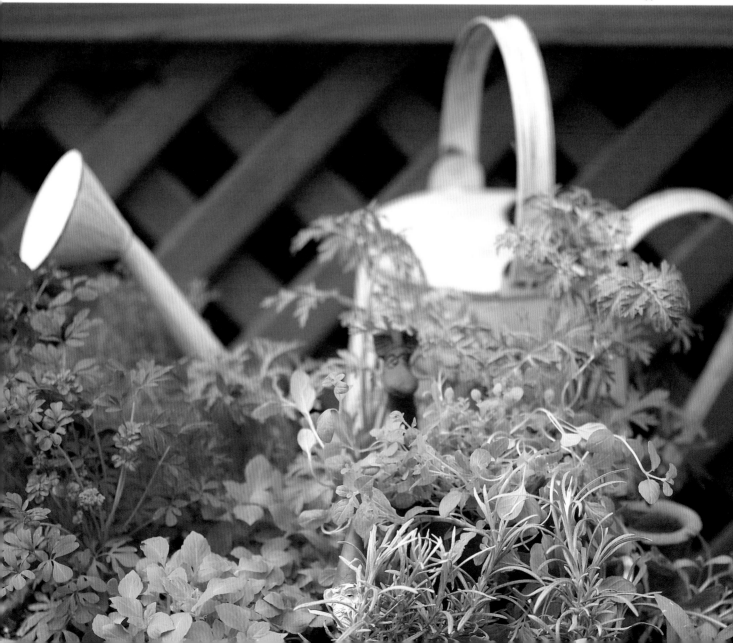

Compost

Now that you are growing your herbs you will be wondering how to fertilize them.

Compost and herbal sprays, if well made, are the only nutrition they will ever need. Compost is a homemade fertilizer made from rotted organic ingredients. It is cheap, natural, and adds humus to the soil. It improves drainage in a heavy soil, and holds moisture in a sandy or light soil. None of these advantages is to be gained by using any of the artificial fertilizers.

For neatness, compost can be processed in a special bin. You can make it yourself or buy a ready-made version.

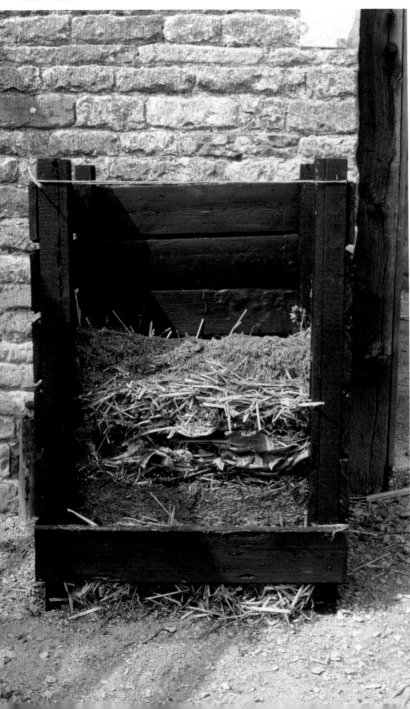

If you are trying to avoid the use of chemicals or other pollutants in your garden, you should be very careful about the raw materials you use in the compost heap. The fragrant grass clipping from your local lawn-mowing man could well be from lawns which have been sprayed with weed killers or other poisons. The rich, wholesome-looking animal manure you buy from a farmer may be from animals which have been treated with antibiotics or chemical drenches. Seaweed washed up after a storm may contain heavy metals or other undesirable elements introduced into the ocean from factory effluent or ships.

There is no need to become paranoid about this problem, but you should maintain an awareness and where possible ask potential suppliers what "additives," if any, have been used. It has been my experience that no offense is caused if the questions are asked diplomatically. In fact, the people concerned show a great deal of interest, as it frequently hasn't occurred to them that the recycling of these raw materials could cause a problem.

If you become a "compost addict" (a very easy addiction to form), there are many books available on compost making. I am a rather lazy gardener and an impatient one as well, so I look for both the quickest and the easiest way. The methods that follow have been working well for me for many years.

Aerobic composting

With this method, the heap is turned regularly, allowing oxygen into the mix to speed up the decomposition process and keep the compost smelling sweet. If an aerobic heap smells nasty or isn't heating up then it's not working properly and you need to consider what you may be doing wrong. It could be too much or too little water or sun, not enough nitrogenous matter (such as manure or grass clippings), or you may not be turning it enough. The most common error is overwatering. Adding more dry

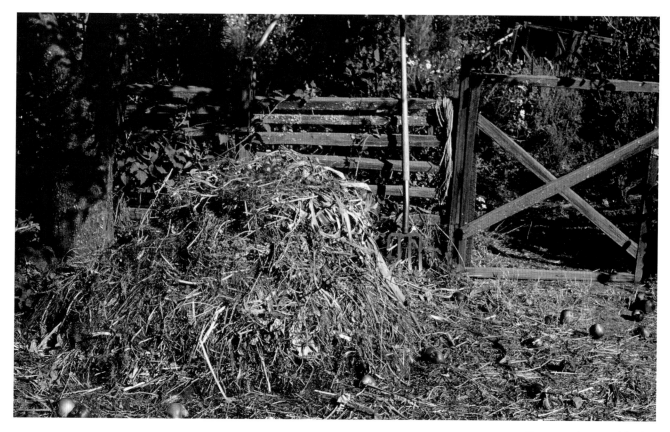

Compost can be processed directly on the ground, but some people find it a bit messy.

material, such as sawdust or straw, easily rectifies this.

Collect the materials in separate piles or bins. Use grass clippings, manure (dog and cat manure is okay if left to mature for a long time), weeds, leaves (from deciduous trees), food scraps, vacuum cleaner contents, hair, hay, straw, sawdust, to name just a few. Avoid adding fat of any description, as it takes a long time to decompose. Chop the materials with a spade or compost shredder: The finer they are, the quicker the compost pile will be complete and ready to use.

When you have enough, choose a partly shaded area (filtered light under a tree is ideal), near a tap and not too close to the house. I arrange for lawn clippings and horse manure to be delivered on the same day if possible. All household scraps and green waste from my garden have been accumulating in bins with some soil sprinkled over the piles to deter marauding animals. When everything is ready I can begin.

The following method has the advantage of not using bins as the basis of its construction, but be warned that it could make a neat, small garden look a bit messy. This may not bother you if, like me, you are so proud of your compost that guests are led down the garden path to admire the compost heap before they get to eat!

* Dig over the soil and insert a central stake for later aeration and watering.
* Put down a layer of loose material (such as leaves or straw) for aeration, and then spread a 2 in (5 cm) layer of manure on top.
* Next add 12 in (30 cm) of grass clippings, vegetable scraps, or other organic waste, plus some finely chopped herbs.
* Cover with about 1 in (2.5 cm) of soil. Repeat layers until pile is 3–6 ft (1–2 m) high, finishing with a thicker layer of soil.
* The minimum size for a heap is 3 ft (1 m) square. Any smaller and it won't heat up. Try to have the base of the pile the same size as its height for optimum efficiency.

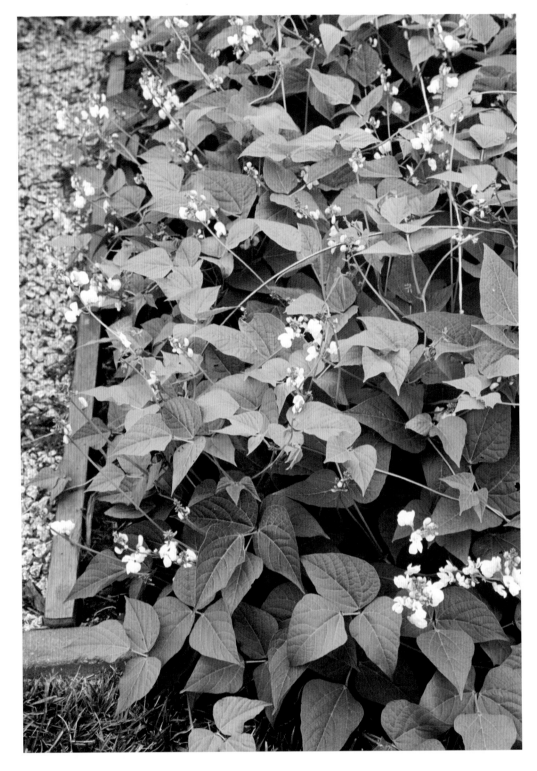

Legumes such as beans are useful as a "rotation crop" to "fix" nitrogen back into garden soil that needs rejuvenating.

Remove the stake and water the pile. It is impossible to tell you how much water to add, other than to say that the pile needs to be as moist as a squeezed-out sponge. Cover with a sheet of black plastic in which a few holes have been punched and secure with rocks or bricks. During the next week, turn the pile twice. Have an identical patch of soil dug next to it ready for turning the pile onto, and then watch it go. It will begin to heat up very quickly (it is possible for a heap to reach a temperature of 170°F [75°C], which will kill disease organisms and seeds). Don't forget to keep it moist. After the first two weeks, turn only about once weekly.

After about two weeks the pile will have cooled and it is at this stage that you add the "ingredient" that will give you a perfect compost heap. Poke holes in the pile and introduce as many worms as you can beg, borrow, or buy. They will do miraculous things in a very short time. They chew up the raw materials and pass them out as fine castings full of nitrogen, phosphorus, potassium, magnesium, and calcium. Look in your local telephone directory for "Worm Farms" and the owners will be able to advise you as to how many you will need.

If the raw materials were finely cut and the weather is warm, you should have compost in about six weeks. The pile will end up about a quarter of its original size. Mix a few handfuls of dolomite through the pile to sweeten it and there you have it: sweet-smelling, rich compost.

This compost is what you are going to use for potting and to pile on your garden, adding humus and nutrients to the soil and plants.

Herbs to use in the compost heap

There are several herbs which will enrich your compost when they are added to the mix.

* Comfrey adds calcium, nitrogen, and potassium
* Yarrow—just one chopped leaf will accelerate decomposition of the pile. Yarrow contains copper, nitrates, and phosphates
* Nettle adds iron, copper, and calcium
* Dandelion adds iron, copper, potassium, sulphur, and manganese
* Chamomile "sweetens" the pile and is rich in calcium

There's no need to restrict yourself to these herbs, but they are particularly rich in the minerals needed. All herbs will add vital nutrients. I often trim herbs and scatter the clippings directly onto the garden to rot. They act as a mulch, humus, and fertilizer.

BIODYNAMIC HERBAL FERTILIZER

Its best to use dried herbs, but if you don't have dried herbs in stock you can use double the quantity of fresh herbs. Spray or scatter this solution on your garden every two weeks during spring and autumn.

1 teaspoon cow or horse manure, dried
1 cup each chamomile, dandelion leaves, nettle, plantain, sage, and yarrow

To make

Mix the manure well with about 1 1/2 gallons (5 liters) of water and leave in the sun for two days. To one cup (250 ml) of this liquid add the herbs plus nearly 6 gallons (22 liters) of water. Leave in the sun for a further two days. Strain before using.

If you don't need the remaining manure liquid for further treatments, you can pour it over your compost heap, along with the strained herbs.

We also "stockpile" manure. For a long time we lived close to a horse stable that fed its horses well with oats and lucerne hay. We would collect several trailer loads of manure at one time, pile it in the corner of the garden, cover it with a tarpaulin and leave it for about a month. After the first couple of days there is no smell at all. We use this to mulch the garden and, as we are on sand, which is very "hungry" for humus, we need to replenish the top manure dressing frequently. This is quick and easy to do and the results are spectacular in regard to the size and quality of crops grown.

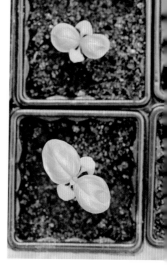

When you buy seedlings, keep the small pots. They can be used later to raise seeds such as basil.

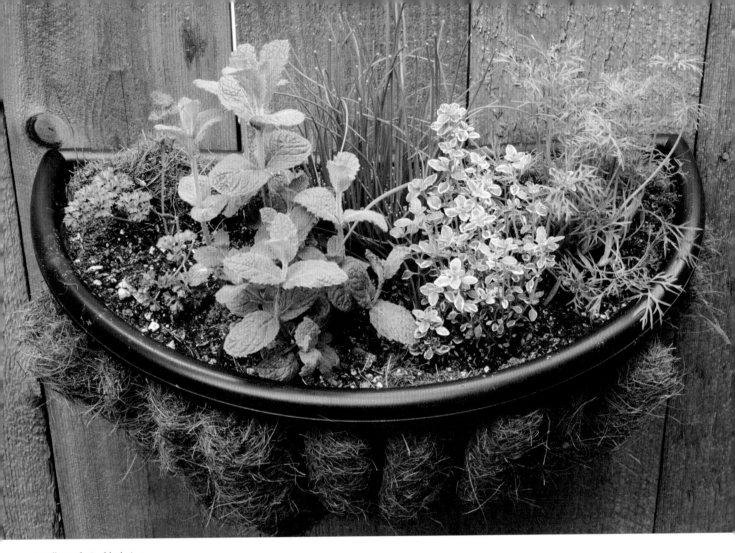

A wall pot of mixed herbs is a good way to grow them when space is limited.

Companion planting

It is well known that some plants like to dislike each other. The reasons for these preferences are many, though sometimes it's impossible to know why they exist.

Some plants exude such strong essential oil perfumes that they disguise the smell of other neighboring plants, thus protecting those plants from predators. Other herbs give off secretions from their roots which benefit nearby plants, or their roots penetrate the soil to such a depth that nutrients are brought to the upper soil. These deep-rooted plants have the additional benefit of helping to break up heavy soil. Tall plants protect smaller plants from wind and sun. Some plants are visited by bees and other insects, thus helping to attract pollinating insects to the vicinity.

A lot of companion planting is plain common sense—part of knowing your herbs and what conditions they like. I make every effort not to move self-sown plants, which often appear, seemingly from nowhere, in my garden. These plants are almost always stronger and bigger than the plants which I put into the garden with such care! When I go for walks, I find it of great interest to see where plants choose to grow in the wild. I learn a lot from these observations.

The average garden is a far cry from the forests of Europe, the dry, hot cliffs of Greece, or the lush meadows and hedgerows of Britain. The best we can do is to be as sensitive as possible to the herbs we plant. They will repay us many times over for our efforts.

The table lists the good and bad companion herbs for different plants.

Good companions, bad companions

Apple trees	Good companion: Chives, horseradish, garlic, nasturtium, tansy
Apricot tree	Good companion: Basil, horseradish, southernwood, tansy
Asparagus	Good companion: Anise, basil, parsley
Beans, all	Good companion: Anise, calendula, savory Bad companion: Fennel, garlic
Brussels sprouts	Good companion: Anise, chamomile, cilantro (coriander), dill, hyssop, mint, nasturtium, oregano, rosemary, sage, tansy, thyme Bad companion: Garlic, rue
Cauliflower	Good companion: Anise, nasturtium, tansy, thyme
Carrots	Good companion: Anise, chives, cilantro (coriander), rosemary, sage
Celery	Good companion: Anise, dill
Cucumber	Good companion: Anise, chives, marjoram, nasturtium, oregano
Grapes	Good companion: Basil, hyssop, nasturtium, tansy
Lettuce	Good companion: Anise, calendula
Parsnips	Good companion: Anise, garlic
Peach trees	Good companion: Garlic, nasturtium, tansy
Potatoes	Good companion: Calendula, horseradish Bad companion: Rosemary
Radishes	Good companion: Anise, nasturtium Bad companion: Hyssop
Raspberries	Good companion: Tansy
Roses	Good companion: Calendula, chives, garlic, parsley, tansy
Silverbeet	Good companion: Anise, lavender
Strawberries	Good companion: Anise, borage, sage Bad companion: Garlic
Tomatoes	Good companion: Anise, basil, calendula, chives, dill, parsley, fennel, rosemary Bad companion: Garlic
Zucchini	Good companion: Anise, nasturtium

INSECT-ATTRACTING HERBS
PLANT THE FOLLOWING HERBS THROUGH YOUR VEGETABLE GARDEN, UNDER FRUIT TREES, OR ANYWHERE YOU WANT POLLINATION TO TAKE PLACE:
ANISE
BASIL
BERGAMOT
BORAGE
CATNEP
DANDELION
LAVENDER
LEMON BALM
MALLOW
MARJORAM
MINTS
ROSEMARY
SAGE
THYME
VALERIAN
YARROW

Insect-repellent herbs

The term "insect repellent" is rather misleading, as it suggests the aim of the gardener is to rid the garden of insects. What a disaster that would be! Pollination would slow down dramatically if there were only the wind to rely on. I suppose, if we are truthful about what we really want, we are asking for the pest-free garden, undamaged fruit and vegetables, aphid-free roses and baby plants growing free from the threat of slugs and snails—all this without resorting to the use of poisonous sprays.

What we need to aim for is not to kill insects but to discourage them from destroying the plants. This can be achieved with time, effort, a few "tricks," and a lot of fresh herbs.

Snails and slugs are a real threat only to young seedlings, and these are fairly easy to protect. I cut out and discard the bottoms of a number of plant pots, push the top parts into the soil around each young plant and remove them only when the plant is well established. I also use the inner cardboard tubes from toilet paper rolls pushed around the base of small seedlings. They get plenty of light and seem to appreciate the protection, not only from snails but also from wind. Fresh grass clippings or wood cinders around young plants also deter snails, as well as providing mulch to keep their tender roots as cool as possible.

Some herbs can be used to repel certain insects. This is not going to work if you plant a solitary basil near a rose bush and trust that every aphid in the vicinity is going to leave. You need to plant enough of the herb you have chosen to form a reasonable barrier near the plant you want to protect. For instance, if a border of feverfew is planted around a bed of carrots, the strong scent will mask the smell of the carrots and the carrot fly will fly over your garden to your next-door neighbor's!

I have noticed that insects and disease rarely bother self-sown plants. There is a valuable lesson to be learnt here. A strong,

Butterflies don't do any harm, but their larvae (caterpillars) can be a pest.

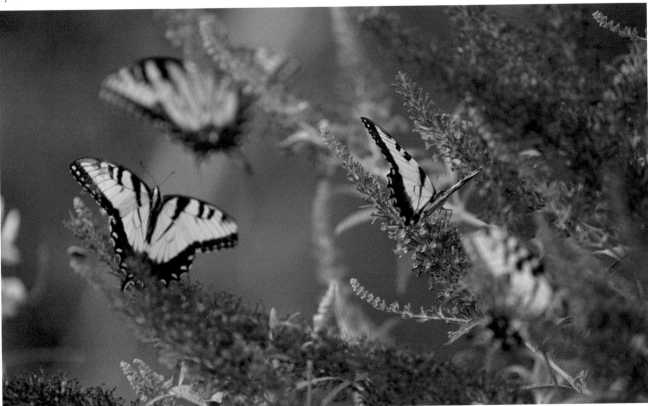

healthy plant, growing in the right position in good soil, can put up its own resistance.

If you want a good vegetable garden you need to avoid growing crops in the same position more than once every four years. This is known as crop rotation. It has the double benefit of discouraging insect pests from reaching plague proportions by breeding in the same patch, and preventing the ground from being depleted of the particular nutrients taken from it by that crop.

Some herbs are of general benefit and protection to most plants. These include anise, feverfew, garlic, hyssop, southernwood, and yarrow. Borage increases resistance to disease, and lemon balm and nettle are ideal to use in general-purpose sprays. It's good to plant these among your vegetables and flowers and also to use them in sprays. For small gardens a small spray bottle will often do. This can be a recycled, well-washed kitchen or bathroom cleanser bottle, with a spray nozzle on it.

The following pests can be kept at bay by inter-planting or surrounding the garden bed with the recommended insect-repellent herb or herbs to mask the odor of the plants you wish to protect.

* Ants: Marjoram, mint, oregano, pennyroyal, rue, tansy
* Aphids: Basil, calendula, caraway, chives, cilantro (coriander), elder, nasturtium, tansy
* Apple scab: Chives horseradish
* Beetles: Catnep, lavender, nasturtium, rosemary, tansy, wormwood
* Black fly: Thyme
* Cabbage moth: Cilantro (coriander), dill, hyssop, rosemary
* Cabbage worm: Chamomile, cilantro (coriander)
* Carrot fly: Cilantro (coriander), rosemary, sage, wormwood
* Caterpillars: Elder, mint
* Eelworm: Calendula
* Fleas: Fennel, pennyroyal, rosemary, rue, tansy
* Flies: Caraway, lavender, rue

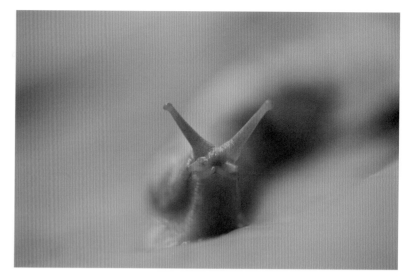

Snails and slugs can quickly devastate young seedlings.

* Fungus: Chamomile
* Mice: Catnep, mint, tansy
* Mosquitoes: Basil, caraway, elder, feverfew, garlic, pennyroyal
* Moths: Bay, chamomile, feverfew, tansy
* Potato bug: Horseradish
* Snails and slugs: Horseradish, pennyroyal, rue, sage, wormwood
* Silverfish: Bay, tansy, wormwood
* Tomato worm: Borage
* Weevils: Bay

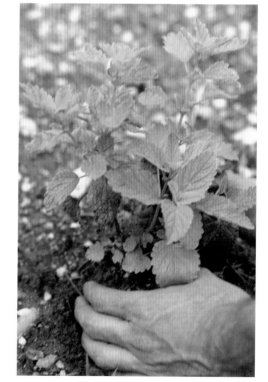

Lemon balm (Melissa officinalis), planted through your garden will help to protect against disease. It is also good used in a general-purpose spray.

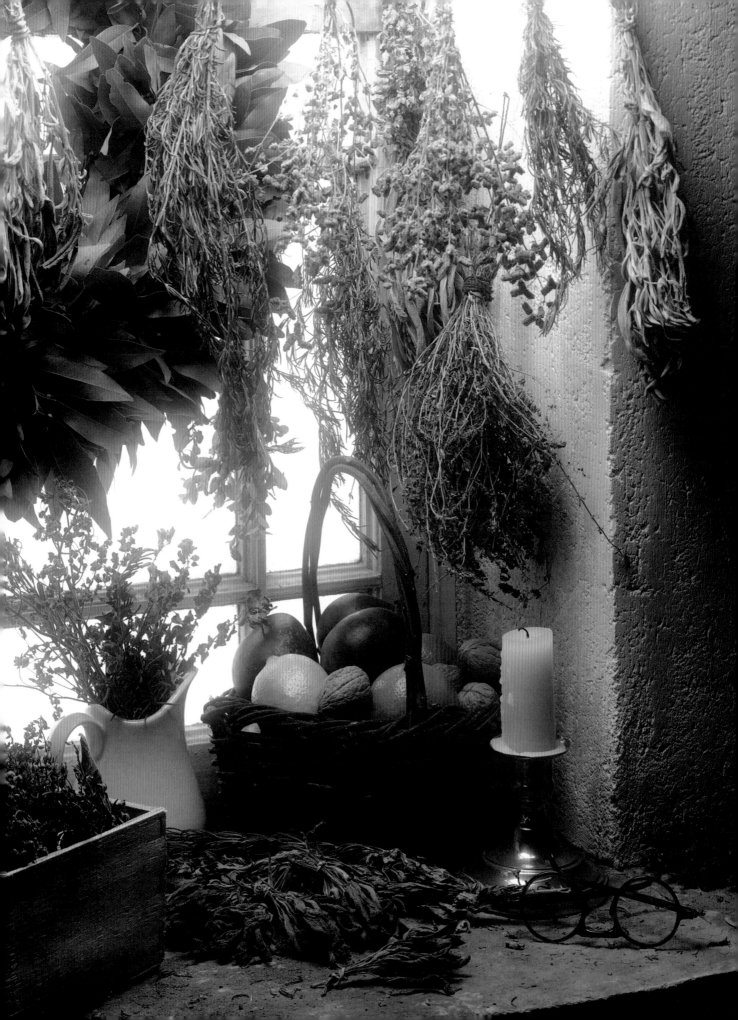

Harvesting and drying herbs

The difference to the tastebuds between shop-bought dried herbs and your own carefully dried or freshly picked herbs is very pronounced. You also have the satisfaction of knowing they are as uncontaminated as you could possible manage to make them. To ensure a regular supply of herbs you will need to harvest and preserve your own as they reach their prime. This is usually just as they come into flower.

Harvesting your herbs

Choose a warm, sunny morning to harvest—before the sun is too strong, but after every trace of moisture has dried from the plant. The picking time is critical, as the sun causes the plant to "expire" its precious essential oils. These oils are what gives the plant most of its perfume and flavor and must be protected at every stage, from picking to using.

Gathering leaves

Cut a whole branch or stem just as the plant is coming into flower, cutting the stem just on or above the leaf node. Take only as much as you can process quickly as the leaves can deteriorate very soon after picking. Pick over the material, discarding all dead or discolored plants, its pointless storing anything but the best.

Gathering flowers

Cut these just before they are fully open.

Gathering seeds

Cut whole heads as they turn from beige to brown. If there is a danger of the seed falling before you gather it, the head may be enclosed in a paper or muslin bag until the seeds are ripe (see "Drying herbs," page 218).

Gathering roots

The roots are usually best collected in the plant's most dormant season when there is not much leaf growth.

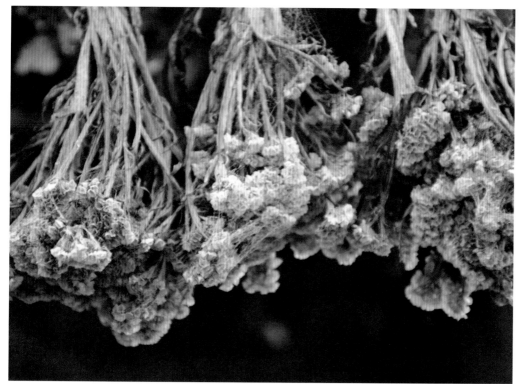

Dry flowers by hanging upside down in bunches over fine mesh.

Using herb flowers in your cooking

The flowers of the aromatic herbs may be used in many ways for taste and visual appeal. Sprinkle in salads, or soups, fold into cheese dips, rice or pasta dishes, or herb butters.

Basil	has spikes of white flowers. Use the whole spike as decoration, or the individual flowers in salads.
Bergamot	flowers are delicately flavored and are a striking blood red. Use the petals in salads.
Borage	boasts exquisite blue stars with black stamens. Lovely in punches, lemonade, sorbets, chilled soups, and cheese dips.
Calendula (*Calendula offficinalis*, not African or French marigolds)	has golden orange petals. Sprinkle on soups, pasta or rice dishes, herb butters, and salads.
Chives	have lovely star-shaped flowers ranging from bright pink to lavender hues. Great with any savory dish.
Cilantro (coriander)	flowers look like white or pink lace and are decorative and tasty. Great with any savory dish.
Dill and fennel	have charming umbels of tiny yellow flowers. The whole head can be used for decoration in the center of a salad or a cold meat plate, or the individual flowers may be picked off.
Geranium flowers	are often scented and come in a variety of colours and fragrances. Sprinkle the flowers over the desserts, and use in cold drinks or freeze in ice cubes. Some geranium leaves are also delicious. Try dipping small leaves of peppermint geranium in chocolate and serving as after-dinner mints.
Hollyhocks	have bold flowers in a variety of colours to decorate trays of sandwiches.
Lavender	flowers are lovely sprinkled over chocolate cake, or as a garnish for sorbets, or ice creams.
Lemon verbena flowers	are tiny and cream colored, and are citrus scented and flavored—fresh and pretty in a jug of iced lemonade on a summer's day.
Nasturtiums	have brilliant coloured and peppery flavored flowers to garnish platters, salads, soups, cheese dips, open-faced sandwiches, and savory appetizers. Nice when stuffed with a flavored cream cheese.
Pineapple	sage has brilliant scarlet plumes that make elegant and fragrant garnishes for platters of food. The individual flowers add color, scent, and flavor to sorbets, ice cream, and cakes, and are ideal for refreshing cold drinks.
Rose petals	can garnish salads, ice cream and desserts. Freeze tiny rosebuds in ice cubes and float them in punches and clear glass jugs of lemonade. Crystallized petals or entire miniature roses are lovely. Remove the bitter white piece at the bottom of the petals before using.
Rosemary	blooms come in delicate shades of pale to dark blue and white are tasty in cheese dips.
Sage flowers	are a delicate purple. They are delicious in salads and sandwiches and make attractive garnishes.
Violets, pansies, and viola flowers	either crystallized or fresh, taste as good as they smell. Eat both the young leaves and flowers in salads, and use the flowers to decorate cakes, biscuits, desserts, and iced drinks. Freeze them in ice cubes to drop in summer drinks and punches.
Zucchini (courgette), squash, and pumpkin flowers	are tasty and decorative when dried, lightly crushed, and sprinkled over foods such as salads and soups.

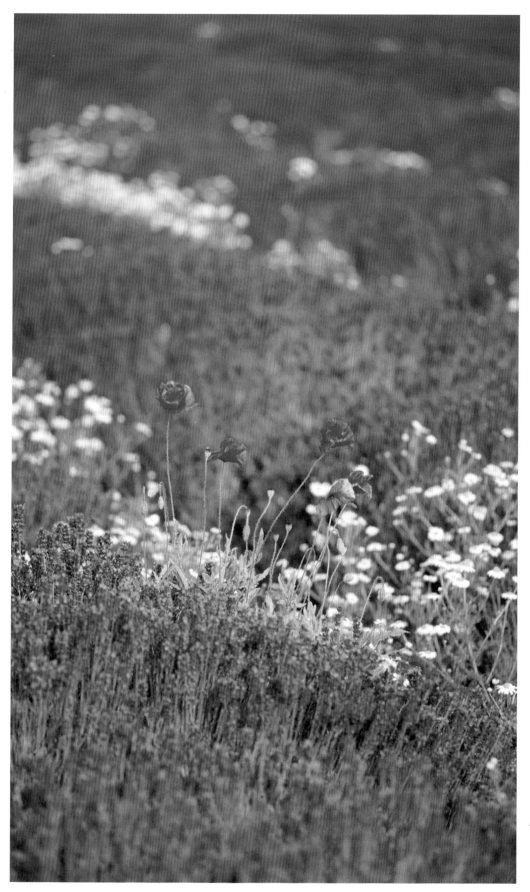

Poppies in the middle of a lavender field in Norfolk, UK.

Drying herbs

Unless your herbs are dirty there is no need to wash them (I'm assuming that you don't use chemical sprays). If, however, they are dusty or have soil clinging to them, they will need a quick rinse. Fill the sink with cold water and immerse the herbs. Lift the whole lot in and out of the water several times and then lift out onto the draining board or into a colander. (Drain the water out of the sink after removing the herbs and not before, or the dirt will just settle back onto the herbs as the water drains away.) Pat the herbs gently between tea towels or towels until dry.

The quicker you dry your herbs, the better the color and flavor will be. However, they must never be dried in direct sunlight or high temperatures, as this destroys the plants' special properties.

Choose an airy, dust-free area, or an oven set at its lowest temperature with the door open. If using the oven method, keep the herbs on the lowest rack and turn them regularly. If you have a wood stove in your kitchen you can create a wonderful drying area by making screen racks to fit above the stove. This is the method we used most at our farm, as it could be utilized all year round.

Manufacturers maintain that herbs can be dried using microwave ovens. I feel that while the plants may dry satisfactorily, the essential oils will be lost. These oils are very sensitive to heat and need to be treated with the utmost respect. I would not recommend this form of drying.

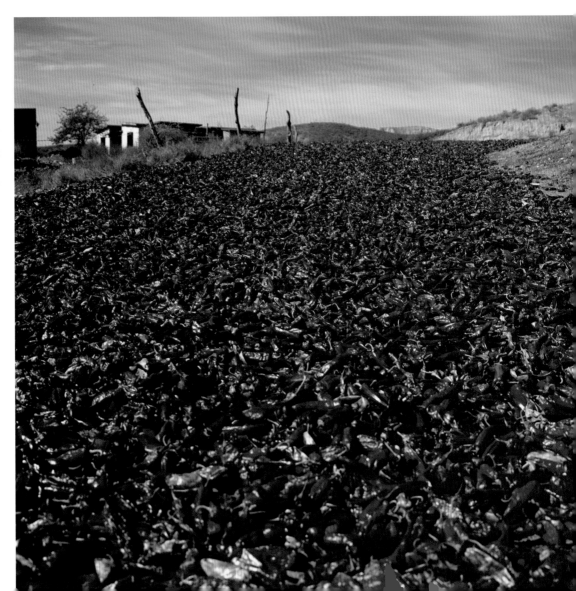

Commercially grown chilies drying next to Highway 1, Baja, Mexico, Central America.

An electric dehydrator is excellent for drying herbs, but be sure to buy a model with a fan for circulating air and also a temperature control which can be set to about 95°F (35°C). This may sound hot, but if there is air circulating constantly, the herbs stay cool.

Leaves and flowers

These can be tied in small bunches and hung in a suitable area. If dust or flies are a problem, enclose the bunches in muslin bags. Alternatively, they can be spread on insect screens or dried in the oven as described above. The leaves may be stripped from the stems.

The material is dry when it is just becoming crisp. If you are using an oven, watch the herbs carefully to prevent overdrying.

Roots, barks, and stems

These parts of the plant usually need to be washed and thoroughly dried, then chopped as finely as possible to speed up the drying process. I find the oven or dehydrator methods best for roots but, unlike leaves and flowers, roots may be dried in the sun. If you are drying them in summer, spread them on old flyscreens or some other suitable type of mesh, cover them with cheesecloth and put them in a sunny place away from dust. (On top of a water tank or shade house will do nicely.)

Roots, bark, and stems are dry when they easily snap.

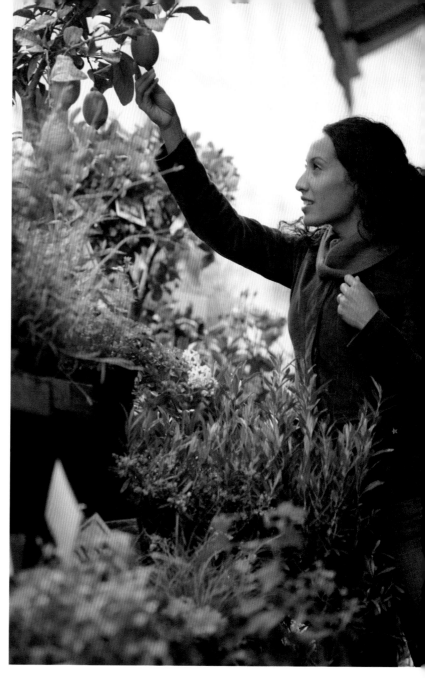

Home-grown produce, free of pesticides, is your best raw material.

Seeds

The best way to dry seeds is to enclose the seed head in cheesecloth while still on the plant. If this isn't practicable cut the seed heads off, enclose them in a muslin or cheesecloth bag, hang them in an airy place out of the sun and forget about them for about two months. If you prefer, you can strip the seeds off the head first. Do search the seed heads for insects first or you may have provided a tasty larder for creepies!

Large leaves and pods

The way to deal easily with large leaves such as borage, comfrey, and mullein, and with pods such as chilies, is to thread a large needle with tough linen thread or dental floss and push the needle through the stem of the leaf of pod. Hang them in such a way that they won't touch each other.

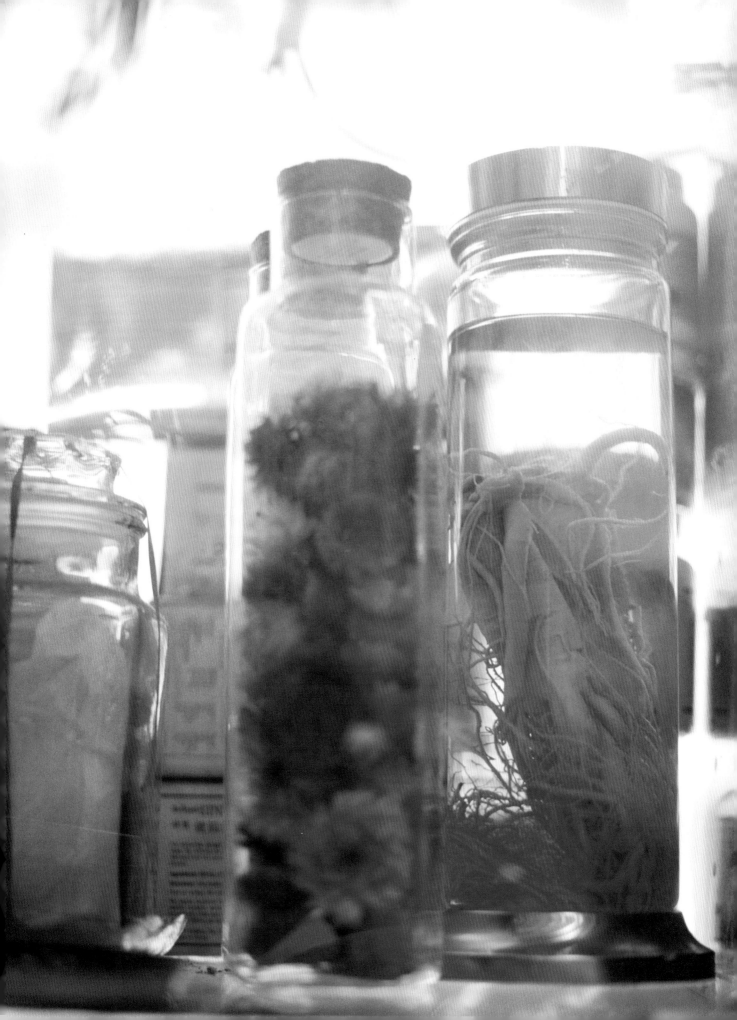

Storing herbs

Over the years I experimented with several methods of storage and finally settled on glass jars. These give protection from damp, insects, and dust, and have the advantage of allowing you to keep a close eye on the contents. It's very important to check the jars regularly, particularly in the first few weeks, as any moisture left in the herbs could cause mold to develop.

Choose a jar that fits the amount of herb. A lot of air in the jar will detract from the keeping qualities of the herbs being stored. Collect sizes from very large to very small.

I particularly like small instant coffee jars that I soak to remove the printed labels, and then put through the dishwasher. It's very important if using second-hand jars, to make sure they are spotlessly clean and dry. Sometimes even glass can seem to hold a residual smell if the old contents have been

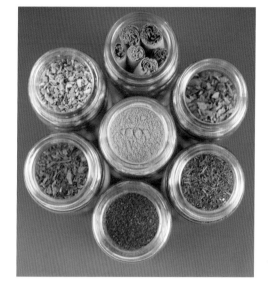

Clockwise from top: *Cinnamon, cilantro (coriander), thyme, paprika, basil, sage, and turmeric.*

strong smelling. It always goes but make sure the lids are clean as well, as I have found that they are the source of odd smells, more than the glass jars.

Label your jars carefully with the common name, Latin name, and date of storage. Don't trust your memory, as many

French farmer gathering large bundles of lavender, St Remy de Provence, France

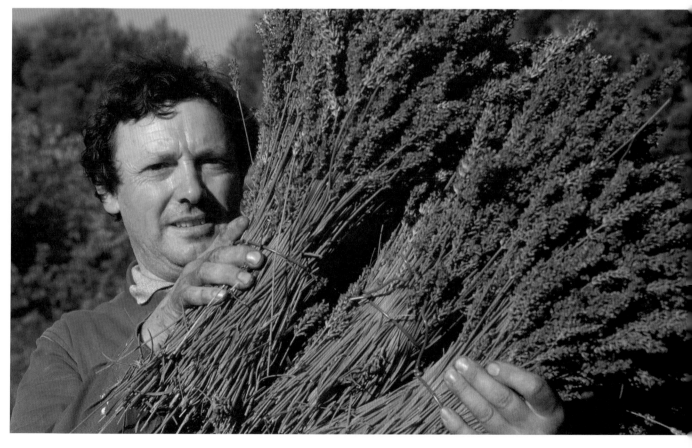

herbs smell and look very similar after they are dried. It's often a good idea to label the lid as well, as if you take the tops of two or more similar jars, you won't remember which lid belongs to which.

Store the jars in a dark cupboard in a cool area of your home.

Oil

I'm not happy about storing fresh herbs in oil as I feel there is always a danger of botulism occurring. If you want herb-flavored oil, use dried herbs and remove from the oil once the flavoring process is finished.

Other ways of preserving herbs

Many herbs lose both color and flavor when dried, and these may be preserved by other methods.

Herbs drying in the sun on a hand-made, cane drying rack.

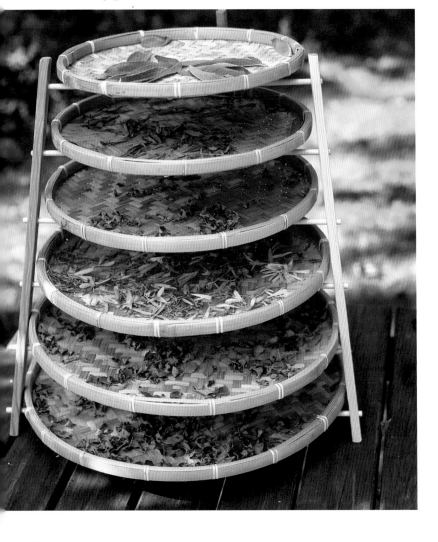

Freezing

This is one of my favorite ways to store my everyday herbs. They are the ones I use in cooking and in lots of my lotions and creams.

Strip the leaves and petals from the stems and pack them flat in zip-top plastic bags or freezer containers. Press bags to remove as much air as possible, then seal and mark with the name of the herb and date packaged. I find that herbs keep their flavor for about six to nine months, by which time the next crop is growing in the garden.

When you want to use the frozen herbs, take as much as you want from the bag and chop as quickly as possible while the leaves are still frozen. If allowed to defrost they can get very tough or soggy.

Another way to get full use of your herb crop is to freeze them in cubes. I often blend leaves with olive oil or water and press the pulp into ice cube trays ready for dropping into soups, stews, and so on. Basil is particularly good when prepared in this way, as you can add garlic, ginger, chili (or other herbs of your choice) to the leaves while processing, and have instant flavoring to add to stir-fries, beans, or other dishes.

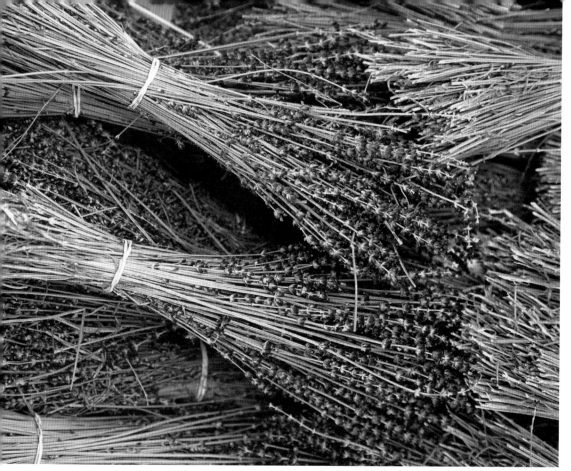

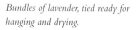

Bundles of lavender, tied ready for hanging and drying.

Below: Dried lavender flowers packaged in voile sachets ready for sale.

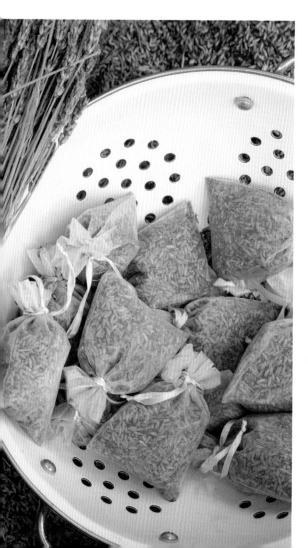

Storing herbs for cooking

Herb	Method	Use
Basil	Freeze flat in plastic bag	Use frozen
Bay	Airtight container	Use whole
Chives	Freeze flat in plastic bag or chop and freeze in water ice cubes	Use frozen or drop cubes into soups or casseroles
Cilantro (coriander)	Chop and freeze in water ice cubes	Drop cubes into soups or Asian dishes
Dill	Chop and freeze in water ice cubes	Drop cubes into soups or casseroles
Mint	Chop and freeze in water ice cubes	Drop cubes into soups or casseroles
Parsley, curly and flat	Freeze flat in plastic bag or chop and freeze in water ice cubes	Use frozen or drop cubes into soups or casseroles
Rosemary	Freeze flat in plastic bag	Use frozen
Sage	Freeze flat in plastic bag	Use frozen
Tarragon	Chop and freeze in water ice cubes	Use frozen or drop cubes into soups or casseroles

HERBS IN THE GARDEN

GARDEN SPRAYS

Sprays are best used in the morning before the sun gets too hot. If applied in the evening the moisture might encourage fungal diseases to grow. The following sprays need to be used at least once a week and more often if the problem is a serious one.

NETTLE SPRAY

Nettles add vitamins and minerals to the soil.

To make and use

Place bunches of nettles in a large container with a lid and cover with water.
Put the lid on the container and leave until rotted and fermenting.
Strain before use.
Spray the entire plant including the underside of the leaves.

GENERAL SPRAY

This will repel insects and give health to plants.

To make and use

Use southernwood, mint, tansy, feverfew, chamomile, nettle, parsley, sage, and borage.
Place equal quantities of as many of these herbs as possible in a large container with a lid and cover with water.
Put the lid on the container and leave until rotted and fermenting.
Strain before use.
Spray the entire plant including the underside of the leaves.

CHAMOMILE SPRAY

Use to give a lift to sick plants or water onto young seedlings to prevent "damping off."

To make and use

Make a triple-strength tea of chamomile flowers.
Stand for 24 hours.
Strain, then dilute to a weak tea.
Spray the entire plant including the underside of the leaves.

ELDER SPRAY

Spray on young plants to protect from insects and caterpillars.

To make and use

Make a triple-strength tea of elder leaves.
Stand for 24 hours.
Strain, then dilute to a weak tea.
Spray the entire plant including the underside of the leaves.

WORMWOOD SPRAY

Wormwood makes a good caterpillar spray.

2 cups finely chopped wormwood leaves
1 teaspoon soap flakes

To make and use

Simmer wormwood leaves in 1 quart (1 liter) of water for 30 minutes with the pan covered.
Stir, strain through a sieve, and then through coffee filter paper.
Dissolve the soap flakes in the water while it is still warm.
Spray the entire plant including the underside of the leaves.

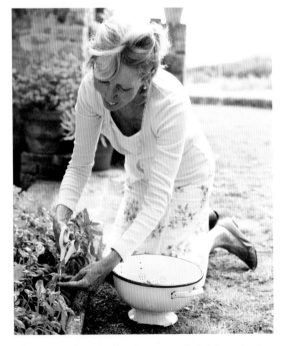

The most rewarding part of growing your own herbs is harvesting them and adding them fresh to your meals.

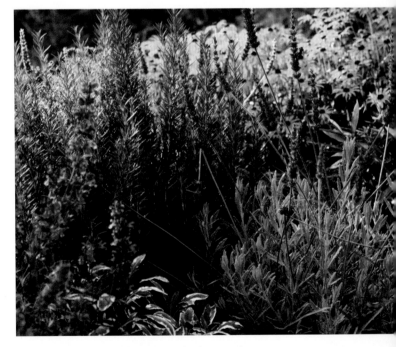

Herbs work well when planted in amongst other decorative plants.

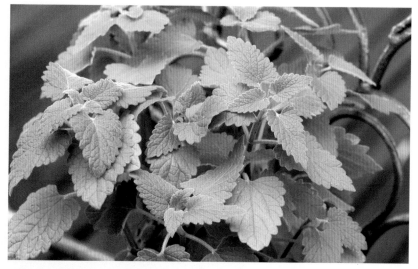

Catnep flourishing in a small pot.

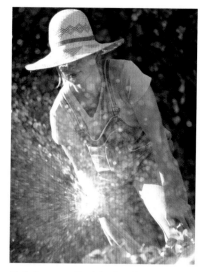

Herbs love water. Don't let them dry out.

SPRAY FOR FUNGAL DISEASES AND APHIDS

6 large rhubarb leaves, finely chopped
1 teaspoon soap flakes

To make and use

Place the chopped rhubarb leaves in a saucepan, add 1 quart (1 liter) of water, cover, and bring to the boil.

Remove from the heat, and leave to steep overnight.

Strain solution through a sieve, and then through coffee filter paper.

Dissolve the soap flakes in a little hot water, and add to the infusion. Mix well.

Store in a labeled glass jar or bottle.

Use as required, in a spray bottle, on plants for fungal diseases and aphids.

BICARBONATE OF SODA SPRAY

Use this solution for powdery mildew and blackspot.

Choose a large container, as the mixture will form froth when the vinegar is added.

4 teaspoons bicarbonate of soda
3 teaspoons soap flakes
1 cup (250 ml) warm water
3 teaspoons vegetable oil
40 drops tea tree oil
4 teaspoons vinegar

To make and use

Mix the bicarbonate of soda and soap flakes with the water.

Add the vegetable oil, tea tree oil, and vinegar. Store in a bottle and for use add 3–4 tablespoons to 2 quarts (2 liters) of water. Spray plants, covering tops and bottoms of leaves.

SLUG SPRAY

To 1 cup (250 ml) of ammonia add 1 cup (250 ml) of water.

To make and use

Mix slowly to avoid creating froth.

Pour the liquid into a spray bottle and spray where slugs are active.

This will kill the slugs but will not hurt the plants, as the ammonia breaks down into nitrogen.

MEALYBUG-KILLER SPRAY

Spray with neat rubbing alcohol.

GARLIC SPRAY

$3\frac{1}{2}$ oz (100 g) garlic cloves
6 onions
6 red chilies
liquid paraffin oil, to cover
4 cups (1 liter) water
1 cup (250 g) dried skim milk powder

To make and use

Blend the garlic, onions, and chilies well in a food processor. Add paraffin oil and leave to stand for two days.

Add four cups of water, and the skim milk powder, and mix well. Strain through a fine cloth.

Dilute one part solution to 50 parts water (stronger if needed) and use to spray against aphids, ants, spiders, and caterpillars.

BUG-OFF BLEND

This blend may be used both on the body and in the air to keep mosquitos, fleas, and other "biters" at bay.

$2\frac{1}{2}$ teaspoons lemon-scented tea tree oil
1 teaspoon cedarwood oil
1 teaspoon patchouli oil
$\frac{1}{2}$ teaspoon manuka oil

To make and use

Mix all the oils in a labeled 1 fl oz (30 ml) bottle and shake well. Leave for four days to synergize.

Store in a cool dark place.

To use on the body

Put 25 drops in a 2 fl oz (60 ml) bottle

Add 2 teaspoons of vodka or witch hazel extract, and fill with grape seed or almond oil.

Shake well before rubbing onto exposed parts of the body.

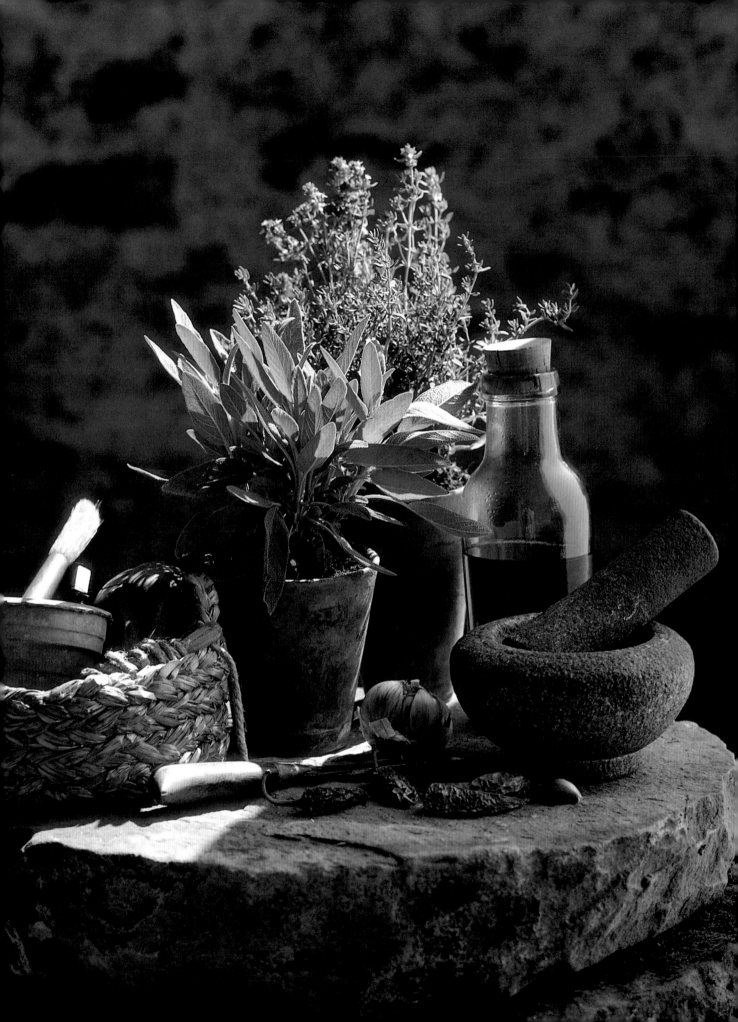

Herbal gifts from the heart of the home

When you want to give a gourmet herbal gift, why not a beautiful basket or box of home-made oils, vinegars, marinated vegetables, or sweet treats complete with gift tags and even paper you have created yourself with stencils or stippling?

Flavored vinegars and oils are quick and simple to make. They can be used for sprinkling on food, marinating, making dressings, and brushing on vegetables, fish, poultry, or meats, before or after cooking, and can transform a simple meal into a gourmet experience.

Home-made dressing and mayonnaise are also popular gifts along with marinated vegetables, cheeses, or olives, although these need to be kept in the refrigerator.

And for a sweet finish, don't forget the delights of candied herbs and flowers.

Herb vinegars, oils, dressings, and marinated vegetables

Keep a look out for beautiful bottles and jars in which to store your flavored oils and vinegars. If giving as a gift, delay the final addition of sprigs of herbs until the last minute, as the vinegar quickly strips the color from the plant material.

Use a good quality vinegar as the base, as cheap vinegars are too harsh, and will overpower the flavor of the herbs. Being strongly acid, it is important to use suitable non-aluminum pans. Enamel, stainless steel, and ceramic lined cast iron are all suitable.

Use corks or acid-proof lids or bottle tops (glass, plastic, or plastic lined) for sealing sterilized containers.

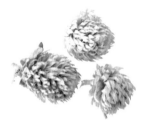

Tiny rose buds collected from the garden and dried create a romantic aroma throughout the home.

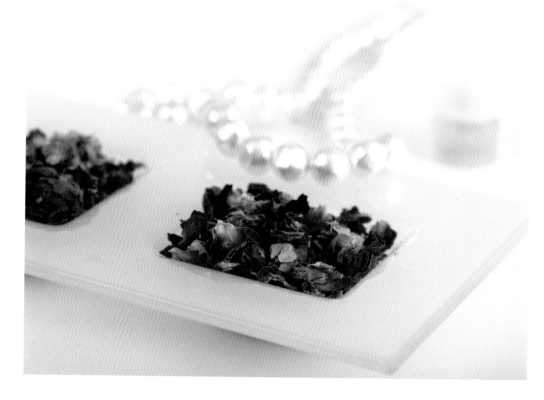

Opposite: A fabulous selection of home-made goodies from the garden for your own use or, if you can bear to give them away, as gifts for friends.

HERB VINEGAR

Makes about 3 cups (750 ml).

Use your favorite mix of herbs for this recipe. A good blend is thyme, savory, basil, oregano, and a bay leaf.

3/4 cup chopped fresh herbs
3 cups cider or white wine vinegar
Sprigs of fresh herbs for bottling

To make

Mix herbs and cider vinegar together in a large jar
Seal and leave in a warm place for two weeks, shaking often.
Strain vinegar through cheesecloth, and then through coffee filter paper. Pour into sterilized, labeled bottles, and add two or three sprigs of fresh herbs to each bottle.
Seal with acid-proof lids or bottle tops.

TARRAGON VINEGAR

Makes about 3 cups (750 ml).

1 cup chopped fresh tarragon leaves
3 cups white wine vinegar
sprigs of fresh herbs for bottling

To make

Mix tarragon and vinegar together in a large jar. Seal and leave in a warm place for two weeks, shaking often.
Strain vinegar through cheesecloth and then through coffee filter paper. Pour into sterilized, labeled bottles and add two or three sprigs of fresh herbs to each bottle.
Seal with acid-proof lids or bottle tops.

LEMON VINEGAR

Makes about 3 cups (750 ml).

3 cups (750 ml) white wine vinegar
juice of 3 lemons
12 black peppercorns
long thin strips of lemon rind

To make

Pour the vinegar and lemon juice into a large jar.
Seal and leave in a warm place for one week.
Strain vinegar through coffee filter paper.
Pour into sterilized, labeled bottles and add some peppercorns to each bottle and a long, twisted strip of lemon rind.
Seal with acid-proof lids or bottle tops.

RASPBERRY VINEGAR

Makes about 3 cups (750 ml).

1 lb (500 g) raspberries
3 tablespoons (45 ml) honey
2 cups (500 ml) red wine vinegar

To make

Mash the raspberries and place in a large jar, then mix in the honey.
Heat the vinegar, then pour it over the raspberries.
Cover and leave to stand for two days.
Strain through a double cheesecloth, then through coffee filter paper.
Pour into a sterilized, labeled bottle.
Seal with acid-proof lids or bottle tops.

GARLIC OIL

Makes about 4 cups (1 quart/1 liter).

This takes only minutes to prepare, tastes delicious and will save you a lot of time if you use garlic often. It's a very useful oil as a garlic flavor is needed in so many dishes. I use extra virgin olive oil for this as I don't store it in the refrigerator, but keep it by the stove.

4 cups (1 quart/1 liter) oil
8–10 cloves garlic, peeled and finely sliced
fresh, whole, peeled garlic cloves, optional

To make

Place the oil of your choice and the garlic in a screw top jar.
Cover securely and leave for a week in the refrigerator to allow the flavor to develop.
Strain the oil (use the garlic in your cooking).
Pour into clean bottles.
If you wish, add three fresh, whole, peeled garlic cloves to each bottle before giving as a gift.

When serving a home-made tea always choose a beautiful tea pot and matching cups.

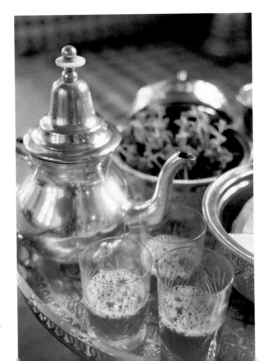

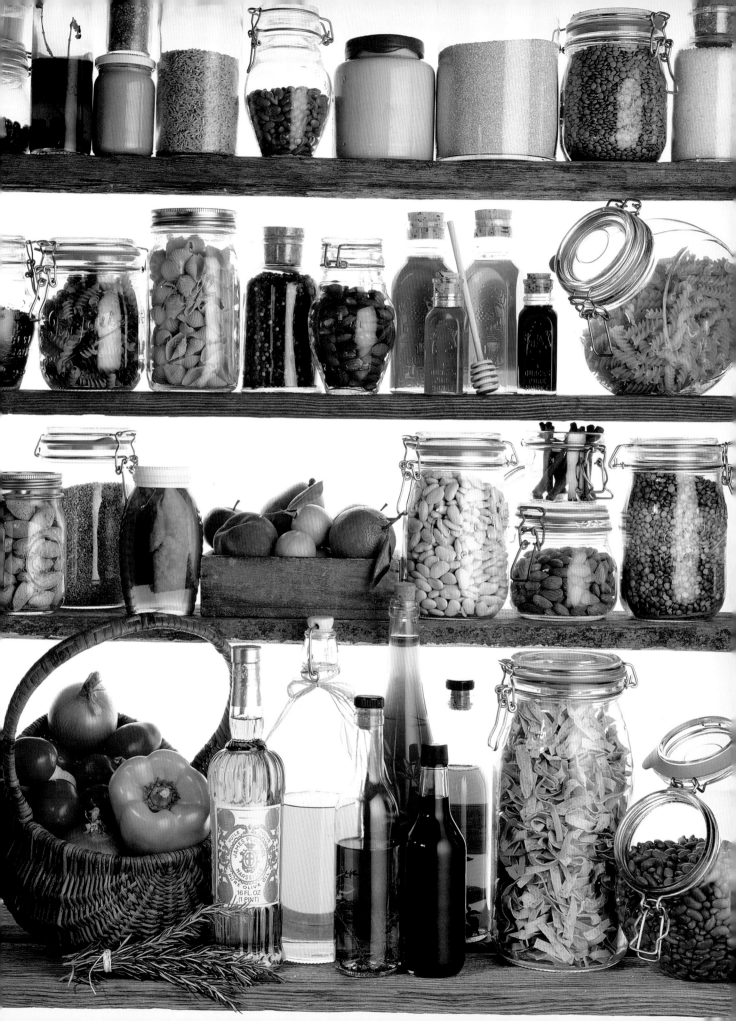

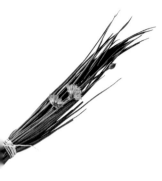

HERB OIL

Makes about 2 cups (500 ml).

It's best to make small quantities of this oil to make sure it keeps fresh. I would use about 2 cups (500 ml) of combined oils with this quantity of herbs.

$^1/_2$ cup chopped fresh tarragon
$^1/_4$ cup chopped fresh thyme leaves
$^1/_4$ cup chopped fresh chives
2 teaspoons celery seeds, crushed
1 cup (250 ml) olive oil
1 cup (250 ml) another oil of your choice
whole pink and green peppercorns, optional

To make

Half fill a jar with the herbs and celery seeds.

Top with an equal mixture of the two oils.

Cover and leave in a warm place for two weeks, shaking the jar often.

Strain the herb-flavored oil and rebottle.

If you wish, add whole pink and green peppercorns, then top securely and label.

HOT CHILI OIL

Makes about 2 cups (500 ml).

Don't treat this oil lightly—it's a good servant but a cruel master! If sautéing, mix it with some plain oil. Add in very small quantities to dips, dressings, bastes, and marinades.

2 cups (500 ml) oil
$^1/_2$ cup (15 g) chopped dried chilies (or to taste)
1 teaspoon chili powder (or to taste)
2 in (5 cm) piece fresh ginger, grated or finely chopped
24 black peppercorns, bruised
6 cloves garlic, crushed
1 medium onion, finely chopped

To make

Heat the oil until quite hot, then add the remaining ingredients to the hot oil and remove from the heat.

Cover and stand overnight.

Strain the oil through double cheesecloth .

Pour into bottles and seal well. Label.

Herbal vinegar capped professionally with a cork and wire tie.

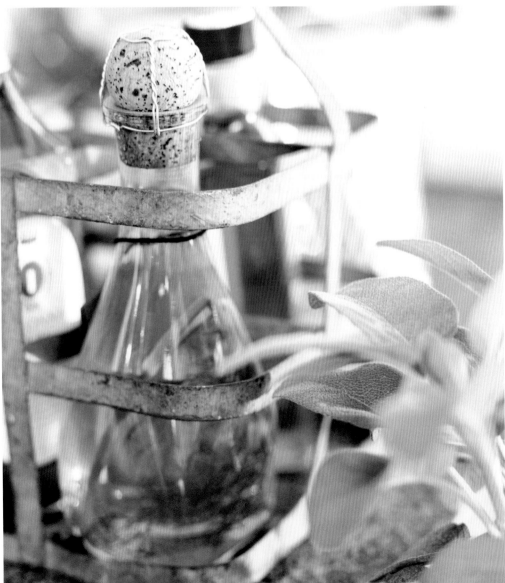

HERB VINAIGRETTE

Makes about 2 cups (500 ml).

If refrigerated, this keeps for several weeks. The herb leaves should be fresh, all stems and stalks removed.

$^1/_2$ cup fresh parsley leaves, finely chopped
1 tablespoon fresh basil leaves, finely chopped
$^1/_2$ cup fresh oregano leaves, finely chopped
1 cup (250 ml) olive oil
3 tablespoons (45 ml) lemon juice
3 tablespoons (45 ml) white wine vinegar
1 clove garlic, crushed
1 cup (2$^1/_4$ oz/60 g) chopped green onions (scallions)
1 teaspoon French mustard
salt and freshly ground black pepper to taste
1 tablespoon honey

To make

Place the chopped herbs in a jar with a well-fitting, acid-proof lid.

Add all the remaining ingredients, cover securely, and shake until well blended and thick.

Store dressing in the refrigerator. If the olive oil solidifies on chilling, stand at room temperature until it clears before using the dressing.

MARINATED FETA CHEESE

I like to use low-salt feta for flavor and health reasons. Other cheeses may be preserved in this manner. Other varieties of goat's cheese are particularly nice.

2 lb (1 kg) feta cheese cut into 1 in (2.5 cm) cubes
4 teaspoons black mustard seeds
4 teaspoons white mustard seeds
2 tablespoons black peppercorns
2 bay leaves
2 whole red chilies
olive oil, to cover

To make

Layer the feta cheese with all the remaining ingredients, except the oil, in a wide-necked, sterilized jar with a well-fitting lid.

Pour sufficient oil into the jar to cover the contents.

Seal well, label, and store in the refrigerator for at least one week before serving.

MARINATED OLIVES

1 lb (500 g) pickled olives (black Greek olives are best)
$^1/_2$ red bell pepper (capsicum), thinly sliced
$^1/_2$ green bell pepper (capsicum), thinly sliced
2 cloves garlic, sliced
2 sprigs fresh lemon thyme
2 bay leaves
2 sprigs fresh oregano
3 strips lemon peel (with no pith)
olive oil to cover

To make

Rinse and drain the olives.

Combine all the ingredients in a wide-necked, sterilized jar with a well fitting lid.

Add the oil, covering the olives by 1 in (2.5 cm). Seal the jar securely. Label.

Store the olives, allowing the flavor to develop for at least one week before using.

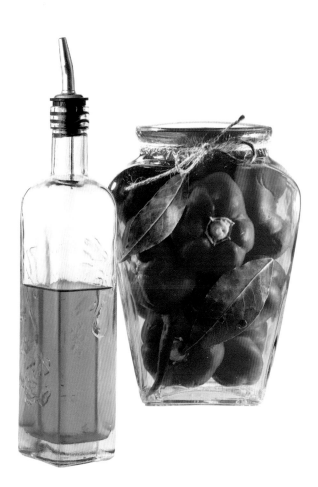

Sweet treats

The skill of candying and crystallizing is quite easy to master, however, it requires patience and a delicate touch. The best whole flowers to crystallize are violets and borage; the best petals are carnations and rose. The latter need to have the white pithy bit at the base of the petals removed as this is quite bitter.

PRESERVED ANGELICA STEM

I have tried lots of methods and find this old recipe to be the best. It's worth a bit of bother and stored properly it will last about 12 months.

To make

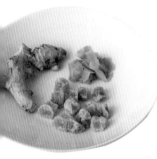

Cut young angelica stems into 2 in (5 cm) lengths and simmer in water until tender.

Remove from the water and peel when cool enough to handle.

Return to the water and simmer gently until very green.

Drain, cool, then weigh.

Measure an equal weight of sugar to angelica.

Sprinkle the sugar over the angelica and leave for two to three days.

Bring to the boil, simmer for 10 minutes, then drain.

Spread the angelica stems on a wire rack over a baking tray.

Place in a cool oven set as low as your oven will go to dry out the stems

Store in a single layer in a labeled, airtight container in a cool place.

HERB SUGAR

This sugar is a way of adding a subtle herb flavor to cakes, desserts, and cookies.

1 cup tightly packed, unsprayed herbs of your choice (for example, rose petals, lavender leaves or buds, lemon verbena), bruised but not chopped
$1\frac{1}{2}$ cups (170 g) granulated sugar

To make

Layer the herbs and sugar alternately in 1 in (2.5 cm) layers in a wide-necked, sterilized jar with a well-fitting lid. Cover securely and let stand for two or three weeks in a warm place.

Sieve the herbs from the sugar and place a layer of new, dried herbs in the bottom of the jar. Pour the sugar on top of the dried herbs and store in a cool place for up to nine months.

Herbal tea lends itself to a glass teapot where it's possible to see the soft color of the herbs.

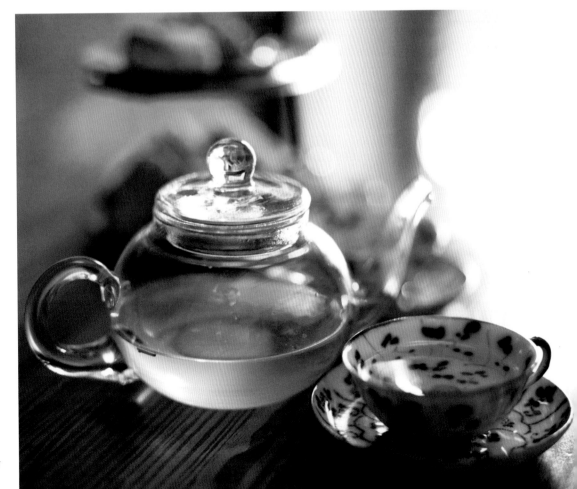

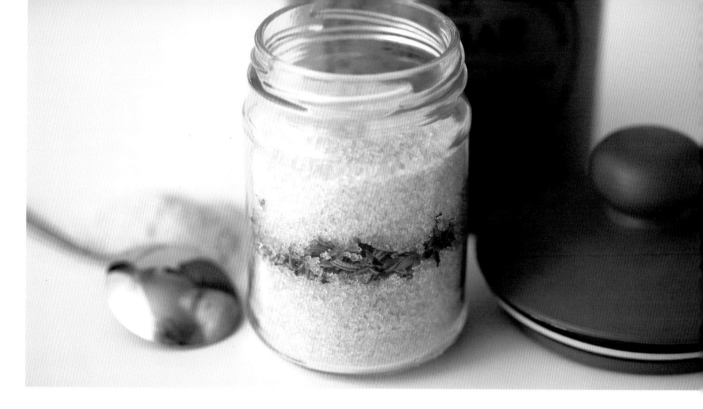

CRYSTALLIZED FLOWERS

1 egg white
fresh flowers or petals
powdered (caster) sugar

To make

Whisk the egg white until it is broken down, but not too frothy.

Using a very fine paintbrush, coat each petal with a thin layer of egg white and sprinkle with powdered (caster) sugar making sure that the petal is totally covered.

Place on a fine wire rack or fine mesh, cover with greaseproof paper and leave to dry.

Store in layers separated by greaseproof paper in airtight, labeled containers.

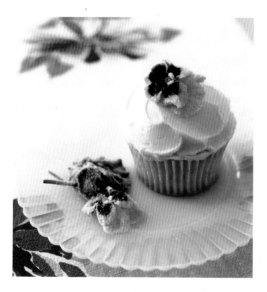

PRESERVED GINGER

This ginger will keep for many months and makes a delicious gift for ginger lovers.

2 lb (1 kg) fresh ginger
1 rounded teaspoon bicarbonate of soda
4 cups (880 g) granulated white sugar

To make

Wash and scrape the skin from the ginger. Cut the ginger into $1/2$ in (1 cm) cubes (or a little larger if you prefer).

Cover with water in a non-aluminum pan, bring to a boil and simmer for 10 minutes. Drain.

Add the bicarbonate of soda, cover again with water and boil for 20 minutes. Drain, add more water, then boil again for 3–4 minutes, or until the ginger is tender.

Combine half the sugar with 1 cup (250 ml) of water in a saucepan. Stir over a low heat until the sugar is dissolved. Simmer gently for 5 minutes, then add the ginger. Cover and simmer for 10 minutes.

Pour into a dish, cover and leave for two to three days.

Strain the syrup into a saucepan.

Add one cup of the remaining sugar to the syrup, stir over a low heat until the sugar is dissolved and simmer gently for 5 minutes. Pour over the ginger and leave for 24 hours. Strain and repeat this process with the remaining cup of sugar and the syrup.

Pack into labeled jars and seal securely.

Herb sugar is a geat ingredient for cakes and cookies.

Cup cakes look cute and yummy when topped with crystallized flowers.

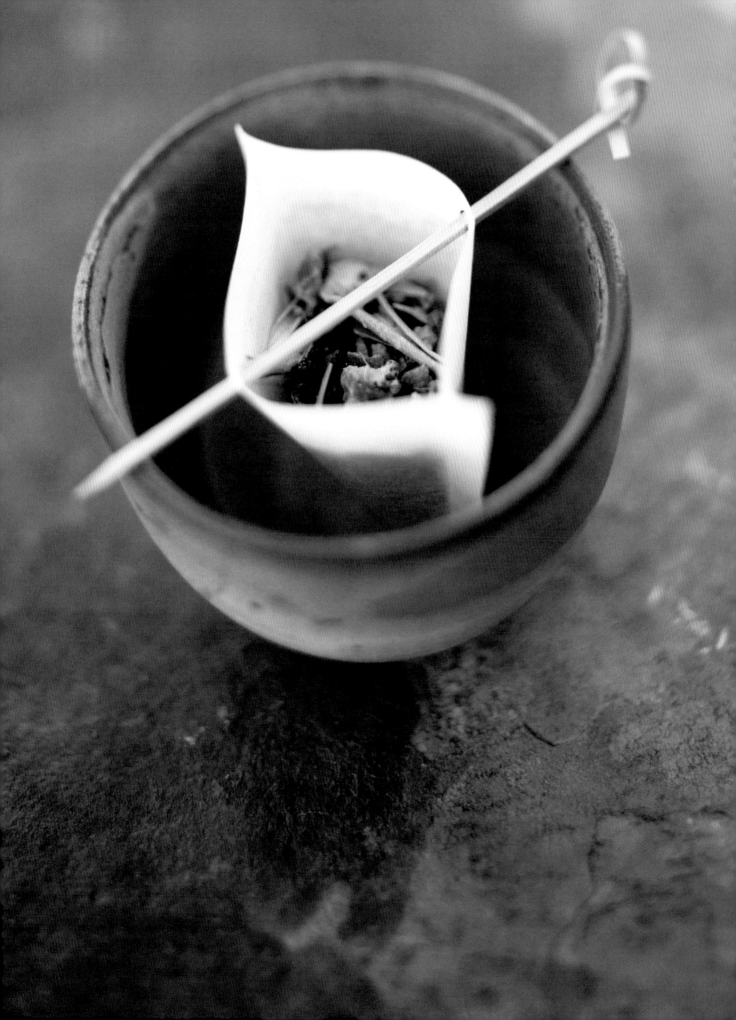

Herbal teas and wines

We drink for many reasons: To quench thirst, to warm or cool ourselves, to share companionship with friends, and to comfort ourselves. In the case of herb teas, there is the additional benefit of the therapeutic properties to be gained. Tea and coffee have a valuable role as stimulants and tea is a useful antioxidant but, unfortunately, we often drink them to excess and the stimulating properties can be destructive to the nerves and body, leaving us feeling "jumpy" and with an "acid" stomach. If we try to limit the intake of regular tea and coffee to about three cups a day while drinking herbal infusions or decoctions the rest of the time, we are getting the best from both types of drinks.

It can be unwise to stick to one single herb or blend of herbs until you are absolutely sure of what you are doing. Continual use of any particular herb may aggravate the very symptoms which

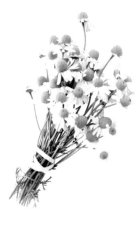

you are trying to alleviate. If you don't thoroughly understand the properties of the herbs you are using, you may unwittingly overstimulate certain organs or functions of the body, so try to vary the types of drinks you consume, especially at first. Making mixtures of the herbs helps overcome the problem and creates the excitement of discovery as you make and taste a new and unique blend.

To create herbal mixtures you will need to know the individual taste of each herb. As with any experiments you make, you might like to keep records if you want to repeat your successes. I work in a fairly haphazard way, using a quarter of a cup of boiling water and adding pinches of herbs until the taste is to my liking. You can be more scientific if you like. The important thing is the end result, but don't forget to note down what you used, whichever way you do it.

You can also make delicious, medicated wines which act as tonics, digestive aids, sedatives, and breath sweeteners as well as tasting good. In fact, by choosing your herbs you can devise wines for many different complaints.

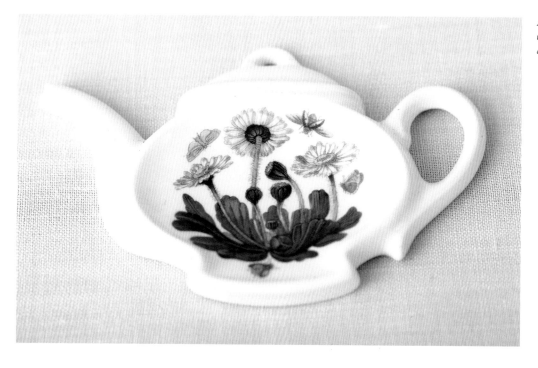

An English porcelain tea bag rest used to stop staining on furniture and table linen.

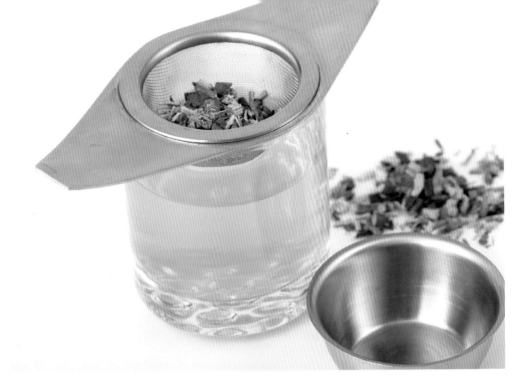

Licorice root tea is an excellent remedy for tummy problems.

Which herbal tea?

The following list will help you to make blends of tea to remedy particular ailments or problems. Try small amounts at first. Make these drinks using fresh or dried herbs, but remember, if you want a specific mix, dried herbs will ensure that you have the same blend throughout the year.

Antacid	Alfalfa sprouts, lemon juice, nettle leaves, red clover sprouts
Antidepressant	Chamomile flowers, sage leaves
Appetite depressant	Anise or fennel seeds, crushed, parsley leaves
Appetite stimulant	Alfalfa or red clover sprouts, calendula flowers, ginger root, lemon rind or juice, nettle, tarragon, thyme leaves.
Blood cleanser	Alfalfa or red clover sprouts, bergamot, elder, peppermint, nettle or yarrow leaves, lemon juice or rind.
Body warmer	Anise seeds, bergamot, lemon balm, peppermint or sage leaves, calendula or elder flower, ginger root, lemon rind or juice, yarrow leaves or flowers.
Bowel toner	Calendula flowers, dill or fennel seeds, ginger root, lemon rind or juice, raspberry leaves, red clover sprouts.
Breath freshener	Anise seeds, cilantro (coriander), dill or fennel seeds, lemon rind or juice, orange peel, peppermint, rosemary, sage or thyme leaves.
Coughs	Lemon rind or juice, mullein, raspberry or sage leaves, red clover sprouts.
Digestion aid	Angelica leaves or root, anise or caraway seeds, lemon juice, mallow root, marjoram or savory leaves.

Herbal teas

Herbs for tea-making should be chopped or crushed until the pieces resemble Indian tea in size. Store the mixtures in glass jars away from the light (if you have space, it's a good idea to freeze them), keeping out only enough for immediate use. In this way you will preserve the flavor, color, and goodness for as long as a year.

Keep a separate teapot or infuser for herbal drinks, as tannin residue from other teas can alter the delicate flavor of the herbs. Lemon zest and juice and orange peel can be added to any tea to improve flavor, and increase vitamin and mineral content.

Some teas can be made like conventional tea, just by pouring boiling water over the flowers and leaves and leaving it to stand, covered, for a few minutes. Others, such as seeds or roots, need to be simmered, as a decoction, to draw out enough flavor and goodness from the herb. Either way, much of the therapeutic value of herb teas is in the essential oils that will evaporate off in steam. It's important, therefore, to cover the mug or pot to prevent loss of these oils.

Some of the recipes are teas for particular conditions, others for pleasure. You may like to try each tea and then add or substitute your own flavors. All these teas are made using the infusion method.

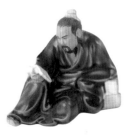

Herbal teas can be purchased in bulk from supermarkets that specialize in Asian products, as well as specialty tea stores.

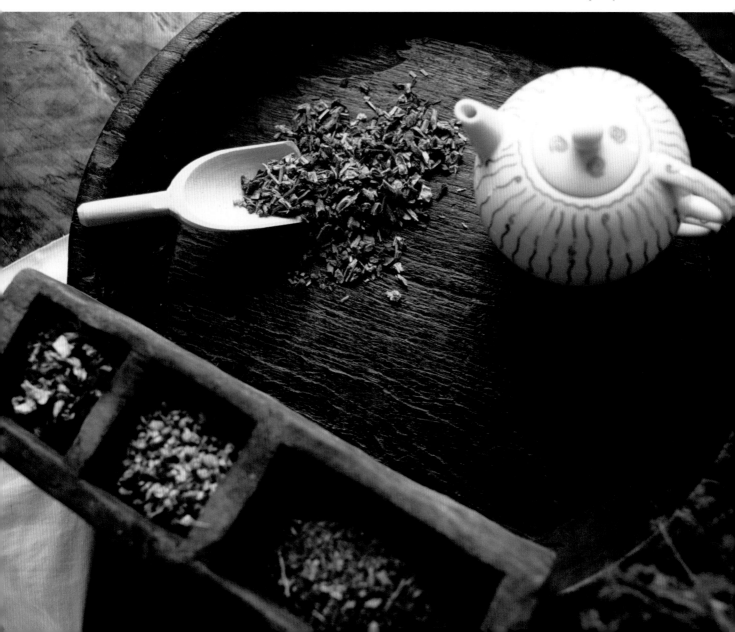

WATCHPOINTS

Borage/mullein: The hairs on the leaves of these plants can cause contact dermatitis and also stomach problems. Use gloves to pick the leaves if you are sensitive. Strain the tea through a coffee filter to avoid ingesting the hairs.

Nettle: Old plants need to be well cooked, as they contain a substance which could cause kidney damage if eaten raw.

Parsley: Avoid using as a tea if pregnant or if the kidneys are inflamed. The small amount normally used in cooking and salads is safe.

Rosemary/sage/thyme: Not to be used in large quantities or for an extended period of time.

Yarrow: Extended use may make the skin light-sensitive, resulting in pigmentation.

Valerian: Extended use may have a depressant effect. Take no more than twice a day for six days. Repeat for three weeks only.

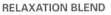

REFRESHMENT BLEND
Bergamot, lemon balm or lemongrass leaves, borage leaves or flowers, lemon rind or juice, orange peel.

RELAXATION BLEND
Aniseed, chamomile or elder flower, lemon balm, marjoram, oregano, sage or tarragon leaves.

STOMACH UPSET BLEND
Alfalfa sprouts, angelica leaves or root, caraway seeds, chamomile, mallow root, orange peel, peppermint, spearmint, savory or thyme leaves.

THIRST QUENCHER BLEND
Basil or borage leaves, lemon grass leaves, peppermint leaves, lemon rind or juice.

TONIC BLEND
Alfalfa or red clover sprouts, angelica leaves or root, anise seeds, basil, bergamot, peppermint, nettle, parsley, raspberry, rosemary, sage, savory leaves.

VITAMIN AND MINERAL SUPPLEMENT BLEND
Alfalfa or red clover sprouts, anise seeds, catnep, lemon grass, nettle, parsley, raspberry, sage, tarragon, thyme, yarrow leaves, lemon rind or juice, orange peel, mallow root.

Lavender ready for chopping on a board reserved just for herbs.

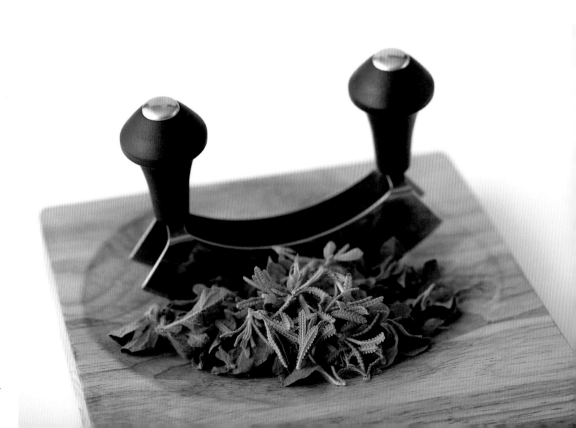

PREGNANCY TEA BLEND

1 part ginger root
1 part licorice root
2 parts nettle leaves
1 part mallow, roots or leaves
1 part yellow dock root
4 parts raspberry leaves

SLEEPY TIME BLEND

2 parts chamomile flowers
2 parts lemon balm leaves
2 parts nettle leaves
2 parts licorice root or anise seeds
1 part catnep leaves
1 part elder flowers

COMFORTER BLEND

2 parts peppermint leaves
1 part lemon balm leaves
2 parts chamomile

SUMMER QUENCHER

For a delicious chilled drink, strain after 10 minutes, chill and add lemon juice and ice cubes.

3 parts lemon grass leaves
2 parts lemon balm leaves
2 parts borage leaves
2 parts lemon peel
1 part dill seed

POSTNATAL BLEND

4 parts raspberry leaves
2 parts fennel seeds
1 part borage leaves and flowers
$\frac{1}{2}$ part dandelion root or leaf
1 part nettle leaves
1 part dill
$\frac{1}{2}$ part mallow, roots or leaves

ELDER TISANE

6 parts elder flowers
1 part caraway
2 parts red clover
1 part dried orange peel
1 part lemon balm leaves

USING HERBAL HONEYS

I like to use unprocessed honey in herbal drinks and as often as possible in cooking. Flavored honeys are delicious and healthy and they also make attractive gifts. To make them, be sure not to use wild honey (usually dark-colored) or "blended honey" (a mixture of honey which usually includes wild honey). These honeys tend to have a strong taste that could overpower the herbs.

- Heat the honey gently until it's runny—don't let it get too hot or the medicinal properties will be destroyed. Add half a cup of chopped herbs to each cup of honey, stir thoroughly and leave for a couple of weeks in a warm (not hot) place.
- Reheat and strain, pressing the herbs to get as much honey as possible, and pour into a jar.
- These honeys need refrigerating, as the heating seems to destroy some of the natural keeping properties.

GINGER HONEY

This ginger honey is good for cooking or for a hot herb and lemon drink (when you are cold and shivery or are coming down with a cold). It is also wonderful for desserts, marinades, and many other dishes.

To make
Peel and chop a 3–4-in (7.5–10 cm) piece of ginger root.
Put in a small pan and cover with honey.
Bring to the boil. Lower the heat and barely simmer for one hour.
Strain and pour into a sterilized jar. Seal securely and label.

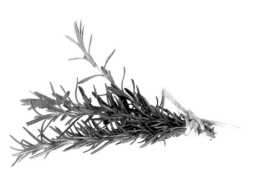

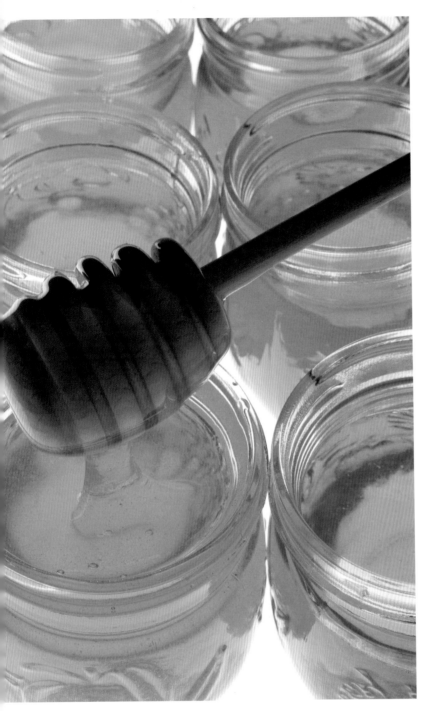

Choose a pure honey to sweeten herbal teas.

Herbal wines

If you want a really mellow wine, let it mature for a month or so after straining, Store in a cool, dark place. If you want your wine to last a long time, it's best to choose a full-bodied wine as a base. For tonics I use a good muscat, as the flavor seems to blend well with herbs.

HONEY SYRUP FOR LIQUEURS

Honey syrup is suitable for adding to any drink which has a spirit base, such as whiskey, brandy, or vodka. It you add honey syrup, the liqueur needs to be matured for a further two to three months at room temperature.

To make

Mix together equal quantities of water and honey, bring slowly to a boil, remove from the heat and stir until the honey is melted. Cool.

CALMING AND DIGESTIVE WINE

This simple, effective recipe has been around for at least a century. Sip a glass to calm you down after a stressful day.

1 tablespoon chopped fresh rosemary leaves
4 whole cloves
1 tablespoon honey
1 in (2.5 cm) piece cinnamon stick
1 bottle dry white wine

To make

Place the rosemary, cloves, honey, and cinnamon into a sterilized bottle and top up with wine.
    Shake daily until the honey is dissolved, then strain well. Drink after a week.

TONIC WINE

This wine is great any time you feel "under the weather" or "down in the mouth!" It is a good pick-me-up after illness to stimulate the appetite, or can be drunk just because you like it. Use fresh herbs if you can get them, and bruise them (don't completely crush them) one at a time by pounding gently two or three times in a mortar and pestle.

1 teaspoon each wormwood, rosemary, thyme, and sage
1 in (2.5 cm) piece fresh ginger
1 in (2.5 cm) piece cinnamon stick
2 whole cloves
peel of 1 lemon, pared thinly and sliced
2 teaspoons anise seeds, bruised
2 cups (500 ml) muscat

To make

Place the herbs and spices into a sterilized bottle and top up with the wine (if pouring from a measuring jug, it must be very clean).

Cork and store in a cool, dark place for two weeks. Strain and filter the wine and pour back into the bottle. Label.

Leave in a cool, dark place for one month before use.

Sweeten with Honey Syrup (page 240) if you like.

DIGESTIVE LIQUEUR

1 tablespoon each crushed caraway seed and fennel seed
1 in (2.5 cm) piece fresh ginger, crushed
1 tablespoon chopped peppermint leaves
2 strips lemon peel, about 2 in (5 cm) each
2 cups (500 ml) brandy
$^1/_2$ cup (125 ml) Honey Syrup (page 240)

To make

Place the herbs and spices into a sterilized bottle and top up with the brandy (if pouring from a measuring jug, it must be very clean).

Cork and store in a cool, dark place for three to four weeks.

Strain and filter the liqueur and pour back into the bottle. Label.

Leave in a cool, dark place for three months in a cool, dark place before drinking.

MINT LIQUEUR

3 tablespoons fresh peppermint leaves, bruised
3 tablespoons fresh spearmint leaves, bruised
4 strips orange peel, about 2 in (5 cm) each
4 strips lemon peel, about 2 in (5 cm) each
$2^1/_2$ cups (625 ml) brandy
$^1/_2$ cup (125 ml) Honey Syrup (page 240)

To make

Place the herbs, peels, and brandy in a large, sterilized jar.

Shake once daily for two weeks. Strain and filter.

Add the Honey Syrup, then bottle, label and store in a cool, dark place for two to three months.

Buy the best brandy you can afford as a base for your herbal liqueurs. Here, barrels of Armagnac brandy are stored in a cellar in the Gascogne district of France.

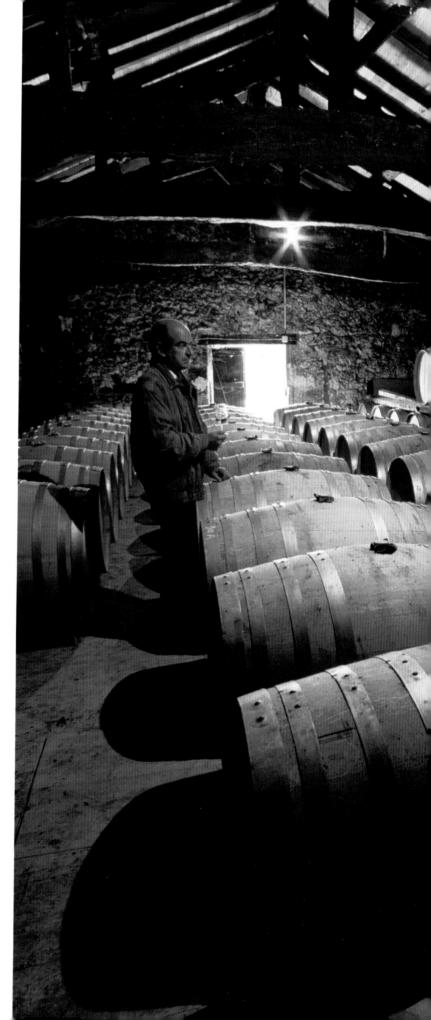

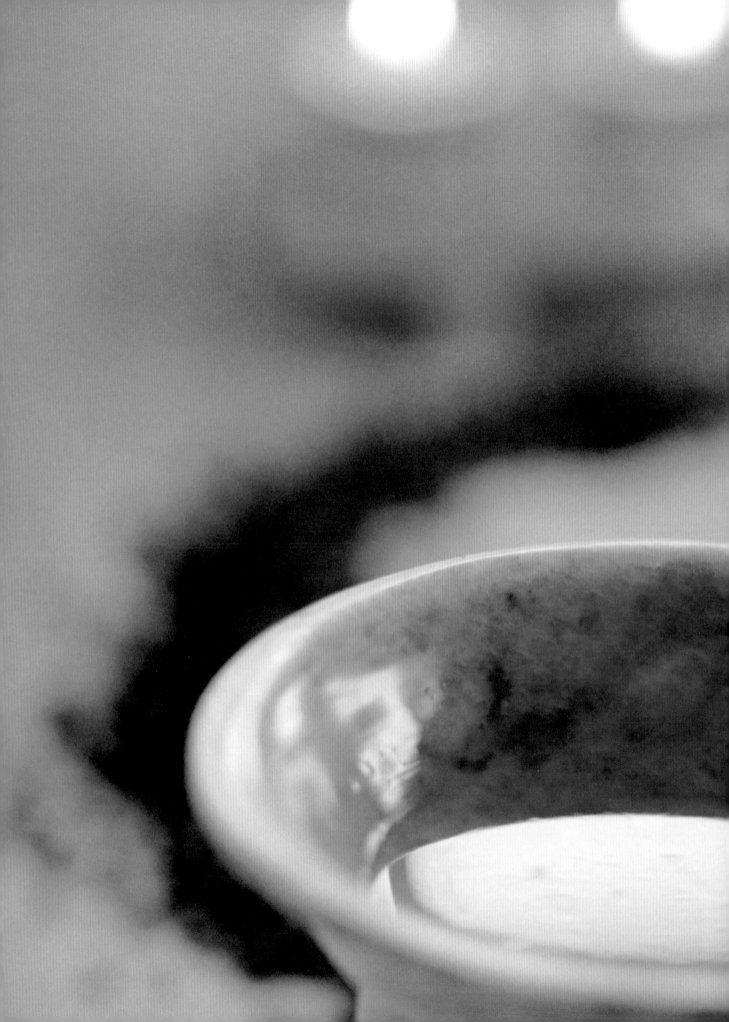

PART 3

CHERISH

In an increasingly hectic world, where we have little time for ourselves, it is nourishing and empowering to allow yourself a brief break to create something beautiful for your family and yourself. By making and using the recipes in this chapter you will feed the outside of your body as lovingly as you feed the inside. By using the best quality ingredients you can find, such as herbs, cold-pressed oils, essentials oils, cider vinegar, honey and beeswax, you will create creams and lotions far superior to almost all of those found on the shelves of stores.

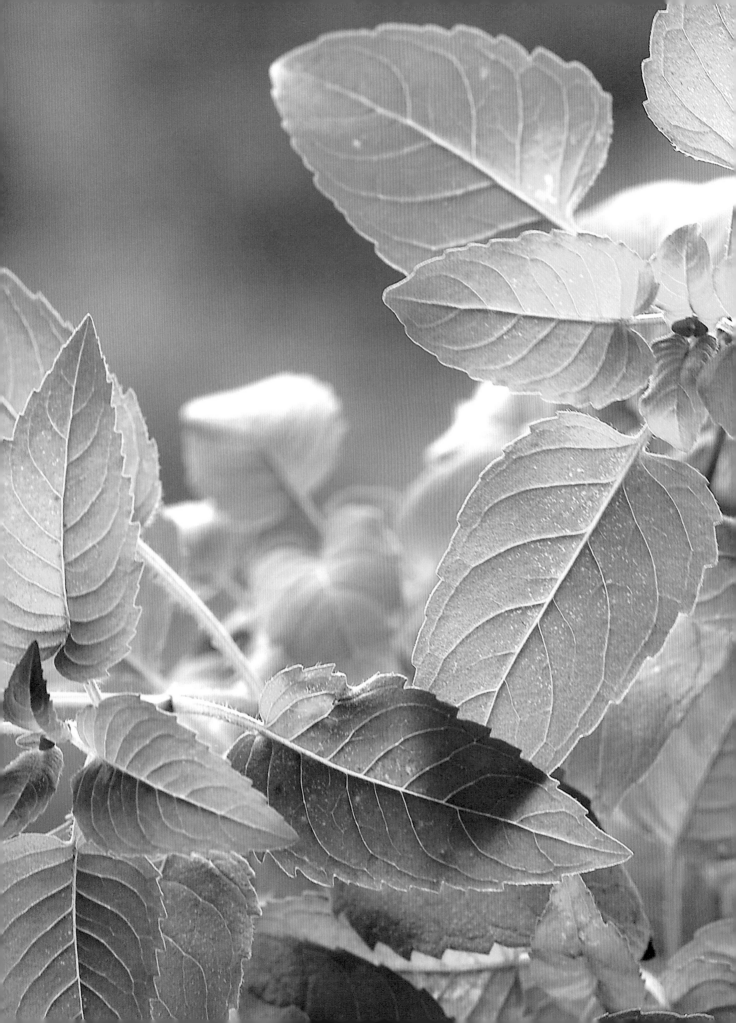

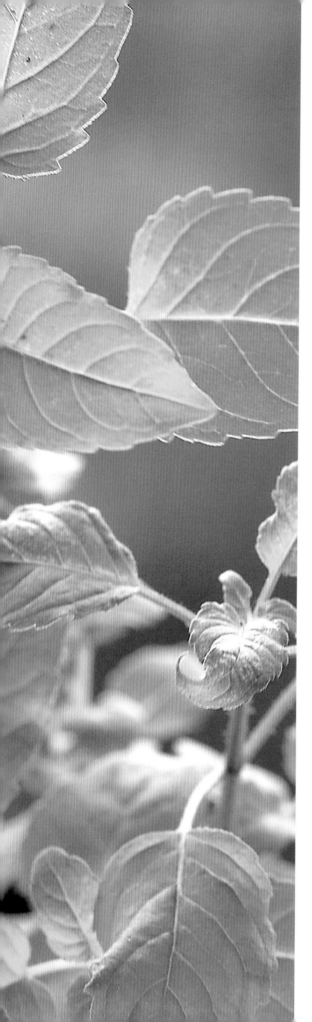
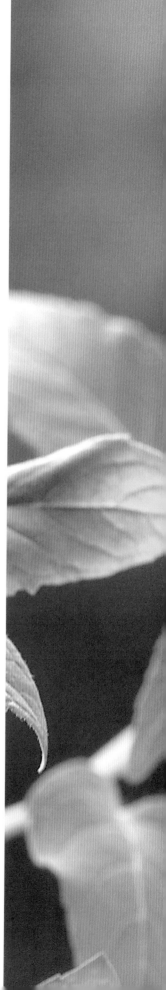

NATURAL HEALTH

Home-made products, which you can make using natural ingredients and pure essential oils, will be a pure pleasure to your nose and will also benefit your body. I hope that you enjoy making and using them as much as I do. Once you begin to use the essential oils, they fast become a daily delight and their therapeutic benefits become obvious. You will find, as I do, that your essence is nourished by the use of essential oils.

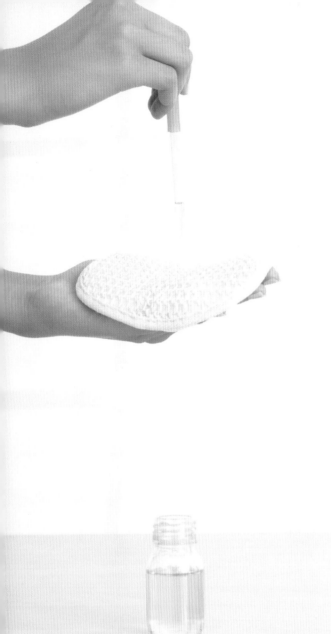

There couldn't have been a more unlikely place to have a mini factory than in the middle of our herb gardens overlooking the hills and the river. Yet we only had to step out of the door, basket in hand, to collect our magical ingredients from the garden.

We are now so used to the luxury of our own luscious toiletries, that we can no longer bear to use artificial, expensive chemical soups that pass as skin- and hair-care treatments. The following recipes are easy and inexpensive to make and a joy to use. I have created and made them in my laboratory, in the minute kitchen of our motor home, camped in the splendor of Australia's Snowy Mountains and in the silence of the desert, during the six years we spent being gypsies—beautiful and unlikely places to make moisturizers and shampoos.

The recipes in this chapter will pamper your skin and hair. Many of them won't feel or look like the shop-bought variety but you will quickly become used to the difference. Don't feel intimidated by the thought of making your own toiletries—it's no different from cooking a meal (much easier in some cases), and the quantities are not usually too critical. Many will need to be refrigerated but I have found that some of these recipes will freeze really well too.

Essential oils must be diluted with fixed or carrier oils before applying directly to the skin. Do not disregard the advisory percentages.

Getting started

People often ask me how I began making natural beauty and skin-care products. More than 30 years ago when we had our herb farm, a friend came to visit and asked if I could make cruelty-free toiletries using herbs and other natural ingredients. I said that I would try. One year later, Rivendell Skin and Hair Products was registered as a company. That sounds as though I waved a magic wand, but in truth, there was a great deal of both anguish and triumph between the faltering experiments in the kitchen and the launch of the laboratory and the business.

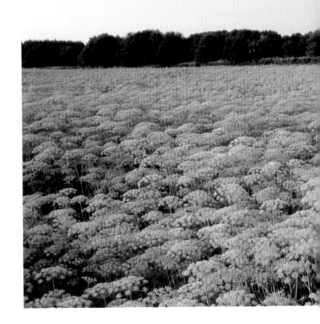

Equipment

To make the following recipes you will need equipment, kept separate from your kitchenware. If you have small children it's important that you be able to lock the store room or area in which you keep your essential oils and equipment.

It's wise to set aside special equipment (measuring spoons and cups, bowls for mixing, pans for heating) for making the recipes, as the powerfully perfumed essential oils are absorbed into wooden spoons and utensils and can ruin food with their strong perfume. Tea tree-flavored cheese can make a novelty but isn't gourmet! Beeswax and wool fat are difficult to clean off pans and dishes so it's best to save those pans for ointment making.

If you are making very small quantities of creams and lotions you can make them in the jar in which they will be stored.

Make sure that the equipment is scrupulously clean before you begin. This is important, as the cleaner your equipment and storage containers, the longer your aromatic products will keep fresh and uncontaminated.

All glass containers should be washed in hot soapy water, rinsed well, and dried at the bottom of an oven which is set on low.

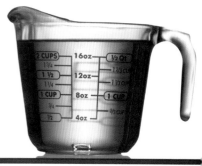

Alternatively, the bottles or jars can be boiled in water for 20 minutes—place a folded cloth in the bottom of the pan to keep them stable.

To make many of the recipes in this book you will need a double boiler, which is simply a pan in a pan. The mixture is in the top pan and the water in the bottom pan. The mixture is protected from burning by having no contact with direct heat and the temperature is easier to control.

Small amounts of the mixture may be made in a little jar that the preparation will be stored in, by standing the jar in warm water in a small shallow pan.

If you get involved in making many recipes you may find that you need some more sophisticated heat-resistant glass measuring flasks. These are expensive but you can add them to your collection of equipment one at any time.

GUIDE TO MEASURES

18–20 drops = 1 ml
90–100 drops = 5 ml = 1 teaspoon
$\frac{1}{4}$ (quarter) teaspoon = 1.25 ml
$\frac{1}{2}$ (half) teaspoon = 2.5 ml
1 teaspoon = 5 ml
1 tablespoon = 15 ml

See Practicalities for a more extensive conversion chart

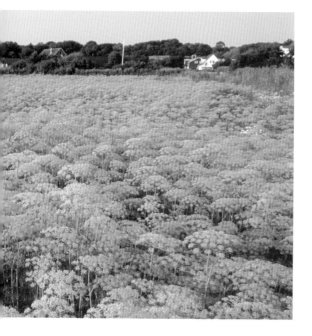

Dill plants in bloom form hundreds of tiny yellow cushions across fields in Bjare, Sweden.

* Essential oils must be measured very accurately as they are immensely powerful. If a recipe says to use two drops, then four drops will certainly not be better! Droppers or syringes and glass or plastic measures may be bought from pharmacies.
* The strength of herbal oil or liquid to be used is indicated by the terms "double-strength" or "triple-strength."

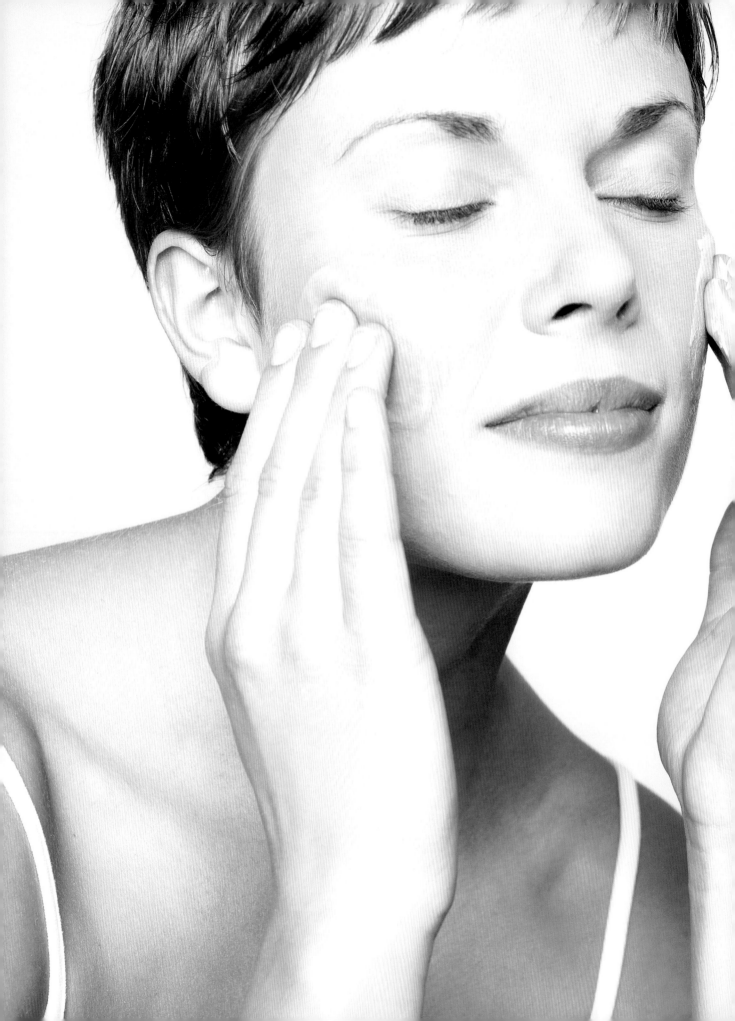

Skin care

Your skin deserves the best treatment you can give it.

As babies, we usually have perfect skin: Smooth, close-textured, moist, and with enough oil to protect but not cause problems. As we get older, hormonal changes, heredity factors, and the ageing process all begin to change the texture of our skin. We need to know how to care for our individual skin type in order to keep it looking as good as possible, and for as long as possible.

Skin is a complex structure that serves us well. It acts as an efficient envelope, a temperature regulator, a toxin excreter, and a sensory connector between the nervous system and outside stimuli. Our skin is made up of three layers: the epidermis, the dermis, and subcutaneous tissue.

Epidermis

This is the outer, visible layer. It is made up of flattened, dead and dying cells that overlap to form an elastic, water-resistant surface. New cells from beneath are constantly replacing these cells, the layer being renewed every month. All the layers are gradually replaced over a period of seven years.

Dermis

This layer produces the new cells that make their way up to the epidermis. The dermis contains oil glands, blood vessels, hair follicles, and nerves and is connected to the epidermis by collagen fibres.

Subcutaneous tissue

This is a fatty layer that provides a protective pad for underlying bone and organs, and also contains sweat glands.

Along with your hair, your skin usually shows the condition of your health. Stress, lack of sleep, poor diet, and illness are some of the conditions that can show in the skin. To keep your skin in the best possible condition, there are a few simple steps you can take. The rest is up to nature!

* Eat lots of fruit and vegetables.
* Drink six to eight glasses of water daily.
* Get six to eight hours sleep a night.
* Do some form of exercise daily, whatever you enjoy.
* Use the purest skin preparations that you can make or buy.
* Keep out of the sun during the hottest part of the day, use a good sunblock whenever you are outside in the summer, and wear a hat.
* Cultivate a positive attitude. Stress is about the worst thing for skin, giving it that lined, drawn look.

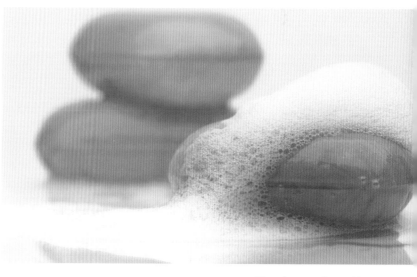

Natural, unscented, vegetable glycerine soaps are best for sensitive skin.

Following are recipes and treatments for every type of skin. If you do not have the essential oils listed in a particular recipe, consult the "Which essential oils to use when and where" table on page 250 and choose another oil with similar properties.

The recipes are suitable for both men and women. Men suffer from skin problems just as often as women do, but it is usually assumed that men "just have skin." In the recipes where fragrance lingers on the skin, I have suggested different oils for men, as the perfume of some of the essential oils might be perceived as too feminine.

Which essential oils to use when and where

Condition	Use
Acne and dermatitis	Chamomile, galbanum, geranium, immortelle, juniper, lavender, litsea cubeba, palmarosa, patchouli, rosewood, sandalwood
Ageing skin and hair	Carrot seed, frankincense, galbanum, geranium, lavender, rose, neroli, palmarosa, ylang-ylang
Allergies	Chamomile
All skin types	Geranium, jasmine, lavender, neroli, palmarosa, rose, rosewood
Antiseptic	All essential oils, to some degree, especially benzoin, geranium, lavender, juniper
Astringent	Benzoin, carrot seed, geranium, juniper, lemon, patchouli, rose, sandalwood
Balancer	Frankincense, geranium
Cell growth	Frankincense, geranium, immortelle, lavender, neroli, palmarosa, Peru balsam, rose
Cellulite	Grapefruit, juniper, lemon
Cracked, dry skin	Benzoin, sandalwood
Dehydrated skin	Carrot seed, sandalwood
Deodorant	Benzoin, bergamot, cypress, geranium, lavender, litsea cubeba, neroli, patchouli, rosewood
Dry skin and hair	Jasmine, rose, rosewood, palmarosa, lavender, sandalwood
Eczema	Chamomile, geranium, immortelle, juniper, lavender, palmarosa, Peru balsam
Elasticity	Benzoin, carrot seed, chamomile, neroli
Emollient	Chamomile, geranium, jasmine, lavender, rose, sandalwood
Fixative (perfume)	Benzoin, patchouli
Fungal infections	Benzoin, lavender, myrrh, patchouli, tea tree
Inflammation	Benzoin, chamomile, rose, sandalwood
Normal skin	Geranium, lavender, jasmine, neroli, palmarosa, rose, rosewood, ylang-ylang
Oily skin	Cypress, juniper, lemon, litsea cubeba, patchouli, rosewood, ylang-ylang
Preservative	Benzoin
Puffiness	Chamomile, geranium, rose
Scars	Carrot seed, chamomile, frankincense, geranium, juniper, lavender, lemon, patchouli, rosewood
Sebum regulator	Cypress, palmarosa
Sensitive skin	Chamomile, jasmine, neroli, rose
Thread veins	Chamomile, cypress, lavender, lemon, neroli, rose, rosewood
Wrinkles	Carrot seed, frankincense, lavender, palmarosa, patchouli, rose, rosewood

Caring for your face

Normal skin

Normal skin is fine-textured, smooth and soft with no large pores, blackheads, spots, flakes, or broken veins apparent. If a tissue is pressed to this skin first thing in the morning there will be only a trace of oil showing. If you are blessed with this type of skin you certainly are among the fortunate few, and should protect it with loving care. Protect it from wind, sun, dry air, and air conditioning by using light and gentle moisturizers, cleansers, and toners.

Oily skin

If you have oily skin, a tissue pressed to the face first thing in the morning will show quite a lot of oil. The texture of the skin is coarse with large pores and a tendency to blackheads and spots due to the pores being blocked with excessive sebum. The bonus of having oily skin is that it has less of a tendency to wrinkle than any other skin type—and will become less oily as you get older.

It is a mistake to use harsh soaps and strong astringents containing lots of alcohol in an attempt to control excessive oiliness, as these tend to stimulate the skin to produce more sebum and in the long run they make the situation worse.

Oily skin needs an oil-free moisturizer, except on the areas around the eyes, throat, and lips, where a richer moisturizer is needed. This type of skin benefits from regular use of masks and steams to help unblock pores and prevent blackheads from forming.

Combination skin

This type is a combination of normal/dry and oily skin. Press a tissue on your face first thing in the morning; if there is a greasy "T" shape on the tissue this will indicate combination skin. There may be a tendency to blackheads around the nose and pimples on the forehead or chin. There are often small greasy areas on the jaw line.

The program for this skin has to be oily/normal or oily/dry.

Dry skin

Dry skin is fine textured, delicate and thin with a tendency to line easily. I have skin of this type and rarely use soap and water as it makes my skin feel tight and as if it is going to crack!

All masks and steams need to be used with great care as they could encourage broken veins to which this type of skin can be prone.

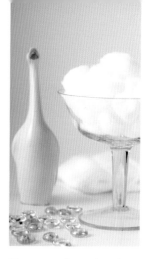

Use cotton wool to gently apply facial products.

Oil poured on the forehead—part of an Ayurvedic treatment.

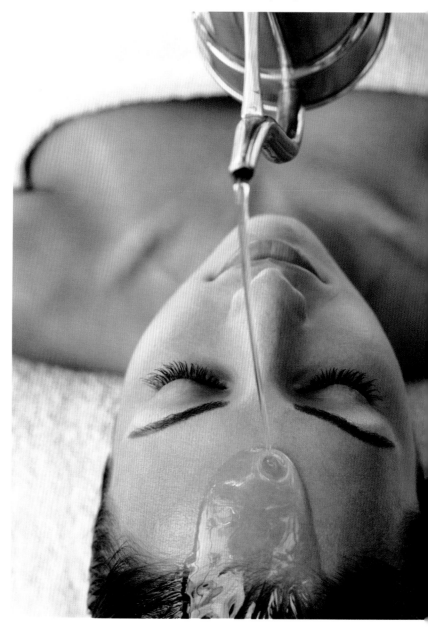

Fixed oils for skin types

Different oils react in different ways with the skin. For instance, grape seed and rice bran oil are good "all-rounders"—light, nourishing, almost dispersible in water and quickly absorbed into the skin. Wheat germ oil acts as a preservative, so it's good to include some in all massage oils. As a rule of thumb, you will find that the following oils are good for these skin types.

Dry skin: Almond, castor, cocoa butter, grape seed, olive, peanut, rice bran, wheat germ

Normal skin: Almond, corn, grape seed, peanut, sesame, rice bran, sunflower, safflower

Oily skin: Soybean

Oils which are easily absorbed into the skin (use for cosmetics) are: Corn, grape seed, rice bran, sesame, sunflower, and wheat germ.

Less easily absorbed oils (use for massage oils) are: Sweet almond, avocado, coconut, olive, apricot, and peanut.

Your skin-care routine

It's good to develop a skin-care routine to keep the skin in good condition, or to improve it if it's in poor condition. This needn't be time-consuming but it is as necessary as cleaning your teeth.

Two factors determine the number of times a day you need to follow this routine: The work you do (whether dusty or clean), and whether you live in the city with polluted air or in the country. Also, if you spend much time in air-conditioned rooms your skin will need more moisturizing.

The way you apply treatments to your face and throat is very important. Remember that skin loses its elasticity as it gets older, so use two fingers only, in gentle, non-stretching movements. Gravity is working against us as well, so always use upward movements in an effort to counteract this.

The therapist is pouring warmed oil onto the back in preparation for massage.

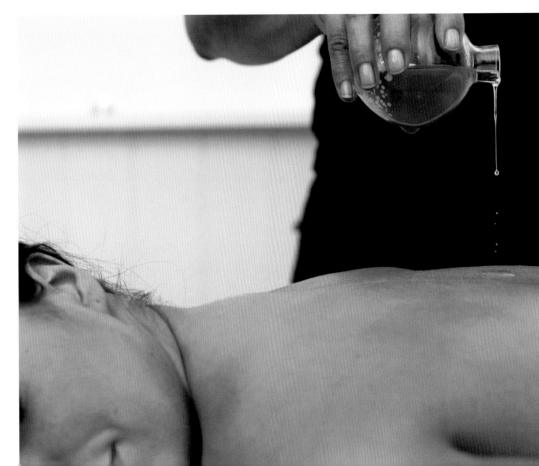

Herbs and ingredients for natural skin care

To care for normal skin

Cleanse with lotions or creams containing chamomile, dandelion, elder flower, honey, dried milk, oatmeal, or sage.

Deep cleanse with masks containing aloe vera, anise, caraway, castor oil, chamomile, egg yolk, elder flower, fennel, honey, lavender, dried milk, oatmeal, parsley, vinegar, or plain yoghurt.

Steam with chamomile, comfrey root, fennel, or red clover.

Nourish with moisturizers and masks of aloe vera, comfrey root, egg, honey, or plain yoghurt.

Tone with calendula, chamomile, cider vinegar, comfrey root, dandelion, elder flower, lavender, lemon balm, lemon grass, lemon juice, distilled witch hazel, or yarrow.

Caution: Overuse of yarrow can cause the skin to become sensitive to sunlight, making it more likely to pigment, often unevenly.

To care for dry skin

Cleanse with lotions or creams containing chamomile, dandelion, elder flower, honey, lemon balm, lemon grass, dried full-cream milk, or oatmeal.

Deep cleanse with masks containing aloe vera, anise, castor oil, chamomile, egg yolk, elder flower, fennel, honey, dried full-cream milk, oatmeal, parsley, or plain yoghurt.

Steam occasionally with chamomile, comfrey root, elder flower, mallow root, or red clover.

Nourish with moisturizers and masks of aloe vera, comfrey root, egg yolk, honey, or mallow root.

Tone with borage, chamomile, cider vinegar, elder flower, marjoram, or rosewater.

To care for sensitive skin

Cleanse with lotions or creams containing chamomile, elder flower, honey, dried full-cream milk, or oatmeal.

Deep cleanse—cleansing masks are not recommended for sensitive skin.

Steam with chamomile, comfrey root, fennel, or red clover.

Nourish with moisturizers and masks of aloe vera, comfrey root, or honey.

Tone with aloe vera, chamomile, comfrey root, mallow root, or rosewater.

To care for oily skin

Cleanse with lotions or creams containing borage, elder flower, honey, marjoram, oatmeal, parsley, peppermint, raspberry, or sage.

Deep cleanse with masks of bergamot, brewer's yeast, catnep, dandelion, whole egg, fennel, honey, lavender, lemon grass, lemon juice, marjoram, dried skim milk, oatmeal, parsley, plantain, sage, or yarrow.

Steam with anise, fennel, lavender, lemon grass, marjoram, plantain, raspberry, red clover, or yarrow.

Nourish with moisturizers and masks of aloe vera, comfrey, or honey.

Tone with bay, bergamot, calendula, cider vinegar, fennel, lavender, lemon balm, lemon grass, lemon juice, thyme, distilled witch hazel, or yarrow.

Caution: Overuse of yarrow can cause the skin to become sensitive to sunlight, making it more likely to pigment, often unevenly.

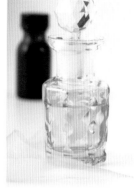

Essential oils are diluted for use in natural perfumes and colognes.

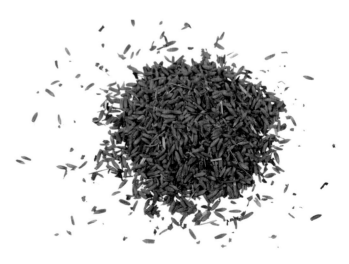

Cleansing

If you have oily skin in a dirty environment, you will need to cleanse at least twice a day. If your skin is normal or dry, then once a day should be sufficient. The evening is the best time to cleanse, to rid the skin of the grime and oil accumulated during the day.

The aim of cleansing is to rid the skin of excess grease, dead skin cells, and dirt. Some people don't feel clean unless they use soap and water on their face. This is fine if you are careful to use good-quality, vegetable glycerine soap and follow with a rinse designed to restore the skin's natural acid balance. For those who don't like soap (many people prefer not to use it on their faces), use oil, cleansing cream, or a lotion. Recipes for various types of cleansers are given.

Soaps

Soap-making from scratch is quite time-consuming. For most people, it is easier to use ready-made soap as the base, and the following recipes use this method. Buy the

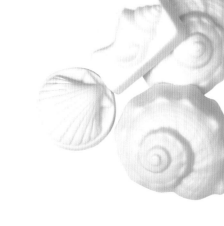

simplest, least expensive soap in your supermarket, preferably unperfumed and with no fancy additives. It is the ideal base to make a range of soaps which are inexpensive, cleansing, moisturizing, sweetly scented, and always a pleasure to use.

The amount of infusion or decoction needed in these recipes varies because the soap you buy can contain varying amounts of water. The less water you use, the better, as too much will cause a lot of shrinkage as the soap is maturing.

The soaps will dry more quickly if plenty of air can circulate around them. Drying time will be about six weeks.

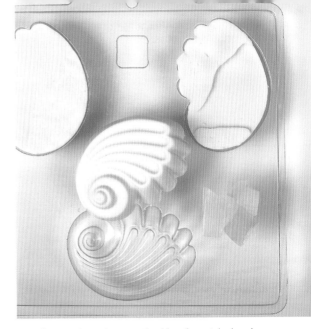

Press the soap mixture into greased molds to form nicely shaped bars of therapeutic soap.

LEMON AND CORN SOAP

This is a gently exfoliant soap, good for oily or combination skins.

4 cups (400 g) very finely grated soap
$1/2$ cup (125 ml) hot, triple-strength tea or decoction of your favorite herbs, strained
4 teaspoons vegetable glycerine
$1/4$ cup (40 g) fine polenta
$1/2$ teaspoon lemon essential oil

To make

In a double boiler, melt the soap into the tea or decoction and add the vegetable glycerine. Cool to lukewarm, add the polenta and essential oil and work in well.

Form into balls or press into greased molds such as soapboxes, small jelly molds, or baskets lined with cheesecloth. When set, remove from the molds and leave to dry.

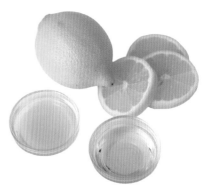

GENTLE TOUCH SOAP

This soap smells and feels wonderful on the skin. If you have very fine, dry skin, use this soap on your body. On the face it suits all skin types. I use orange peel, comfrey root, and mallow root decoction, and add orange oil to finish.

4 cups (400 g) finely grated soap
$^1/_2$ cup (125 ml) hot, triple-strength tea or decoction of your favorite herbs, strained through a sieve and then through coffee filter paper
2 teaspoons honey
2 teaspoons vegetable glycerine
$^1/_2$ teaspoon orange essential oil

To make

In a double boiler, melt the soap into the tea or decoction and add the honey and vegetable glycerine.

Cool to lukewarm, add the essential oil and work in well.

Form into balls or press into greased moulds such as soapboxes, small jelly molds, or baskets lined with cheesecloth.

When set, remove from the molds and leave to dry out completely.

LAVENDER DREAM SOAP

Suitable for normal or dry skins.
This soap has little lather but is so gentle on your skin that you will overlook the lack of froth. A good face or body cream or any of the "oil-in-water" moisture cream recipes in this book will be suitable for this recipe. Don't use a "water-in-oil" emulsion, as the effect won't be the same.

2$^1/_2$ cups (250 g) finely grated soap or soap flakes
$^1/_2$ cup (125 ml) warm water
$^1/_4$ cup (60 g) moisture cream
6 drops lavender essential oil
3 drops geranium essential oil
2 drops rosemary essential oil

To make

In a double boiler, melt the soap into $^1/_2$ cup (125 ml) warm water and add the moisture cream. Remove from heat, cool to lukewarm, add the essential oils, and work in well.

Form into balls or press into greased molds such as soapboxes, small jelly molds, or baskets lined with cheesecloth.

When set, remove from the molds and leave to dry out completely.

CITRUS GLORY

This soap suits all skins except the very dry or sensitive.

2$^1/_2$ cups (250 g) finely grated soap or soap flakes
$^1/_2$ cup (125 ml) warm water
$^1/_2$ cup (100 g) finely ground almonds
2 drops grapefruit essential oil
2 drops lavender essential oil
2 drops lime essential oil
2 drops lemon essential oil
2 drops orange essential oil

To make

In a double boiler, melt the soap into $^1/_2$ cup (125 ml) warm water

Remove from the heat and add the ground almonds, mixing thoroughly.

Cool to lukewarm, add the essential oils, and work in well.

Form into balls or press into greased molds such as soapboxes, small jelly molds, or baskets lined with cheesecloth.

When set, remove from the molds and leave to dry out completely.

FOREST SPICE

This is one for the boys.

2$^1/_2$ cups (250 g) finely grated soap or soap flakes
$^1/_2$ cup (125 ml) warm water
$^1/_4$ cup (50 g) ground oats
1 drop nutmeg essential oil
1 drop pine essential oil
2 drops cedar essential oil
4 drops lemon essential oil
2 drops sandalwood essential oil

To make

In a double boiler, melt the soap into $^1/_2$ cup (125 ml) warm water

Remove from the heat and add the ground oats, mixing thoroughly.

Cool to lukewarm, add the essential oils and work in well.

Form into balls or press into greased molds such as soapboxes, small jelly molds, or baskets lined with cheesecloth.

When set, remove from the molds and leave to dry.

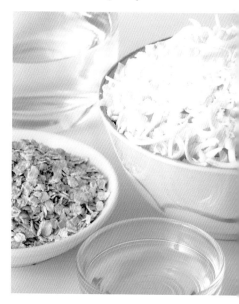

The raw ingredients ready to make Forest Spice soap.

Lotion and cream cleansers

Those of you who prefer not to use soap on your face will find the following cleansing lotion and cream cleansers to be non-drying and gentle.

ROSEWATER CLEANSING LOTION

Those troubled with pimples or acne will benefit from this oil-free cleanser.

$1/3$ cup (80 ml) rosewater
1 cup (250 ml) distilled or purified water
$1/4$ teaspoon glycerine
12 drops essential oil (suitable for your skin type)

To make and use

Mix all ingredients together in a 7 fl oz (200 ml) bottle and shake well to blend thoroughly. Leave for 4 days to synergize, shaking occasionally.

Filter mixture through coffee filter paper.

Store in a dark-colored glass bottle and shake well before use.

Take a palm-sized piece of absorbent cotton (cottonwool), dip it in warm water and squeeze out well.

Flatten it out into a pad, sprinkle with Rosewater Cleansing Lotion and use to cleanse throat and face. Repeat if necessary.

There is no need to use a toner after this treatment as it is quite mild.

WASHING LOTION

Use a special washing lotion to cleanse the face if the skin is very sensitive, or if it is troubled with acne, pimples, or other skin problems. This water may also be used as a moisturizing lotion with the addition of one teaspoon of sweet almond oil, or other fine-textured oil.

$2 1/2$ tablespoons (40 ml) rosewater
$1/4$ cup (60 ml) purified water
$1/4$–$1/2$ teaspoon glycerine (try $1/4$ teaspoon first, and increase to $1/2$ teaspoon if you like it)
6 drops essential oil (suitable for your skin type)

To make and use

Mix all ingredients together in a $3 1/2$ fl oz (100 ml) bottle and shake well to blend thoroughly. Leave for 4 days to synergize, shaking occasionally.

Filter mixture through coffee filter paper.

Store in a dark-colored glass bottle and shake well before use.

Take a palm-sized piece of absorbent cotton (cottonwool), dip it in warm water and squeeze out well.

Flatten it out into a pad, sprinkle with Washing Lotion and use to cleanse throat and face. Repeat if necessary.

There is no need to use a toner after this treatment as it is quite mild.

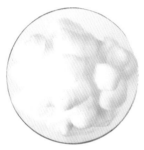

Tinted plastic or glass jars make home-made products look really professional—and they make perfect gifts!

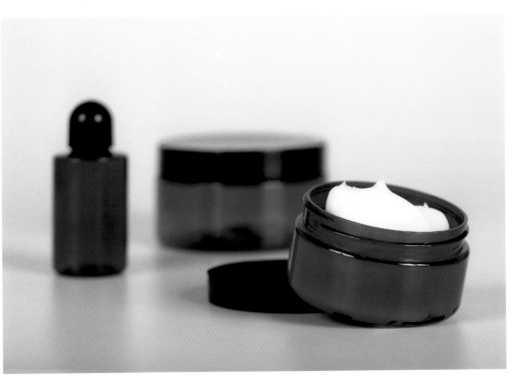

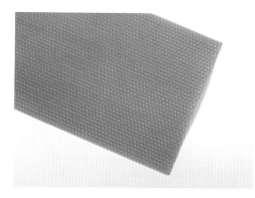

OLIVE AND ROSEWATER CLEANSER

Olive oil is very softening to the skin and rosewater gives a delicate and well-loved perfume to the cream. It is suitable for dry and normal skins.

1 oz (30 g) beeswax
$3^1/_2$ fl oz (100 ml) olive oil
2 tablespoons (30 ml) rosewater
1 level teaspoon borax

To make

In a small double boiler, gently melt the wax and oil together.

Cool to just above hand heat but still liquid.

Heat the rosewater in a separate double boiler to just above hand heat and dissolve the borax into the warm rosewater.

Add slowly to the wax mixture, stirring constantly. If the mixture begins to solidify, heat a little to soften it.

Stir until no separate drops of water can be seen in the solution.

Pot and label. Store in a cool, dark place.

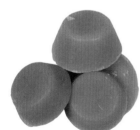

MILK AND HONEY CLEANSER

This is a quick and stimulating cleanser for all skin types. It removes dead skin, oil, and grime.

1 teaspoon dried milk powder
1 teaspoon finely ground almond meal
2 teaspoons honey
$^1/_2$ teaspoon rosewater
3 drops almond or sunflower oil

To make and use

Mix all the ingredients together in a small bowl.

Pat on from the base of the throat up to the hairline (but not around the eyes).

Massage gently into the skin and rinse off with lukewarm water.

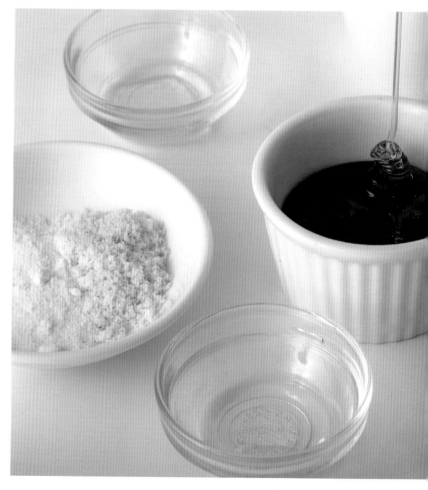

Milk and Honey Cleanser—ready to mix.

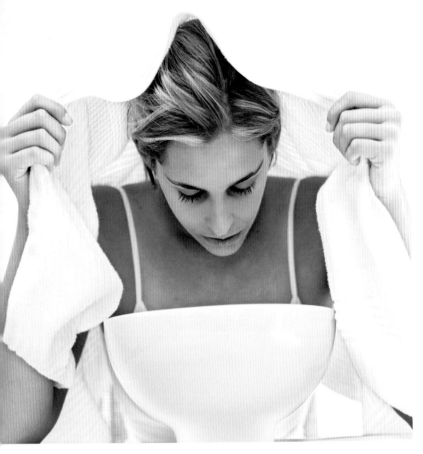

Facial steaming cleanses the skin of impurities in a gentle way.

Facial steaming

Facial steaming causes the skin to perspire, which in turn helps to loosen grime, dead skin cells, and hardened sebum. The heat increases the blood supply to the surface of the skin and also hydrates it, giving a more youthful, softer skin tone with a clearer, brighter color.

If thread veins are a problem, you will need to be very careful when steaming. Apply a thick layer of moisturizer, or night cream, over the veined area and hold your face about 16 in (40 cm) away from the steam—no closer. Do not steam your face more than once every two weeks.

People with normal, oily, and combination skin types may use facial steaming as often as twice a week, if liked.

If your water is chlorinated, it's wise to use either rain or distilled water for steaming, or, failing this, expose a bowl of tap water to the air for 24 hours to evaporate away the chlorine. The steam from chlorinated water carries chlorine gas, which can be harmful.

TIP REMEMBER THAT IN AN EMERGENCY, LAVENDER FIXES ALMOST ANYTHING.

MAKING AND USING FACIAL STEAMS

Place all ingredients listed for the blend in a bottle and shake to combine.

If possible leave for four days to synergize. Store in a dark, cool place.

Shake well before use. Use one teaspoon of the selected blend for each facial steam treatment.

HAVING A FACIAL STEAM

Have ready a shower cap, a large towel, and a heatproof pad for the table. Wash or cleanse the face. Put on the shower cap.

Place 2 quarts (2 liters) of boiling water in a bowl; set the bowl on a heatproof, non-slip mat on the table.

Add two drops essential oil, or one teaspoon of one of the steaming blends (recipes follow) on the surface of the water. Quickly form a tent with the towel over the bowl and your head.

Keep your face about 12 in (30 cm) away from the steam (for skin with no thread veins only), close your eyes and enjoy the facial steam for about 5–10 minutes.

Next, splash your face with cool (not cold) water and finish with a face tonic and some moisturizing cream.

FACIAL STEAM FOR NORMAL AND COMBINATION SKIN

$\frac{1}{4}$ cup (60 ml) sweet almond oil
8 drops geranium essential oil
6 drops palmarosa essential oil
6 drops lavender essential oil

FACIAL STEAM FOR DRY SKIN

$\frac{1}{4}$ cup (60 ml) light olive oil
8 drops rose essential oil
8 drops palmarosa essential oil
6 drops lavender essential oil

FACIAL STEAM FOR OILY SKIN

$\frac{1}{4}$ cup (60 ml) rice bran oil
12 drops cypress essential oil
4 drops patchouli essential oil
4 drops ylang-ylang essential oil

FACIAL STEAM FOR AGEING AND MATURE SKIN

$\frac{1}{4}$ cup (60 ml) grape seed oil
12 drops chamomile essential oil
6 drops frankincense essential oil
2 drops lavender or rose essential oil

Facial scrubs

Facial scrubs exfoliate the skin, meaning they clear excessive oiliness, refine, and unplug pores, improve circulation, and generally nourish the skin. They leave the skin looking fresh and rosy.

The frequency with which you use scrubs and masks depends entirely on your skin type. If you have oily, blemished skin, you will be able to use these preparations once or twice a week but if your skin is fine and dry, choose only the most gentle treatment, and use it maybe once every two weeks.

Scrubs should never be used where there are thread veins, as they would stimulate the area, and possibly aggravate the condition.

You can use many ingredients such as oat flakes, sugar, wheat germ, bamboo powder, dried herbs, nuts, or dried legumes as the exfoliant, but any of these need either grinding in a coffee grinder, or pestle and mortar, to a fine consistency. If too coarse they can cause small cuts in the skin.

I like to use some oil in a scrub as it makes it easier to apply and feels gentler.

Cider vinegar is a useful addition as it maintains the natural acidity of the skin. Orange juice is a good substitute for dry skins. Yeast stimulates the circulation, bringing blood to the surface of the skin. Use for oily skin only. Yoghurt nourishes and balances skin pH. Honey deep cleanses, hydrates, and has a natural antiseptic action. No more than two drops of essential oil should be used in a single application scrub.

MAKING AND USING FACIAL SCRUBS

Mix all the ingredients together to form a paste.

Massage gently into the skin of the face and throat, rinse off with lukewarm water, and pat dry.

Apply moisturizing cream or lotion.

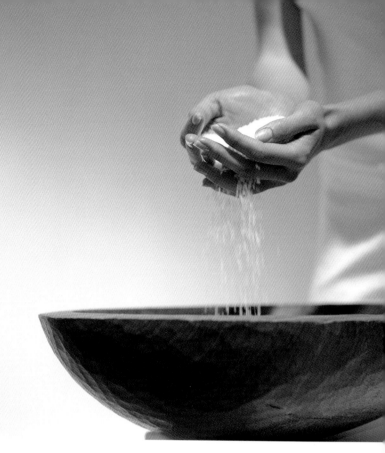

Gently mix the dry ingredients for your scrub before storing in an airtight container.

BASIC SCRUB MIX

Mix the dry ingredients for this scrub in bulk and store in a labeled, airtight container and use as needed in scrub recipes such as the Milk and Honey Scrub or similar.

4 parts fine oatmeal
1 part fine polenta
2 parts ground almonds
$\frac{1}{2}$ part kaolin
$\frac{1}{2}$ part raw sugar

MILK AND HONEY SCRUB

1 teaspoon honey
1 teaspoon vegetable glycerine
2 drops lavender or palmarosa essential oil
1–2 teaspoons Basic Scrub Mix
milk, to mix

To make and use

Mix the honey, glycerine, and essential oil together in a small bowl.

Blend in one or two teaspoons of the Basic Scrub Mix and enough milk to make a soft paste.

Wet your face, put a little mixture into the palm of your hand and massage the scrub onto the skin in a gentle, circular motion.

Splash off with cool water.

Apply moisturizing cream or lotion.

Masks

Masks are very beneficial treatments for all skins. They can improve color and texture, deep cleanse, remove dead cells from the surface, and bring fresh color and life to sallow skin.

MAKING AND USING MASKS

Spread the mask over your face and neck (if you have dry skin or broken veins be very careful as masks may be overstimulating).

Lie down on your bed or in the bath with pads of absorbent cotton (cottonwool) soaked in distilled witch hazel, or cooled chamomile tea, or cucumber slices on your eyes.

Now, relax, and let your mind drift for 15–20 minutes.

Wash the mask off in lukewarm water followed by a cool splash.

Apply a moisturizer.

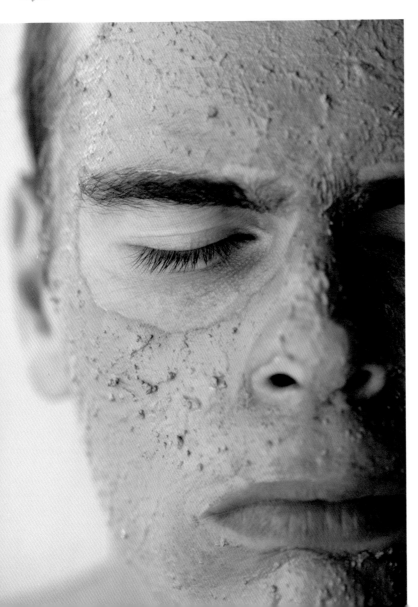

Green herb mask is especially useful for men as it exfoliates the different skin types present on the face.

BASIC MASK

The Basic Mask may be made in advance and stored in an airtight jar ready for mixing one tablespoon to a soft paste with water. Add yoghurt, honey, fruit juice or pulp, vinegar, egg, or oil if liked.

2½ oz (75 g) Fuller's Earth or kaolin
2 tablespoons cornstarch (cornflour)
1 tablespoon finely ground oats
1 tablespoon finely ground almond meal
15 drops essential oils suitable for your skin type

To make

Combine all dry ingredients together well in a small bowl. Add the essential oils a drop at a time, stirring well to prevent lumping.

Mix well, bottle, label, and store in a tightly covered jar.

MILK AND ORANGE MASK FOR NORMAL SKIN

1 egg, beaten
1 teaspoon olive oil
2 teaspoons orange juice
1 teaspoon honey
1 drop rose or geranium essential oil
1 drop rosewood or jasmine essential oil
dried milk powder, to mix

To make and use

Mix all the ingredients together in a small bowl, adding just enough dried milk powder to make a smooth paste.

Smooth over your face and neck and leave for 15 minutes.

Rinse off and apply a moisturizer.

YEAST AND YOGHURT MASK FOR OILY AND COMBINATION SKIN

4 teaspoons brewer's yeast
1½ teaspoons yoghurt
1 teaspoon distilled witch hazel
1 teaspoon olive oil
1 teaspoon wheat germ oil
1 drop palmarosa essential oil
1 drop lemon essential oil
finely ground rolled oats or kaolin clay powder

To make and use

Mix all the ingredients together in a small bowl, using just enough rolled oats or kaolin to make a soft paste.

Smooth over your face and neck and leave for 15 minutes.

Rinse off and apply a moisturizer.

EGG AND ALMOND MASK FOR SENSITIVE SKIN

1 egg yolk, beaten
1 teaspoon jojoba oil
$^1/_2$ teaspoon honey
1 drop chamomile essential oil
1 drop carrot seed essential oil
1 teaspoon powdered milk or cornstarch (cornflour)
water or rosewater, to mix

To make and use

Combine the egg yolk, jojoba oil, honey, and essential oils in a small bowl.

Add the powdered milk or cornstarch and mix well.

Add enough water or rosewater to make a smooth paste.

Smooth over your face and neck and leave for 15 minutes.

Rinse off and apply a moisturizer.

ARROWROOT MASK

This is a very useful mask, as the honey attracts, and holds moisture in the skin. By choosing your own herbs, this recipe can be adapted for any skin type or problem. For a thicker or thinner mask, vary the amount of arrowroot. The mixture thickens as it cools.

2 teaspoons arrowroot
2 teaspoons honey
$^3/_4$ cup (180 ml) double-strength infusion or
    decoction of your favorite herbs
1 teaspoon infused oil

To make and use

In a saucepan, mix the arrowroot and honey to a smooth paste with a little of the infusion.

Stir in the remaining infusion and cook, stirring, until thickened. Add the infused oil.

Smooth over your face and neck and leave for 15 minutes.

Rinse off and apply a moisturizer.

This mask keeps well without refrigeration except in very hot weather.

ARROWROOT OR CORNSTARCH MASK BASE

Make this jelly to suit your own needs, adding only a little water at first and thinning if you find the mixture too thick. Slowly add $^1/_2$–$^2/_3$ cup (125–160 ml) of cold water to two teaspoons of either arrowroot or cornstarch. Bring to the boil in a small saucepan, stirring all the time. Cool until lukewarm. Now add your choice of mashed herbs, fruit, vegetables, or any other nutrient-filled mask ingredient.

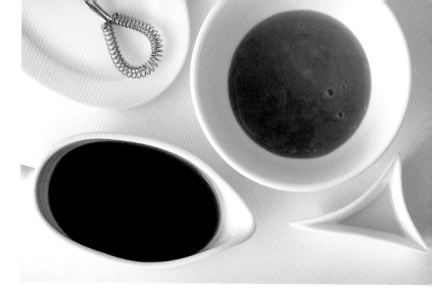

Double-strength infusion and infused oil ready to add to arrowroot and honey mix to make Arrowroot Mask.

GREEN HERB MASK

This is suitable for all skin types, depending on the herbs chosen.

2 handfuls fresh herbs, finely chopped
$2^1/_2$ tablespoons (40 ml) distilled or purified water
1 teaspoon honey
dried milk powder or wheat germ

To make and use

Blend or mash the herbs, water, and honey together until pulpy and very fine.

Add enough dried milk or wheat germ to make a soft paste.

Pat onto your face and throat and lie down for 10–20 minutes.

Rinse off with lukewarm water and apply a moisturizer.

OILY SKIN MASK

1 tablespoon dried and powdered lemon grass
$^1/_4$ teaspoon brewer's yeast
1 tablespoon plain yoghurt
kaolin or oat flour, to mix

To make and use

Mix together the lemon grass, yeast, and yoghurt in a small bowl. Add enough kaolin or oat flour to form a soft paste.

Pat onto your face and throat and leave for 10–20 minutes. Rinse off with lukewarm water and apply a moisturizer.

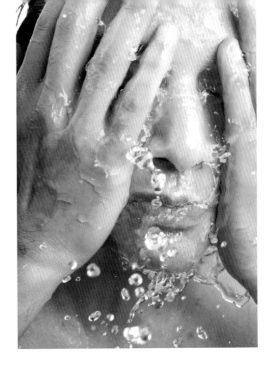

Toners and astringents

Toners and astringents remove surplus oil from the skin, gently stimulate the circulation, restore the skin's acid mantle, and leave it feeling fresh and clean.

Toners and astringents may also be used to remove makeup or as a freshener during the day.

Toners which contain alcohol, or a large amount of distilled witch hazel, are called astringents and they should not be used on dry, sensitive, or ageing skin. Even very oily skin types should avoid too-frequent applications of astringents containing a lot of alcohol, as this stimulates the oil glands.

There are two basic methods for applying toners and astringents.

1. Wet some absorbent cotton (cottonwool) with water and squeeze dry (this prevents waste of your precious lotion). Sprinkle with a few drops of the lotion and gently stroke the absorbent cotton (cottonwool) upward over your throat and face.

2. Press the damp absorbent cotton (cottonwool) flat and fold in half. Pour on a little toner, hold a corner of the wool and slap your face quite briskly (avoiding the cheeks where those delicate veins break really easily). This treatment brings a nourishing, cleansing, blood supply flowing to the skin and gets rid of a sluggish, pasty appearance.

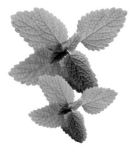

A splash of natural aftershave first thing in the morning tones the skin and closes the pores.

When making the Gentle Rose Toner, witch hazel can be substituted for purified water, if your skin is oily.

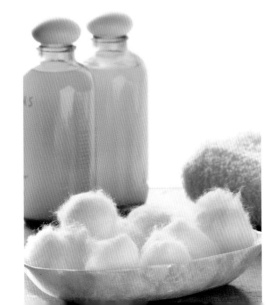

"TOP OF THE MORNING" ASTRINGENT OR AFTERSHAVE

For oily and combination skin.

$1/2$ cup (125 ml) distilled witch hazel
$1/4$ cup (60 ml) distilled or purified water
4 teaspoons cider vinegar
5 drops sandalwood essential oil
2 drops spearmint essential oil
$1/4$–$1/2$ teaspoon glycerine

To make
Place all the ingredients in a bottle and shake to blend.

If possible leave for four days to synergize. Label and store in a dark, cool place.

Shake well before use.

GENTLE ROSE TONER

For dry and ageing skin. If your skin is normal or combination, you can substitute witch hazel for the water content.

This is a simple and effective toner made from rosewater—one of the gentlest and best known skin tonics.

$3/4$ cup (180 ml) rosewater
$1/4$ cup (60 ml) distilled or purified water
3 drops rosewood or rose essential oil
3 drops palmarosa essential oil
$1/2$ teaspoon glycerine

To make
Place all the ingredients in a bottle and shake to blend. If possible leave for four days to synergize.

Label and store in a dark, cool place. Shake well before use.

COSMETIC VINEGAR

This vinegar may be used not only as a skin toner but as a deodorant, hair rinse, wound wash, and bath additive. The dilution rate is a matter of personal preference. I would never use more than two teaspoons in 1 cup (250 ml) of water as a facial rinse or after-shower splash, but would use it neat as a deodorant. Your skin type also determines the dilution, oily skins being able to tolerate a much stronger mix.

$2^{1}/_{4}$ oz (60 g) fresh herbs
2 cups (500 ml) cider vinegar
4 teaspoons vegetable glycerine

To make

Chop the herbs very finely.

Heat half the vinegar to just below boiling point and immediately add the herbs. Remove from heat, cool.

Pour into a jar, close with a non-metal lid and leave for a week, shaking several times a day.

Strain through a sieve and then through coffee filter paper and add the remaining vinegar.

If you want a very strong vinegar you can repeat the process of heating the vinegar and adding fresh herbs once, or even twice more.

Add the vegetable glycerine, then bottle and label. This vinegar keeps well without refrigeration except in very hot weather.

ROSE PETAL SKIN TONER

The following is a simple and effective toner for all skins. If your skin is dry you can increase the rosewater and decrease the witch hazel. If your skin is oily you can do the reverse.

Rosewater is a gentle skin tonic and may be bought from any good pharmacy. Witch hazel is another well-known tonic. It is stronger than rosewater and should be tested on a small area before use on sensitive skin.

$^{1}/_{2}$ cup (125 ml) rosewater
$^{1}/_{4}$ cup (60 ml) distilled witch hazel
$^{1}/_{2}$–1 teaspoon vegetable glycerine

To make

Mix all the ingredients together in a small bowl.

Bottle, label, and store in a cool dark place. Shake well before use.

SUNRISE AFTERSHAVE

For normal and combination skin.

Use this gentle but thorough aftershave to help contract the skin after shaving without drying it out.

$^{1}/_{4}$ cup (60 ml) distilled witch hazel
$^{1}/_{4}$ cup (60 ml) distilled or purified water
5 drops sandalwood essential oil
3 drops benzoin essential oil
2 drops rosemary essential oil
$^{1}/_{4}$ teaspoon glycerine

To make

Place all the ingredients in a bottle and shake to blend. If possible leave for four days to synergize.

Label and store in a dark, cool place. Shake well before use.

MINT ZINGER

Another blend for men that can be used as an aftershave or toner. It will leave the face feeling cool and clean.

$^{3}/_{4}$ cup (180 ml) distilled or purified water
$^{1}/_{4}$ cup (60 ml) witch hazel
3 drops peppermint essential oil
2 drops spearmint essential oil
2 drops lemon essential oil
2 drops lavender essential oil
2 drops clove essential oil
1 teaspoon glycerine
$^{1}/_{4}$ teaspoon tincture of benzoin

To make

Mix all the ingredients in a jar. Leave for one week, shaking often.

Strain through coffee filter paper before bottling in amber glass bottles.

Label and store in a cook, dark place. Shake well before using.

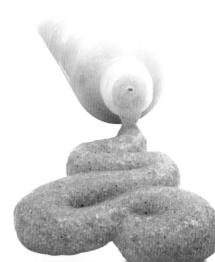

KEEPING NATURAL PREPARATIONS FREE FROM BACTERIA AND MOLD

Unless you add a preservative, most home-made preparations such as moisturizers made with oil-in-water formulas and containing liquid ingredients (herb teas, juices, and decoctions in particular) will last for only a couple of weeks or so, even with refrigeration.

To keep your preparations free from mold and bacteria, you need to use some form of preservative that either kills or inhibits the growth of bacteria and acts as an antioxidant to slow down oxidation.

If you choose to go "natural," there are ways in which you can guard against contamination and also boost the activity of your chosen "natural" preservative and antioxidant. The first point to make is that you must be constantly vigilant about cleanliness when making preparations.

OILS

Choose oils and essential oils that have a long shelf life but that also contain the skin-care properties that you seek.

- Many essential oils have antibacterial and antifungal properties that can be used to boost the action in conjunction with other natural preservatives. Be sure not to exceed the allowed percentages and check that the oils are suitable for the product in which you will be using them.
- Cold-pressed oils contain vitamins that also help to act as a preservative.

HERBS

Almost all herbs have an antibacterial action, some more than others; and many also have an antifungal and antioxidant action.

Filter herbal infusions through filter paper to remove any solid plant matter, use as quickly as possible and re-boil before use.

WATER

Always use distilled water, not tap water.

PACKAGING AND STORING

The containers you use can also determine for how long your creams and lotions will remain fresh. Jars are the most at risk as they are being constantly exposed to air and bacteria on fingers. Bottles, particularly those that stand on their caps (Malibu tubes for example) are ideal as air contact is minimal.

- Fill bottles to the top and tap to get rid of trapped air.
- Store finished products and raw materials under dry, dark, and cool conditions.

USING PRESERVATIVES

Without preservation, creams and lotions can become very dangerous very quickly and although I have successfully used natural preservatives, you must have absolutely sterile lab conditions and a large range of antibacterial and antifungal essential oils.

There are many, many synthetic preservatives on the market but the only one that I can recommend is phenoxyethanol (brand names Optiphen or Optiphen Plus). And this is the preservative I have used in the recipes in this book.

Caution: Avoid the paraben family of preservatives, and also those that are formaldehyde releasers.

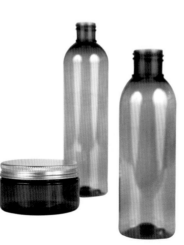

Phenoxyethanol

Phenoxyethanol, also known as phenoxetol (Optiphen) is clear, viscous, glycol ether. Although effective against bacteria, it has limitations against fungus, and for this reason should be combined with a co-preservative that is active against fungus. It is used by many dermatologists to preserve their topical creams and also as a fixative in perfumes.

Phenoxyethanol is used at a concentration of one percent; that is, 2–3 drops to every $3^1/_3$ oz (1 g to every 99 g) of other ingredients.

It isn't a very strong fungicide so I recommend using it in conjunction with potassium sorbate at 0.1–0.2 percent (Optiphen Plus).

Potassium sorbate

This is a white crystalline powder, with no odor, that is easily soluble in cold water. It is a very effective against molds, yeast, and aerophile bacteria. In water, potassium sorbate releases sorbic acid, the active agent. It is widely used as preservative in foods and cosmetics. It's even more effective used in conjunction with grapefruit seed extract.

Use 0.1–0.2 percent (in combination with phenoxyethanol)

BUYING PRESERVATIVES

The trade names for phenoxyethanol and phenoxetol are Optiphen or Optiphen Plus. They are available from either: www.theherbarie.com or www.heirloombodycare.com.au

Read the notes that come with your preservative very carefully, or ask your supplier for directions for use. Most preservatives need to be added at a particular temperature and phase. They may lose their efficacy if added too soon. Always ask your supplier for details about your purchase, percentage to use, safety precautions, etc.

If you are proposing to sell to the public you will need to get your products tested by a laboratory to ensure that your preservative system is effective.

Moisturizing

In order to introduce moisture to the skin we need to use both oil and water. Used alone, water evaporates—but when it is used in combination with oil, the water is held on the skin until it is massaged in. The following range of moisturizing recipes includes something for all skin types.

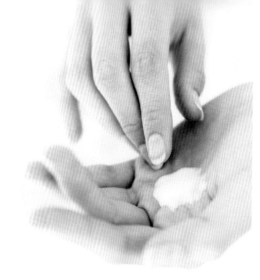

Warming the moisturizer in your hand before applying will help absorption.

PRIMROSE PATH MOISTURIZING OIL

For dry skin.

2$\frac{1}{2}$ tablespoons (40 ml) sweet almond oil
2$\frac{1}{2}$ tablespoons (40 ml) olive oil
1 teaspoon avocado oil
1 teaspoon wheat germ oil
60 drops evening primrose oil
20 drops borage seed oil
10 drops jojoba oil
10 drops palmarosa essential oil (sandalwood for men)
5 drops carrot seed essential oil
5 drops rosewood essential oil
5 drops lavender essential oil
2 drops sandalwood essential oil (benzoin for men)
2 drops patchouli essential oil (neroli or frankincense for men)

To make

Place all the ingredients in a bottle and shake to blend. If possible leave for four days to synergize.

Label and store in a dark, cool place. Shake well before use.

DEW DROPS MOISTURIZING OIL

For normal and combination skin.

$\frac{1}{3}$ cup (80 ml) sweet almond oil
1 teaspoon avocado oil
1 teaspoon wheat germ oil
30 drops evening primrose oil
10 drops jojoba oil
10 drops palmarosa essential oil (sandalwood for men)
5 drops carrot seed essential oil
5 drops rosewood essential oil
5 drops geranium essential oil (benzoin for men)
5 drops ylang-ylang essential oil (neroli or frankincense for men)

To make

Place all the ingredients in a bottle and shake to blend. If possible leave for four days to synergize.

Label and store in a dark, cool place. Shake well before use.

SATIN SKIN GEL

For oily, combination and normal skin.

This gel provides a lovely oil-free treatment for oily skin.

8 drops carrot seed essential oil
6 drops litsea cubeba or patchouli essential oil
8 drops lavender essential oil
3 drops juniper essential oil
3$\frac{1}{2}$ oz (100 g) 95% or 100% aloe vera gel

To make

Add all the oils to the gel in a small bowl and mix well.

Blending might take a little time and needs to done very thoroughly.

If possible leave for four days to synergize.

Bottle, label, and store in a dark, cool place. Shake well before use.

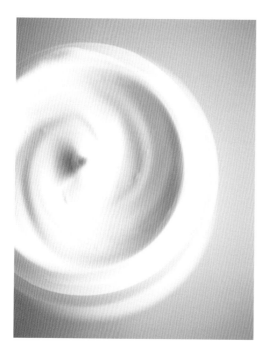

Glass jars are good for face creams and gels.

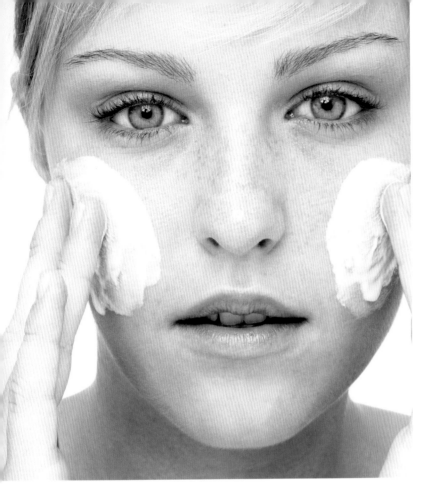

Apply Skin Mayo in an upward motion on your cheeks.

Opposite: Make sure all your bottles, brushes, towels, and bowls are perfectly clean when making and applying your own moisturizer.

SKIN MAYO

Skin Mayo is a simple, wholesome moisturizer that is nourishing for all skins. It is suitable for men, women, and children. (Children's skin needs protection as much as that of adults if the climate is harsh, but this protection needs to be very light and non-clogging to those fine pores.)

This is basically a mayonnaise, although the taste isn't as good as the action! It moisturizes, feeds, balances, and leaves your skin soft. As well as moisturizing, you can use it as a pre-shampoo treatment, bath oil, after-shower oil, or hand cream.

1 egg yolk, or 1 whole egg if you have oily skin
$\frac{1}{2}$ teaspoon white wine vinegar
1 cup (250 ml) infused oil (this is approximate—it depends how thick you want the moisturizer)
$1\frac{1}{2}$ tablespoons plain yoghurt
30 drops essential oil

To make

Beat the egg and vinegar in a blender until well mixed. Add the oil slowly in a thin trickle until the mixture is very thick.

Mix the remaining ingredients in very well.

Bottle, label, and store in a covered container in the refrigerator, where it will keep for several weeks.

ORANGE MOISTURE LOTION OR NIGHT CREAM (OIL-IN-WATER EMULSION)

This is a lovely moisturizer, rich and creamy. Very little is needed. It suits dry, normal, and combination skins. Massage gently into the skin until absorbed. It may feel a little greasy at first, but is very soothing, especially to dry skin.

In very hot weather the lotion may separate, so shake well until blended again. It is particularly good with orange peel used in the infusion and infused oil mix.

1 cube ($\frac{1}{2}$ oz/14 g) beeswax
4 teaspoons coconut oil
$\frac{1}{2}$ cube ($\frac{1}{4}$ oz/7 g) cocoa or shea butter
$\frac{1}{2}$ cup (125 ml) infused orange oil
$\frac{1}{2}$ teaspoon borax
$\frac{1}{2}$ cup (125 ml) triple-strength orange peel (zest only) infusion
15 drops orange essential oil

To make

Melt the wax in a small saucepan over a pot of simmering water or in a double boiler.

Add the coconut oil, and cocoa or shea butter, and stir until melted.

Slowly add the infused orange oil, stirring. Remove from heat.

Dissolve the borax in the orange peel infusion, strain and add slowly to the oil mixture, stirring and heating again if necessary to 110°F (45°C).

Stir in the orange essential oil and bottle the mixture. Shake the bottle occasionally until the mixture is cold.

Label and store in a cool, dark place.

SILK SKIN AND HAIR MOISTURIZING OIL FOR OILY SKIN

$\frac{1}{3}$ cup (80 ml) grape seed or fractionated coconut oil
30 drops evening primrose oil
10 drops carrot seed essential oil
10 drops lemon essential oil
10 drops lavender essential oil
5 drops juniper essential oil

To make and use

Place all ingredients in a bottle and shake to blend.

If possible leave for 4 days to synergize.

Label and store in a dark, cool place. Shake well before use.

Use this oil on the throat, around the eyes and the lips, and also apply a thin smear of it over the whole face last thing at night.

MOST PRECIOUS MOISTURE LOTION
(OIL-IN-WATER EMULSION)

This is the moisture lotion that I make for my family, friends, and myself. It's rich but not greasy and you can create your own perfume blend to make it especially yours.

You'll notice that I have used grams even for liquid measures. In the making of skin-care products it's far more accurate to use weight rather than volume as most people don't possess accurate volume measures. The only exception to the rule is essential oil. Laboratories throughout the world use the metric weight system as the scales can measure amounts less than 1 g, which doesn't have a sensible conversion to parts of an ounce.

1 oz (30 g) emulsifying wax NF
$\frac{1}{2}$ oz (15 g) stearic acid
2$\frac{1}{2}$ oz (75 g) infused calendula/elder flower oil
$\frac{1}{2}$ oz (15 g) jojoba oil
1$\frac{1}{4}$ cups (310 ml) aloe juice
2 cups (500 ml) infusion of calendula/elder flower, strained through coffee filter paper
4 teaspoons (20 ml) glycerine
2 teaspoons (10 ml) Optiphen Plus (very accurately measured)
2 x 500iu capsules vitamin E d-alpha-tocopherol
1 teaspoon essential oil blend

To make

Melt the wax and oils together in a small double boiler and heat to 150°F (65°C).

In a separate pan, heat the aloe juice, herbal infusion, glycerine and Optiphen Plus to 160°F (70°C).

Pour the aloe mixture into the melted wax and oil, stirring continuously until it is 110°F (45°C).

Add the squeezed oil from the vitamin E capsules and essential oil blend, mix in really well and pour into bottles.

Label and store in a dark, cool place.

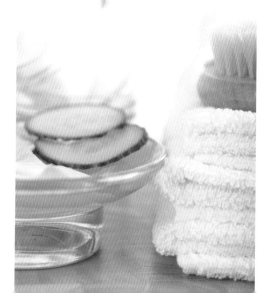

APRICOT AND AVOCADO MOISTURIZING OIL
FOR SENSITIVE SKIN

$\frac{1}{3}$ cup (80 ml) apricot kernel oil
1 teaspoon borage seed oil
60 drops evening primrose oil
1 x 500iu capsule vitamin E d-alpha-tocopherol
5 drops chamomile essential oil
5 drops rosewood or rose essential oil
2 drops lavender or neroli essential oil

To make and use

Place all ingredients in a bottle and shake to blend.

If possible leave for four days to synergize.

Label and store in a dark, cool place.

Shake well before use.

Although this blend contains only the gentlest essential oils, test each of them on your skin before using on your face.

TIP USING A LITTLE MORE INFUSION WILL GIVE YOU A LOTION RATHER THAN A CREAM. EXPERIMENT UNTIL YOU FIND WHICH IS THE BEST FOR YOUR SKIN.

Moisturizer is best absorbed when the skin is warm after a bath or shower.

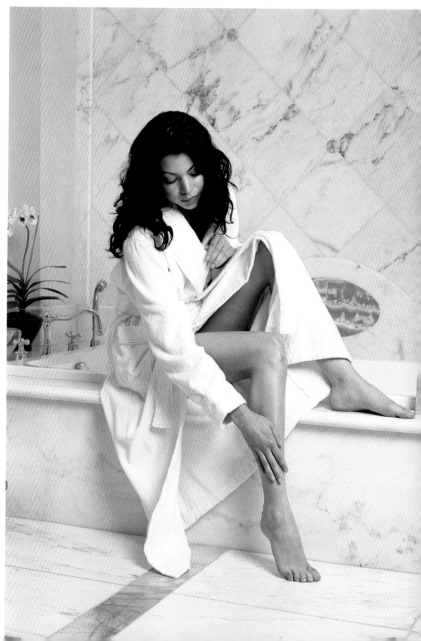

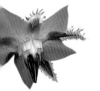
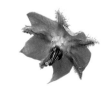

Around the eyes

The skin around the eyes shows early lines in the same way as the neck. Crow's feet, bags under the eyes, and dark circles can be very demoralizing—laughter lines are a different matter. Remember that the skin around the eyes is fragile, and harm can be done if you are heavy-handed. Here's the basic method for caring for the skin around your eyes.

Moisten the skin around and under the eyes. Then pat a few drops of the oil onto the skin, using the middle finger of your right hand (left, if you are left-handed). This is the weakest finger and so it exerts the least pressure. Keep patting gently to help the oil be absorbed.

Leave for 20 minutes and then very gently blot off any surplus oil.

Do not allow the oil to go in your eyes as it might sting.

Under Eye Oil will inhibit the occurrence of "crow's feet" around the eye.

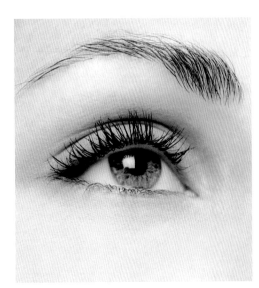

UNDER EYE OIL

1 x 500iu capsule vitamin E d-alpha-tocopherol
2½ tablespoons (40 ml) sweet almond oil
15 drops evening primrose oil
5 drops carrot seed essential oil
5 drops borage seed essential oil

To make and use

Puncture the vitamin E capsule. Squeeze the liquid into a small bowl, combined with the other oils.

Mix together and pour into a 1½ fl oz (50 ml) bottle. Shake well.

Label and store in a dark, cool place.

One drop under each eye is enough.

Apply the oil at night, leave for 10 minutes and carefully blot the excess with a tissue. Avoid getting this oil into the eye itself or it will sting and could be harmful.

PRECIOUS NIGHT OIL

This extremely rich and luxurious oil is suitable for all skin types. The essential oils will help to regulate and balance the sebum content, and to smooth, soothe, and soften the skin.

2 teaspoons sweet almond oil
1½ teaspoons apricot kernel oil
1 teaspoon hazelnut or rice bran oil
1 teaspoon borage seed oil
1½ teaspoons olive oil
1 teaspoon jojoba oil
1 teaspoon avocado oil
2 x 500iu capsules vitamin E d-alpha-tocopherol
5 drops evening primrose oil
5 drops carrot seed essential oil
5 drops palmarosa essential oil
5 drops rosewood or rose essential oil
5 drops geranium essential oil
5 drops ylang-ylang or jasmine essential oil

To make and use

Place all ingredients in a bottle and shake to blend.

If possible leave for four days to synergize.

Label and store in a dark, cool place. Do not refrigerate.

Shake well before use. Apply a few drops of this oil to slightly damp skin.

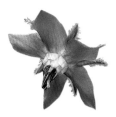

Skin problems

Acne

This distressing and disfiguring complaint is mainly a teenage problem but can occur in older people as well. Teenage acne usually starts at puberty. There are many hormonal changes happening within the body at this time. As with most skin problems, acne treatment begins within the body. Following are some choices you can make for yourself for a healthy body and a healthy skin.

* Make sure that your bowels are regular.
* Eat lots of raw and cooked vegetables and fruit daily.
* Cut out, or certainly cut down on, eating junk foods.
* Think about taking the following daily supplements—multi vitamin/mineral capsule, extra vitamin B6, vitamin E (d-alpha-tocopherol), vitamin C plus 15 mg zinc, evening primrose capsules.
* Exercise every day as this increases circulation, which brings healing nutrients and oxygen to the skin.
* Drink six glasses of purified water daily.
* Treat your face to 10 minutes of sunlight a day, preferably early in the morning or late afternoon.
* Reduce salt intake.
* Talk to a doctor about Retin A therapy.
* Before breakfast, drink a glass of water containing the juice of one lemon, with no sweetener.
* Learn to relax. Join a stress management or meditation group; spend time peacefully alone; make sure you budget time for fun.
* Wash the face two times a day using very mild soap which contains glycerine, then rinse well with lukewarm water, and pat dry using a fresh towel each time if there are any weeping spots.
* Try to avoid using makeup. I know that this is hard but you stand a better chance of healing if you do this. Use only the Herbal Healing Day Oil and Herbal Healing Night Oil on your skin.
* Have a facial steam once or twice a week, see page 272.
* Never, but never, be tempted to squeeze a pimple. The result of this type of interference will be scarring and a spread of infection.

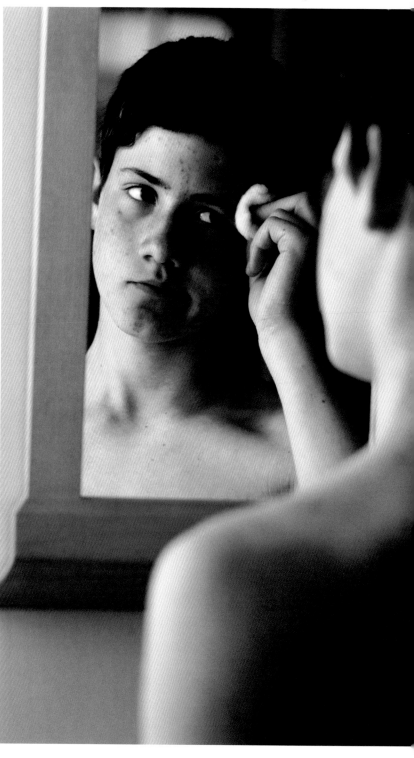

Skin problems during adolescence can be greatly helped by the use of natural astringents.

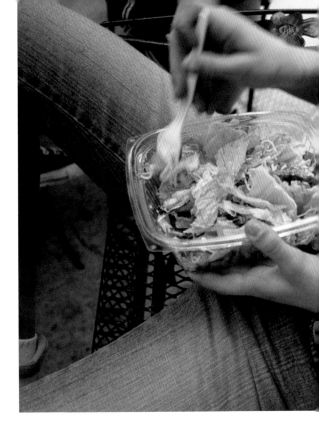

"MAGIC THREE" TONER

$\frac{1}{2}$ cup (125 ml) rosewater

$\frac{1}{4}$ cup (60 ml) purified water

1 teaspoon cider vinegar

$\frac{1}{4}$–$\frac{1}{2}$ teaspoon glycerine

5 drops juniper essential oil

3 drops sandalwood essential oil

2 drops chamomile essential oil

To make and use

Place all ingredients in a bottle and shake to blend.

If possible leave for four days to synergize.

Label and store in a dark, cool place. Shake well before use.

Pour a little on dampened absorbent cotton (cottonwool) and use frequently to freshen skin.

PALMAROSA RINSE LOTION

$\frac{1}{3}$ cup (80 ml) cider vinegar

15 drops palmarosa essential oil

15 drops tea tree essential oil

2 teaspoons tincture of myrrh

To make and use

Place all ingredients in a bottle and shake to blend.

If possible leave for four days to synergize.

Label and store in a dark, cool place.

Shake well before using.

Add 1 teaspoon to 1 cup (250 ml) warm water and use as a facial rinse after washing.

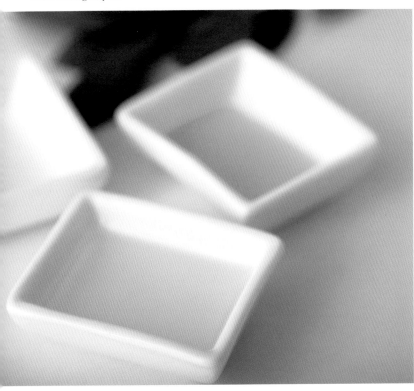

Essential oils ready to combine for Herbal Healing Day Oil

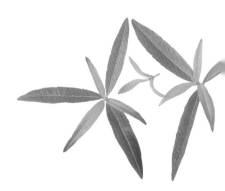

HERBAL HEALING DAY OIL

This gentle but powerful oil is for day treatment of acne, pimples, or otherwise infected skin. Use morning and midday.

$2\frac{1}{2}$ tablespoons (40 ml) sweet almond oil

10 drops carrot seed essential oil

10 drops palmarosa essential oil

5 drops tea tree essential oil

5 drops geranium essential oil

To make and use

Place all ingredients in a bottle and shake to blend.

If possible leave for four days to synergize.

Label and store in a dark, cool place. Shake well before using.

Place three to four drops of the blend on the palm of your hand, dip the fingers in, and gently smooth over the skin.

Don't get any in your eyes as it will sting. Leave on for 5–10 minutes, blot surplus off with tissue.

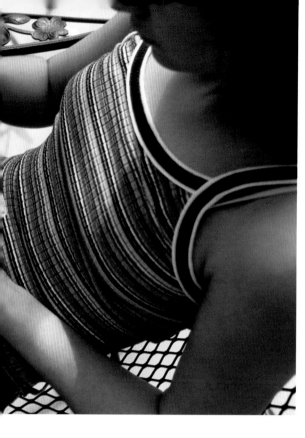

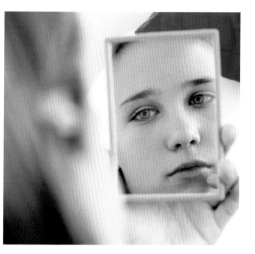

Despite the temptation, encourage your teen not to squeeze pimples.

HEALING MASK FOR ACNE, ECZEMA, AND OTHER SKIN PROBLEMS

4 teaspoons finely ground almonds
2 teaspoons cornflour or kaolin clay
1 teaspoon honey
1 drop juniper essential oil
1 drop chamomile essential oil
1 drop lavender essential oil
water to mix

Healthy eating is the best treatment to gain healthy skin.

To make and use

Mix all the ingredients together, adding enough water to the mixture to form a soft paste.

Gently spread the mask mixture over your face and neck, keeping it away from your eyes. Lie down with pads of absorbent cotton (cottonwool) soaked in distilled witch hazel or cooled chamomile tea over your eyes for 10–15 minutes.

Wash mask off in lukewarm water followed by a splash of cool water.

HERBAL HEALING NIGHT OIL

This blend feels a little oilier than its daytime companion. Don't worry—these oils heal and regenerate while you sleep.

$^1/_4$ cup (60 ml) sweet almond oil
20 drops evening primrose oil
10 drops carrot seed essential oil
5 drops tea tree essential oil
5 drops palmarosa essential oil

To make and use

Place all ingredients in a bottle and shake to blend.

If possible leave for four days to synergize.

Label and store in a dark, cool place. Shake well before using.

Place three to four drops of the blend on the palm of your hand, dip the fingers in, and gently smooth over the skin.

Don't get any in your eyes as it will sting. Leave on for 5–10 minutes, blot surplus off with tissue.

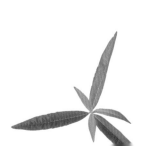

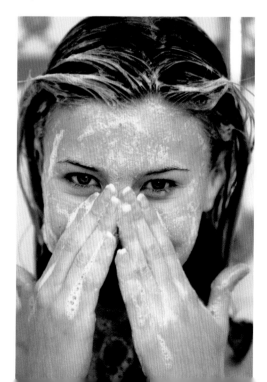

Good skin hygiene will stop the spread of acne.

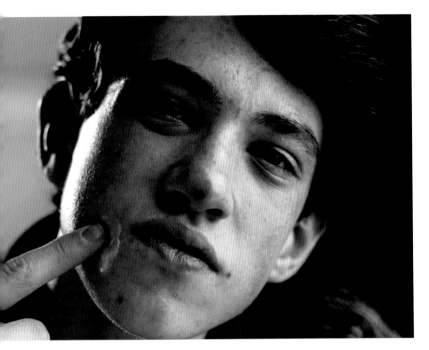

Apply astringents and anti-acne treatments topically rather than over the whole face.

A daily routine for your teen's skin is the ideal start in life.

Blackheads

When the sebaceous glands oversecrete and the excess sebum doesn't move out of the duct, a blackhead results. This can become a problem if not properly dealt with, as the pore can become infected if the blackhead is carefully removed, but the area isn't disinfected.

Facial scrubs are useful in the prevention of the formation of blackheads. The safest way to remove blackheads is to steam the skin, using boiling water and antiseptic oil to prevent infection. This loosens the sebum and relaxes the pores. Basic steam procedure for blackheads is as follows:

* Three-quarters fill a large bowl with boiling water.
* Place one drop tea tree essential oil and two drops geranium essential oil on the water, and cover your head with a towel, forming a tent around the bowl and your head.
* Steam for about 10 minutes, keeping your face about 12 in (30 cm) away from the bowl of water.
* Pat your skin dry.
* With absorbent cotton (cottonwool) wrapped around your nails, gently press the skin on either side of the blackhead

until it pops out, or use a little tool for extracting blackheads, available from cosmetic counters and pharmacies.
* Splash the skin with the following mixture, which will help to shrink and disinfect the pore.

ASTRINGENT LOTION

$2\frac{1}{2}$ tablespoons (40 ml) purified water
2 teaspoons witch hazel
2 drops cypress essential oil
1 drop palmarosa essential oil

To make and use

Place all ingredients in a bottle and shake to blend. If possible leave for four days to synergize.

Label and store in a dark, cool place. Shake well before using.

Pour a little on a damp absorbent cotton (cottonwool) pad. Pat over the skin.

BLACKHEAD REMOVER

Never attempt to squeeze blackheads until the skin is soft, moist, and warm—as after one of the following treatments. Use a special tool for extracting blackheads or cover your nails with absorbent cotton (cottonwool) before squeezing.
* Steam the face using a blend of bay leaves, fennel seeds, lemon grass, and nasturtium leaves.
* Make and use a scrub using oatmeal.

BROKEN VEINS COMPRESS

Make a triple-strength tea of borage leaves and flowers, calendula petals, and chamomile flowers. Strain through coffee filter paper and apply daily as a cool compress.

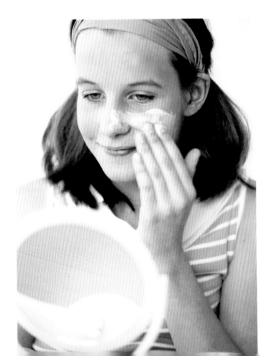

Dermatitis

Dermatitis is inflammation and/or irritation of the skin. It is usually caused by sensitivity to a substance or substances with which the skin has come in contact. Barworkers and hairdressers often suffer from dermatitis due to daily skin contact with beer and the chemical used in hairdressing. Obviously, the condition won't clear until the irritant is removed and in extreme circumstances this can mean giving up work. Stress is another factor that can aggravate the condition. The following eczema treatment is appropriate for dermatitis.

Eczema

This is an inflammatory condition of the skin that manifests variously as itching, skin inflammation, dry, thickened skin, and tiny blisters that burst, weep, and can become infected. It is a very difficult problem to treat—particularly if the cause isn't found. Look for the cause among allergies, low stomach acid, stress, poor or inadequate diet, dysfunctional immune system, or build up of toxins.

Initially, the aims of aromatherapy treatment are to lower stress, ease the itching, and so prevent scratching, and to promote healthy new skin tissue. Various oils should be tried until suitable ones are found. The following list may be used, choosing one to two from each list to use in blends.

Condition	Oils
Anti-stress essential oils	Cedarwood, chamomile, cypress, geranium, juniper, lavender
Detoxifying essential oils	Juniper
Anti-inflammatory essential oils	Chamomile, lavender, lemon, myrrh
Healing essential oils	Calendula infused oil, carrot seed, rosehip

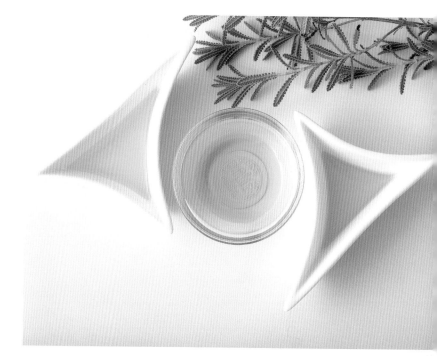

Oil Blend for Eczema—oils ready to mix, and a sprig of lavender.

COMPRESS BLEND

1 cup (250 ml) cold water
2 drops geranium or lavender essential oil
2 drops lemon or myrrh essential oil
1 drop chamomile or cypress essential oil

To make and use

Place all ingredients in a bottle and shake to blend.
If possible leave for four days to synergize.
Label and store in a dark, cool place. Shake well before using.
Use for a compress twice a day.

OIL BLEND FOR ECZEMA

2$\frac{1}{2}$ tablespoons (40 ml) sweet almond oil
10 drops evening primrose oil
10 drops chamomile essential oil
5 drops myrrh essential oil
5 drops lavender essential oil

To make and use

Place all ingredients in a bottle and shake to blend.
If possible leave for four days to synergize.
Label and store in a dark, cool place.
Shake well before using.
Pour a little on a damp absorbent cotton (cottonwool) pad.
Smooth gently over the affected areas.

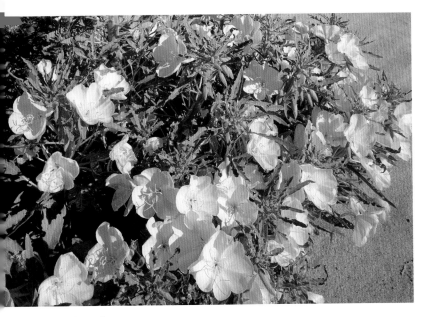

Evening primrose flowers.
The distilled oil is used in
Psoriasis Massage Oil Blend.

CREAM BLEND FOR WEEPING ECZEMA

1³/₄ oz (50 g) aloe vera gel
10 drops chamomile essential oil
5 drops patchouli essential oil
5 drops myrrh essential oil

TIP USE EIGHT DROPS OF
CHAMOMILE ESSENTIAL
OIL AND TWO DROPS
MYRRH ESSENTIAL
OIL MIXED WITH ONE
TEASPOON SWEET
ALMOND OIL IN A
WARM BATH.

To make and use

Decant the gel into a small bowl and mix the oils
in very thoroughly.

Apply frequently and gently all over the
affected areas.

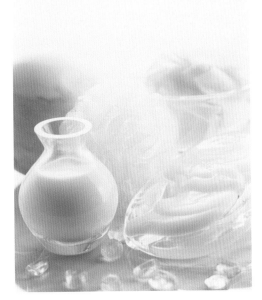

Weeping eczema should be treated
with aloe vera gel and essential oils
in a cream blend.

Psoriasis

Psoriasis is a skin condition characterized
by thick, scaly, pink patches of cells with
overlapping, silvery scales. It usually appears
on the scalp, back of the wrists, elbows,
knees, and ankles. The condition is difficult
to treat and patience may be needed. Stress
or an underfunctioning liver may be the
cause, and until the cause is found and
addressed there will be no permanent cure.

The following suggestions will
certainly help but I would suggest that
aromatherapy is used in conjunction with a
stress management course and a good liver
cleansing program.

PSORIASIS MASSAGE OIL BLEND

¹/₂ cup (125 ml) sweet almond oil
30 drops borage seed oil
30 drops evening primrose oil
15 drops lavender essential oil
10 drops bergamot essential oil
10 drops rosemary essential oil
10 drops tea tree essential oil

To make and use

Place all ingredients in a bottle and shake to blend.

If possible leave for four days to synergize.

Label and store in a dark, cool place. Shake well
before using.

Float one teaspoon of the blend on warm water
in a small bowl and use for a massage.

Pour two teaspoons into a bath or foot bath,
agitate to disperse and soak in the bath for
30 minutes, massaging any floating oil droplets
into the affected parts.

Pour a little into the palm of the hand and
massage over the body after showering while the
skin is still damp.

Use the blend topically several times a day.
If it causes any discomfort increase the amount of
almond oil.

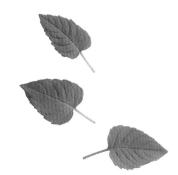

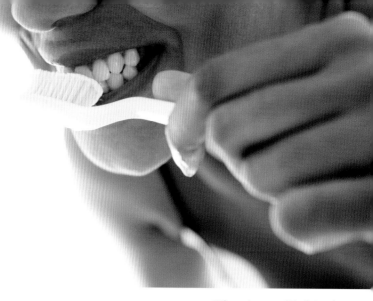

Caring for your mouth and teeth

When we are young we are invincible. We are confident that we will keep our teeth until the day we die. We crack nuts, remove bottle tops (I'm cringing as I write!), and break tough cotton thread with our teeth. We forget to floss, eat sweets between meals, and generally treat them in a very cavalier fashion.

It is hopefully never too late to change our ways. Herbal products can help you keep your mouth sweet and your lips in good condition. In addition to the following recipes you will find that bergamot, fennel, lavender, and lemon grass are good for a mouthwash, while you can heal mouth ulcers with tincture of myrrh and sage mouthwashes. The Tooth Powder recipe is also good for cleaning dentures—even dentures need care—and also your gums.

When using natural Tooth Powder keep a separate jar for each member of the family.

TOOTH POWDER

½ cup (60 g) fine sea salt
½ cup (150 g) bicarbonate of soda
8 drops peppermint essential oil
5 drops lemon essential oil
2 drops myrrh essential oil

To make

In a small bowl, combine the sea salt and bicarbonate of soda until well mixed.

Add the essential oils very slowly, a drop at a time, stirring constantly to prevent the mixture from lumping.

Keep in separate jars—one for each member of the family.

PEPPERMINT AND MYRRH MOUTHWASH

A mouthwash helps to sweeten the breath, and to heal sores, ulcers, and gum problems. If bad breath is an ongoing problem it would be wise to look for the source of the problem. A visit to the dentist may be needed or, if the cause is a digestive one, eating one to two cups daily of yoghurt which contains an acidophilus culture will create a healthier digestive system.

The myrrh essential oil in this recipe helps to heal mouth ulcers.

⅓ cup (80 ml) cider vinegar
4 teaspoons brandy
1 teaspoon glycerine
10 drops peppermint essential oil
10 drops lemon essential oil
5 drops myrrh essential oil

To make and use

Pour all the ingredients into a 3½ fl oz (100 ml) glass bottle. Stand for four days shaking occasionally. Strain.

Label and store in a dark, cool place. Shake well before using.

Add one teaspoon to ½ cup (125 ml) of warm water. Rinse mouth thoroughly with mixture, but do not swallow it.

QUICKIE MOUTHWASH

One teaspoon of cider vinegar and one drop of peppermint essential oil in a glass of water will freshen the mouth. Rinse the mouth and spit out. Don't swallow.

Cider vinegar and peppermint essential oil swished through the mouth make a perfect quick mouthwash.

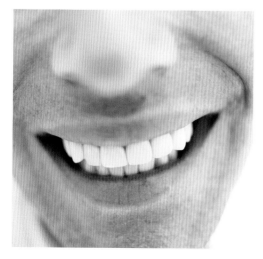

TIP TESTING FOR
SOFTNESS/HARDNESS:
A SMALL KNIFE MAY BE
KEPT IN THE FREEZER
AND DIPPED INTO THE
FINISHED BUT STILL
WARM AND LIQUID
MIXTURE. THE TEXTURE
WILL BE IMMEDIATELY
APPARENT ON THE
KNIFE AND CAN BE
ADJUSTED EITHER WAY
BY THE ADDITION OF
EITHER MORE OIL OR
MORE WAX.

Lips

Lips have much thinner, drier skin than the rest of the face. Dry, cracked lips can be painful and unsightly. Regular use of the following lip salve will help to keep the skin soft and moist. If you don't use lipstick, carry a little pot of this lip salve in your pocket or handbag, and use it often during the day.

BREATH AND LIP SWEETENER
This is a delicious mouthwash. Use fresh herbs if possible.

2 cups (500 ml) sherry
1 teaspoon finely chopped spearmint
1 teaspoon finely chopped peppermint
1 teaspoon finely chopped lemon thyme
1 teaspoon finely chopped sage
4 cloves, bruised
1 teaspoon ground cinnamon
15 drops peppermint essential oil
5 drops lemon essential oil

To make and use
Measure the sherry in a clean jug.
    Put all the herbs, spices, and oils in a bottle and top up with the sherry.
    Cork, label, and store in a dark, cool place for two weeks. Strain, filter, and rebottle.
    Add two teaspoons to a glass of water and use to rinse the mouth.

LIP SALVE
This will make three $^1/_2$ oz (20 g) pots or twelve $^1/_8$ oz (5 g) tubes.

$^1/_2$ oz (15 g) beeswax
$^1/_2$ oz (15 g) cocoa butter (or olive butter)
1 tablespoon (15 ml) infused calendula oil
1 tablespoon (15 ml) castor oil
1 tablespoon (15 ml) jojoba or rice bran oil
6 drops vitamin E oil
4–6 drops essential oil such as peppermint, orange or mandarin

To make
Cut or grate the beeswax into very small pieces and melt in a small container standing in hot water on the stove.
    Add the grated cocoa (or olive) butter and melt; don't overheat the waxes.
    Add the calendula, castor, and jojoba or rice bran oils slowly, stopping if the waxes begin to harden and restarting as the waxes melt again.
    Remove from the heat.
    Feel the outside of the container and add the vitamin E when the temperature is just above blood heat and the mixture is still liquid.
    Test for firmness/softness.
    If more wax is needed, you will need to melt some extra beeswax in a separate small container and, when melted, add the already-made salve and heat gently until all are combined but not overheated.
    If more oil is needed, heat some more oil until it's a little hotter than the made salve and slowly but thoroughly mix the extra oil through the salve.
    Pour quickly into little pots and cover with lids.
    If using tubes, fasten them together with an elastic band and stand them in a clean, small bowl in case of drips. With a steady hand! fill the tubes three-quarters full. Scrape down the side of the jug and put it back in the pan of hot water to help to melt remaining salve. When the salve in the tube is set, top up with the remaining salve. This prevents a "pit" from forming on top of the salve.

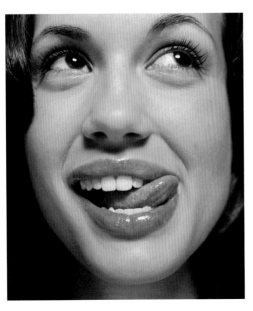

Breath and Lip Sweetener freshens the breath and has a yummy taste.

Opposite: Lip Salve and all other lip creams should be dabbed on not rubbed into the lips.

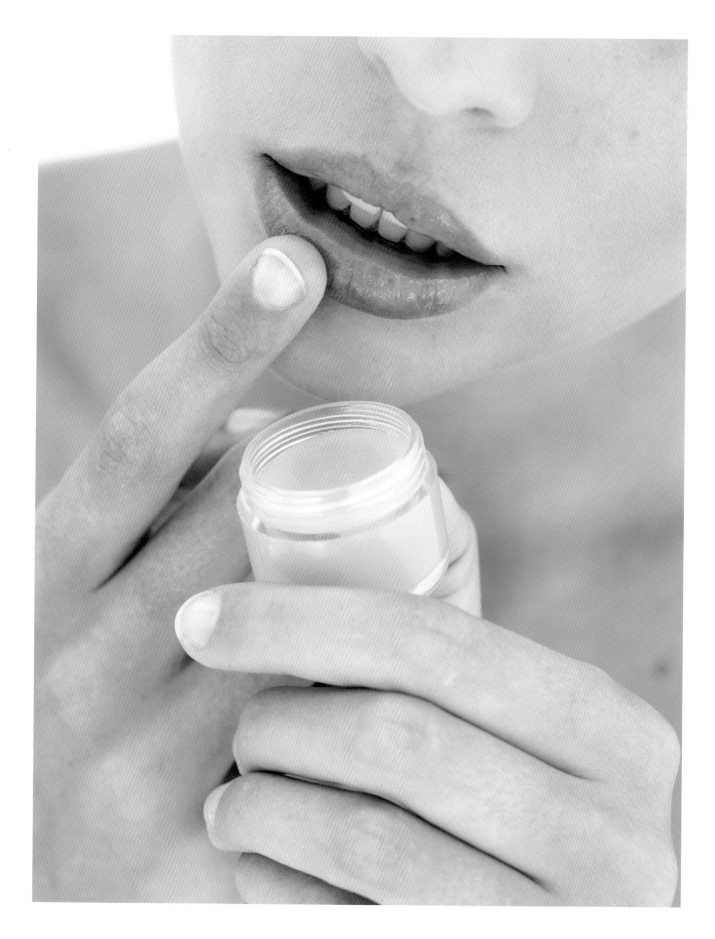

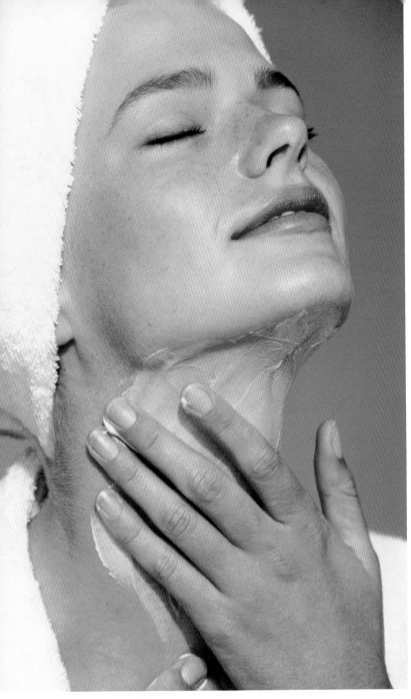

Ensure that neck cream is blended over the whole surface of the neck and upper chest.

"The first feminine feature that goes, with advancing age, is the neck."
GLORIA SWANSON

Water, olive oil, and kaolin clay, mixed to a paste, ready for the addition of lavender essential oil to make Lavender Barrier Cream.

The neck

The skin on the neck is usually drier than on our faces, and it is often very neglected, resulting in a crepey, dry texture. Also, if the hair is short, the back of the neck is very exposed to the sun, so it's particularly important to keep the whole area supple, not just the throat.

The special neck blend should be used night and morning, but don't forget sunblock during the day.

SPECIAL NECK BLEND

This oil blend is gentle and rich. If used regularly, it can help to keep wrinkles at bay and to soften and smooth those that have already appeared.

2 x 250 iu vitamin E capsules
2 teaspoons jojoba oil
1 teaspoon avocado oil
1 teaspoon wheat germ oil
$\frac{1}{2}$ teaspoon evening primrose oil
5 drops carrot seed essential oil
5 drops lavender essential oil
5 drops palmarosa essential oil
5 drops rosewood essential oil

To make and use

Pierce the vitamin E capsules and mix with all ingredients in a bottle and shake to blend.

If possible leave for four days to synergize.

Label and store in a dark, cool place. Do not refrigerate.

Shake well before use.

Spray or splash a little water on the throat.

Sprinkle a few drops of the oil onto the palm of your hand and massage gently into the throat in an upward direction until it has been absorbed.

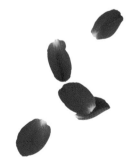

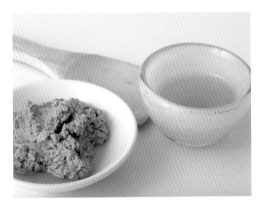

Hands

These hard-working parts of our bodies need all the love and care we can give them.

It is very common to spend a great deal of time and money on our hair and faces, and to neglect our poor hands. They are exposed to the weather just as our faces are, and they also have to contend with gardening, washing clothes, and dishes, and all the other jobs which are so hard on skin.

Essential oils are particularly good for hands as they work very quickly and are readily absorbed without leaving a greasy feeling. The following oil is a luxurious treat for the tools we use most often and usually appreciate the least.

LEMON AND LAVENDER HAND SOFTENER

This is a cream for dry, rough, work-worn hands.

3 cubes (about 1 1/4 oz/36 g) beeswax
1/3 cup (80 ml) almond oil
1/2 cup (125 ml) olive oil
2 1/2 tablespoons (40 ml) glycerine
2 drops lemon essential oil
2 drops lavender essential oil

To make and use

Melt the beeswax into the sweet almond and olive oils gently in a double boiler.

Stir in the glycerine until completely blended. Remove from heat.

Drip the essential oils into the slightly cooled mixture.

Stir mixture very well then pot.

Label and store in a cool, dark place.

Massage it into the hands before doing dirty jobs.

If your hands are really rough, use this rich cream during the evening while talking or watching television, or massage a goodly amount on before bedtime, and cover the hands with cotton gloves to protect the bedding.

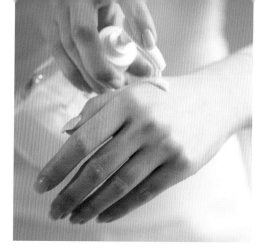

The back of the hands are exposed to more sunlight than any other part of the body. Apply hand cream at least three times a day.

LAVENDER BARRIER CREAM

4 teaspoons purified water
2 1/2 tablespoons (40 ml) olive oil
2 teaspoons kaolin clay
10 drops lavender essential oil

To make and use

Mix the ingredients together thoroughly in a small bowl.

Pot up in a clean glass jar.

Label and store in a cool, dark place.

Massage cream well into hands before doing dirty jobs.

HEALING HAND CREAM

If you do not have the time or energy to make a cream from scratch, this blend is for you.

Buy aloe cream, not aloe ointment, from a health-food store, making sure you get one containing the largest amount possible of aloe.

The combination of the aloe cream and essential oils will heal and soften sore, dry, or cracked skin.

1 3/4 oz (50 g) jar aloe vera cream
1/2 teaspoon benzoin tincture or 5 drops benzoin essential oil
10 drops sandalwood essential oil
10 drops palmarosa or lavender essential oil
10 drops lavender essential oil

To make and use

Decant the aloe vera cream into a small bowl.

In another bowl, mix all the oils and tincture together.

Add the combined oils slowly to the cream, a drop at a time, mixing constantly.

When the oils are thoroughly incorporated, spoon the cream back into the jar.

Label and store in a cool, dark place.

Use it after washing your hands and at bedtime.

TIP: THE SKIN ON THE HAND CONTAINS VERY LITTLE OIL. USE SUITABLE GLOVES FOR GARDENING, HOUSEWORK, ETC., AND USE A RICH HAND CREAM WHENEVER POSSIBLE.

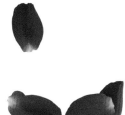

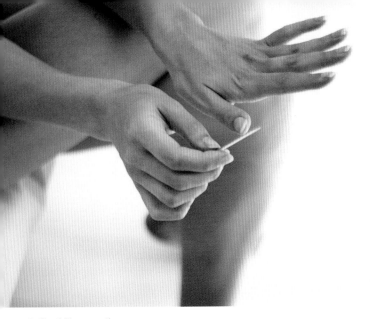

Buff and file your nails once a week before applying moisturizer.

HAND-CARE TIPS

- Manicure your nails every week.
- Wear gloves when doing the dishes, hand-washing clothes, and gardening.
- Keep a cut lemon close to the kitchen sink. Lemon juice removes stains, whitens the skin, and cleans the nails.
- Use a hand cream after doing dishes, gardening, or any DIY work about the house.
- Use a sunblock cream on your hands in summer.

HAND AND NAIL OIL

The combination of the aloe cream and essential oils will heal and soften sore, dry, or cracked skin.

5 x 250iu vitamin E capsules
4 teaspoons sweet almond oil
2 teaspoons avocado oil
2 teaspoons olive oil
1 teaspoon jojoba oil
20 drops evening primrose oil
5 drops benzoin essential oil
10 drops sandalwood essential oil
10 drops lemon essential oil

To make and use

Prick the vitamin E capsules and squeeze the contents into a 2 fl oz (60 ml) bottle.
Add all the other oils and shake to blend.
If possible, leave for four days to synergize.
Label and store in a cool, dark place.
Pour four to six drops into the palm of your hand.
Massage oil into the skin and around the nail bed until absorbed. Repeat.

HAND LOTION

This lotion keeps well without refrigeration except in very hot weather.

1 teaspoon distilled witch hazel
4 teaspoons vegetable glycerine
5 teaspoons cologne (see "Colognes," pages 320–1)

To make and use

Mix all the ingredients together in a small bowl.
Pour into a small bottle or clean glass jar.
Label and store in a cool, dark place.
Apply a few drops and massage in well.

LUSCIOUS LOTION BAR

Lotion bars look like a bar of soap but melt into your skin. They are great for moisturising work-worn hands, feet, or anywhere that the skin is very dry.
If you are giving these bars as a gift, they can be wrapped in either cellophane or greaseproof paper.

4 oz (120 g) cocoa butter
1 oz (30 g) shea butter
1 tablespoon (15 ml) almond oil
1 teaspoon calendula infused oil
30 drops phenoxitol
30 drops essential oils of your choice

To make

Place the cocoa butter, shea butter, and the almond and calendula oils in a double boiler and heat until just melted.
Remove from the heat and stir well to mix.
Allow to cool until the outside of the pan is just above hand heat.
Add the phenoxitol and essential oils and stir really thoroughly to incorporate.
Pour into small soap or chocolate molds and freeze for a few minutes until hard, then tap from the molds.
These bars are best kept in a covered container in the refrigerator, unless your storage area is very cool.

Hair

Take a good look at hair next time you are in a crowd of people and you will see that the average person has perfectly ordinary hair. Some people have thick hair, others have dull hair. Despite the fact that they regularly use shampoo and conditioners, only one in a thousand will have hair that looks like the hair on the television commercials.

Now take a look at the people in old photographs and paintings—was their hair worse than ours is? Chances are that their hair was considerably stronger and in better condition.

Hair type is mostly inherited. Learn how to make the best of what nature and your parents blessed you with, and stop attempting to achieve the impossible.

In this section I have included many treatments, which will add natural body and shine to dry hair, control grease and dandruff, and gently and fragrantly care for all hair types.

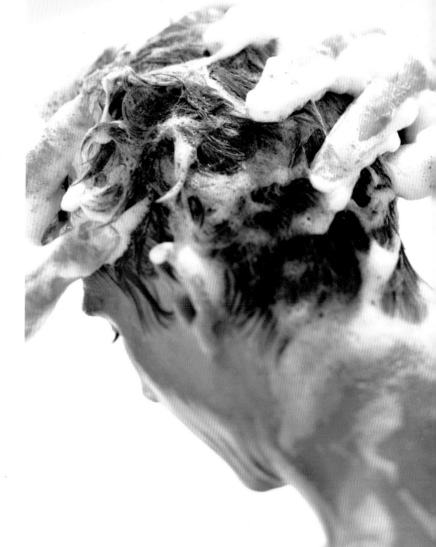

Lather shampoo especially around the hairline to make sure the whole head is cleansed.

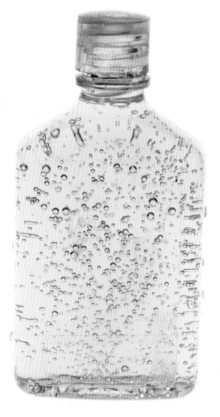

Commercial shampoos aren't magic potions

Commercial shampoos and conditioners are comparatively new. When I was a child we used a block of soap and rainwater to shampoo, with vinegar rinse to finish the job. I have photographs of myself and my mother with shining dark hair that owed nothing to a bottle of bought shampoo. Most people had a reasonable head of hair unless they were sick or had been handed a poor deal by their genes!

I have spent time in India and noticed that even the poorest men and women have sleek, shining hair that has never been washed with bottled shampoo. I once became friendly with a very poor Indian woman who only used mashed, cooked lentils to shampoo her hair. She shared the

Commercial shampoos are often full of detergent so it's best to make your own from natural ingredients that suit your hair type.

lentils with me and the result was gratifying and astonishing!

If we are credulous, we will believe that a beautiful head of hair can only be achieved by using extravagantly advertised products. These promise hair that miraculously will be transformed from being dry, dull, and tangled to being shiny, healthy, and tangle-free within a week of starting to use a particular shampoo.

Despite using such products, I have rarely met a person who is content with their hair, and a "bad hair day" has become a catch phrase. The discontent is sometimes because their hair is straight instead of curly or vice-versa but it's usually the hair's actual "condition" that gives rise to the most repeated moans.

Commercial shampoos aren't magic potions, they are merely a chemical blend of detergents, waxes, and other ingredients that make our hair thick, shiny, and healthy. There are even "strippers" available now to rid the hair of the "build-up" of the shampoo and conditioner that cost us so much money to apply in the first instance!

Cosmetic labels list content in order of percentage—the highest being the first and smallest last. Take a look at the average bottle of herbal shampoo and you will find the herbal content is generally last on the list.

For a luxurious afternoon, try and convince a friend to exchange head massages. There is nothing more soothing or relaxing.

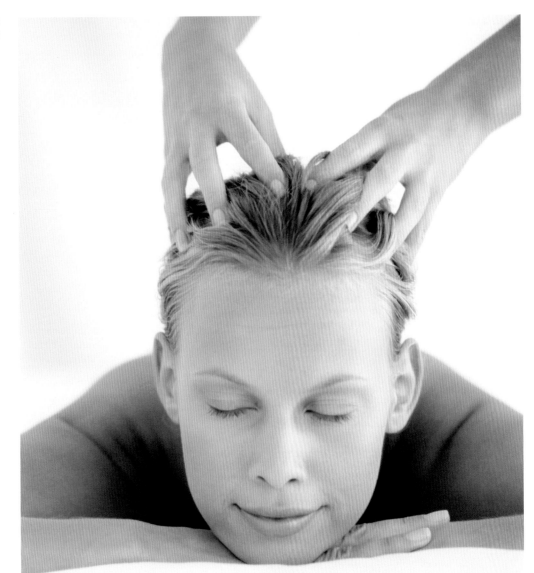

HAIR TYPES

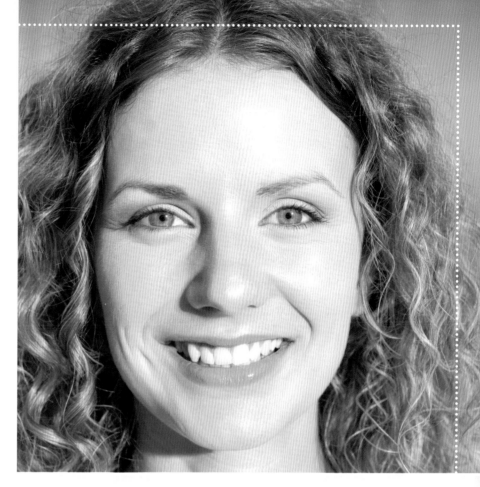

FINE HAIR

Despite the fact that fine hair may be limp and lack body, it can look very lovely if it is treated with natural pre-shampoo and after-shampoo conditioners, as these give added thickness and "body" to the strands.

Fine hair needs to be treated very gently. Use a soft bristle brush with rounded ends on the bristles. Don't expose it to too much wind or strong sunlight. Don't overcolor, overperm or overbleach as fine hair becomes brittle and breaks easily.

Avoid frequent use of hair rollers or styles where the hair is tightly pulled back or fastened into elastic bands as this can stress the delicate structure of the hair.

THIN HAIR

Thin hair is often fine as well. Treat the hair gently, never use harsh shampoo, and avoid overcoloring or overperming. Don't brush excessively and use a soft brush with rounded ends on the bristles. Use pre-shampoo and after-shampoo treatments that contain protein, such as egg and milk, to add the fullness, which this hair lacks.

COARSE HAIR

Be happy if you have coarse hair. Thick, strong, and wiry, this hair will resist a lot of abuse without splitting or breaking. You may not need to condition this type of hair but if it's not as shiny as you would like, an after-shampoo conditioner and/or between-shampoo hairdressing will help.

OILY HAIR

Overactive subcutaneous glands are responsible for the excessive oil on this type of hair. Shampooing every day can aggravate the problem, as the glands become more active in response to the

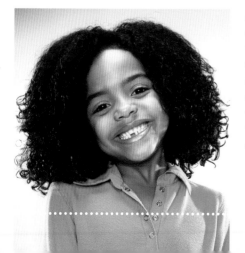

constant stimulation. Dry shampoos are a compromise as they remove oil between shampoos. Don't brush too hard or for too long. Twenty to thirty strokes will be sufficient to distribute the oil evenly down the hair shaft. Don't use very hot water for shampooing or rinsing, as the heat will encourage the production of more oil. A vinegar rinse will strip the excessive oil and leave the hair shining and manageable.

DRY HAIR

Dry hair is dull, has a tendency to split and break, and is difficult to style. And all of the above (except oily) types of hair may be afflicted with dryness under certain circumstances. Dry hair may be the result of ill health, harsh shampoo, overuse of hair dryers, and/or straightening or curling wands, too much exposure to wind and sun, neglecting to wash the hair after swimming, or too much brushing. The treatment for this type of hair should begin with an analysis of the cause. Once you know this, apply the appropriate remedy.

GRAY HAIR

Gray hair is a mixture of your natural color and white hairs. Hair color is decided by melanin structure and by genetics. The lessening of melanin production causes grayness; as you age it is almost inevitable that your hair will lose its color or, if your mother or father went white or gray when young, the chances are that you might also.

Commercial hair colorants carry poison warnings and some people react very badly to the chemicals contained in hair dyes. On a long-term basis it has yet to be shown what damage may be done to the health by the continual use of these products.

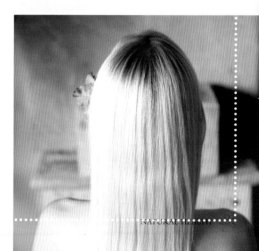

I believe that the shampoo and conditioner that you can make at home using pure, natural ingredients is infinitely superior and you aren't paying for packaging, advertising, and marketing. The contents of the bottles themselves are usually only worth a few cents (I know because I have worked for some of the biggest multinational cosmetic companies) because there has to be plenty of "margin" to pay everyone along the line from manufacturer to wholesaler and retailer. I have also owned a business that made skin and hair products and know how small a profit margin there is when you use expensive, natural products.

Hair and health

Remember that our hair and nails are very useful as "barometers of health" and are frequently the first parts of our bodies to warn us that we may have a health problem. Hair can become thin, dull, and lifeless; nails can become brittle with ridges and sometimes white spots. The external attention and money that we spend to gain a good head of hair is going to be largely wasted if our nutrition is inadequate, we are unduly stressed, or not getting sufficient sleep.

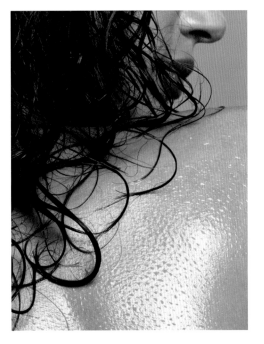

Keep the ends of your hair well conditioned and trimmed to prevent split ends.

The best way to condition your hair is to comb it through before rinsing in lots of fresh water.

How to have healthy hair

Commercial shampoos

If buying commercial shampoos, choose the most natural one you can find in a health-food shop. You can then easily improve it and make it last longer by adding concentrated herbal teas or essential oils (see tables on pages 286 and 288).

Washing your hair

Hair only needs washing once a week unless you have been doing something that has made it really dirty. Too much washing makes dry hair drier and oily hair oilier! Clean hair shouldn't be "squeaky"—that's an old wives' tale as they say. If hair squeaks it means that every trace of oil has been removed and it's this natural oil that gives hair its shine. One shampoo is sufficient; two will leave hair unmanageable.

Brace yourself! One of the best ways to ensure thick, healthy hair is to use only lukewarm water to shampoo and to use cold water (or herbal vinegar in cold water) for the final rinse.

Don't do anything rough to your hair while it is wet. After shampooing, towel lightly and run your fingers through to arrange it. Wet hair is very elastic and can be badly damaged by rough handling—and that includes brushing and combing.

Chlorinated water and seawater are both very damaging to hair. Rinse your hair immediately after swimming, and shampoo as soon as possible, using a conditioning treatment before and after shampooing.

Hairbrushes

Buy the best hairbrush that you can afford. Pure bristle is the best but even these need checking. Tap the bristles on the palm of your hand to make sure that the ends of the bristles are rounded and not sharp. Gentle washing once a week will extend the life of your brush.

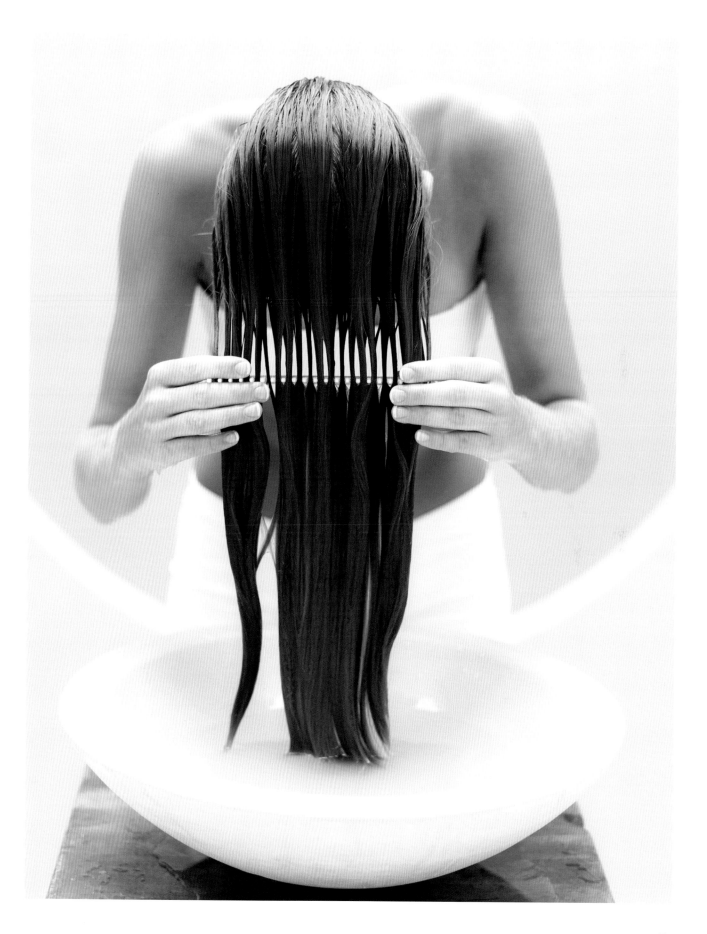

Choosing herbs for your hair

Condition/ treatment	Herbs
Cleansing	Bay, clover, lemon balm, lemon grass, and thyme to shampoos.
Conditioning	Lavender, nettle, lemon grass, rosemary, and sage to shampoos and rinses.
Treating dandruff	Nettle, rosemary, and lavender in tonics. Comfrey, mallow root, and willow bark are good to use in shampoos and rinses. Add one tablespoon of cider vinegar to each liter of rinse.
Dry scalp	Comfrey root, mallow root, and nettle.
Scalp irritation	Chamomile, comfrey, and mallow in shampoos. Bay, elder flower, parsley, rosemary, southernwood, and wormwood are suitable in rinses and scalp tonics. Add one tablespoon of cider vinegar to each liter of rinse.
Dark hair	Nettle, rosemary, sage, and thyme.
Fair hair	Chamomile and calendula.
Normal hair	Basil, bay, comfrey root, clover, lavender, lemon balm, nettle, southernwood, and wormwood.
Oily hair	Lemon grass, lemon peel, and witch hazel bark.
Dry hair	Comfrey root, mallow root, and orange peel to use as a pre-shampoo treatment. Use triple-strength teas of chamomile, elder flower, and lavender in shampoos and rinses.
Loss of hair	Nettle, rosemary, southernwood, thyme, and wormwood.
Fragrant hair	Basil, lavender, lemon balm, lemon grass, lemon peel, orange peel, rosemary, and thyme.
Shiny hair	Calendula, chamomile, lemon peel, nettle, rosemary, and sage.

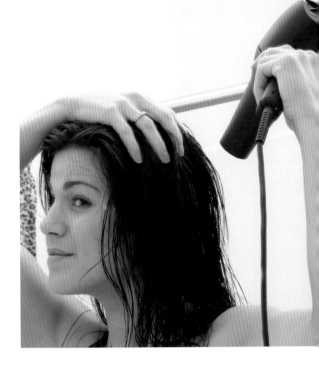

About 30–40 strokes are enough when brushing (20–30 for oily hair). Bend over and brush from the scalp to the ends of the hair to distribute the oil evenly. Bending over also increases the blood supply to the scalp, which is beneficial to the hair follicle.

Use a wide-toothed comb. Teeth that are too close together can pull out a lot of hair.

Hair styles and coloring

If you pull your hair back in a style that causes tension for long periods of time you could develop a condition called traction alopecia. This means that you are losing your hair because you are pulling it out!

Overuse of chemicals to color your hair and using heat to dry your hair could result in brittle hair that breaks. If you don't do either of these and your hair is still brittle, look to your diet.

Essential oils can also help to repair damage and keep colored, bleached, or dyed hair in good condition. Use the following oils in shampoo, rinses, vinegar rinses, and tonics. Never use more than one percent—20 drops in 100 ml (that's just under $1/_2$ cup) fluid. Use half this amount of essential oils in shampoos for children aged 5–12 and two drops only for pre-schoolers aged 2–5.

Scalp massage

Regular scalp massage can increase the flow of blood to the hair follicle and greatly improve the condition of your hair. Place all your fingers and both thumbs firmly on the scalp and move the skin on the scalp. Don't rub or you will merely pull hairs out, which is rather counter-productive!

Pre-shampoo treatments

If your hair is naturally dry or has become dry due to overshampooing, overbleaching, overcoloring, or too much sun or illness, both hair and scalp will benefit from the following treatments.

EGG AND HONEY TREATMENT FOR DRY, DAMAGED, OR FINE HAIR

1 egg yolk, beaten
2 teaspoons castor oil
1 teaspoon runny honey
dried milk powder, to mix
2 drops sandalwood essential oil
2 drops clary sage essential oil

To make and use

Mix the egg, castor oil, and honey together then add enough dried milk to make a very soft paste. Add the essential oils and mix well.

Rub the paste thoroughly into the hair and scalp.

Cover hair with a plastic shower cap and then wrap the whole head in a hot towel. Alternatively, wrap the head in a towel wrung out in very hot water.

Leave for 20 minutes.

Shampoo with a mild herbal shampoo.

EGG AND LEMON PRE-SHAMPOO TREATMENT

This one is for oily hair.

1 beaten egg
1 teaspoon runny honey
1 teaspoon lemon juice
3 drops lemon essential oil
dried milk powder, to mix
1 tablespoon water

To make and use

Combine all the ingredients in a bowl with one tablespoon of water using enough dried milk powder to make a very soft paste.

Rub the paste thoroughly into the hair and scalp.

Cover hair with a plastic shower cap and then wrap the whole head in a hot towel. Alternatively, wrap the head in a towel wrung out in very hot water.

Leave for 20 minutes.

Shampoo with a mild herbal shampoo.

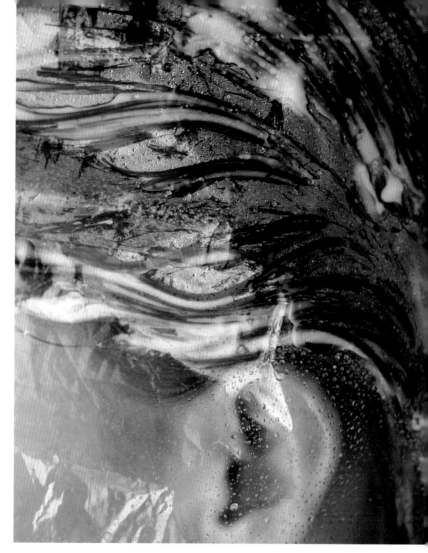

HOT OIL TREATMENT

The quantities in this recipe may need to be doubled if your hair is very long or thick.

$2\frac{1}{2}$ tablespoons (40 ml) castor oil
4 teaspoons olive oil
10 drops lavender essential oil
5 drops clary sage essential oil
5 drops sandalwood essential oil

To make and use

Mix all the oils together and warm to blood heat (no hotter).

Massage the blend into your hair and scalp.

Cover hair with a piece of toweling wrung out in very hot water, and then with a shower cap. Wrap the whole head in a hot towel.

Reheat this towel when it cools two or three times. Do not shampoo for at least one hour.

Follow with a herbal shampoo.

Cover your hair with plastic after applying conditioner and leave for a few minutes before rinsing to increase the shine.

Opposite: Tinting and coloring your hair is very fashionable, but don't overdo it. Consistently putting chemicals on your hair will make it brittle, and it may even break off.

Choosing essential oils for your hair

Condition/ treatment	Oils
Alopecia	Bay laurel, carrot seed, clary sage, evening primrose, lavender, rosemary, thyme
General haircare	Cedarwood, clary sage, geranium, lavender, rosemary, ylang-ylang
Dry hair	Geranium, lavender, rosemary, sandalwood, ylang-ylang
Oily hair	Bay laurel, clary sage, cypress, lavender, lemon, rosemary
Normal hair	Lavender, lemon, geranium, rosemary
Dandruff	Bay laurel, bergamot, cedarwood, clary sage, lavender, rosemary, sandalwood
Fragile hair	Chamomile, clary sage, lavender, sandalwood
Loss of hair	Cedarwood, juniper, lemon, rosemary
Scalp tonic	Bay laurel, cedarwood, chamomile, clary sage, lemon, rosemary, tea tree, ylang-ylang
Split ends	Rosewood, sandalwood

SIMPLE HOT OIL TREATMENT

This simple treatment works well on dry, damaged hair and is also a good treatment for dandruff as it loosens the scaly dried sebum from the scalp.

Heat a mixture of olive oil, coconut oil, and castor oil to lukewarm. Massage gently into the hair and scalp.

Cover the head with a piece of toweling wrung out in hot water and a plastic shower cap. Wrap the head in a separate hot towel. Change the towel when it cools.

Reheat a few times, using the treatment for at least an hour. Follow with a herbal shampoo.

PROTEIN TREATMENT

Use lukewarm water to shampoo this out or you will end up with scrambled eggs in your hair!

1 beaten egg
1 teaspoon glycerine
4 teaspoons rice bran oil

To make and use

Combine all the ingredients in a bowl.

Rub the mixture thoroughly into the hair and scalp. Cover hair with a shower cap and then wrap the whole head in a hot towel. Alternatively, wrap the head in a towel wrung out in very hot water.

Leave for 20 minutes.

Shampoo with a mild herbal shampoo.

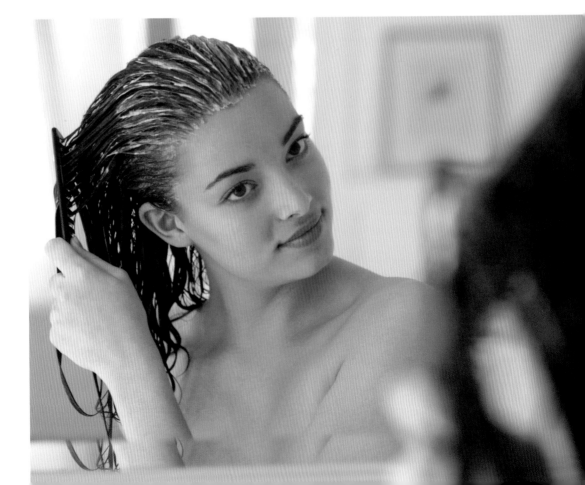

Use only a wide-toothed comb when applying treatments to your hair.

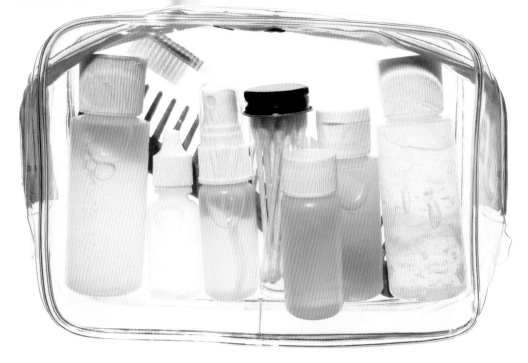

It's good to keep all your different hair products together for ease of use and cleanliness.

Real shampoos, rinses, and dressings

Commercial shampoos are, basically, the same formula as carpet shampoo. One of the main ingredients is a foaming agent. We have been conditioned to believe that seeing plenty of foam means that the product is cleaning well, when in fact the foam has nothing to do with the product's cleaning capacity—it is purely for our gratification.

Detergent-based shampoo strips the hair of all its natural oil and that is why wax conditioners are needed. The following recipes are for natural herbal shampoos based on soap. This is the type of shampoo our grandmothers used before the advent of detergents. Their hair was certainly no worse than ours, and frankly, I think it was much better. Soap-based shampoo will not strip your hair of its natural oils, but you will need to use an acid rinse afterwards as soap is alkaline.

At first, using this Basic Herbal Shampoo may feel completely different from your regular purchased brands, but persevere—your hair and hip pocket will both thank you! After about three weeks (it takes this long to get rid of wax conditioners, fillers and other chemical ingredients from the hair shafts) you will really begin to enjoy your new hair treatment.

BASIC HERBAL SHAMPOO

$2^1/_2$–$3^1/_2$ oz (80–100g) pure soap flakes (such as Lux)
Blended oils or single essential oil of your choice
1 quart (1 liter) rain or purified water, heated
2 teaspoons borax

To make and use

Stir soap, water, and borax together until completely dissolved.

Reheat if necessary. Cool.

Add the blended oils or single essential oil of your choice.

Stir until completely incorporated. This shampoo may go lumpy after standing. It doesn't matter—just give it a good stir until it is blended again.

"QUICKIE" SHAMPOO

If you don't have the time or inclination to make your own shampoo then choose one that claims to be mild and "customize" it.

Add 50 drops of single or mixed essential oils suitable for your hair type (see table, page 288) to 1 cup (250 ml) shampoo. (10 drops of oil for children from 5–10 years old; five drops only for children from 2–5 years old.)

Mix the oils in very thoroughly.

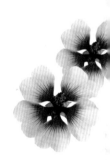

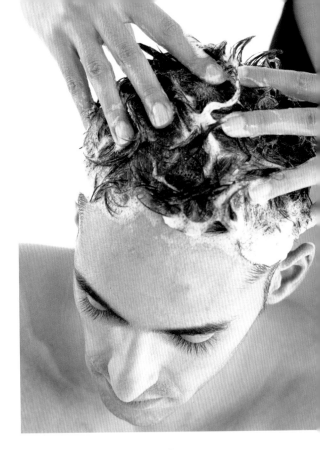

Opposite: There is nothing more inviting than a luxurious bathroom. I try to make mine a sanctuary.

AFTER SHAMPOO RINSE

2 cups (500 ml) cider vinegar
2 teaspoons appropriate mixed or single
   essential oils

To make and use

Mix all the ingredients together in a 17 fl oz
(500 ml) bottle.

Leave for four days to synergize.

Label and store in a cool, dark place.

Add $1/2$ cup (125 ml) of the rinse to 1 quart (1 liter)
of warm water.

Rinse hair, using a bowl to catch the drips.

Repeat rinsing as often as you like, or until your
arms are too tired.

DRY SHAMPOO

The more you wash your hair the oilier it will
become, as you overstimulate the subcutaneous
glands. You can use a dry shampoo to remove
excess oil or if, for some reason, you can't wash
your hair.

Sprinkle one teaspoon of cornmeal, oatmeal,
orris root, or bran through your hair and massage
into the scalp.

Brush out well.

For perfectly clean hair use the After Shampoo Rinse to rid the hair of any residual shampoo.

Rinse your hands and fingers well after shampooing.

ECONOMY HERBAL SHAMPOO

For this recipe you will need a bottle of the best
natural shampoo you can find, plus an empty bottle.
I use a mixture of half herbs and half shampoo
because I don't mind the thin consistency and want
as much herbal content as possible. Try for yourself
and see which proportion you like best.

Empty one-quarter of the shampoo into the
empty bottle and save for another time.

Put four heaped teaspoons of dried (or eight
teaspoons fresh chopped) herbs into a saucepan
with 1 cup (250 ml) of water.

Cover and simmer very gently for 10 minutes.

Allow to stand for 30 minutes.

Strain, pour back into the saucepan, and simmer
until enough remains to top up the three-quarters-
full shampoo bottle.

Cool the liquid before adding to the bottle.

Shake very gently to mix well.

Alternately, add 20 drops of lavender and 10 drops
of rosemary essential oil to a 9 fl oz (250 ml) shampoo
bottle. Proportionately less if your shampoo bottle
is smaller.

Invert the bottle before use to thoroughly mix
in the oils.

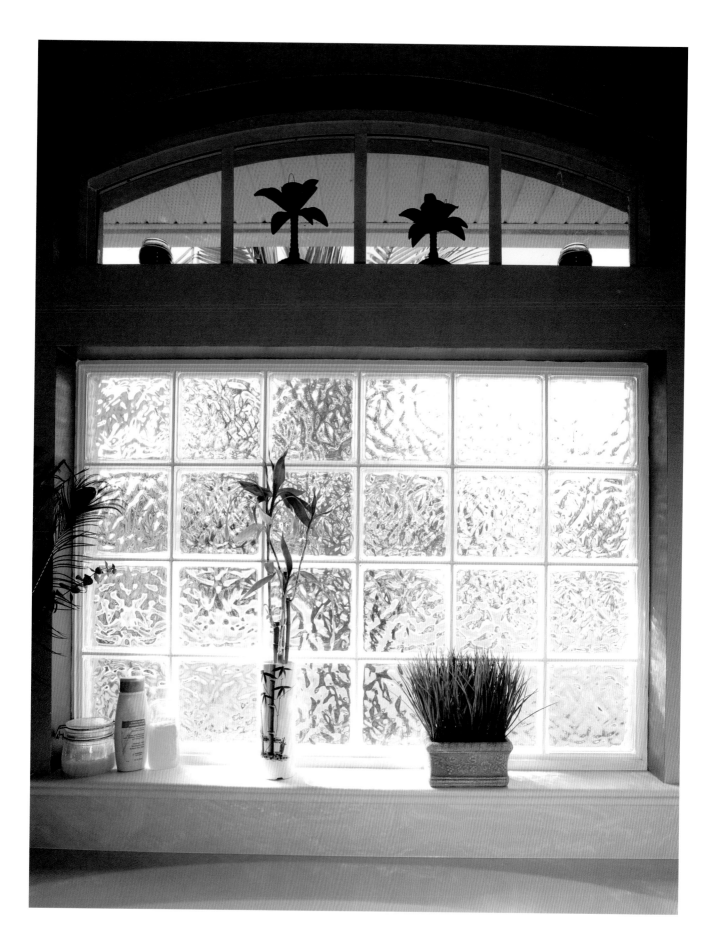

CASTILE SHAMPOO

Liquid Castile soap is readily available in health-food stores. It comes in a bottle with a handy pump dispenser. I like to add essential oils to the soap. It can also be diluted with a little purified water. If you choose to make and use this shampoo you will need a vinegar rinse or a herbal conditioner to restore the acid balance to your hair.

A bottle of Castile soap usually contains 17 fl oz (500 ml) and you will need to decant about one quarter (about $^1/_2$ cup/125 ml) to make room for the herbal infusion.

It's difficult to make a mixture of herbs in the small amount required. To overcome this I make up 1 oz (30 g) of mixed dried herbs and rub them down to the size of a tea leaf. I save what I'm not using immediately in a jar labelled "Shampoo Herbs."

1 teaspoon (about 5 g) finely chopped dried herbs
$1^1/_4$ cups (300 ml) distilled water
2 teaspoons vegetable glycerine
30 drops lavender essential oil
30 drops rosemary essential oil
$1^1/_2$ cups (425 ml) liquid Castile soap (unperfumed or rosemary is best)

To make and use

Gently simmer the herbs and water in a covered saucepan for 30 minutes.

Stand for one hour.

Strain through a sieve and squeeze the herbs well to get every drop of liquid out.

Discard the herbs.

Return the infusion to a pan, simmer, covered, until reduced to $^1/_2$ cup (125 ml).

Strain the extract through coffee filter paper.

Mix the vegetable glycerine and essential oils together in a small bowl. Add to the Castile soap.

Pour into a clean 17 fl oz (500 ml) squeezy bottle. Slowly add the herbal extract to the mixture in the bottle, shaking gently to blend.

Gently upend the bottle a couple of times before use.

Use an acidic rinse following the shampoo.

Castile Shampoo can be made from any of your favorite herbs.

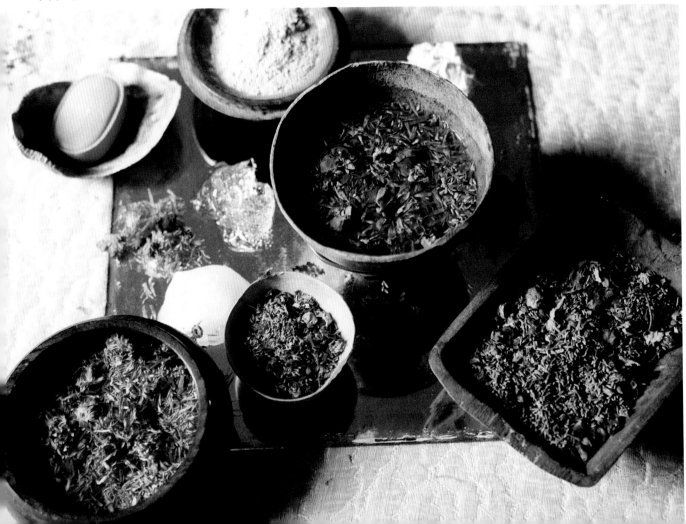

HERBAL VINEGAR RINSE

Choose herbs from the table on page 286.

To make and use

Fill a jar with chopped fresh herbs or half-fill with dried herbs.

Cover with warm cider vinegar, then with a non-metal lid.

Stand the jar in the hot sun or another warm place for 24 hours.

Strain the vinegar, add more fresh herbs and repeat the above process.

Repeat once more if a very strong vinegar is desired.

Strain through a sieve and then through coffee filter paper.

Add 2 teaspoons of glycerine to each cup of vinegar.

To use, add 1–2 tablespoons (15–30 ml) vinegar to a 10 fl oz (300 ml) spray bottle.

Rinse the hair with water after shampooing then spray thoroughly with the vinegar rinse. Don't rinse out.

HAIR TONIC

This tonic will keep for three to four weeks in the refrigerator in a screwtop bottle or jar, but some of it may be frozen to extend its life.

Herbs to use could include: Basil, red clover, lavender, lemon grass, nettle, rosemary, southernwood, thyme, or wormwood, or you may choose herbs from the table on page 286.

To make and use

Make a triple-strength tea using as many as possible of the above herbs. Strain into a jug.

For every 2 cups (500 ml) of infusion add three teaspoons of borax and two teaspoons of glycerine and dissolve together.

Add 40 drops of lavender oil and 40 drops of rosemary oil.

Bottle and shake well. Label the bottle.

To use, shake the bottle well, apply a few drops to your scalp and, using the pads of the fingers, massage in briskly with a zigzag movement.

Don't pull your hair while massaging.

Use once or twice a day.

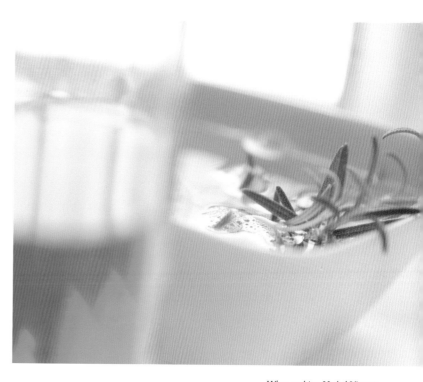

HAIR OIL

This oil will give health and sheen to your hair without making it greasy. It also gives your hair a wonderful fragrance.

To make and use

Mix together equal parts of rosemary, lavender, and either basil or juniper oils, with jojoba oil.

Put a few drops on the palm of one hand and rub your hands together.

Now rub the oil from your palms through your hair.

This can be done as frequently or as infrequently as you like.

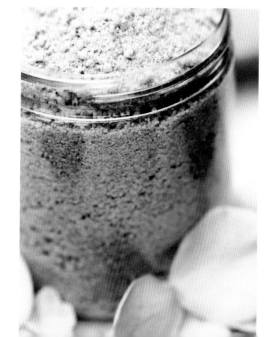

When making Herbal Vinegar Rinse, choose the very freshest and aromatic herbs that you have on hand. Rosemary makes a nice spicy scent for men.

Keep clear jam jars for storing bath products. Scrub them and finish the cleaning by a good wash in the dishwasher.

Conditioners

You may find that after using the shampoo and vinegar rinse your hair doesn't need a conditioner. If, however, you have very fine, limp hair or if your hair has been overpermed or overcolored or otherwise abused you may need a protein conditioner. Leave the conditioner on for at least 10 minutes after shampooing, rinse off, and finish with a vinegar rinse or spray.

The following conditioners don't put layers of silicon on the hair shaft and they will leave your hair full-bodied, soft, and glossy.

A body brush made of natural bristles with a wooden handle is not only good for the body but it looks good too.

ROSEMARY CONDITIONER

For all hair types except oily.

1 beaten egg
1 teaspoon glycerine
2 drops castor oil
2 drops rosemary essential oil
2 drops lavender essential oil
skim milk powder

To make and use

Beat all ingredients together adding enough milk powder to form a soft paste.

Use immediately; massage into the hair after shampooing.

Leave on for a few minutes then rinse hair lightly with lukewarm water.

Keep plenty of fresh clean towels in your bathroom to increase the pampered feel.

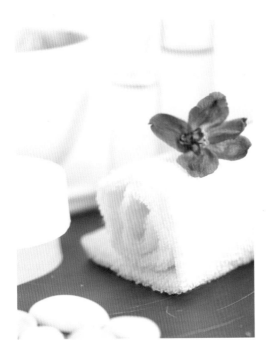

BRANDY LEMON CONDITIONER

For oily hair.

2$\frac{1}{2}$ tablespoons (40 ml) brandy
1 teaspoon runny honey
1 beaten egg
2 drops lemon grass essential oil
1 drop rosemary essential oil
skim milk powder

To make and use

Beat all the ingredients together with enough milk powder to form a soft paste.

Use immediately; massage into the hair after shampooing.

Leave on for a few minutes then rinse hair lightly with lukewarm water.

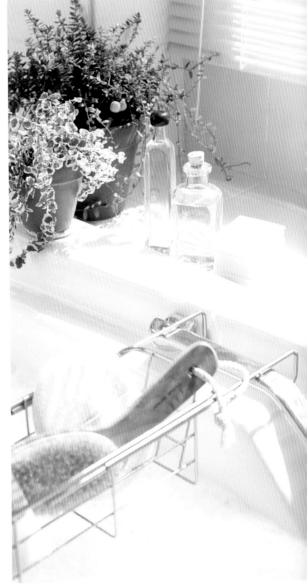

HAIR DRESSING

This treatment can be used as often as you like.
Hair dressing is used between shampoos to keep
hair glossy, smooth, and healthy. The non-greasy
essential oils are absorbed into the hair shaft,
making it suitable for all hair types.

2 teaspoons lavender essential oil
2 teaspoons rosemary essential oil
$^1/_2$ teaspoon geranium essential oil
$^1/_2$ teaspoon jojoba oil (for dry or damaged hair only),
    or $^1/_2$ teaspoon juniper essential oil (for other
    hair types)

To make and use

Mix all ingredients together in a dropper bottle.
    Label the bottle and shake before using.
    Put a few drops in the palm of one hand and
then rub your hands together.
    Now, rub your palms through your hair.

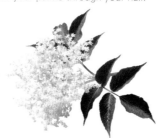

*Luxurious Brandy Lemon
Conditioner contains lemon grass
essential oil, which leaves the hair
with a fresh citrus smell.*

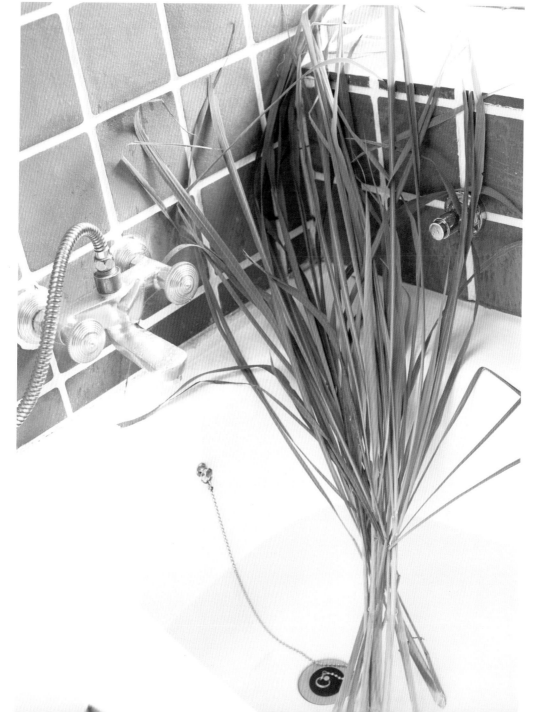

Pre-treating your hair before washing or coloring will help prevent the onset of serious hair loss. Reducing stress will also help.

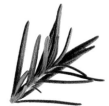

Hair problems

Alopecia

Alopecia (temporary baldness) can be the result of illness, thyroid or pituitary deficiency, poorly functioning ovaries, or stress. The hair loss is usually gradual but severe and sudden hair loss has been known if there has been sudden traumatic shock or grief.

Alopecia can often be helped considerably by treatment with essential oil but it as also necessary to visit a health practitioner who can run tests to determine the reason for the condition.

Scalp massage is of great benefit as it increases the blood supply to the hair follicle. Use in conjunction with the vinegar treatment below.

Essential oils for alopecia: Carrot seed, clary sage, evening primrose, lavender, rosemary, thyme.

HAIR LOSS

This treatment is for hair loss other than from alopecia. There are many reasons why hair begins to fall out at a faster than usual rate. The following drugs can cause mild to major hair loss: Two or more aspirin a day; birth control pills (see your doctor for a change of pills if you notice your hair falling out), diet pills, cortisone (this can make your hair grow on your face and fall out of your head!), anticoagulants, amphetamines, and chemotherapy. Major trauma such as serious accident, or stress such as death of someone close, divorce, prolonged illness, or liver disease caused by years of heavy drinking, can all cause hair loss. If the situation is remedied and the stress brought under control, the hair loss is not usually permanent and the follicles will usually begin to grow hair again within a few weeks.

If you are pregnant or a new mother the nutritional demands on your nerves and body are heavy, and the hair loss may be a combination of stress and nutritional deficiencies such as iron. Very heavy periods can also cause iron deficiency and accompanying hair loss. A blood test is indicated in these three physical conditions if the hair loss is great and you are very tired. Hypo- or hyper-hydroidism is another condition where the hair loss is considerable and blood test is indicated.

Take heart. Unless the hair loss is genetic, it will slowly grow again when the reason for the loss has been eliminated. Use the treatment and oils for alopecia.

ALOPECIA PRE-WASH TREATMENT

1 tablespoon castor oil
1 tablespoon olive oil
10 drops jojoba oil
10 drops lavender essential oil
5 drops carrot seed essential oil
5 drops clary sage essential oil

To make and use
Mix all the oils together and warm to blood heat (no hotter).
Use immediately; massage into the hair and scalp.
Cover hair with a piece of old toweling wrung out in very hot water, and then with a shower cap. Wrap the whole head in a hot towel. Reheat the towel when it cools.
Repeat a few times, and do not shampoo for at least an hour.
Follow with Alopecia Shampoo.

ALOPECIA SHAMPOO

1/2 cup Basic Herbal Shampoo
14 drops jojoba oil
10 drops lavender essential oil
4 drops rosemary essential oil

To make and use
Mix ingredients together thoroughly.
Bottle and label.

ALOPECIA VINEGAR TREATMENT

3 1/2 fl oz (100 ml) cider vinegar
45 drops appropriate mixed or single essential oils

To make and use
Mix all the ingredients together in a bottle.
Label and leave for four days to synergize.
Shake the bottle before using.
Add one teaspoon of the rinse blend to one tablespoon warm water and use for a scalp massage.

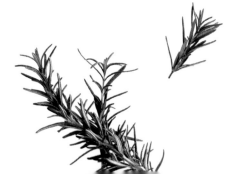

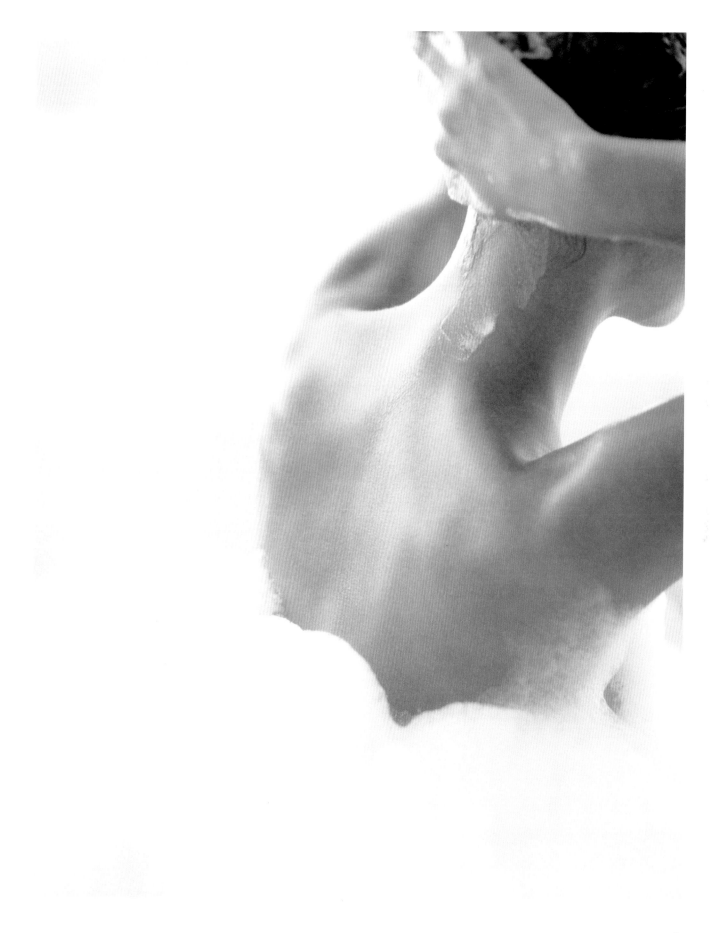

Dandruff

Dandruff (seborrheic dermatitis) is a miserable and common complaint causing embarrassment to the sufferer. The creamy white flakes that are shed from the scalp can ruin the appearance of an outfit. The scalp is sometimes itchy, sore, and irritated which causes the sufferer to scratch, and this in turn loosens more flakes. There is still debate as to the cause of dandruff—one theory is that it is caused by excess sebum blocking the pores. Others are now of the opinion that it is caused by a fungal infection. A third school of thought blames inadequate nutrition.

Beware of commercial dandruff shampoos, they keep the problem at bay but I've never heard of a user being permanently cured. It's possible to treat excess sebum and fungus simultaneously by the use of herbal and essential oil remedies. The Hot Oil Treatment described previously is excellent as the oils dissolve the hardened sebum while the essential oils attack the fungus.

Dandruff is hard to treat and is often recurring but it seems that a moist scalp and well-conditioned hair are the best treatments.

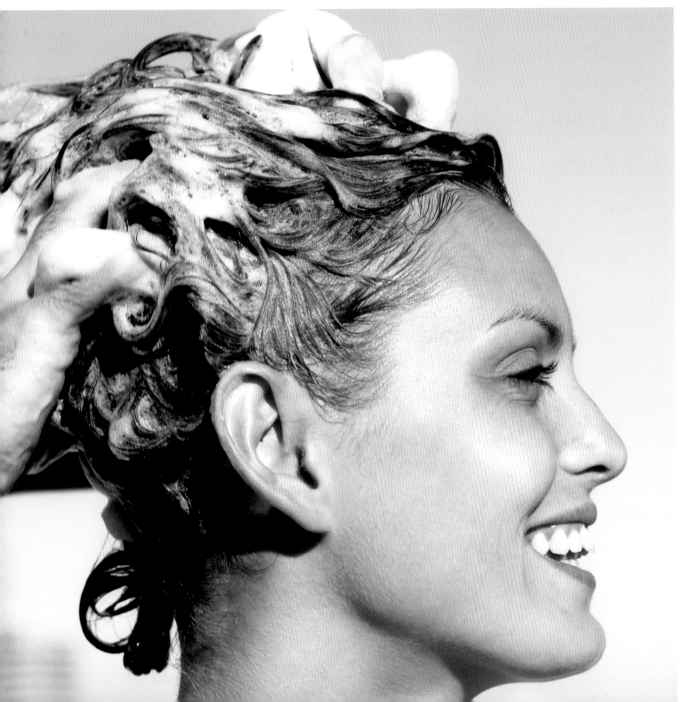

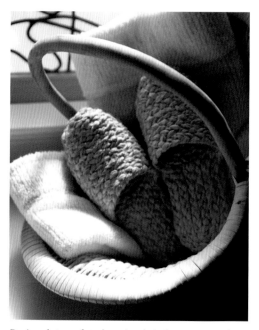

Don't neglect your feet when using the bathroom as some viruses, bacteria, and fungi thrive in moist conditions. Keep a special pair of slippers for use in the bathroom.

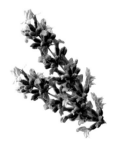

Nothing eases stress or sets a better mood than a candle made from your favorite essential oil.

Here are some tips for treating dandruff:

* Eat plenty of fruit and vegetables daily.
* Start the day with the juice of a lemon in a glass of water.
* Shampoo twice weekly using lavender and tea tree essential oils in the shampoo. Follow with a Herbal Bath Vinegar rinse (page 315). Massage the vinegar onto the scalp (cider vinegar has effected cures using no other treatment).
* Massage the scalp with Anti-Dandruff Tonic every night.
* Hats and other head coverings encourage dandruff. Keep the head exposed as much as possible.
* Take a B-complex capsule daily.
* Use the Simple Hot Oil Treatment on page 288 once a fortnight.

ANTI-DANDRUFF TONIC

This is a very good hair tonic that will both attack fungus and help to remove excess sebum.

1 cup hot distilled water
1 teaspoon borax
2 teaspoons witch hazel (optional)
2 tablespoons cider vinegar
20 drops lavender essential oil
20 drops tea tree essential oil

To make and use

Dissolve the borax in the hot water and allow to cool.

Add the remaining ingredients and bottle and label. Shake well before use.

Part the hair with a comb and apply the tonic with an absorbent cotton (cottonwool) ball making sure that all the skin on the scalp has been treated.

Massage the scalp gently before bedtime.

To add to the scent, it's always nice to add some of the original herb to an essential oil bath.

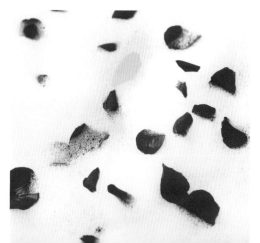

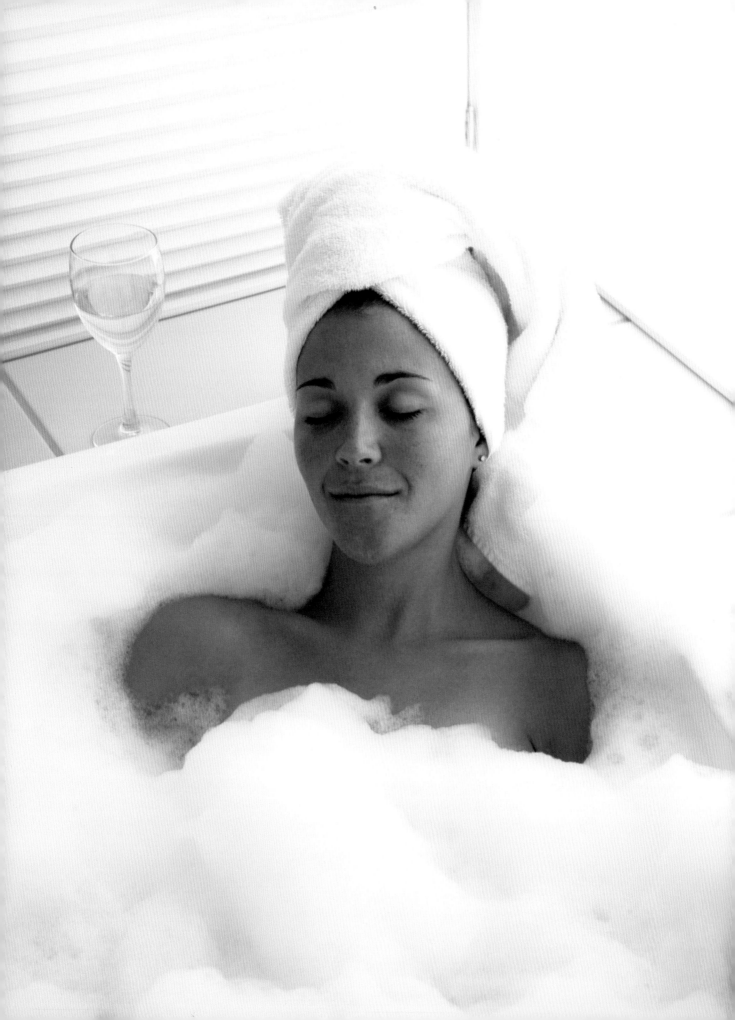

Baths

We take water for granted and overlook the precious gift it is. Our bodies need it inside and outside. Water stimulates, relaxes, heals, and purifies.

Everyone knows the clean, relaxed feeling after a long, leisurely bath, but the benefits can be infinitely greater in terms of health. Bathing is an "anti-stress" aid. Run a deep bath, pour something pleasant into the water, light a perfumed candle or oil burner, spread a soothing mask on your face, and lie back against a bath pillow, or a hot-water bottle filled with warm water, sipping a warm drink and listening to soft music. Your stress will run down the drain with the bath water and you will leave the bathroom ready to take on the world again. Don't forget the "Do Not Disturb" sign to hang on the doorknob!

There are few people who do not enjoy a bath. One the reasons they are so relaxing is that the water gets rid of all the prickly positive ions which make us feel so stressed and tired. It's not generally realized that the skin (which is the largest organ in the body), given optimum conditions, can be responsible for one-third of the excretion of waste matter from the body. By so doing, the liver, kidneys, and lungs are relieved of quite a load. In order to work efficiently, the skin needs to be clean and free from dead cells, which can block the pores. Using a body brush before bathing or showering helps to get rid of these dead cells.

The luxury of a jet spa bath can now be enjoyed in your own home.

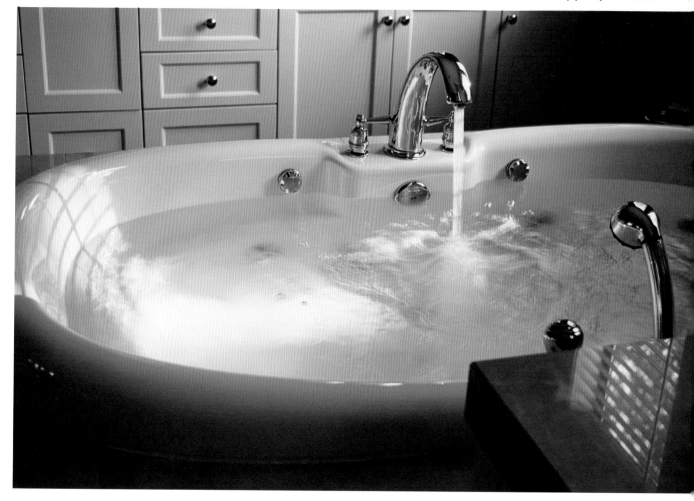

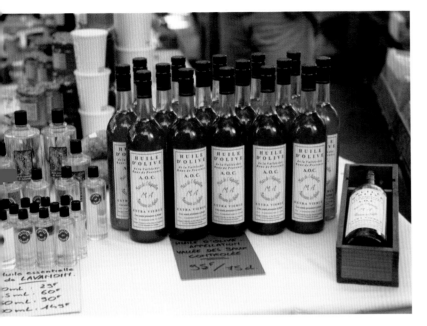

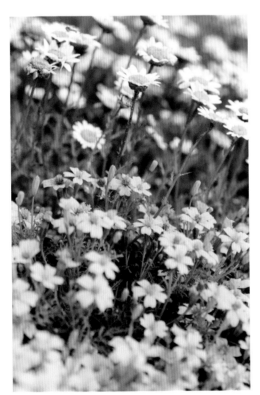

Maurice Messegue, the famous French herbalist, used hot herbal foot and hand baths in preference to administering herbs internally. He found that the infusion, which is absorbed by the skin into the bloodstream, works faster and more efficiently than the same infusion taken internally and absorbed through the digestive system.

Luxury bath products can easily be made in your kitchen and at a fraction of the price of the bought variety. Most of the treatments suggested for the bath may also be used in the shower.

Do be careful when using essential oils directly in the bath water. I once sprinkled a few drops of rosemary oil on the water but didn't "swoosh" the water around. As I climbed in I must have collected the oil on my calf and the outside of my thigh. After a few moments I experienced a burning sensation and after the bath I was very red and lightly blistered in these areas. I had been using these oils for decades and should have known better!

The recipes given here can also be used if you prefer a shower. The bag containing the herbs or oatmeal mixture may be used as a washcloth and, instead of putting infusions in your bath water, you can splash them onto your body after a shower.

If you do not have access to a bath, you can sprinkle a drop or two of the appropriate essential oil on a very wet face cloth, partially wring it out and wipe it over your body. Another option is to make an air spray using essential oils for your particular problem—no more than 6 drops in a 1 cup (250 ml) pump spray bottle—and shake the bottle well. Spray your body lightly after you have finished washing, massage into your skin, then pat dry.

There are many ways of getting maximum value from your bath: Use pre-bath treatments, bath oils, after-bath colognes, powders, and oils. You will find recipes for all these in the following pages.

Essential and culinary oils for sale at a market in Aix-en-Provence, France.

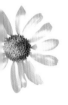

Yellow marigolds and white chamomile in bloom.

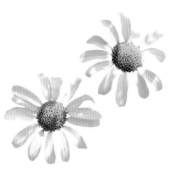

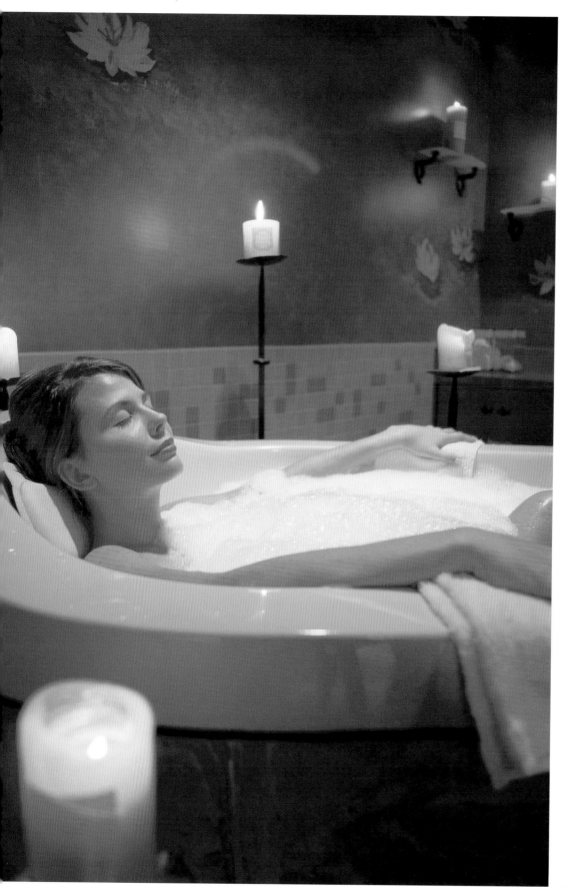

*Dim the lights, light the candles,
and put out a "Do not disturb!"
sign before taking your "Me" time.*

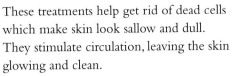

Pre-bath treatments

These treatments help get rid of dead cells which make skin look sallow and dull. They stimulate circulation, leaving the skin glowing and clean.

Dry-brush massage

You will need a body brush with a long, preferably removable handle. These are quite inexpensive and can be bought at health-food shops or pharmacies. You can use a long loofah, but I find a brush easier.

Brush the whole body from the neck down, being gentle on delicate areas such as the thighs, abdomen, and breasts. Pay particular attention to the areas where there are glands—that is, the groin, armpits, and side of the neck. Brush these areas gently but thoroughly with a circular motion.

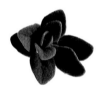

Ground oats and a natural sea sponge are the perfect combination for smooth soap-free skin.

SALT RUB

Stand in the bath or shower recess to use this rub, as it's pretty messy. It's even better if you share this with a friend so you can do each other's backs! Don't use salt rub on the genital regions, however.

To make and use

Mix together four teaspoons of coarse salt and four teaspoons of the infused oil of your choice. Add two drops of essential oil.

Lightly oil your body first with sweet almond oil or your infused oil and then, using a firm circular motion, rub the mixture onto the skin. You will be astonished to see the amount of dirt that comes off.

Shower or bathe and use some herbal massage oil to finish.

OAT CLEANSER

This cleanser may be used instead of soap. It makes a good facial scrub by mixing a small amount to a paste with water, gently massaging it into the skin, and rinsing off with cool water. When used in the bath, it is very soothing to itchy, sore skin. It's excellent for babies' baths but only the gentlest herbs should be used. Make large quantities of this mixture as it keeps indefinitely if stored in the refrigerator.

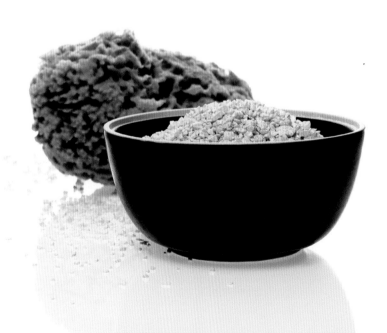

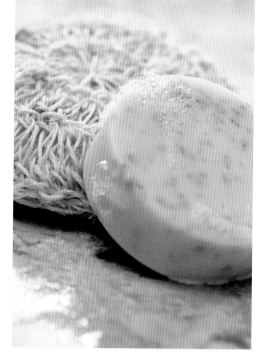

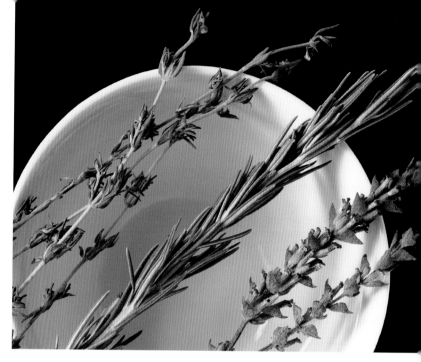

Bathing with herbs

Herbs in the bath hydrate and soothe the skin, but it's not much fun having a bath with twigs and leaves floating around in it; they will clog your plumbing if not laboriously picked out at the end of your relaxing bath, destroying the mood and mystique. Much better to use one of the following methods.

Put a handful of herbs in a pan, cover with water, add one to two tablespoons of cider vinegar, cover with a lid and simmer on a low heat for 20 minutes. Strain (put the herbs in your compost bucket) and pour the wonderfully rich herb soup into the bath, or sponge it over your body when you have finished showering. The cider vinegar creates the correct acid balance and also extracts more properties from the herbs than water alone.

An alternative is to chop the herbs and tie them in a piece of fine cloth or a muslin bag, hang the bundle under hot water as it's running and then use it as a washcloth.

If you are in a hurry or don't have access to fresh herbs, you can use herbal tea bags, either dropped into the bath and squeezed well, or made into a strong infusion as in the first method above.

Bath mitts accompanied by a big jar of herbal mix make a nice gift for family and friends to use in the bath or shower. To make a mitt you will need a piece of toweling about 8 in × 20 in (20 cm × 50 cm). Blanket stitch or machine zigzag along one long edge (this becomes the wrist edge, or the mitt's opening). Cut into three mitt shapes then stitch the three shapes together around three sides, leaving the previously zigzagged edges free. You now have a mitt with two pockets— one for the herb mixture and one for your hand. You can sew a loop on one corner for hanging the mitt up to dry.

Less glamorous but just as effective are bags made from the feet of an old pair of tights (pantyhose).

The following preparations are for mixtures of crumbled, dried herbs to use in the bath. The quantities are quite large so that you can keep them on hand ready to use. Fresh herbs are lovely to use, as the perfume is usually more intense, but unless you intend to dry the surplus, the recipe should be reduced to an amount suitable for only one bath.

The measures are in cups. You can use a teacup or coffee cup that holds 1 cup (250 ml) of water if you don't have a set of measuring cups.

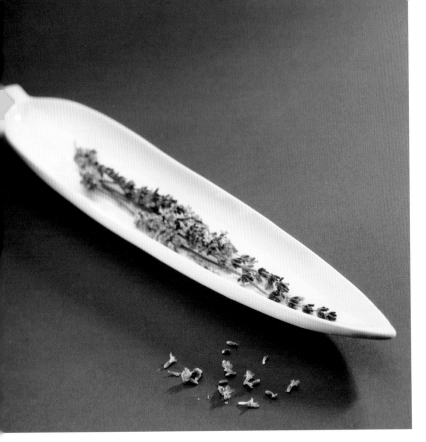

The saying goes: "Lavender fixes anything." It is definitely the favorite herb for bathing.

The essential oils are optional but they intensify both the perfume and the therapeutic effect of the bath. Mix the dried herbs thoroughly and sprinkle the essential oil evenly through the herbs, then mix again. Powdered dried orris root or clary sage added to these mixtures helps to fix the perfume.

QUICKIE HERBAL BATH

Use herbal tea bags to make a very strong brew. Tip the tea in the bath and fold the used bags in a piece of cheesecloth to use as a body washer.

It's hard to resist brushes and scrubbers made from natural products.

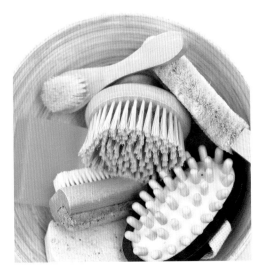

SPIRIT OF YOUTH

If you are feeling jaded, older than your years, or need a "pick me up," try the following bath mixture of dried herbs.

3 cups dried, crumbled lavender
1 cup dried, crumbled rosemary
2 cups dried, crumbled peppermint
1 cup dried, crumbled comfrey
1 dropperful peppermint essential oil

To make and use
Mix the crumbled herbs and oil together well to combine.
    Store in a tightly sealed, labeled container.
    Use $1/4$–$1/2$ cup of the mixture (about a handful) for each bath.

SOFT TOUCH

When your skin feels sore and dry and your mind feels "scratchy," this bath will make your skin feel like silk, and will calm your mind and soothe the heart.

$1/2$ cup bicarbonate of soda
4 cups rolled oats or oatmeal
2 cups bran
2 heaped tablespoons wholemeal flour
1 cup dried milk powder
1 dropperful lavender essential oil

To make and use
Combine all the dry ingredients and mix together well.
    Drizzle the essential oil over the mixture while stirring well to combine.
    Store in a tightly sealed container.
    Use $1/4$–$1/2$ cup of the mixture for each bath.

DEODORANT BATH

This is gently deodorising for a sweet-smelling body.

2 cups dried lovage root, finely chopped
2 cups dried lavender, crumbled
$1/2$ cup dried rosemary, crumbled
1 cup dried sage, crumbled
$1/2$ cup dried thyme, crumbled
$1/4$ dropperful patchouli essential oil
$1/4$ dropperful orange essential oil

To make and use
Mix the herbs well and drizzle the combined oils over the mixture while stirring.
    Store in a tightly sealed, labeled container.
    Use $1/4$–$1/2$ cup of the mixture for each bath.

QUICK DEODORANT BATH

This is a simple infusion bath. The herbs can be used fresh but if you don't have them straight from the garden, you can use dry herbs. They will not have quite the same feel but they will still freshen the body. Use 2–3 tablespoons of dry herbs for each $\frac{1}{2}$ cup fresh herbs.

$\frac{1}{2}$ cup chopped lavender (stems and flowers if
   possible)
$\frac{1}{2}$ cup chopped thyme leaves
$\frac{1}{2}$ cup chopped rosemary leaves
1 muslin bag
1 quart (1 liter) water

To make and use

Use a small muslin bag or the toe end of an pair of tights (pantyhose). Add the fresh or dried herbs to the bag and tie off well.

Bring the water to the boil and add the bag to the water and put on the lid. Allow to simmer for 15–20 minutes.

Remove the bag from the water and allow it to cool slightly. Do not discard the water as this is the infusion.

Add the infusion and bag to your bath and top up with hot water. You can use the bag of herbs as a washcloth if you wish.

RELAXATION BATH

This one is just for lying in until the water goes cold and you have to top it up. It's hard to get out of.

$\frac{1}{2}$ cup dry chamomile flowers
$\frac{1}{2}$ cup dry lemon balm
2 cups (500 ml) boiling water

To make and use

Sprinkle the herbs over the boiling water and cover. Leave to simmer for 20 minutes. Remove from heat and allow to cool slightly.

Strain through a very fine sieve and then add the infusion to your bathwater.

GODDESS OF SLEEP

This will help to ensure a good night's sleep. The bath should be warm, not hot. Sip a cup of chamomile or catnep tea sweetened with honey while relaxing in the bath. Add the following to the bath water: 3 cups dried and crumbled catnep; 2 cups dried and crumbled chamomile; $\frac{1}{2}$ cup dried and crumbled hop flowers; and 1 tablespoon bicarbonate of soda. After you have soaked for 20–30 minutes, dry your body gently and slip between the sheets.

Below left: Lavender essential oil and cologne have very little color—a shame considering the scent.
Below: At least you can buy beautiful towels to remind you of the glorious fields of Provence, France.

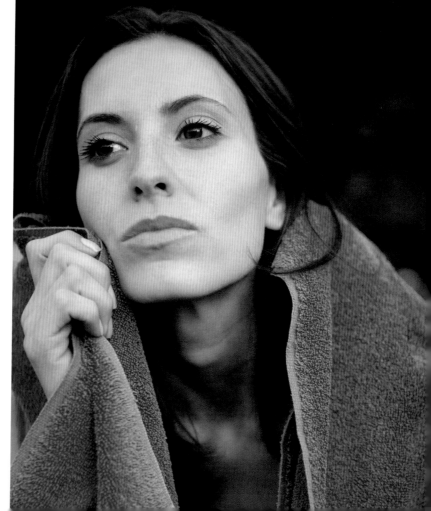

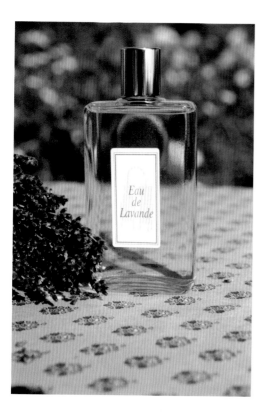

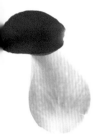

"FLORA AND THE COUNTRY GREEN"

This deliciously fragrant mixture can be used in bath bags or made into cologne. Packaged in a beautiful bottle, the cologne makes a lovely gift.

$\frac{1}{4}$ cup dried and crumbled peppermint
$\frac{1}{4}$ cup crushed bay leaves
$\frac{1}{2}$ cup dried and crumbled lemon balm
$\frac{1}{2}$ cup dried and crumbled lavender
2 tablespoons dried and crumbled wormwood
$\frac{1}{4}$ cup dried and crumbled marjoram
$\frac{1}{4}$ cup dried and crumbled thyme
$\frac{1}{4}$ cup dried and crumbled lemon thyme
$\frac{1}{4}$ cup dried and crumbled angelica
$\frac{1}{2}$ cup perfumed rose petals
$\frac{1}{2}$ dropperful lavender essential oil
$\frac{1}{2}$ dropperful peppermint essential oil
1 cup (250 ml) vodka

To make and use

In a large bowl, combine the dried and crumbled herbs.

Gently simmer about half the herb mix in a covered saucepan for 10 minutes in 1 quart (1 liter) of water. Strain. Repeat the process, using the remaining herb mix in the strained infusion.

Add extra water to bring the amount of infusion back up to 1 quart (1 liter).

Allow to stand for 24 hours

Strain through a sieve and then through coffee filter paper.

Add the essential oils and vodka to the infusion. Bottle and label.

To use, pour $\frac{1}{4}$ cup (60 ml) into the bath while the water is running.

Tea lights are inexpensive and create a romantic ambience.

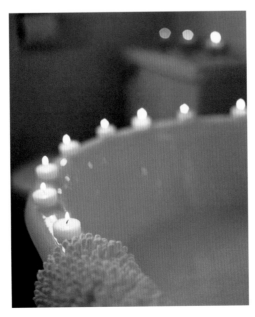

DRY SKIN BATH

Depending where you live, you will usually find that one season in particular, causes the skin to be drier than at other times. Where I live it's usually winter because we get very little rain compared to summer. Whatever that season is for you, here is a marvelous mix to smooth out dry skin. It is also quite quick to make and requires no special bags for infusing.

1 quart (1 liter) boiling water
$\frac{1}{4}$ cup fresh calendula flowers
$\frac{1}{4}$ cup fresh chopped thyme

To make and use

Bring the water to the boil and toss in the flowers and herbs. Cover and simmer for 10–15 minutes.

Remove the pot from the heat and allow it to cool until it is lukewarm. Strain out the flowers and herbs and add the infused water to the bath. Top up with hot water and enjoy.

FRAGRANT BATH

This bath is all about scent. The bathroom will be beautifully scented as well as your skin. You can use dry herbs for this bath; about half the quantity of fresh herbs.

2 tablespoons fresh lavender flowers
2 tablespoons fresh chopped sweet marjoram
2 tablespoons fresh chopped peppermint
1 muslin bath bag
1 quart (1 liter) boiling water

To make and use

Add the lavender buds and herbs to the muslin bag and tie tightly. You can also use the toe of an old pair of tights (pantyhose). Place the bag in the boiling water and cover with the lid on for 15–20 minutes.

Remove from the heat and allow to cool to lukewarm. Add the bag and the water to the bath and top up with hot water.

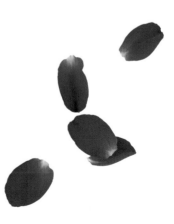

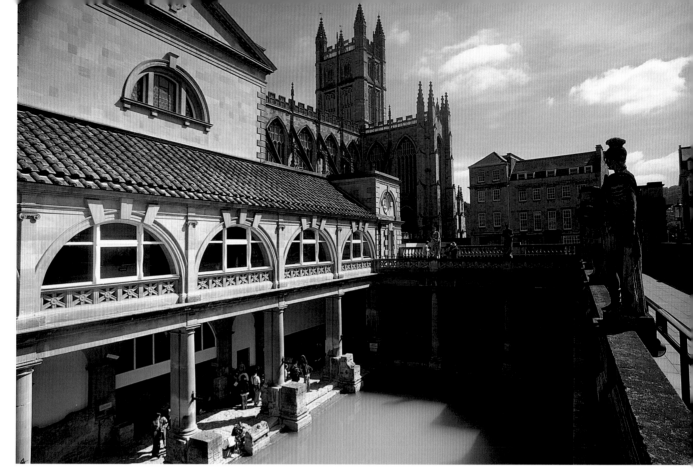

Essential oil bath blends

The following essential oil blends are for baths for adults only. To make, mix 5–10 drops of the bath blend with one tablespoon or so of either full-cream milk or vegetable oil (this helps the oil to disperse more evenly into the water). Add to the bath directly before or just after entering the water or the precious essences may evaporate before your can get full benefit. Agitate the water to disperse the oils thoroughly before getting in.

ANTIBACTERIAL BATH OIL BLEND
3 drops tea tree essential oil
3 drops eucalyptus essential oil
2 drops thyme essential oil
1 drop lemon essential oil
1 drop clove essential oil

ANTIVIRAL BATH OIL BLEND
3 drops tea tree or manuka essential oil
3 drops eucalyptus essential oil
3 drops lavender essential oil
1 drop thyme essential oil

DEODORIZING BATH OIL BLEND
4 drops clary sage essential oil
2 drops eucalyptus essential oil
2 drops patchouli essential oil
2 drops peppermint essential oil

DRY SKIN BATH OIL BLEND
4 drops chamomile essential oil
4 drops palmarosa essential oil
2 drops patchouli essential oil]

OILY SKIN BATH OIL BLEND
5 drops lemon essential oil
3 drops ylang-ylang essential oil

SPOTTY SKIN BATH OIL BLEND
2 drops eucalyptus essential oil
2 drops thyme essential oil
4 drops lavender essential oil
2 drops chamomile essential oil

HEAD-CLEARING BATH OIL BLEND
2 drops peppermint essential oil
2 drops lemon essential oil
1 drop thyme essential oil
2 drops rosemary essential oil
3 drops lavender essential oil

The Roman Baths in the center of Bath, United Kingdom.

Fed by the "Sacred Spring," with water at a temperature of 115°F (46°C), the Great Bath was the centerpiece of Roman bathing, dating back to the late first century. It was designed to cater for the needs of the local people, as well as travelers and pilgrims from across the Empire. The bath is lined with 45 thick sheets of lead and is 5 ft (1.6m) deep and was originally covered by a timber roof.

The benefit of bathing was recognised in the early nineteenth century, when the mineral qualities of the waters were said to benefit recuperation from illness. Most also drank the waters (not from the actual bath) even though the taste was abhorrent.

Bath features in Jane Austen's Pride and Prejudice.

Opposite: Dried rosebuds and lavender flowers in bowls for potpourri.

HYDRATING BATH OIL BLEND
2 drops chamomile essential oil
2 drops lavender essential oil
2 drops carrot seed essential oil
2 drops geranium essential oil
2 drops rose essential oil (optional)

"JUST-AHHHHH" BATH OIL BLEND
1 drop lavender essential oil
2 drops grapefruit essential oil
2 drops geranium essential oil
2 drops ylang-ylang essential oil
2 drops patchouli essential oil

ENERGY RENEWAL BATH OIL BLEND
3 drops rosemary essential oil
2 drops lemon essential oil
2 drops frankincense essential oil

REJUVENATING BATH OIL BLEND
4 drops lavender essential oil
3 drops rosemary essential oil
2 drops peppermint essential oil

Below right: Moist herbal tea bags sooth tired eyes and also relieve pain after tooth removal!

It doesn't seem to matter where you put lavender, it always looks and feels luxurious.

RELAXING BATH OIL BLEND
4 drops chamomile essential oil
3 drops lavender essential oil
3 drops ylang-ylang essential oil

RISE AND SHINE BATH OIL BLEND
2 drops bergamot essential oil
3 drops orange essential oil
3 drops lemon essential oil
1 drop peppermint essential oil
1 drop cinnamon essential oil

MILD SUNBURN BATH BLEND
8–10 drops lavender essential oil

CALMING BATH OIL BLEND
3 drops lavender essential oil
2 drops bergamot essential oil
2 drops cedarwood essential oil

ANTI-STRESS BATH OIL BLEND
4 drops geranium essential oil
2 drops peppermint essential oil

SLEEP WELL BATH OIL BLEND
3 drops chamomile essential oil
2 drops neroli essential oil
3 drops lavender essential oil
2 drops marjoram essential oil

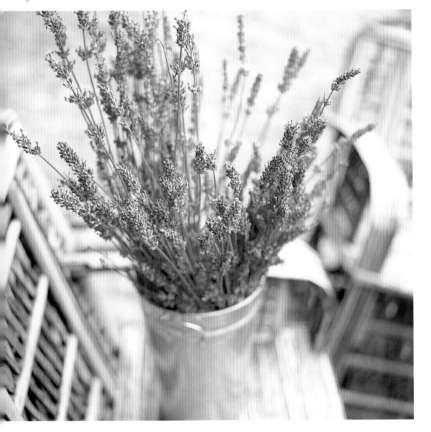

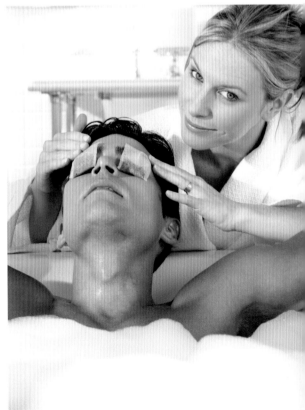

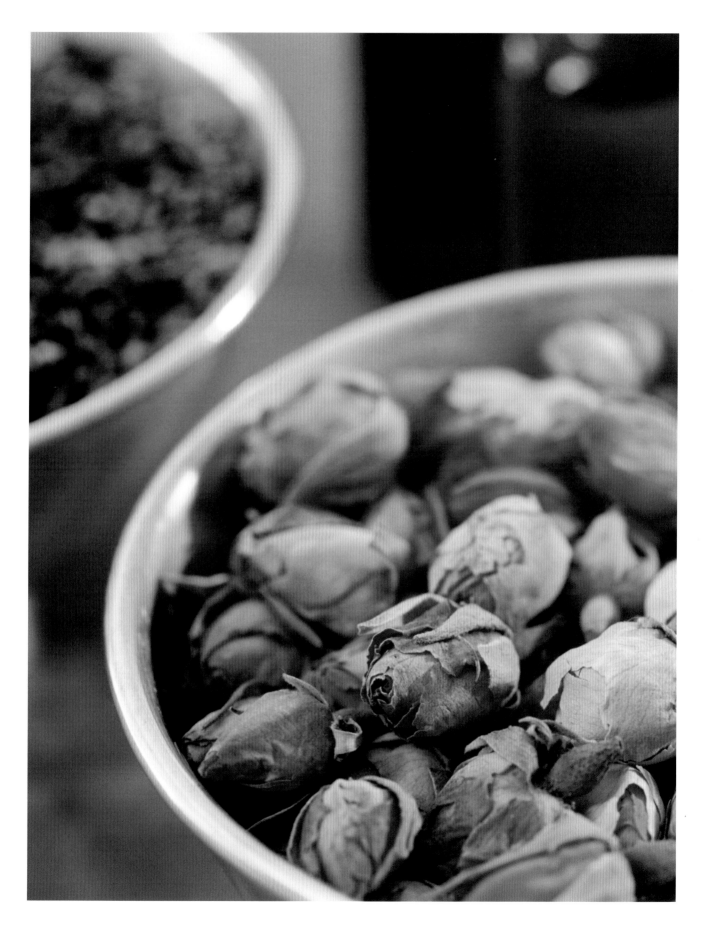

Bath oils

Bath oils are dispersible, semi-dispersible and floating. As the names suggest, the dispersible oils dissolve entirely into the bath water, semi-dispersible ones mostly dissolve into the water, and non-dispersible ones float on the top.

CITRUS GROVE MOISTURIZING BATH OIL

This bath oil is dispersible and keeps well without refrigeration.

60 drops lemon essential oil
40 drops orange essential oil
30 drops grapefruit essential oil
10 drops essential oil of cloves
1 tablespoon tincture of benzoin
$\frac{1}{2}$ cup (125 ml) vodka
$\frac{1}{4}$ cup lanolin
1 tablespoon runny honey
$1\frac{1}{2}$ cups (375 ml) infused oil

To make and use

In a small bowl, dissolve the essential oils and tincture of benzoin in the vodka.

Heat the lanolin, honey, and infused oil in a small saucepan until warm and melted (be careful not to get the mixture hot).

Take off the heat, cool slightly and slowly add the essential oils mixture while stirring constantly.

To use, add $\frac{1}{4}$–$\frac{1}{2}$ cup to the bath as the water is running.

DEMETER BATH OIL

This is a semi-dispersible bath oil.

1 cup (250 ml) infused oil
$2\frac{1}{2}$ tablespoons (40 ml) good quality shampoo
40 drops lavender essential oil
40 drops grapefruit essential oil
40 drops geranium essential oil
30 drops ylang-ylang essential oil
20 drops patchouli essential oil
1 teaspoon vegetable glycerine

To make and use

Bottle all the ingredients, label, and shake gently to combine.

Invert the bottle a few times before use.

Add 1–2 tablespoons of the bath oil to the bath.

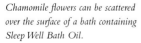

Chamomile flowers can be scattered over the surface of a bath containing Sleep Well Bath Oil.

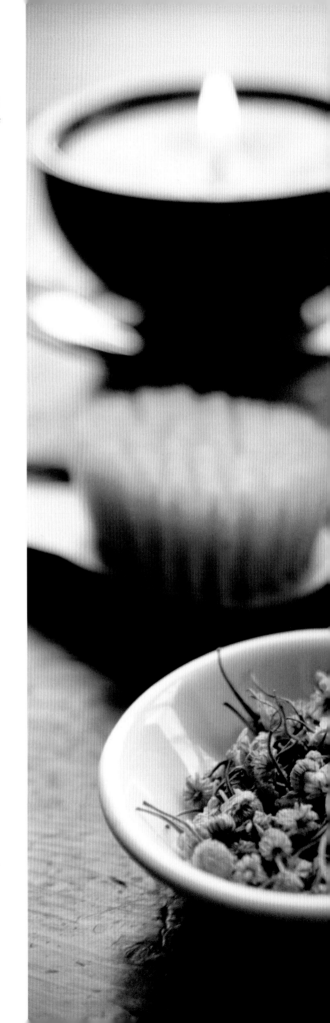

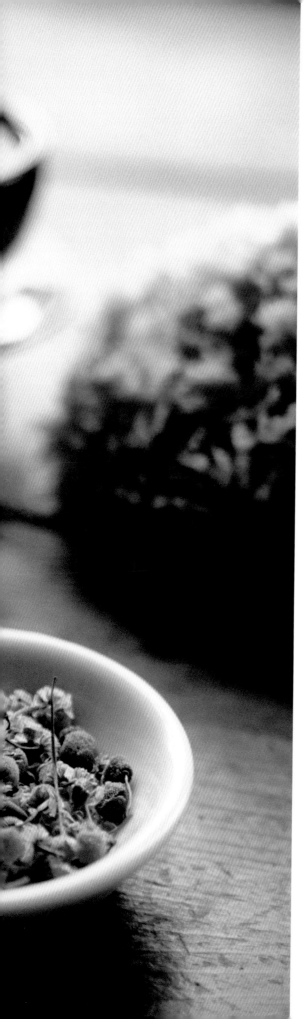

SLEEP WELL BATH OIL

This oil is semi-dispersible.

1 cup (250 ml) brandy or vodka
2 teaspoons chamomile essential oil
1 teaspoon lavender essential oil
1 teaspoon marjoram essential oil
1 teaspoon sandalwood essential oil
3 teaspoons glycerine

To make and use

Mix all the ingredients together in a bottle and label.
Invert several times to mix well.
Shake before using.
Add $\frac{1}{2}$–1 teaspoon of the blend to the bath; any more and you might overdose on the powerful fragrance, or you may even become so enlightened you float off the planet! You'll find your sleep will be refreshing.

BASIC SEMI-DISPERSIBLE BATH OIL

This oil will almost disperse in the bath water.
Vodka is expensive, but as this recipe makes enough for about 30 baths, each luxury bath becomes extremely affordable. My personal choice, cider vinegar, adds its own distinctive aroma to the oils and also has the benefits of being inexpensive and therapeutic.

$\frac{1}{2}$ cup (125 ml) vodka or cider vinegar
$2\frac{1}{2}$ tablespoons (40 ml) good quality shampoo
3 teaspoons glycerine
3 teaspoons essential oils for adults (use only
$1\frac{1}{2}$ teaspoons for children or if you have oily skin) (see blends following)

To make and use

Mix all ingredients together in a bottle.
Invert several times to mix well.
Leave for 4 days to synergize, inverting several times again.
Add $1\frac{1}{2}$ teaspoons of the mixture to the water after the bath has been drawn.
Agitate the water to disperse the mixture thoroughly.
Lean back and enjoy!

Essential oil blends for adding to Basic Semi-Dispersible Bath Oil

CHILDREN
$\frac{1}{2}$ teaspoon chamomile essential oil
$\frac{1}{2}$ teaspoon lavender essential oil
$\frac{1}{2}$ teaspoon mandarin essential oil

DRY SKIN
1 teaspoon lavender essential oil
1 teaspoon rosewood or rose essential oil
1 teaspoon palmarosa essential oil

NORMAL SKIN
1 teaspoon geranium essential oil
1 teaspoon rosewood essential oil
1 teaspoon ylang-ylang essential oil

OILY SKIN
$\frac{1}{2}$ teaspoon juniper essential oil
$\frac{1}{2}$ teaspoon lemon essential oil
$\frac{1}{2}$ teaspoon patchouli essential oil

SLEEP WELL
$\frac{1}{2}$ teaspoon chamomile essential oil
1 teaspoon lavender essential oil
1 teaspoon marjoram essential oil
$\frac{1}{2}$ teaspoon sandalwood essential oil

ANTI-CELLULITE
2 teaspoons juniper essential oil
$\frac{1}{2}$ teaspoon grapefruit essential oil
$\frac{1}{2}$ teaspoon lemon essential oil

Geraniums growing in a flower box in Sicily. Geranium oil is a much-loved essential oil.

A few times in my life I have been fortunate enough to visit Provence, France, where I have spent hours browsing the beautiful "marchés."

Bath lotions and vinegars

Inexpensive, easy, and satisfying to make and use is a way to describe herbal vinegars. Bath vinegars may be used in a variety of ways as you can see in the table.

Bath vinegar

Vinegar restores the acid mantle to skin, relieves dryness, itching, and the pain of sunburn. Cider vinegar seems to have the most therapeutic properties but any good quality white vinegar can be used.

For skin tonics, white wine vinegar is more gentle and refined. If you really hate the smell of vinegar you can substitute vodka (mixed half and half with purified water) or white wine. These last two are more expensive but the perfume of the essential oils is more apparent.

To make the following bath vinegar blends, mix 2 cups (500 ml) cider or white wine vinegar with 100 drops mixed or single essential oils. Choose from the following oil blends.

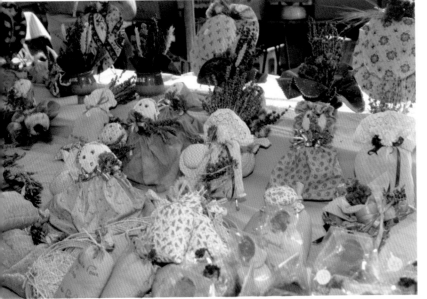

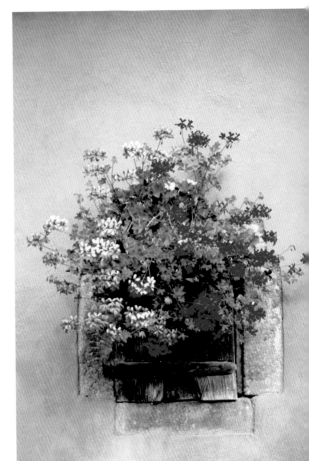

LAVENDER

100 drops lavender essential oil

CITRUS SENSATION

30 drops lemon essential oil
25 drops petitgrain essential oil
20 drops bergamot essential oil
20 drops orange essential oil
5 drops clove essential oil

MINT TANG

40 drops peppermint essential oil
40 drops spearmint essential oil
15 drops lavender essential oil
5 drops clove essential oil

HERB SPICE

40 drops clary sage essential oil
40 drops rosemary essential oil
10 drops fennel essential oil
10 drops anise essential oil

FOREST FANTASY

40 drops pine essential oil
20 drops hyssop essential oil
20 drops lemon essential oil
10 drops cypress essential oil
10 drops peppermint

HERB BLENDS FOR BATH VINEGARS

Lavender: Traditional, simple, and delicate.
Citrus Sensation: Lemon verbena, lemon thyme,
    powdered lemon peel, powdered orange peel.
Mint Tang: Peppermint, spearmint, apple mint,
    bruised cloves.
Herb Spice: Sage, rosemary, fennel seeds,
    star anise.
Forest Fantasy: Pine needles, white oak bark,
    hyssop, cedar, lemon gum, peppermint.
Deodorant: Lovage, witch hazel bark, rosemary,
    sage, white willow bark.
Itchy Skin Soother: Calendula, chamomile, mallow,
    comfrey root.
Flesh Firmer: Horsetail, nettle, honey.
Sleepy Time: Valerian root, hop flowers, lime
    flowers, passionflowers, chamomile.

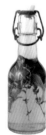

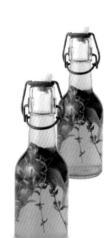

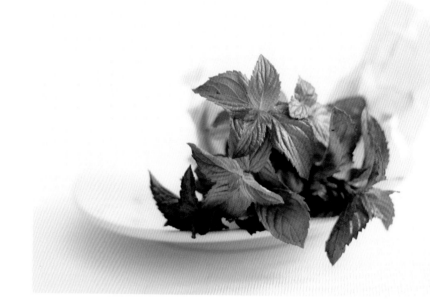

Using bath vinegars

Purpose	Use
Bath	Add $\frac{1}{4}$ cup (60 ml) of vinegar to a full bath
Hair rinse	Add $\frac{1}{2}$ cup (125 ml) of bath vinegar to 4 cups water
Skin and hair tonic	Add 4 teaspoons of bath vinegar to 1 cup (250 ml) water
After–shower friction rub	Add $\frac{1}{4}$ cup (60 ml) of bath vinegar to $\frac{1}{2}$ cup (125 ml) water
Deodorant	Use undiluted

HERBAL BATH VINEGARS

Fill a screw-topped jar loosely with chopped leaves
or flowers of your choice, using the list on the left
as a guide. Pour in enough vinegar or vodka to cover.

Leave for two weeks, shaking twice daily (this
is important, as it releases the properties from the
plant into the liquid).

At the end of the two weeks, strain. If it is
not strong enough, repeat the process and strain
through several layers of cheesecloth, then bottle.

Add a dropperful of an appropriate essential oil
if desired. If giving as a gift you can put a sprig of
the plant in the bottle as decoration.

To use, add $\frac{1}{4}$–$\frac{1}{2}$ cup of bath vinegar to the
bath water.

A fabulous bath vinegar can be made from peppermint, spearmint, and apple mint, to which you add a few bruised cloves.

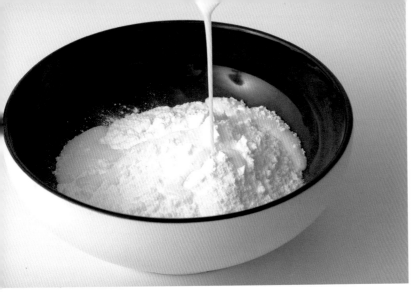

Coconut oil being added to the dry ingredients of Desert Island Dream.

Bath salts

Bath salts soften the water and are a safe way of using essential oils in the bath as there are no floating drops of oil that could burn the skin. Food coloring can be added to the salts to produce pretty bath water.

These bath salts make excellent gifts when packaged in cellophane bags or attractive jars with very well fitting lids (if steam gets into the jar the salts absorb the moisture and go rock hard). Add a label or tag that gives instructions for use.

TROPICAL HEAVEN FIZZY SALTS
1 cup (250 g) cornflour
2 cups (500 g) bicarbonate of soda
1 cup (250 g) citric acid
50 drops ylang-ylang essential oil
50 drops patchouli essential oil
50 drops sandalwood essential oil
20 drops lemon grass essential oil

To make and use
Sieve the cornflour and bicarbonate of soda, add the citric acid and mix together thoroughly.

Drip in the mixed essential oils, stirring constantly.

Store in a labeled jar with a well-fitting lid.

Sprinkle $^1/_4$–$^1/_2$ cup in a drawn bath.

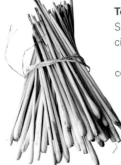

Don't be rushed out of the bathroom. We all need time to ourselves, for grooming and pampering.

DESERT ISLAND DREAM
If you like the scent of coconut, this is truly luscious. Use the type of coconut oil used for flavoring chocolate (not the same as coconut fixed oil, which has no scent).

$3^1/_2$ oz (100 g) tartaric acid
$3^1/_2$ oz (100 g) bicarbonate of soda
$2^1/_4$ oz (60 g) arrowroot powder
coconut oil as required

To make and use
Mix the powders together really well.

Drip on coconut oil, stirring constantly until the scent is as strong as you desire.

Put it all in a labeled jar and shake daily for a few days.

Sprinkle $^1/_4$–$^1/_2$ cup in the bath as the water is running.

TEMPLE CHIMES BATH SALTS
$3^1/_2$ oz (100 g) tartaric acid
$3^1/_2$ oz (100 g) bicarbonate of soda
$1^3/_4$ oz (50 g) arrowroot powder
1 dropperful lavender essential oil
2 drops clove essential oil
4 drops sandalwood essential oil

To make and use
Mix the dry ingredients together very thoroughly

Add the essential oils drop by drop, stirring all the time to prevent caking.

Put it all in a labeled jar and shake daily for a few days to blend the scents.

Sprinkle $^1/_2$ cup in the bath as the water is running.

OLD-FASHIONED GIRL
$3^1/_2$ oz (100 g) tartaric acid
$3^1/_2$ oz (100 g) bicarbonate of soda
$1^3/_4$ oz (50 g) arrowroot powder
8 drops lavender essential oil
8 drops sandalwood essential oil
4 drops clove essential oil

To make and use
Mix the powders together well.

Add the oils drop by drop, stirring all the time to prevent caking.

Place all in a labeled jar and shake daily for a few days.

Sprinkle $^1/_2$ cup of the blend into the bath as the water is running.

Bath milks and creams

Bath milks and creams need refrigeration and should be used within two weeks. They are easy to make and leave the skin soft and moisturized. Don't add them to very hot water or the egg will set and go stringy. The oil disperses in the water and doesn't leave a greasy ring around the bath.

CLEOPATRA'S MILK BATH

The ingredients in this recipe will leave your skin feeling soft and silky.

4 oz (115 g) dried skim milk powder
2$\frac{1}{4}$ oz (60 g) cornflour
2$\frac{1}{4}$ oz (60 g) citric acid
30 drops vitamin E oil
20 drops rose geranium essential oil
10 drops ylang-ylang essential oil

To make and use

Sift the milk powder and cornflour together.
    Place the citric acid in a small bowl.
    Drop the oils onto the citric acid stirring constantly.
    Add the citric acid mixture to the mixed powdered milk and cornflour, stirring constantly until completely blended.
    Store in an airtight labeled jar in the refrigerator.
    To use, sprinkle 1–2 tablespoons in the bath as the water is running.
    Use within two weeks.

LAVENDER CREAM

1 egg
$\frac{1}{4}$ cup (60 ml) olive oil
4 teaspoons glycerine
$\frac{1}{4}$ cup dried milk powder
10 drops carrot seed essential oil
10 drops orange essential oil
20 drops lavender essential oil
2 cups (500 ml) water

To make and use

Beat the egg, olive oil, and glycerine together.
    Add the milk powder while beating to make a smooth mixture.
    Beat in the essential oils and 2 cups (500 ml) of water a little at a time until all the ingredients are well mixed.
    Bottle, label, and store in the refrigerator.
    To use, add $\frac{1}{4}$–$\frac{1}{2}$ cup to the bath water and agitate the water to disperse.
    Use within two weeks.

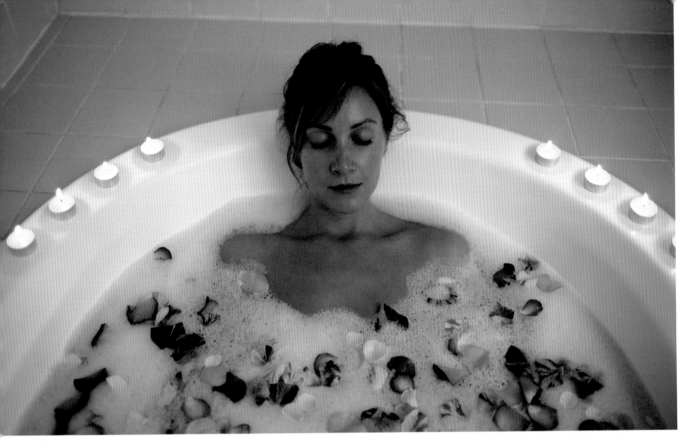

Bubbles are the ultimate luxury, but are even better when you sprinkle in petals.

CINNAMON CREAM

2 teaspoons gelatine powder

2 cups (500 ml) of hot water

1 egg

$1/4$ cup rice bran oil

$1/4$ cup olive oil

1 tablespoon runny honey

20 drops cinnamon oil

10 drops clove essential oil

10 drops vanilla essence

To make and use

In a bowl, dissolve the gelatine in 2 cups (500 ml) of hot water.

In another bowl, beat the remaining ingredients together then slowly add the dissolved gelatine, mixing continuously until well combined.

Bottle, label, and store in the refrigerator.

To use, add $1/4$–$1/2$ cup to the bath water.

Use within two weeks.

Cinnamon and rosemary—two essentials when making your own bath products.

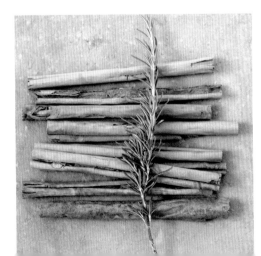

Bubble baths

Bubble baths are fun and have a luxurious feeling but one should not indulge for too long or too often as the base of most commercial bubble baths is the cheapest available detergent and can overdry the skin. Use only the amount recommended and use a massage oil after the bath to counteract the drying effects. The addition of honey, glycerine, or oil to recipes counteracts the drying effect of the detergent. You can make your own superior product by using a good shampoo or the best quality detergent available.

PERFUME OIL BUBBLE BATH

The oils for this recipe can be chosen from the suggestions for Herbal Bath Vinegar, page 315.

$1/4$ cup (60 ml) olive or sweet almond oil

1 cup (250 ml) good quality shampoo

50 drops essential oil

To make and use

Mix all ingredients together very thoroughly.

Bottle and label.

Invert bottle several times to mix contents before using.

Slowly trickle $1/4$ cup (60 ml) of the mixture under fast running water to maximize the bubbles.

Bath bags

Bath bags are the easy way to go. There is nothing to do but add the herbs to a small bag or the toe of an old pair of tights (pantyhose). Add it to the running water in the bath and hop in. You will find the scent of the herbs will fill the bathroom and relax and rejuvenate you as you inhale them and bathe in the lovely water. You can use the bag as a washcloth to complete the experience. It will leave your skin with that subtle scent of fresh herbs and spices.

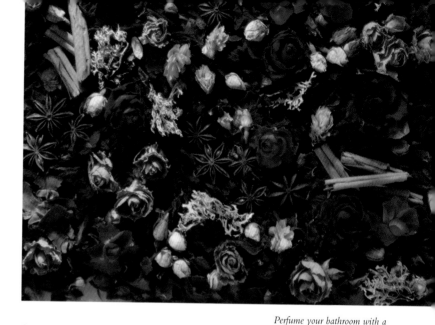

INDULGENCE BATH BAG

This is all about flowers and the best of them at that. It's worth the money to buy these flowers just once in a while and indulge yourself totally. You can use them in a bath bag or just throw the mixture into the bath itself. Of course that way you will be floating in petals but can anything be more extravagant?

$^{1}/_{4}$ cup dried rose petals,
$^{1}/_{4}$ cup dried chamomile flowers,
$^{1}/_{4}$ cup dried lavender flowers
$^{1}/_{4}$ cup oatmeal
2 tablespoons dried orange peel, chopped
2 tablespoons dried lemon peel, chopped
2 bay leaves, crumbled
2 tiny rosemary sprigs, chopped

To make and use

Combine all the ingredients in a large bowl. Mix well. Store in a large sealed jar.

If possible leave for four days to synergize.

Use in a bath bag or sprinkle over warm bath water.

If you wish, you can infuse this mixture into boiling water and strain the water for use in the bath.

RELAXING BATH BAG

$^{1}/_{4}$ cup dried lemon balm
$^{1}/_{4}$ cup dried chamomile flowers
2 cups (500 ml) boiling water

To make and use

Use in a bath bag or add the herbs, loose, to the boiling water and cover. Leave to infuse for 20 minutes.

Strain well if not using a bag and add the infused water to your bath. Otherwise add the bag and the water. Top up with warm water.

SPICY BATH BAG

This is one that men prefer. It's has a lovely scent of the forest. It seems to help sporting injuries.

To make and use

Infuse 1 cup fresh chopped thyme in 2 cups (500 ml) boiling water for 10 minutes.

Add the infusion to your bath water for cramps, bruises, swellings, and sprains.

TENSION-RELIEVING BATH

Steep 1 cup fresh chopped lemon balm leaves in 1 quart (1 liter) boiling water for 20 minutes. Add the infusion to your bath water for any nervous tension problems.

Perfume your bathroom with a dried collection of flowers and spices like rose, star anise, cinnamon, and lavender.

Children love bubbles but don't be tempted by the commercial variety. Make your own Perfume Oil Bubble Bath.

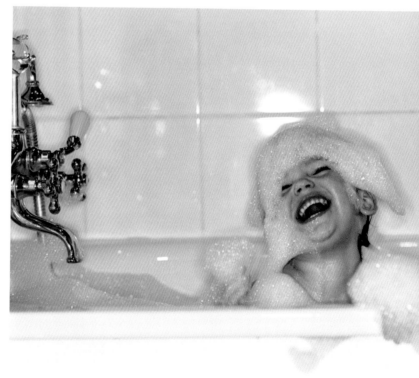

Colognes

I enjoy using colognes more than concentrated perfumes, as they can be sprayed or splashed liberally onto the body to create an "aura" of scent without being overpowering.

Some of the essential oils in the following blends will not be found in the list of essential oils for skin care on page 250 as they are not actually skin oils; they are, however, necessary to create a beautifully balanced perfume.

Colognes are a blend of 60 parts alcohol, 15 parts purified water, 5 parts glycerine and 15 parts essential oil or a combination of oils. Vodka is the best alcohol to use, as it has no smell. The glycerine gives "body" to the blend and counteracts the drying effect of the alcohol. These parts, if converted to quantities, are correct in the Basic Cologne Blend.

Ingredients for Basic Cologne Blend—vodka, water, glycerine, and essential oil..

To make and use the following recipes
Mix all the ingredients together in a 2 fl oz (60 ml) bottle.

Shake well and leave for between two and six months to mature.

The initial scent will bear little resemblance to the final perfume, so patience is needed.

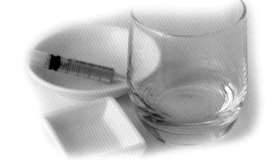

BASIC COLOGNE BLEND
$2^1/_2$ tablespoons (40 ml) vodka
2 teaspoons purified water
$^1/_4$ teaspoon glycerine
$1^1/_2$ teaspoons essential oil—select from the following blends or create your own.

FLOWER GARDEN
$^1/_2$ teaspoon bergamot essential oil
$^1/_2$ teaspoon geranium essential oil
20 drops petitgrain or neroli essential oil
20 drops palmarosa essential oil
2 drops sandalwood essential oil

SWEETHEART
1 teaspoon rosewood essential oil
20 drops ylang-ylang essential oil
10 drops jasmine essential oil
10 drops bergamot essential oil

ENTICEMENT
1 teaspoon ylang-ylang essential oil
15 drops patchouli essential oil
15 drops sandalwood essential oil
5 drops jasmine essential oil
5 drops rose essential oil

LAVENDER LADY
$1^1/_2$ teaspoons lavender essential oil
10 drops lemon essential oil
10 drops palmarosa essential oil

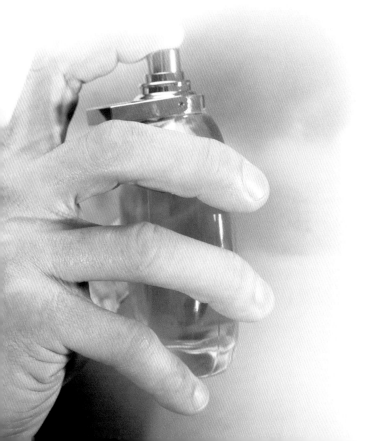

MACHO MAN
1 teaspoon sandalwood essential oil
30 drops cedarwood essential oil
10 drops rosewood essential oil
5 drops lemon essential oil

OCEAN BREEZE
1 teaspoon lavender essential oil
50 drops rosemary essential oil
20 drops bergamot essential oil

SENSUAL
1 teaspoon patchouli oil
40 drops ylang-ylang oil
20 drops sandalwood oil

SILK LADY
1 teaspoon lavender oil
40 drops rose geranium oil
10 drops patchouli oil

FALL MIST
1 teaspoon sandalwood essential oil
40 drops patchouli essential oil
40 drops orange essential oil

MYSTERY
1 teaspoon myrrh essential oil
20 drops sandalwood essential oil
10 drops patchouli essential oil
10 drops frankincense essential oil

SWOON
1 teaspoon patchouli essential oil
$1/_2$ teaspoon ylang-ylang essential oil

MOONLIGHT
1 teaspoon ylang-ylang essential oil
30 drops rose geranium essential oil
20 drops patchouli essential oil

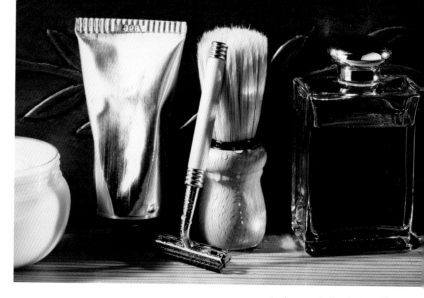

A cologne used after shaving will smooth and tone the skin.

BODY POWDER

If you enjoy using powder after a bath or shower, here is a recipe for a natural one. A word of caution, though: Powder used excessively can block the pores of the skin.

BASIC BODY POWDER
Mix either arrowroot powder or cornflour with an equal quantity of very finely powdered dried herbs, citrus peel, and spices. You can add a few drops of essential oil (not too much or the powder will go lumpy). Mix all the ingredients well, and rub through a sieve. Store in a flat bowl with a lid, and apply with a large wad of absorbent cotton (cottonwool).

BODY POWDER BLENDS
Always check carefully before choosing herbs for powder, (especially for babies), to make sure that the herb will not cause an allergic reaction on the skin. This is particularly important with chamomile.
For babies—chamomile, lemon balm
For a deodorant—rosemary, thyme, sage, lavender, orange peel
For men—licorice, rosemary, lavender, cilantro (coriander) seed

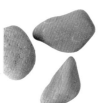

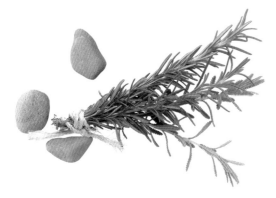

Deodorants

There are only a few areas of the body where the smell of perspiration is a problem—the feet and armpits. The sweat glands in these areas are different from those found elsewhere on the body, and they produce more profuse and stronger smelling sweat.

Fresh perspiration does not smell, but it decomposes very rapidly and becomes really unpleasant. The strength of perspiration odor seems to be determined by many factors: Puberty or other hormonal changes, high intake of meat, junk foods, or alcohol, and stress.

Synthetic clothing doesn't allow perspiration to evaporate and this compounds the problem.

The following deodorants aren't as strong as the commercial varieties but are very pleasant and safe to use. The smell of the vinegar vanishes in a very short time, leaving only the aroma of the essential oils.

FRESH-AS-A-DAISY DEODORANT FOR HER

3$\frac{1}{2}$ fl oz (100 ml) cider vinegar
3$\frac{1}{2}$ fl oz (100 ml) witch hazel
20 drops bergamot essential oil
20 drops lavender essential oil
10 drops patchouli essential oil
10 drops rosewood essential oil
10 drops benzoin essential oil
$\frac{1}{2}$ teaspoon glycerine

To make and use

Combine the ingredients in a labeled bottle and shake well.

Leave for 4 days to synergize, shaking occasionally. Store in a dark, dry, cool place.

Splash or spray on after showering, and as needed.

FOREST FANTASY DEODORANT FOR HIM

3$\frac{1}{2}$ fl oz (100 ml) cider vinegar
3$\frac{1}{2}$ fl oz (100 ml) witch hazel
20 drops benzoin essential oil
20 drops bergamot essential oil
20 drops cypress essential oil
10 drops eucalyptus essential oil
5 drops rosewood essential oil
$\frac{1}{2}$ teaspoon glycerine

Opposite: Crushed flowers and leaves used to make essential oils.

To make and use

Combine the ingredients in a labeled bottle and shake well.

Leave for 4 days to synergize, shaking occasionally. Store in a dark, dry, cool place.

Splash or spray on after showering, and as needed during the day.

DEODORANT POWDER

$\frac{1}{2}$ cup unperfumed talcum powder
$\frac{1}{2}$ cup cornstarch (cornflour)
20 drops lavender essential oil
20 drops myrrh essential oil
10 drops patchouli essential oil
5 drops lemon essential oil

To make and use

Sieve the powder and cornflour together in a bowl. Mix the essential oils together.

Add the oil mixture, a drop at a time, to the powder mixture, stirring constantly to prevent the powder from going lumpy.

Store in an airtight, labeled container.

UNPERFUMED FOOT AND UNDERARM DEODORANT POWDER

1 cup cornstarch (cornflour)
1 cup arrowroot powder
$\frac{1}{2}$ cup bicarbonate of soda

To make and use

Mix the ingredients well together.

Store in a wide-mouthed, airtight, labeled jar, or in a shaker.

QUICKIE DEODORANT

Use witch hazel extract as an underarm splash.

DEODORANT LOTION

$\frac{1}{3}$ cup (80 ml) distilled witch hazel
1 teaspoon glycerine
30 drops clary sage essential oil
20 drops rosemary essential oil
10 drops thyme essential oil
10 drops tea tree essential oil
5 drops sandalwood essential oil

To make

Blend all the ingredients in a 3$\frac{1}{2}$ fl oz (100 ml) labeled bottle.

Shake well to mix and leave for four days to synergize before using.

Shake before use.

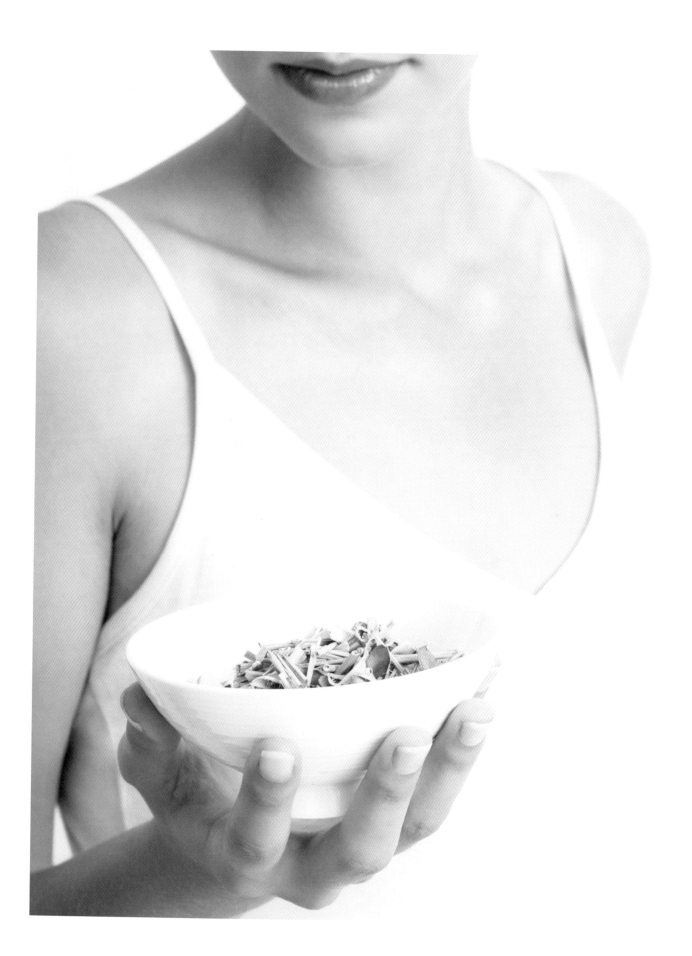

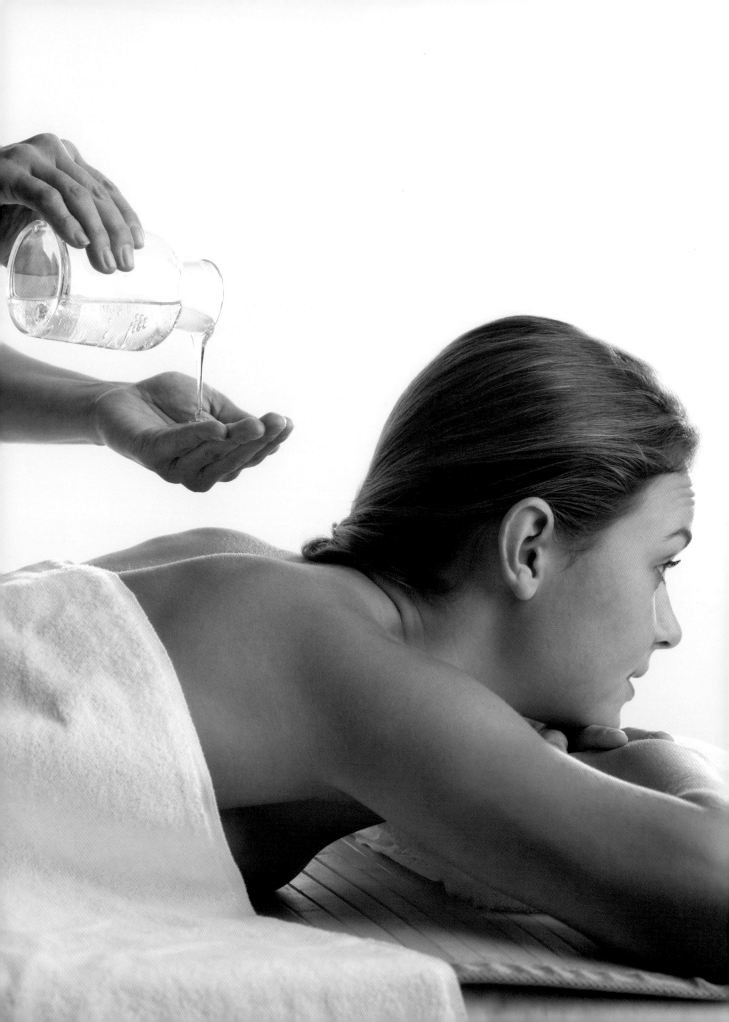

Massage

Massage has been used as a therapy for healing and improving body movement, toning, and general well-being for centuries. It has many benefits, not only to the skin, muscles, and joints of the body, but also on a psychological level, as a massage promotes a wonderful feeling of well-being and lightness.

The feeling of well-being and relaxation you experience after a massage is due partly to the nervous system's many nerve endings being soothed and stimulated. The actual physical touch involved also has a soothing and comforting effect on the mind and body. Increasing the circulation of the blood promotes regeneration and repair of the skin, and also improves muscle tone and general appearance of the skin.

Today, it's possible to experience a variety of different massages from soothing mild touching, to much firmer and rigorous hand movements of a Swedish deep tissue massage. There has also been a huge move towards alternative therapies, along with the addition of such things as warm rocks, suction, and the great trend of using different products from mud, to all sorts of wonderful natural solutions, and scrubs.

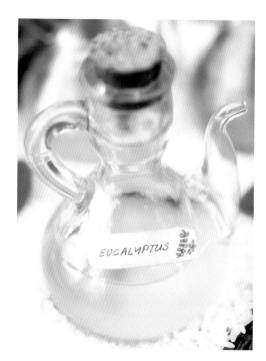

Eucalyptus oil is a traditional muscle soother.

The influence of Asian medicines on our society has also led to many spas offering different kinds of massage such as rhythmic Kodo massage as well as acupressure which is akin to acupuncture but using the hands instead of needles.

The massage treatments described here are more traditional, using essential oils, and a calm, relaxing atmosphere, and touch. I am sure you will find them a great beginning in your journey to a better self.

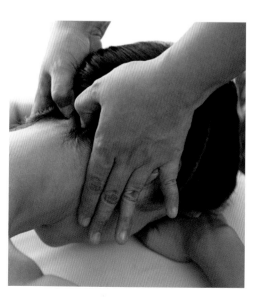

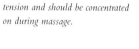

The neck is a major source of tension and should be concentrated on during massage.

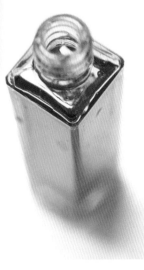

Jasmine, neroli, patchouli, rose, rosewood, sandalwood, and ylang-ylang make a sensual massage oil.

Massage is a very special experience: It can be healing, strengthening, relaxing, sensual, or energizing. And it should always be a loving, sharing, and trusting experience.

The benefits of massage

The many systems within the body respond to therapeutic massage. This helps to improve blood flow through the body, and also increases the elimination of built-up toxins and waste materials.

Muscles respond rapidly to massage, and so it is excellent in sporting situations. Massage helps to stretch the muscles and so reduces aches and spasms; it also helps to speed the healing of strains and sprains.

Tension "knots" are smoothed away, leaving a lighter feeling around the shoulder, upper back, and neck area—an area particularly prone to aches and stiffness for many people. All types of work situations can bring stress to this area, and cause spasms, which can lead to headaches and a feeling of tightness or pressure around the head.

Abdominal massage improves digestion and is beneficial for many digestive disorders, such as constipation and flatulence.

To make sure that you, your family, and friends enjoy the wonderful benefits of massage with these aromatherapy recipes, I recommend that you learn the proper techniques. There are a number of excellent books which give step-by-step instructions, and many places offer courses.

Remember, some essential oils are unsuitable to use if certain conditions exist, such as epilepsy or pregnancy. Please note the cautions contained in the individual herbs and oils, and in the recipes themselves.

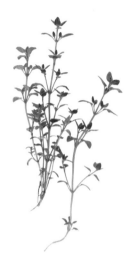

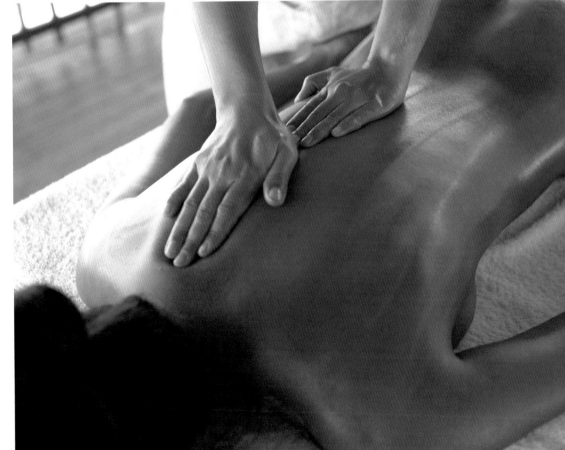

Use firm but gentle pressure on the spine.

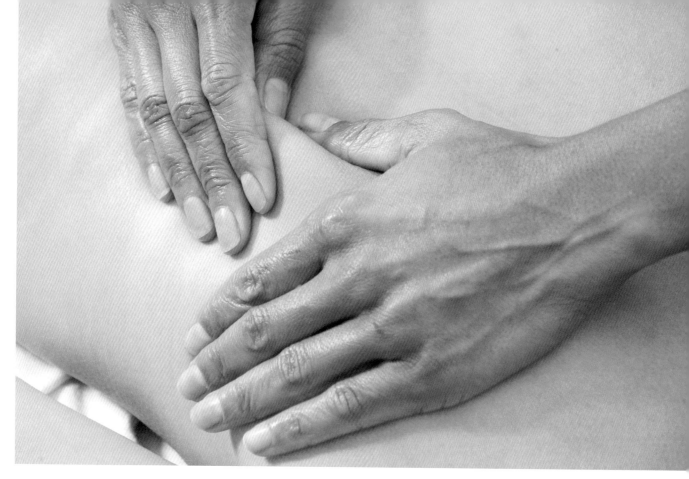

Gentle kneading increases blood flow.

OTHER USES FOR MASSAGE OILS

Massage is probably the best-known way of employing essential oils, and certainly there are few more luxurious and relaxing ways to enjoy the perfume and healing properties of the oils. You don't have to wait for someone to give you a massage—these oils can be used as an after-bath or shower oil, massaged well into the skin over the whole body. Or you can add a few drops to the bath as a bath oil.

Using essential oils for massage

There are few more pleasurable or healing experiences than receiving a massage, but this experience is immeasurably enhanced when essential oils are incorporated into the massage oil, cream, or lotion.

The molecules of essential oils are small enough to pass through the skin. There they dissolve readily into body fat, and are absorbed into the bloodstream, and carried to all the systems of the body.

The aroma of the oil is inhaled during a massage, affecting the limbic portion of the brain; it is also absorbed into the body through the lungs.

Problems associated with the skin, such as poor circulation, muscular and joint problems, or problems associated with digestive, genito-urinary, endocrine systems, immune, and nervous systems may all be alleviated or healed through the use of essential oils.

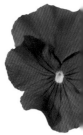

Which oil to choose for massage

Condition	Essential oils
Arthritis and rheumatism	Benzoin, black pepper, cedarwood, chamomile, eucalyptus, ginger, marjoram, rosemary
Asthma	Chamomile, cypress, eucalyptus, frankincense, lavender, peppermint, thyme
Bronchitis, coughs, and catarrh	Cedarwood, eucalyptus, lavender, marjoram, peppermint, pine, rosemary, tea tree, thyme
Circulation and toning	Black pepper, eucalyptus, ginger, rosemary
Colic	Black pepper, chamomile, fennel, ginger, lavender, marjoram, peppermint
Constipation	Black pepper, fennel, marjoram, orange
Fluid retention	Angelica, cypress, fennel, grapefruit, juniper, rosemary
Frigidity	Jasmine, neroli, patchouli, rose, rosewood, sandalwood, ylang-ylang
Immune system	Eucalyptus, lavender, manuka, rosewood, tea tree
Indigestion or flatulence	Aniseed, chamomile, fennel, lavender, orange, peppermint
Muscular aches, pains, and stiffness	Black pepper, chamomile, eucalyptus, ginger, juniper, lavender, marjoram, rosemary
Muscular cramps	Black pepper, cypress, lavender, marjoram, rosemary
Pain relieving	Black pepper
Slack tissue with poor tone	Black pepper, grapefruit, marjoram, rosemary
Sprains and strains	Black pepper, chamomile, lavender, marjoram
Stress, nervous tension, and similar problems	Cedarwood, chamomile, cypress, geranium, juniper, lavender, peppermint
Toxin build-up	Angelica, fennel, grapefruit, juniper
Urinary tract problems	Cedarwood, eucalyptus, lavender, pine

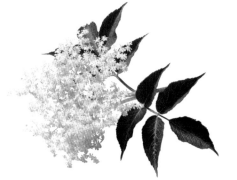

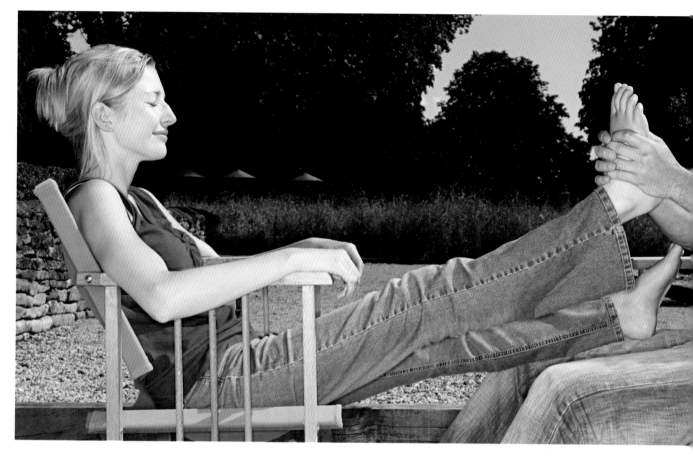

A wonderful foot massage is a perfect end to a busy day.

The benefits of using the oils externally rather than internally are twofold. Firstly, the stomach is bypassed, and the oils are not diluted or affected by gastric juices. Secondly, it is much safer to use the oils externally unless prescribed by an experienced person.

Most essential oils have healing properties, but some are more efficacious than others. I would urge you to make lavender oil the first one that you purchase, followed closely by chamomile and geranium oil.

After you read through the recipes you will notice immediately how often these remarkable oils are used. Lavender, in particular, has the advantage of being gentle and safe enough to use for the whole family.

The following lists contain only the oils most effective for treating the particular problem that you may be dealing with. There are many more oils with similar properties but to give the entire list would be confusing. For a complete profile on the oils refer to the individual oil.

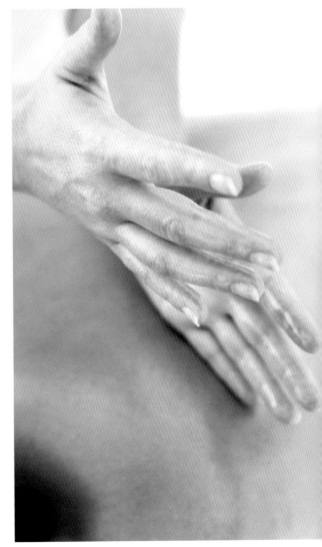

An accurate measuring jug is essential equipment for any massage oil recipe.

Firm rhythmic pressure with the hands gives great relief.

BASIC MASSAGE OIL

For the Basic Massage Oil, choose the appropriate oils from the table or select one of the special blends that follow. The wheat germ oil is an important addition—it helps prevent rancidity. This Basic Massage Oil mix will make 3¹/₂ fl oz (100 ml).

¹/₄ cup (60 ml) grape seed or rice bran oil
3 teaspoons (15 ml) infused oil of your choice
   (if you don't have this, add 3 teaspoons extra
   grape seed oil or rice bran oil)
2 teaspoons (10 ml) sweet almond oil
2 teaspoons (10 ml) avocado oil
1 teaspoon (5 ml) wheat germ oil
40 drops essential oil chosen from the table on
   page 328.

AFTER-SPORT RUB

This oil will help to ease the pain of some muscles after strenuous sport.

1 teaspoon clove oil
1 teaspoon eucalyptus oil
1 teaspoon thyme oil
1 teaspoon black pepper oil
1 teaspoon lavender oil
3¹/₂ fl oz (100 ml) of Basic Massage Oil

To make

Mix the essential oils in a 1 fl oz (30 ml) labeled bottle.
   Shake well. Add 40 drops of the essential oil blend to 3¹/₂ fl oz (100 ml) of Basic Massage Oil.

DEPRESSION LIFTER

This oil will help to lift and calm the spirits. The blend can be used in a warm bath (10 drops) and then followed by a soothing massage.

¹/₂ teaspoon sandalwood oil
¹/₂ teaspoon chamomile oil
2 teaspoons ylang-ylang oil
1 teaspoon lavender oil
1 teaspoon orange oil
3¹/₂ fl oz (100 ml) of Basic Massage Oil

To make

Mix all the oils in a 1 fl oz (30 ml) labeled bottle.
   Shake well. Add 40 drops to 3¹/₂ fl oz (100 ml) of Basic Massage Oil.

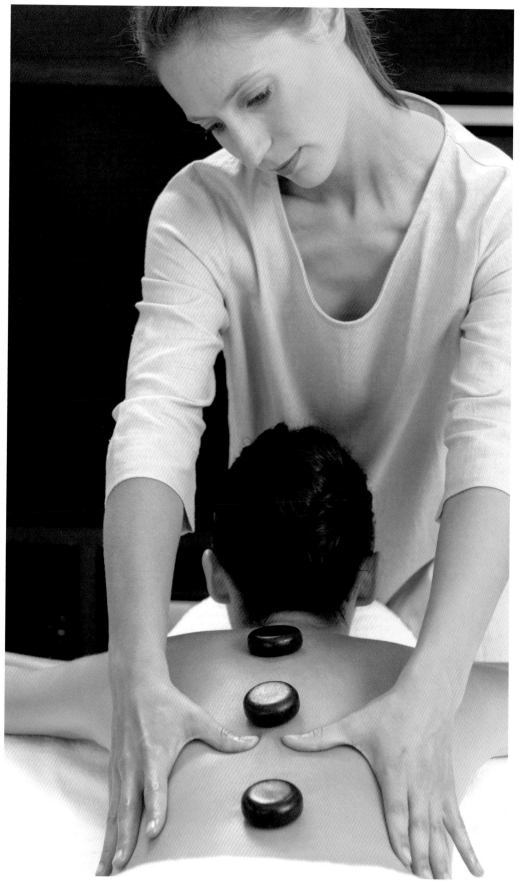

"I don't fear death because I don't fear anything I don't understand. When I start to think about it, I order a massage and it goes away."
HEDY LAMARR

Warm rocks are said to help soothe the body.

POST-VIRAL SYNDROME CHASER

Myalgic encephalomyelitis is a distressing complaint that can cause aching muscles, headaches, extreme exhaustion, mental confusion, loss of memory, and many more symptoms. Ease the misery by using this blend daily as an after-shower or bath massage oil, and by being given a massage as often as possible.

1 teaspoon grapefruit oil
1 teaspoon black pepper oil
1 teaspoon thyme oil
1 teaspoon cypress oil
1 teaspoon rosemary oil
$3^1/_2$ fl oz (100 ml) Basic Massage Oil

To make

Mix the essential oils in a 1 fl oz or 30 ml labeled bottle.

Shake well. Add 40 drops to $3^1/_2$ fl oz (100 ml) of Basic Massage Oil.

WORK-RELATED STRESS EASER

This blend is for those who spend a large part of their lives with workmates, computers, telephones, in traffic, or in stressful environments. Use this blend to help with the "unwinding" process at the end of the day.

2 teaspoons melissa (lemon balm) oil
$^1/_2$ teaspoon benzoin oil
1 teaspoon bergamot oil
1 teaspoon lavender oil
$^1/_2$ teaspoon geranium oil
1 teaspoon ylang-ylang oil
$3^1/_2$ fl oz (100 ml) of Basic Massage Oil

To make

Mix the essential oils in a 1 fl oz (30 ml) labeled bottle.

Shake well. Add 40 drops to $3^1/_2$ fl oz (100 ml) of Basic Massage Oil.

Make sure the room atmosphere is serene before beginning massage.

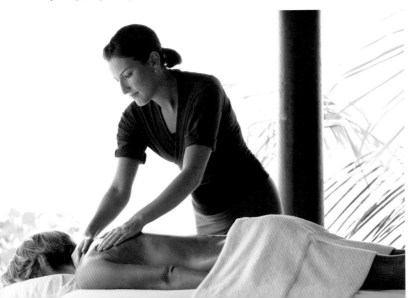

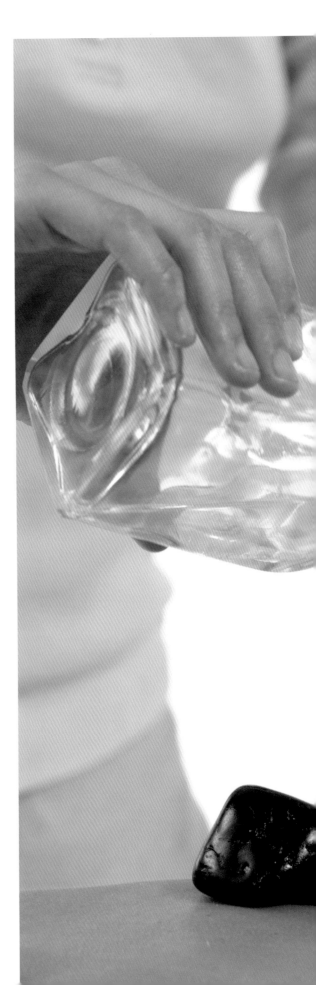

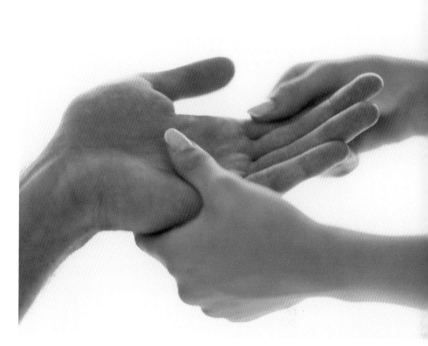

Don't forget the fingertips for a perfect massage.

FAMILY OIL

This blend is suitable for the whole family. After all, the adults aren't the only ones who suffer from stress, or who enjoy a massage. This blend will de-stress, calm, and uplift.

1 teaspoon lavender oil
1 teaspoon lemon oil
1 teaspoon geranium oil
1 teaspoon bergamot oil
$\frac{1}{2}$ teaspoon mandarin oil
$\frac{1}{2}$ teaspoon sandalwood oil
$3\frac{1}{2}$ fl oz (100 ml) Basic Massage Oil

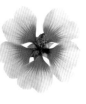

To make

Mix all the oils in a 1 fl oz (30 ml) labeled bottle. Shake well. Add 40 drops to $3\frac{1}{2}$ fl oz (100 ml) of Basic Massage Oil.

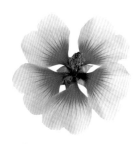

Warm the oil before beginning the massage.

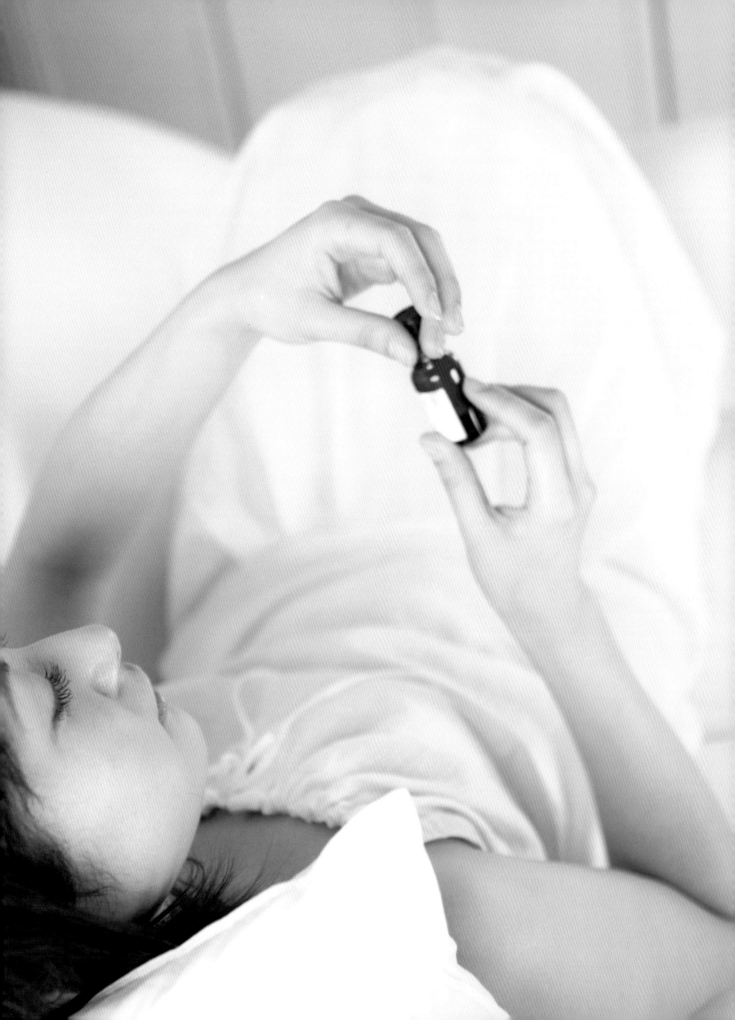

Aromatherapy

Feel stressed? It's not surprising when you consider what you have done before your day officially begins. You have already coped with making breakfast (or nagging others to do it), left the home tidy, organized the children, taken them to school, and then coped with rush-hour traffic to get to the place where you are officially starting work! No wonder you feel permanently tired and edgy.

I have found that, with a little forethought, many of the stresses in our lives can be either reduced or eliminated altogether. We put up with things because that is how they have always been (and, if we are honest, because it is easy to be a martyr). It's time to reorganize. In conjunction with this reorganization, make sure that you are using essential oils, eating well, sleeping well, having fun, exercise, and leisure time, and communicating with your family, and friends.

Essential oils are available everywhere, even the local supermarket, but be careful what you buy, as most of the cheaper ones are blends. It's all a matter of "you get what you pay for" with essential oils. The most expensive are always the most pure. But please try to make your own if you can. Begin by sticking to the simple herbs like lavender, and you will soon find it the most rewarding experience you can have, by treating your family and friends with pure, safe, and lovingly prepared oils.

The following recipes will help to ensure that your life becomes easier and more joyful. I have divided them up into the different realms of our lives making it easier to find exactly what you need.

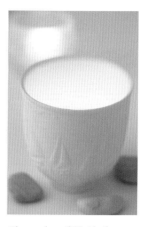

Choose a beautiful holder for candles and oils and you will find the ambience enhances the effects.

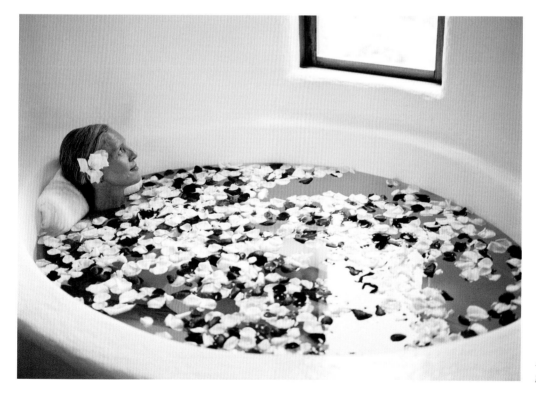

Adding the indulgence of rose petals makes a truly lavish bath.

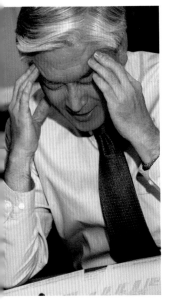

A busy office is always a source of stress, which can cause headaches.

Workplace stress busters

Whether you work alone, as I do, or in a busy, noisy office, or factory, there are stresses with which one has to contend. It is important to first sit down and itemize which parts of your day are the most stressful. For instance, do demands from other people interfere with your own work? Do you have too high expectations of yourself or others? Are you subject to high noise levels, isolation, or being on your feet or on your bottom for excessive lengths of time, and are you in an unhealthily synthetic environment? You will probably be able to add many more stress factors to this list.

Children also have their own stresses to contend with, and essential oils can help to create a productive and happy day at school. It has been my experience that children respond more quickly than adults to essential oils and love having their own special bottle of oils. Any of the following recipes and suggestions may be used by school-age children, but the strength will have to be adapted to suit their age (see opposite). I wouldn't suggest giving a bottle of the oils to children under the age of 10 years, but rather putting a few drops on absorbent cotton (cottonwool) and slipping them into the school bag, pocket, or other convenient place for them to sniff during the day.

Some companies employ therapists to massage staff at work.

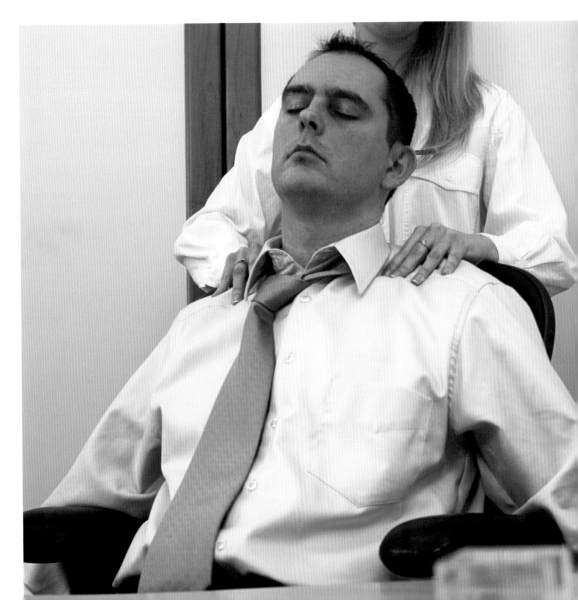

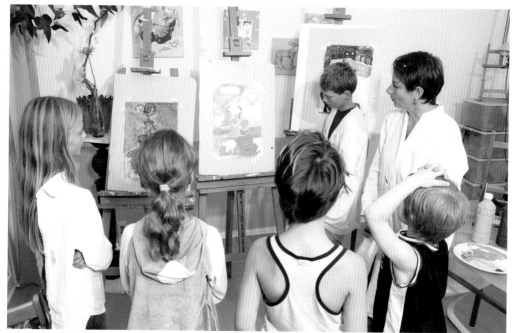

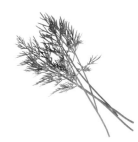

Even school-age children benefit from essential oils.

Oils for school-age children [five to puberty]

All the oils considered safe for adults may be used but in smaller amounts.

In bathwater

5-8 drops of appropriate essential oil with 1 tablespoon olive oil and dispersed thoroughly into the bath water.

Massage

16-20 drops (total) mixed or single essential oils in $^1/_2$ cup mixed olive and almond oils. Shake well before use.

Air sprays

Use one-quarter the adult amount for a 5-year-old, gradually increasing (drop by drop) with child's age.

DAY BREAK FOR GIRLS

The "smooth you out and perk you up" blend to begin your day.

1 teaspoon lavender essential oil
$^1/_2$ teaspoon bergamot essential oil
$^1/_2$ teaspoon geranium essential oil
20 drops peppermint essential oil
20 drops clary sage essential oil

To make and use

Place all ingredients in a labeled, dropper bottle and shake to blend.

If possible leave for four days to synergize. Store in a dark, cool place.

- Add 5 drops of the blend to 1 teaspoon sweet almond oil. Use as a body oil after your shower.
- Put 2–3 drops on a wet wash cloth, squeeze to spread the oils and use to wipe over your body in the shower before drying yourself.
- Put 2 drops on absorbent cotton (cottonwool) and tuck it in the front of your bra where the heat of your body will evaporate the oil.
- Put 2–3 drops on absorbent cotton (cottonwool) or tissue and tuck it in your pocket, handbag, or purse to enliven you each time you open it.
- Put a couple of drops on a tissue to inhale while getting ready for work.
- Wipe a few drops of the blend over the dashboard of the car.
- Add 5 drops to a 2 fl oz (60 ml) atomizer of water. Shake well then spray on the face, avoiding the eye area.

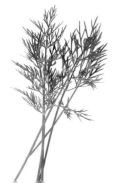

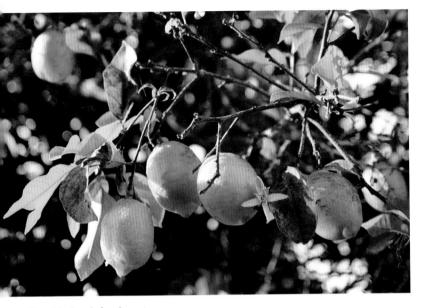

Essential oil made from lemon is the major ingredient in Day Break for Guys.

Commuting

Well! We all know what a drama this can be, so I will not dwell on the traumas which can erupt as soon as you all leave the house. You can help to avoid this sort of stress and create a happy, positive, and calm atmosphere with the following suggestions.

Mix equal amounts of peppermint and lavender essential oils in a labeled, small dropper bottle and store in a little box or bag in the car with some absorbent cotton (cottonwool).

Use a drop or two of this oil blend on the cotton and tuck it around the car—the dashboard, the rear window ledge, on top of the sun visors, and under or down the sides of the seats are all good spots.

Put a drop to two on a handkerchief or tissue for each person, so they can sniff as needed.

DAY BREAK FOR GUYS

1 teaspoon bergamot essential oil
1 teaspoon lemon essential oil
$^1/_2$ teaspoon rosemary essential oil
$^1/_2$ teaspoon cedarwood essential oil

To make and use

Place all ingredients in a labeled, dropper bottle and shake to blend.

If possible leave for four days to synergize. Store in a dark, cool place.

- Use in an aftershave or toilet water splash.
- Add 5 drops of the blend to 1 teaspoon sweet almond oil. Use as a body oil after your shower.
- Put 2–3 drops on a wet wash cloth, squeeze the oils and use to wipe over your body in the shower before drying yourself.
- Put 2–3 drops on absorbent cotton (cottonwool) or tissue, and tuck it in your pocket to give you a reviving lift.
- Put a couple of drops on a tissue to inhale while getting ready for work.
- Wipe a few drops of the blend over the dashboard of the car.
- Add 5 drops to a 2 fl oz (60 ml) atomizer of water. Shake well then spray on the face, avoiding the eye area.

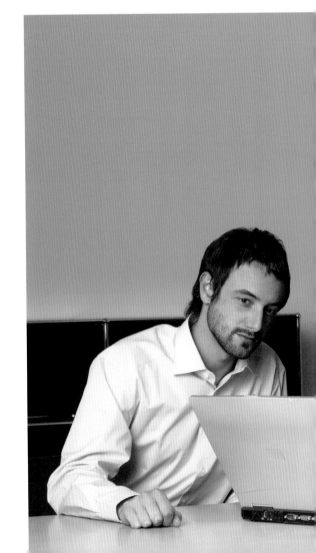

Arriving

It is quite likely that your school or workplace has air-conditioning, computers, synthetic carpets, and synthetic and veneered furniture. These are just a few of the chemical stresses with which we are confronted each day.

Physical stresses involve sitting or standing for long periods of time, using machines or computers, and being exposed to other peoples' airborne germs. Take a minute or two to stretch your muscles at least every 15–20 minutes, and make sure that you are adequately protected with an antibacterial bug buster blend if sick people are thoughtless enough to resume work, and breathe all over their workmates.

In the office

STALE AIR REVIVER

1 teaspoon lemon essential oil
$1/_2$ teaspoon lavender essential oil
$1/_4$ teaspoon grapefruit essential oil
$1/_2$ teaspoon cypress essential oil

To make and use

Place all ingredients in a labeled, dropper bottle and shake to blend.

If possible leave for four days to synergize. Store in a dark, cool place.

Adjust the above blend until it suits everyone in your environment, and use in an air spray and oil burner.

PULSE POINT BLEND FOR BRAIN FATIGUE

3 tablespoons (45 ml) sweet almond oil
10 drops bergamot essential oil
10 drops lemon essential oil
10 drops rosemary essential oil

To make and use

Place all ingredients in a labeled, dropper bottle, and shake to blend.

If possible leave for four days to synergize. Store in a dark, cool place.

Massage onto temples and forehead, and on pulse points inside wrists and throat. Inhale the perfume. Put a few drops on a tissue and inhale as often as needed.

This blend can also be made up in a toilet water, and used to wipe over the hands, arms, and neck to refresh and "de-stress."

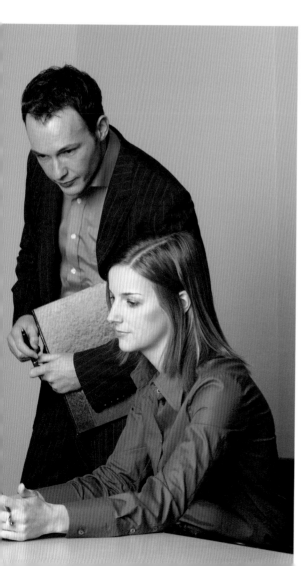

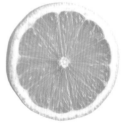

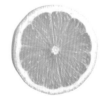

Meetings, meetings, meetings! They are always stress-makers. Carry a tissue with a little essential oil to stay calm.

OIL BLEND FOR COMPUTER USERS

This blend is usually enjoyed by everyone. It brings a fresh atmosphere into a stuffy office.

2 teaspoons lemon essential oil
1 teaspoon cypress essential oil
1 teaspoon cedar essential oil
1 teaspoon pine essential oil

To make and use

Place all ingredients in a labeled, dropper bottle, and shake to blend.

If possible leave for four days to synergize. Store in a dark, cool place.

- Put a few drops of the oil blend on a tissue and wipe over work surfaces.
- Add 10 drops oil blend to 1 teaspoon vodka in a small spray or atomizer. Leave for a day to dissolve. Fill with water and use to spray the air in the vicinity of your desk. Adjust the blend until it suits everyone in your environment.
- Keep an oil burner on your desk with a few drops of the oil blend floating on the water. Don't forget to extinguish the candle before you leave for the day!

Keep a small oil burner on your desk but make sure the oil blend suits everyone.

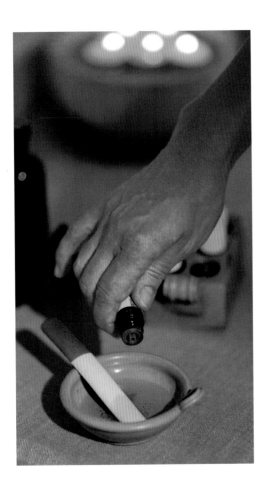

RELEASING THAT TENSION

Driving the kids around or driving to work are probably the most tension-filled parts of our day.

At the same time, they are perfect times to use good relaxation techniques to calm everyone.

When you are waiting at traffic lights, or in traffic jams, and things are getting tense, in spite of the oils, encourage everyone in the car, (including you), to slowly lift their shoulders up to try to touch their ears while they breathe in.

Let the shoulders relax and drop as the breath comes out of the mouth in a long sigh.

Make a great game out of it. Even make a competition to see who can raise their shoulders the highest or who can pull the funniest face while doing it. Children find this good fun without realizing that they are being de-stressed.

Gritting the teeth and jaw on the in-breath and relaxing on the out-breath is another good method of releasing tension.

Just remember to let things go as you drive.

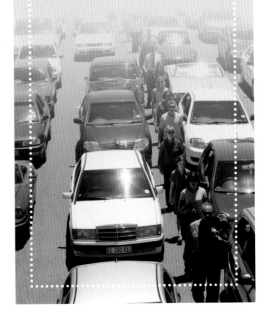

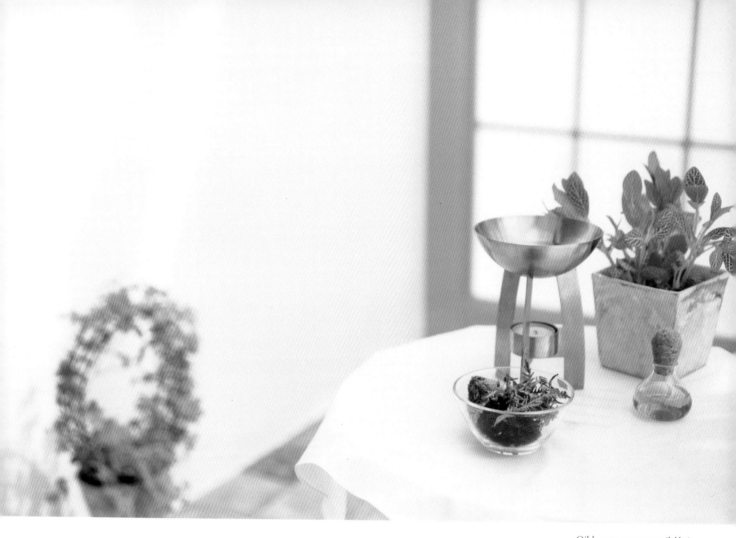

Oil burners are now available in stainless steel for a modern look.

ANTIBACTERIAL BLEND

1 teaspoon lavender essential oil
$\frac{1}{2}$ teaspoon cypress essential oil
$\frac{1}{2}$ teaspoon rosemary essential oil
$\frac{1}{2}$ teaspoon eucalyptus essential oil

To make and use

Place all ingredients in a labeled, dropper bottle and shake to blend.

If possible leave for four days to synergize. Store in a dark, cool place.

- Use in air sprays, or in an oil burner on your desk, or near your work area.
- Put 2 drops of this oil blend on a handkerchief or tissue and inhale the scent as needed.
- Have a shower or at least a wash midway through your day, followed by a toilet water splash containing this blend, to help to disperse the positive ions and increase the negative ion effect.
- Keep a piece of pure wool carpet under your feet, which has been sprayed lightly with a little air spray containing this blend.

AFTERNOON BLEND FOR BRAIN FATIGUE

Ideal for chasing away the cobwebs in the afternoon as you start to feel drowsy after lunch!

3 teaspoons sweet almond oil
6 drops rosemary essential oil
4 drops lemon grass essential oil
2 drops basil essential oil

To make and use

Place all ingredients in a labeled, dropper bottle and shake to blend.

If possible leave for four days to synergize. Store in a dark, cool place.

- Place 1–2 drops on the pulse points of the wrist and throat, massage in and inhale the vapor.
- Place a few drops on a tissue and inhale.

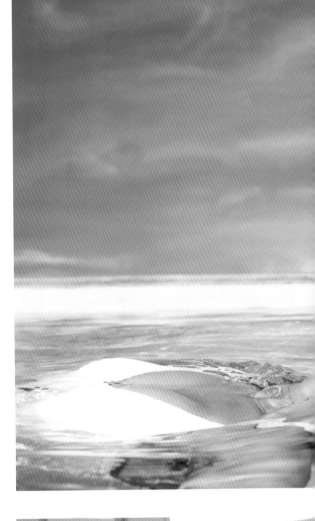

Burn out

Your family and friends have been telling you for weeks, even months to slow down. However, you felt invincible—or at least you felt that if you did not do all the work yourself the whole universe would grind to a halt! And now? You are so mentally and physically exhausted, you have scarcely enough energy to get up in the morning. It is not too late to begin to take care of yourself, but quite a lot of lifestyle changes will be needed. Here are some tips for managing burn out:

* Lessen your workload.
* Make a date with yourself and schedule "Me Time." Put it in your diary or electronic planner. You need time to be alone with no demands being made on your energy.
* Take some sort of exercise every day, such as walking or swimming, or whatever you enjoy most.
* Eat plenty of fresh, unprocessed food, but do not eat if you are upset or overtired. Wait until you are calmer or your body will not be able to cope with digesting the food.
* Get a minimum of eight hours' sleep every night.
* Avoid negative people and situations. Take a rest from reading or watching the news—it will all continue to happen even if you are not monitoring it!
* Do not be embarrassed or afraid to ask for help.
* Learn to meditate.

Swimming is probably the most therapeutic form of exercise.

A beautiful bathroom just makes the sensation of an oil bath more pleasurable.

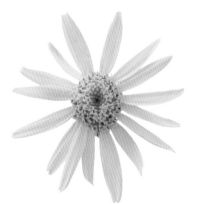

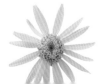

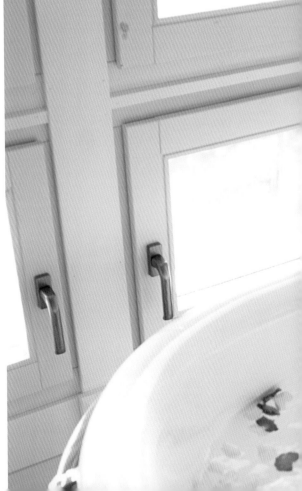

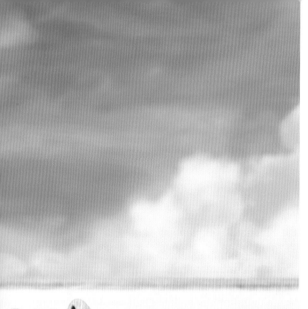
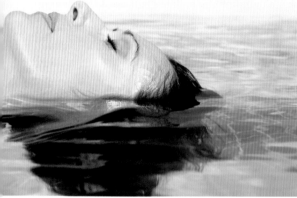
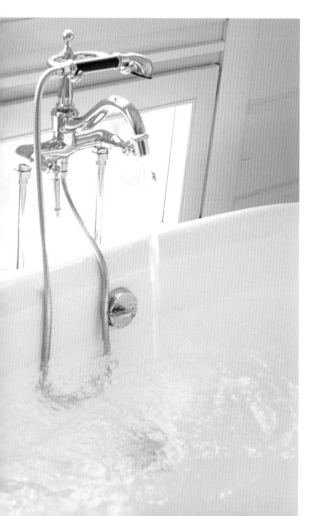

COLDS, INFLUENZA, AND OTHER NASTIES

When you are suffering from any of these, please go to bed and stay there. Keep your germs to yourself. No one is indispensable, and cold cure advertisements that encourage you to "soldier on" are downright antisocial, as very soon many of the people with whom you come in contact each day will, in their turn, be struck down. You can protect yourself from these airborne diseases by carrying some of the Antibacterial Blend, page 341, and using it in the ways suggested in that recipe—along with eating well, exercising, getting plenty of sleep, and "Me Time."

BURN-OUT BLEND

1 teaspoon lavender essential oil
$\frac{1}{2}$ teaspoon grapefruit essential oil
$\frac{1}{2}$ teaspoon lemon essential oil
$\frac{1}{2}$ teaspoon sandalwood essential oil

To make and use

Place all ingredients in a labeled, dropper bottle and shake to blend.

If possible leave for four days to synergize. Store in a dark, cool place.

- Use the blend in the bath and in massage oil, air sprays, oil burners, or in toilet water splashes.
- Arrange to have a once or twice weekly massage using the Burn-Out Blend in the massage oil. If you cannot afford a professional massage, you can trade off with a partner or friend; it is almost as rewarding to give a massage, as it is to receive one!

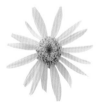

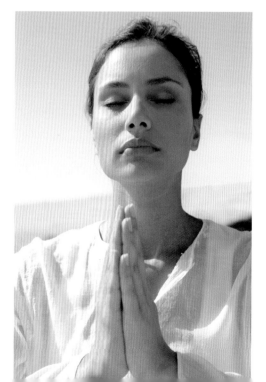

Combine meditation with aromatherapy for the ultimate stress reliever.

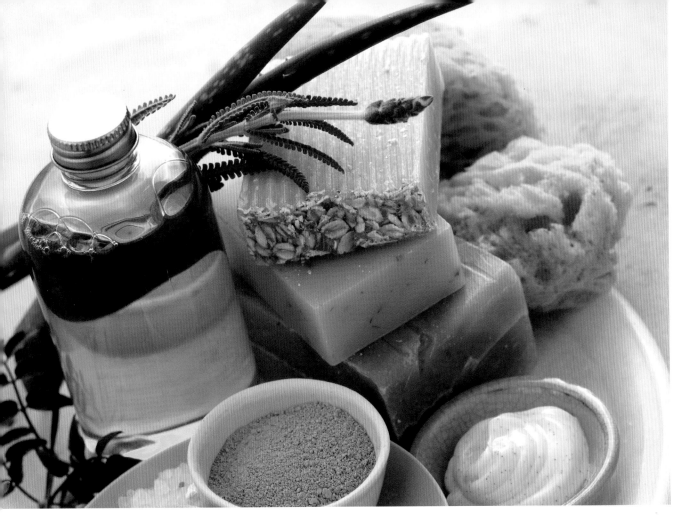

The essentials for a luxury bath experience—soaps, oils, and sponges.

Aromatherapy for travelers

Each year more and more people save money, and plan excitedly, for months in order to have their dream holiday, either in their own country or overseas. A few simple precautions and a small but effective selection of essential oils help to ensure that your holiday is as magical as you anticipated.

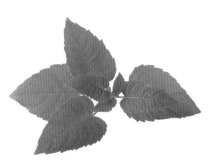

Opposite: Inhalation of essential oils can relieve nerves before flying.

Airplane travel

There are a few simple rules to follow before a flight in order to arrive feeling as bright as possible and, hopefully, to avoid jet lag.

* Drink plenty of water and fruit juice on the plane and try to avoid the temptation of the alcohol cart, whether it is free or not! It you feel nauseous, sip a little of the motion sickness peppermint and honey drink, page 348.
* Do not eat unless you are really hungry.
* Wear loose shoes, or, even better, sandals as your feet might swell on a long journey. If possible wear specialized tights for long haul flights to avoid DVT (Deep Vein Thrombosis). Walk a lot. I resist the temptation to ask for a window seat, as I try to walk at least every half-hour and I do not want to irritate other passengers.
* Sprinkle a tissue with a few drops of eucalyptus essential oil. Breathe the scent deeply if you experience pain as the plane is descending.

PRE-FLYING NERVE TAMER

Many people are nervous of flying, even though statistically it is one of the safest forms of transport. I suppose the fear comes from losing touch with the ground. If this fear is ruining your pre-holiday excitement, use the following essential oil blend for a week before you leave.

1 teaspoon lavender essential oil
$1/2$ teaspoon bergamot essential oil
$1/2$ teaspoon geranium essential oil
40 drops sandalwood essential oil
10 drops chamomile essential oil

To make and use

Place all ingredients in a labeled, dropper bottle and shake to blend.

If possible leave for four days to synergize. Store in a cool, dark place.

- Add 10 drops to 1 teaspoon vegetable oil to use in a deep, warm bath.
- Sprinkle a wet wash cloth with 3 drops, wring out a little and use to rub briskly over the body after a shower or bath.
- Add 4 drops to 1 teaspoon grape seed oil, float on a small bowl of warm water, and use for a massage.
- Use in an air spray and oil burner.
- Sprinkle 1–2 drops of this blend on a tissue or handkerchief, and inhale as needed.

FLYING HIGH

Use this blend once you are airborne to deal with nerves and exhaustion. The blend may be used for adults and children over the age of two years.

60 drops lavender oil
60 drops geranium essential oil
40 drops grapefruit essential oil
1 teaspoon vodka

To make and use

Mix together in a labeled spray bottle or failing this, in a small bottle with a screw top. Shake to blend.

If possible leave for four days to synergize. Store in a cool, dark place.

Spray lightly on a tissue and sniff as needed.

- If you are stressed or nervous, wring a wash cloth out in very hot water, spray very lightly with a little Flying High blend (the equivalent of 1–2 drops), and use to wipe over the face and hands. The heat has a calming effect.
- Holding a hot face cloth on the back of the neck is also soothing and relaxing.
- If using for children, the spray must be very light—only one quick squirt with the spray bottle.

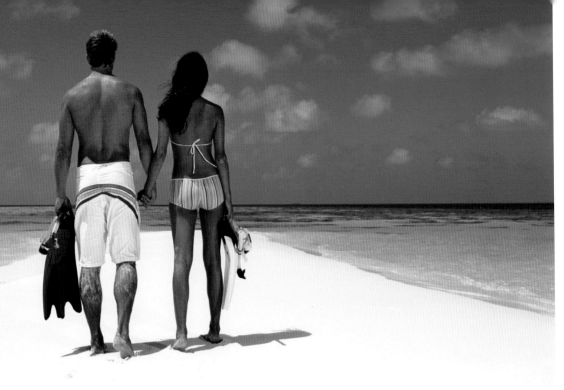

Proper use of essential oils will make your arrival easier.

ACHING, SWOLLEN LEGS, AND FEET

If the blend is to be used for children, use spearmint essential oil in preference to peppermint essential oil.

3 tablespoons (45 ml) unscented gel
10 drops peppermint essential oil
5 drops lavender essential oil

To make and use

Mix the gel and essential oils together really well (you don't want any "hot spots"). Spoon into a labeled jar.

If possible leave for four days to synergize. Store in a cool, dark place.

Pat the gel over the legs and feet whenever you feel the need. Don't massage into the skin.

JET LAG LET GO

Have a shower or bath on arrival, and change your clothes. These suggestions can also be used to recover from your trip when you return home.

60 drops grapefruit essential oil
60 drops lavender essential oil
60 drops rosemary essential oil

To make and use

Place all ingredients in a labeled, dropper bottle and shake to blend.

If possible leave for four days to synergize. Store in a cool, dark place.

- Add 10 drops of the blend to 1 teaspoon of vegetable oil and pour into the bath. Agitate the water to disperse.
- If showering, drip 1–2 drops on a hot, moist wash cloth, squeeze out well, and rub briskly over your whole body (avoiding eyes and genitals).

JET LAG

Flying can get us from one side of the globe to the other in the space of a few hours. A few simple tactics can be helpful to overcome the problems our bodies often experience adjusting to time change.

- Don't go to sleep until local bedtime.

- Sprinkle one drop of chamomile essential oil and one drop of lavender essential oil on a tissue and slip it inside the pillowcase for a good sleep. This method will also soothe overexcited children.
- Drink lots of bottled water, not alcohol.

SLEEP EASY

60 drops lavender essential oil
60 drops geranium essential oil
60 drops chamomile essential oil

To make and use

Place all ingredients in a labeled, dropper bottle and shake to blend.

If possible leave for four days to synergize. Store in a cool, dark place.

- Add 10 drops of the blend to 1 teaspoon of vegetable oil and pour into the bath. Agitate the water to disperse.
- If showering, drip 1–2 drops on a hot, moist wash cloth, squeeze out well and rub briskly over your whole body (avoiding eyes and genitals).
- Also, you could carry an almost full ½ fl oz (15 ml) bottle of Basic Massage Oil, and add 6 drops of the Sleep Easy blend. Either massage the oil all over your body after a shower or ask someone to give you a massage.

"Are we nearly there?"—Traveling with children

If you are traveling with children, the biggest problem will be boredom. I used to say to my children: "The ones who don't ask 'Are we nearly there?' get a present!" Sometimes it worked!

* Stop every hour or so at parks, recreation areas, and other suitable places. The time lost will be amply repaid in what will be much happier journey.

* Make up a little flask or bottle of peppermint tea in case of car sickness or nausea, and read the sections on "Commuting" (page 338) and "Releasing that tension" (page 340) for more suggestions on stress-free car travel.

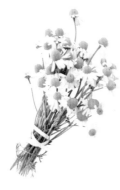

TODDLER TAMER

Children can get very overexcited, tired, and cranky when traveling. This blend is suitable for children over one year old.

For babies up to one year, use two drops chamomile essential oil in one tablespoon grape seed oil.

1 tablespoon grape seed oil
2 drops lavender essential oil
3 drops chamomile essential oil

To make and use

Place all ingredients in a labeled, dropper bottle and shake to blend.

If possible leave for four days to synergize. Store in a cool, dark place.

- Massage the child's arms and legs, using a gentle upward movement towards the heart.
- Put a little on a tissue and encourage them to inhale; this will have a calming effect.

Airplane travel is especially stressful for children. Use essential oils to calm them.

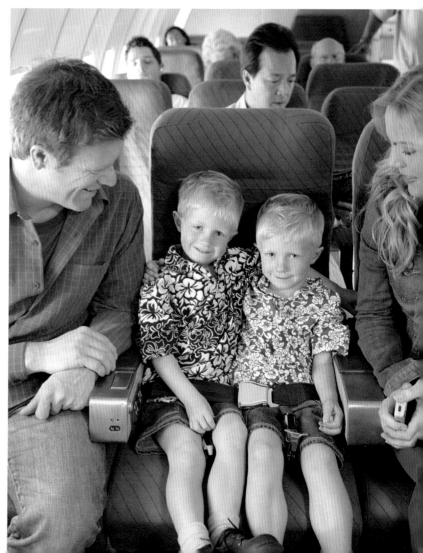

Motion sickness or nausea

Car, boat, or plane sickness can make you regret ever having left home. But don't let it spoil your trip—there are remedies that can overcome this.

Make up a 2 cup (500 ml) bottle containing 2 teaspoons honey and 2 drops peppermint essential oil topped up with water. Shake well and then use it as follows:

Children 2–5: 1 teaspoon mixture in $^{1}/_{4}$ cup (60 ml) water.

Children 5–12: 2 teaspoons mixture in $^{1}/_{4}$ cup (60 ml) water.

Children 12–16: $^{1}/_{4}$ cup (60 ml) undiluted mixture.

Adults: $^{1}/_{2}$ cup (125 ml) undiluted mixture.

When traveling by car, put drops of peppermint and lavender essential oil on absorbent cotton (cottonwool) and place on the back and front window ledges. These will help to prevent nausea and also act as a calmative.

Half to one hour before setting off on a trip, take two ginger tablets or capsules, (available from pharmacies and health food stores) or chew crystallized or glacé ginger.

Use Anti-Infection Hand Wipes because colds, gastroenteritis, hepatitis, influenza, and scabies are just a few of the diseases that can be transmitted by handling door knobs, money, handrails, flush-buttons in toilets, and many other places.

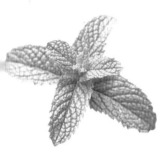

The town of Cassis in Provence, France, is known for its open-air cafés along the foreshores.

ANTI-INFECTION HAND WIPES

$^{1}/_{2}$ cup (60 ml) vodka
20 drops lavender or manuka essential oil
20 drops tea tree essential oil
10 drop bergamot essential oil
10 drops citronella essential oil

To make and use

Place all ingredients in a labeled bottle and shake to blend. If possible leave for four days to synergize.

Make hand wipes out of suitable fabric or kitchen cloths and sized to fit into a small waterproof container that you can carry in your pocket or bag.

Spray the cloths with the blend as often as necessary to keep the oils fresh.

Use after handling money, shaking hands, traveling on public transport, etc.

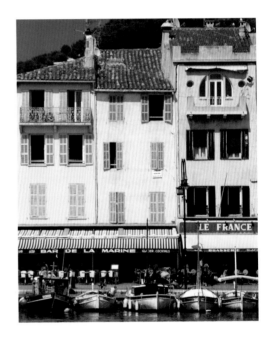

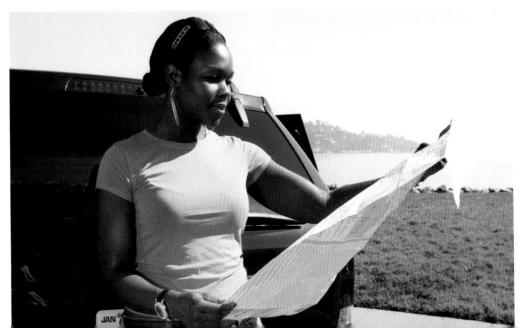

Even when traveling in your own car, you need to keep essential oils with you.

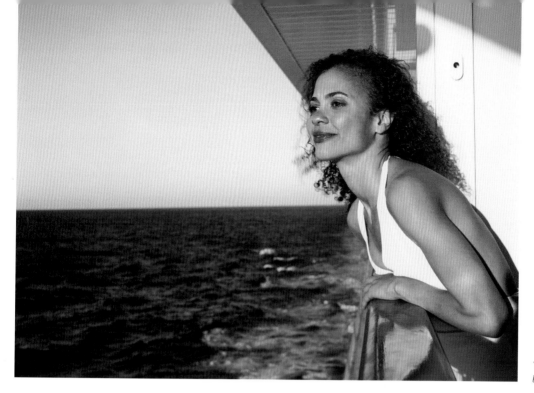

Take ginger tea for motion sickness, before and during travel.

Dysentery

Dysentery is a highly infectious disease caused by bacilli found in contaminated water, and food. It is mainly spread by human contact and flies. Medical help will be needed to treat this condition. Essential oils will be useful to help the patient, to help prevent the spread of the disease, and to protect the carer.

ESSENTIAL OILS

Bergamot, ginger, lavender, thyme.

TREATMENT

- After dealing with the patient, wash your hands with soap and a nailbrush for at least 30 seconds, paying particular attention to the areas around the nails and the wrists.
- Put six drops thyme essential oil and four drops lavender essential oil in a small bowl of water next to the washbasin. Rinse the hands and lower arms thoroughly, and dry on a paper towel.
- Mix 10 drops total of thyme and lavender essential oils with one teaspoon vegetable oil, and add to a warm bath. Make an air spray containing thyme and lavender essential oils and use frequently throughout the whole house and the sick room.
- If the patient has aching muscles and would appreciate a massage—back, hands, feet, or whole body—16 drops of thyme and lavender essential oils can be added to one tablespoon of grape seed oil.

STAYING WELL WHILE TRAVELING

Keep your eating as simple as possible for the first few days. Only eat fruit that can be peeled, and wash the fruit before peeling.

- Take acidophilus tablets as recommended on the packet.
- Drink only bottled drinks. Water that has been stored in a plastic container in a hot place can present hazards of its own. Out-gassing can occur if overheated, and this in turn can result in free radical poisoning. Try to buy water in glass bottles or from an air-conditioned store, or supermarket. You will know as soon as you sip the water if it is contaminated as it will taste of plastic.
- Clean your teeth with bottled water.
- Avoid shellfish, salads, and raw foods
- Avoid fresh milk (use dried), and cream.
- Avoid eating food from roadside stalls.

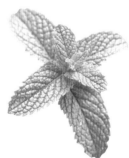

Aromatherapy for the home

Use essential oils as part of your strategy to make and keep your home a safe, calm, and loving place where you and your family can release anxieties, regain strength of purpose, and allow the hectic world to recede until you are ready to "face the pace" once more.

The oils can perfume, deodorize, sooth or stimulate, act as disinfectants, insect repellents, and ionizers. Everyone benefits from the use of essential oils in the home and also from the feeling that something positive and joyful is being created for all, from the tiniest newborn baby to the family elders.

Essential oils can be blended in such a way that the fragrances used in each area of your home will harmonize with each other. Every breath you, your family, and friends take will enhance the quality of health, both physical and emotional. Every part of your home (and everybody living in it) can receive the benefits of essential oils.

The three most important ways to use the oils are:
* Air sprays and oil burners that can be used to safeguard health during times when illness threatens or is present, and create a general calming influence on family members in the living rooms and bedrooms.
* Baths that are deeply therapeutic and stress-reducing—even the most frantic baby is often soothed and calmed by being placed in warm, scented water.
* Massage, which can be a loving, tender, and non-threatening way for family members to draw close to each other. Older people may feel shy or apprehensive about a body massage, but will gain immense pleasure and benefit from a foot or shoulder massage. The following recipes will be a guide to some ways in which you can employ the oils in your home.

Essential oils can be dripped on potpourri or added to candle recipies.

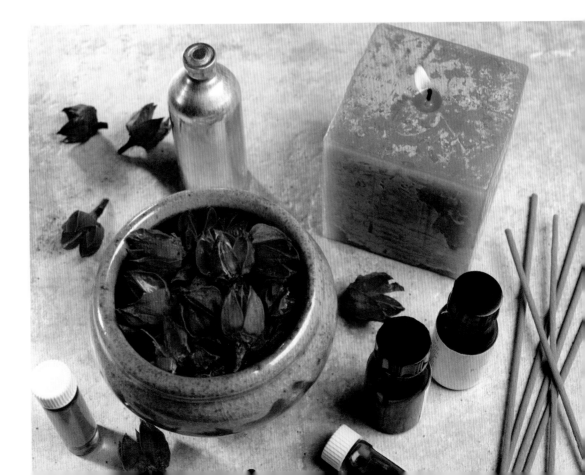

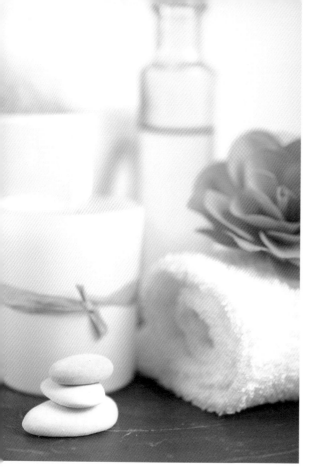

Freshen the bathroom with a candle scented with your favorite essential oil.

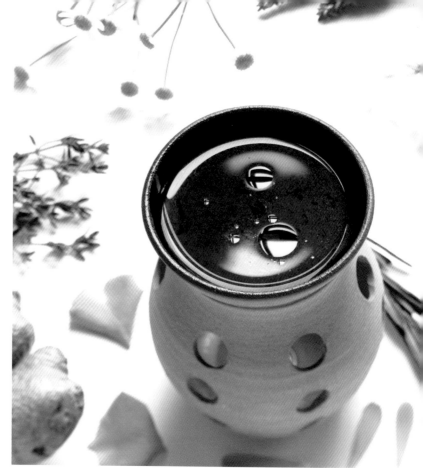

Simple candle-powered oil burners can be used anywhere in the home.

Air sweeteners

The following suggestions and recipes are environmentally friendly, the contents are largely natural, inexpensive, and they work! It might be advisable to make and try small amounts of the blends first to make sure that you like the perfume. They are easy to make and are ideal to use in an air spray or oil burner, on wood for the fire, or other warm places. Don't spray them on polished furniture or delicate fabrics.

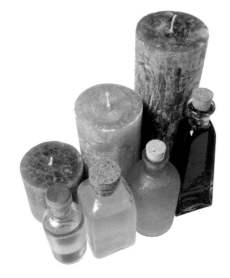

WELCOME HOME

Use this blend to create a happy, restful atmosphere in the living room and dining room. The aroma will give a cheerful welcome to family and friends—but not any bacteria and viruses that they may be carrying!

1 teaspoon geranium essential oil
1 teaspoon bergamot essential oil
1 teaspoon lavender essential oil
1 teaspoon lemon essential oil
50 drops cinnamon essential oil
20 drops clove essential oil
50 ml vodka or brandy
1 cup purified or distilled water

To make and use

Mix all the oils in a 1 fl oz (30 ml) bottle and shake well.

Add $^1/_2$–1 teaspoon of the oil blend to 50 ml vodka or brandy in a labeled spray bottle.

Allow to dissolve and add the water.

Shake well before using as a room spray.

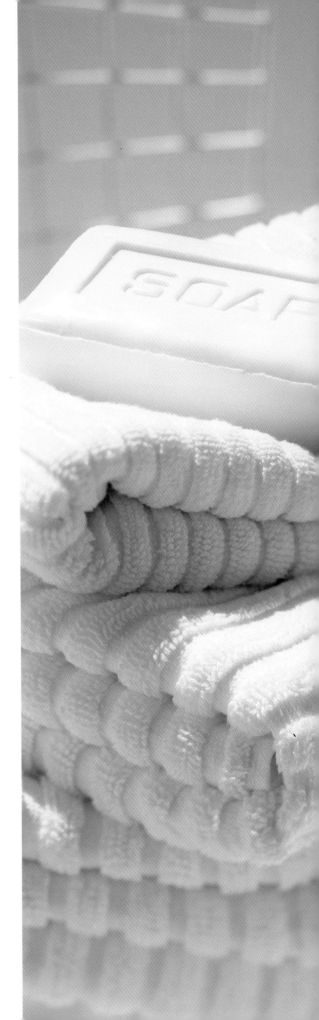

Soap can be purchased from the supermarket scented with essential oil. However, the best perfume will always come from home-made soap.

HAPPY FAMILIES

This blend is joyful and uplifting and useful to counter family stress.

2 teaspoons lavender essential oil
2 teaspoons grapefruit essential oil
$\frac{1}{2}$ teaspoon bergamot essential oil
$\frac{1}{2}$ teaspoon sandalwood essential oil
50 ml vodka or brandy
1 cup purified or distilled water

To make and use

Mix all the oils in a 1 fl oz (30 ml) bottle and shake well.

Add $\frac{1}{2}$–1 teaspoon of the oil blend to 50 ml vodka or brandy in a labeled spray bottle.

Allow to dissolve and add the water.

Shake well before using as a room spray.

ANTI-PLAGUE BLEND

There will be times when visitors or the family have coughs, colds, influenza, or other contagious diseases. You can help protect yourself by using the following blend as a room spray.

1 teaspoon eucalyptus essential oil
1 teaspoon tea tree essential oil
1 teaspoon lavender essential oil
1 teaspoon pine essential oil
$\frac{1}{2}$ teaspoon thyme essential oil
$\frac{1}{2}$ teaspoon cinnamon or clove essential oil
50 ml vodka or brandy
1 cup purified or distilled water

To make and use

Mix all the oils in a 1 fl oz (30 ml) bottle and shake well.

Add $\frac{1}{2}$–1 teaspoon of the oil blend to 50 ml vodka or brandy in a labeled spray bottle.

Allow to dissolve and add the water.

Shake well before using as a room spray.

A few drops of the oil blend can be sprinkled on a tissue and kept in a pocket to take out and sniff from time to time.

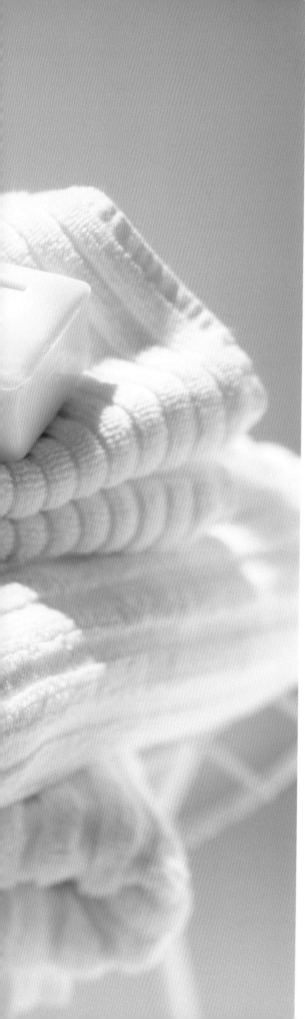

HEAVEN SCENT

TABLE MATS

A few drops of essential oil can be dropped on the underside of cloth tablemats or tablecloths where the heat of the plate will release the perfume. Choose perfumes that won't clash or overpower the scent of the food. Citrus or spice oils are most suitable. Make sure the oil does not come in contact with fine furniture.

NOTEPAPER

Scented notes and letters are a pleasure to receive and also make a gracious gift. The perfume should reflect the personality of the recipient, but be careful not to make it overpowering. Choose a suitable essential oil or blend from this book. Place a few drops of the oil on pieces of blotting paper or thin cloth and interleave them between the writing paper and envelopes. Leave the paper for a week or so for the scent
to permeate.

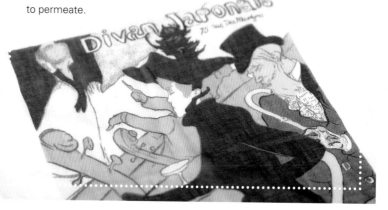

Humidifying rooms

The air in a heated room can get very dry, which in turn can dry the skin. Humidify and freshen the air by putting a few drops of essential oil blend in a small bowl of water and placing the bowl near the heat source.

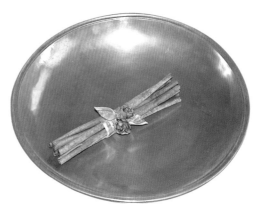

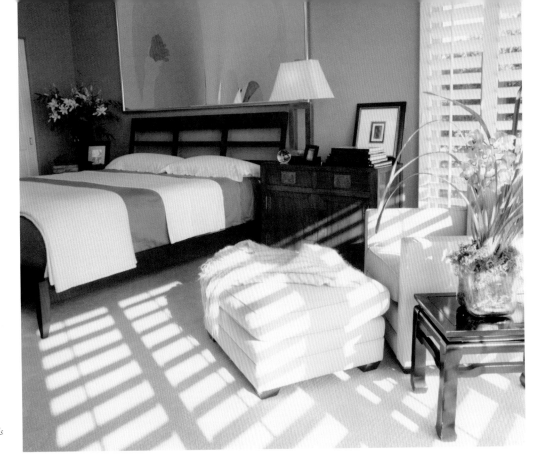

The bedroom should always be a place of tranquility. Enhance this with the subtle use of essential oils on linen and furnishing.

Adults' bedrooms

The bedroom is the place where adults spend about a third of their lives: sleeping, dreaming, talking, and making love. All too often the bedroom can become a battleground, as parents often wait until they are alone in the bedroom to air their grievances. Have disagreements in the car (in the garage!), or down the bottom of the garden, but not in the bedroom, or in front of the children.

Sometimes a partner has a feeling of sexual inadequacy or timidity which can lead to impotence, frigidity, bitterness, and guilt or blame. If the problem is a too demanding partner, a spray containing marjoram essential oil might help to quell the excessive ardor!

Oils have a variety of practical and romantic purposes in bedrooms, from setting the scene for romantic nights, to inducing sweet relaxing sleep, or looking after your clothes with an anti-moth blend for wardrobes! Make sure that the oils used in different areas of the bedroom have the same type of fragrance. It would be disturbing to have a heavy, musky scent in competition with a citrus or floral blend. Try making tiny amounts of the following blends until you find which combinations work best for you.

Here are some ways to use the blends:

* Use in an air spray a few minutes before retiring, or in an oil burner (not near curtains, bedclothes or other flammable materials).
* Sprinkle a few drops on absorbent cotton (cottonwool) and tuck under pillows or under the bed.
* Make a flat sachet out of two handkerchiefs sewn together, sprinkle with 1–3 drops of the blend, and slip inside the pillowcase.
* Sprinkle a few drops on absorbent cotton (cottonwool) and place them between bed linen in drawers and cupboards.
* Add a few drops to the water when washing woodwork and windows in the bedrooms.

ROMANTIC NIGHTS

1 teaspoon ylang-ylang essential oil
$\frac{1}{2}$ teaspoon lime essential oil
$\frac{1}{2}$ teaspoon petitgrain essential oil
20 drops sandalwood essential oil
15 drops patchouli essential oil
5 drops clove essential oil

To make
Place all the ingredients in a labeled dropper bottle and shake to blend.
> If possible leave for four days to synergize.
> Store in a dark, cool place.
> Shake well before use.

SLEEP TIME

This blend will help when, for no particular reason, it's difficult to get to sleep.

$\frac{1}{2}$ teaspoon chamomile essential oil
$\frac{1}{2}$ teaspoon lavender essential oil
20 drops marjoram essential oil
20 drops neroli or clary sage essential oil

To make
Place all the ingredients in a labeled dropper bottle and shake to blend.
> If possible leave for four days to synergize.
> Store in a dark, cool place.
> Shake well before use.

MIND SOOTHER

This blend will help chase away the anxieties and stresses of the day leaving your mind calm and ready for sleep.

1 teaspoon bergamot essential oil
$\frac{1}{2}$ teaspoon lavender essential oil
20 drops mandarin essential oil
20 drops cedarwood essential oil
20 drops sandalwood, peppermint, or juniper
  essential oil

To make
Place all the ingredients in a labeled dropper bottle and shake to blend.
> If possible leave for four days to synergize.
> Store in a dark, cool place.
> Shake well before use.

THE FEMININE TOUCH

1 teaspoon rose geranium essential oil
1 teaspoon orange or mandarin essential oil
$\frac{1}{2}$ teaspoon geranium essential oil
20 drops petitgrain essential oil
10 drops patchouli essential oil
10 drops cinnamon essential oil

To make
Place all the ingredients in a labeled dropper bottle and shake to blend.
> If possible leave for four days to synergize.
> Store in a dark, cool place.
> Shake well before use.

BOY'S OWN BEDROOM

1 teaspoon bergamot essential oil
1 teaspoon lime essential oil
20 drops cinnamon essential oil
10 drops rosemary essential oil
10 drops black pepper essential oil

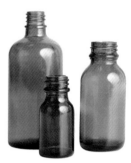

To make
Place all the ingredients in a labeled dropper bottle and shake to blend.
> If possible leave for four days to synergize.
> Store in a dark, cool place.
> Shake well before use.

Wipe furniture with a mild solution of essential oils for a wonderful fresh scent.

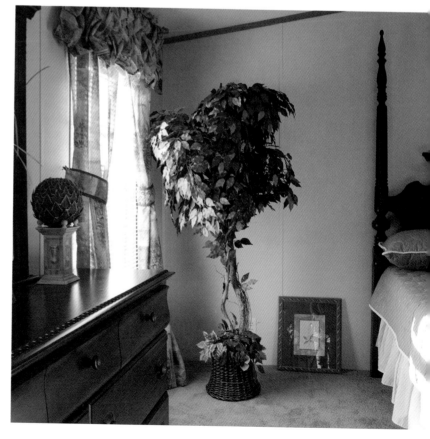

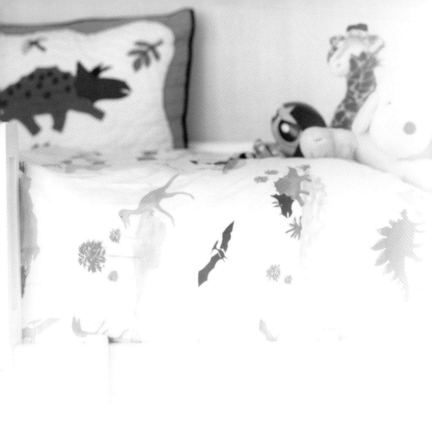

When using essential oils in children's bedrooms, make sure they are out of reach of little fingers.

CHILDREN'S BLEND
1 teaspoon lavender essential oil
1 teaspoon chamomile essential oil
1 teaspoon mandarin essential oil

To make and use
Place all the ingredients in a labeled dropper bottle and shake to blend.

> If possible leave for four days to synergize.
> Store in a dark, cool place.
> Shake well before use.

- Use in an air spray a few minutes before retiring.
- Sprinkle a few drops on absorbent cotton (cottonwool) and tuck under pillows or under the bed.
- Make a flat sachet out of two handkerchiefs sewn together, sprinkle with 1–3 drops of the blend, and slip inside the pillowcase.
- Sprinkle a few drops on absorbent cotton (cottonwool) balls and place them between bed linen in drawers and cupboards.
- Add a few drops to the water when washing woodwork and windows in the bedrooms.

Children's bedrooms

Adults often imagine that they have a monopoly on worry and that children are (or should be) completely carefree. Examination nerves, performance-related stress in sport, fear of the dark, overstimulating movies, peer group pressure, acne and puppy fat, along with many real or imagined fears can make life very difficult for young people.

Try to make the last half hour before bedtime as calm as possible with maybe a warm bath, a glass of warm milk or chamomile tea, and a cuddle while reading a bedtime story. Children need a feeling of security and privacy in their bedrooms. The following oil blend will help to create a bedroom oasis.

Air sprays for children's rooms

Age	Strength
Less than 1 year	Not recommended
1–5 years	Use one-quarter the adult amount
5 years–puberty	As 1–5 years gradually increasing (drop by drop) with child's age

SMELLY SHOES!

If you store shoes in the wardrobe, it can create a less than pleasant ambience in the bedroom! Make up a quantity of Carpet Freshener (opposite). Sprinkle a little in the shoes, shaking to spread it around. Leave overnight and shake out in the morning. Alternatively (and I think better) pour a few spoons of the powder in the cut-off feet of a pair of tights or pantyhose, tie a knot in the top, and slip it in the shoes. These sachets can be used for some time before more oils are needed to refresh them.

Closets, drawers, carpets

Closets

Sprinkle two to three drops of the blend on padded coat hangers. Add two to three drops of the blend to two cups water and wash the inside of the closet.

ANTI-MOTH BLEND

Most commercial moth repellents smell bad enough to repel humans as well. The following oils will keep the closets and drawers fresh and free from insects and moths without interfering with your daytime perfume or aftershave, or clashing with the chosen bedroom blend.

1 teaspoon lavender essential oil
1 teaspoon rosemary essential oil
1 teaspoon lemon essential oil

To make and use

Place all the ingredients in a labeled dropper bottle and shake to blend.
   If possible leave for four days to synergize.
   Store in a dark, cool place.
   Shake well before use.

Drawers

Sprinkle two to three drops of the blend on the lining paper of drawers containing underwear, woolens, sports clothes, or put a few drops on absorbent cotton (cottonwool) and place between the clothes.

Carpets and rugs

This powder is for all carpets and rugs, but those of you with pets will particularly appreciate the bonus of deodorant and disinfectant properties.

CARPET FRESHENER

2 cups bicarbonate of soda
$\frac{1}{3}$ cup unperfumed talcum powder or cornstarch (cornflour)
$\frac{1}{3}$ cup borax
30 drops lemon essential oil
20 drops lavender essential oil
10 drops cinnamon essential oil
10 drops pine essential oil

To make and use

Sift the dry ingredients together in a bowl.
   Mix the oils together in a small bowl and add to the powders one drop at a time while stirring thoroughly.
   Store in a labeled glass jar or a container with a sprinkler lid.
   Stir twice a day for three days before using.
   Sprinkle the mix lightly on the carpet.
   Leave for a few hours or overnight if possible before vacuuming.

TIP THE OILS USED IN THE AIR SWEETENER OR CARPET POWDER MAY ALSO BE USED TO SPRINKLE IN THE BAG OF THE VACUUM CLEANER TO GET RID OF THAT HORRIBLE DUSTY SMELL THAT SEEMS TO BUILD UP.

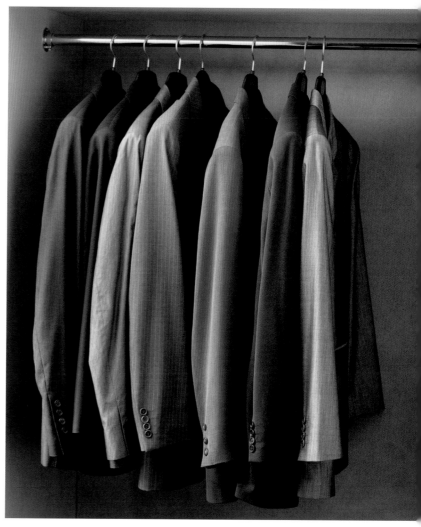

Use padded coathangers to protect clothes and sprinkle the padding with essential oils.

Kitchens

Kitchens can be both a health and a nose hazard! Not only are many of the areas perfect breeding grounds for bacteria, but many of the smells are less than pleasant: Boiled cabbage, fried or grilled meat and fish, trash cans, and drains. The essential oils we use in the kitchen need to be powerful bacteria inhibitors, but they should also smell fresh and clean.

Cleaning kitchen trouble spots

Working surfaces/benchtops	Use All-Purpose Disinfectant Cleaner.
Cupboards	Add 8 drops Bug Buster Blend or 1–2 teaspoons All-Purpose Disinfectant Cleaner to 1 quart (1 liter) warm water.
Kitchen cloths	Add 8 drops Bug Buster Blend or 1–2 teaspoons All-Purpose Disinfectant Cleaner to 2 quarts (2 liters) cold water as a pre-wash soak to sterilize. Leave overnight if possible.
Drains	To sweeten and disinfect, drop 4–6 drops of neat Bug Buster Blend down the drain.
Trash cans	Spray with All-Purpose Disinfectant Cleaner, wipe clean. Sprinkle 4 drops Bug Buster Blend into the can or liner.
Floors	Add 8 drops Bug Buster Blend or 1–2 teaspoons of All-Purpose Disinfectant Cleaner to 1 quart (1 liter) warm water.
Sinks	Wash with 1 teaspoon All-Purpose Disinfectant Cleaner in 1 quart (1 liter) warm water.
Dish washing	Use 1 teaspoon All-Purpose Disinfectant Cleaner in washing-up water in the sink.
Dishwashers	Add 2 drops Bug Buster Blend to dishwasher powder in the powder compartment of the dishwasher.
Air spray	Add 50 drops Bug Buster Blend to 3 tablespoons (45 ml) vinegar. Pour into a 10–14 fl oz (300–400 ml) spray bottle. Add 1 cup (250 ml) water. Shake well before use.

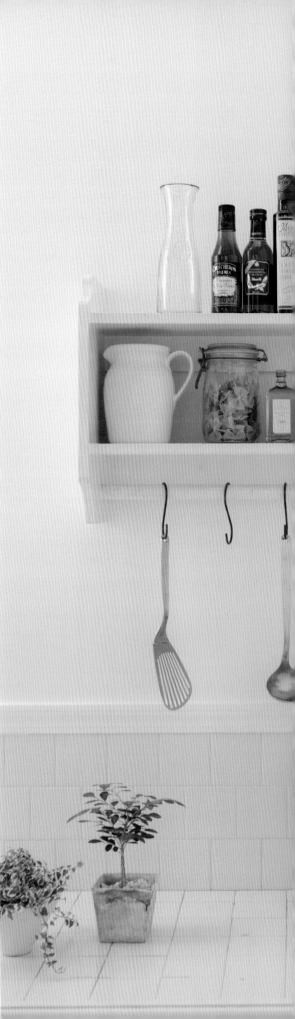

CITRUS FRESH

Use this blend for a calm, confident, cheerful atmosphere during the preparation of food.

1 teaspoon lemon essential oil
$\frac{1}{2}$ teaspoon bergamot essential oil
$\frac{1}{2}$ teaspoon grapefruit essential oil
25 drops sandalwood essential oil
30 drops vanilla essence

To make and use
Place all the ingredients in a labeled dropper bottle and shake to blend.
    If possible leave for four days to synergize.
    Store in a dark, cool place.
    Shake well before use.
- Use in an air spray or an oil burner before cooking begins.
- Sprinkle on a damp cloth and use to wipe work surfaces.

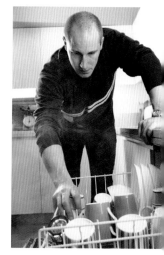

Dishwashers are always a source of strange smells. Eradicate them with Bug Buster Blend.

ALL-PURPOSE DISINFECTANT CLEANER

This cleaner works hard to cut through grease and remove stains. It also acts as a powerful disinfectant. Use on working surfaces, tiles, painted woodwork. Avoid inhaling the ammonia fumes.

2 oz (60 g) bicarbonate of soda
2 quarts (2 liters) hot water
4 teaspoons vinegar
3 teaspoons Bug Buster Blend (below)
4 teaspoons cloudy ammonia

To make and use
Mix together the bicarbonate of soda and hot water. Allow to cool.
    Combine the vinegar and Bug Buster Blend. Allow the oils to dissolve.
    Mix together with the ammonia.
    Mix very well then bottle and shake well.
    Decant some of the mixture into a spray bottle or pour directly onto a cloth to use.

BUG BUSTER BLEND

2 teaspoons lemon essential oil
$1\frac{1}{2}$ teaspoons pine essential oil
$\frac{1}{2}$ teaspoon cinnamon essential oil
$\frac{1}{2}$ teaspoon tea tree essential oil

To make and use
Mix all the ingredients in a 1 fl oz (30 ml) labeled dropper bottle.
    Shake well to blend.
    Allow to stand for four days to synergize before using.

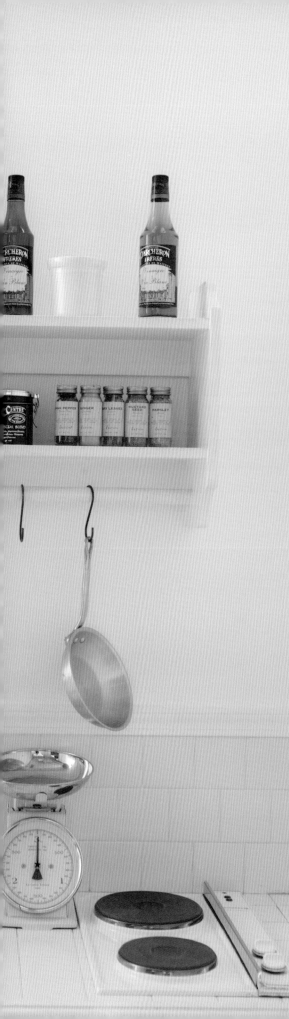

Freshen your kitchen with a fresh blend of citrus essential oils.

Bathrooms

Bugs love bathrooms. Fungus growths love shower stalls. Many diseases (such as tinea) can be transmitted from person to person through the warm, moist bacteria- and fungus-laden floors of the shower stall. No matter how often the shower is cleaned, it can harbor these undesirable bugs unless the appropriate cleaning solutions are used.

BATHROOM OIL BLEND

This blend contains both antibacterial and antifungal oils.

1½ teaspoons lemon essential oil
1 teaspoon bergamot essential oil
1 teaspoon pine essential oil
½ teaspoon citronella essential oil
½ teaspoon thyme essential oil
½ teaspoon tea tree essential oil

To make and use

Mix all the oils together in a 1 fl oz (30 ml) labeled dropper bottle
   Shake well to blend.
   If possible, leave for four days to synergize.
   Store in a cool, dark place.
   Keep the cleaning materials in the bathroom and encourage the family to spray the shower and the air before leaving the room.

Make sure to clean around faucets where bacteria loves to gather.

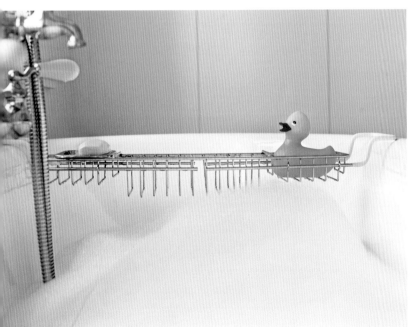

BATHROOM CLEANER

This is basically the same as All-Purpose Disinfectant Cleaner but contains different oils. It works wonderfully in the bathroom. It cleans wall and floor tiles, bath, showers, wash basins, and their surrounds. If extra cleaning power is needed on stubborn stains use bicarbonate of soda as an abrasive in conjunction with the spray.

⅓ cup bicarbonate of soda
2 quarts (2 liters) hot water
4 teaspoons vinegar
3 teaspoons Bathroom Oil Blend
4 teaspoons cloudy ammonia

To make and use

Mix together the bicarbonate of soda and hot water. Allow to cool.
   Mix together the vinegar and Bathroom Oil Blend. Allow the oils to dissolve.
   Mix all together with ammonia.
   Mix very well. Bottle and label clearly.
   Decant some of the mixture into a spray bottle or pour directly onto a cloth.
   Shake the mixture well before use.

Cleaning bathroom trouble spots

Bath and wash basin	Spray with Bathroom Cleaner, leave for a minute or two before wiping.
Vanity surfaces	Spray with Bathroom Cleaner, leave for a minute or two before wiping.
Shower	To disinfect the shower, add 1 teaspoon Bathroom Oil Blend to 3½ fl oz (100 ml) vinegar. Pour into a 10–14 fl oz (300–400 ml) spray. Add 4 teaspoons water. Shake to mix. Spray shower after use.
Floors and tiles	Wash floors and tiles weekly with 2 teaspoons All-Purpose Disinfectant Cleaner in 1 quart (1 liter) warm water.
Air spray	Add 50 drops Bathroom Oil Blend to 3 tablespoons (45 ml) vinegar. Pour into a 10–14 fl oz (300–400 ml) spray bottle. Add 1 cup 250 ml) water. Shake well before use.

The toilet

In the toilet area the two main concerns are bacteria and smell. An essential oil blend can take care of both these problems. It's all very well telling children to wash their hands after going to the toilet, and as adults I'm sure that we automatically do this, but the very actions of pressing the flush button, opening the door, and turning on a faucet is going to spread bacteria from the as yet unwashed hands to many other people. The use of a combined antibacterial and air-freshening spray means that the toilet seat, the flush button, and the door handle are all being cleansed and the air sweetened every time the spray is used.

TOILET BLEND

Label clearly with the following instruction: "After using the toilet, please shake this bottle and spray up towards the ceiling to allow the mist to fall on toilet, door handle, and this container."

2 teaspoons tea tree essential oil
1 teaspoon lavender essential oil
1 teaspoon lemon essential oil
40 drops pine essential oil
40 drops lemon grass essential oil

To make and use

Place all the ingredients in a labeled bottle and shake to blend.

If possible leave for four days to synergize.

Store in a dark, cool place.

Add 1 teaspoon of the blend to 3 tablespoons (45 ml) vodka in a spray bottle. Allow to dissolve and add 1 cup (250 ml) purified water.

Spray up towards the ceiling to allow the mist to fall on the toilet and door handle after using the toilet.

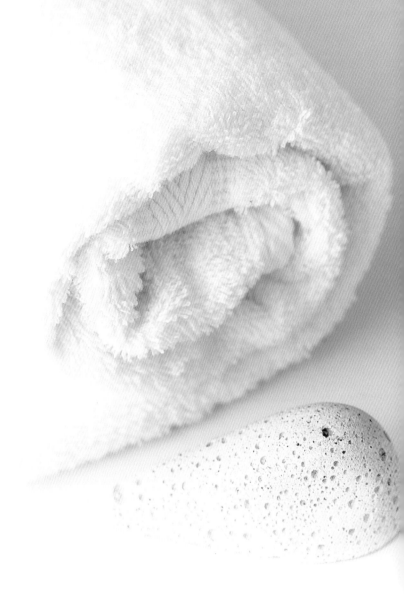

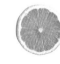

Cleaning trouble spots in the toilet

Toilet cleaning	Sprinkle 10 drops Toilet Blend in the toilet bowl after cleaning, then scrub thoroughly.
Toilet seats and woodwork	Use 1–2 teaspoons All-Purpose Disinfectant Cleaner and 5 drops eucalyptus or tea tree essential oil in 2 cups (500 ml) water.
Floors	Use 1–2 teaspoons All-Purpose Disinfectant Cleaner and 10 drops eucalyptus essential oil in 2 quarts (2 liters) water.

Laundry or utility room

This is often a multi-purpose room. It may be a repository for gardening and sports shoes, dirty laundry baskets, mops, brooms and other cleaning equipment, beach towels, and dog and cat beds. The smells which can build up and become interesting are often not the ones with which you want your home to be associated! The quality to be aimed at in the laundry room is fresh and clean. The oils to use are the ones that are antibacterial, antifungal, and deodorizing. The following blend will leave the room and the wash fresh and lightly fragrant.

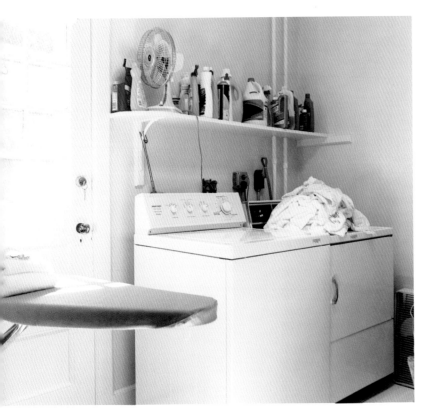

Laundry or utility rooms are a constant battle of clean and dirty. Follow the table to keep the room fresh and clean.

LAUNDRY BLEND

1 teaspoon lavender essential oil
$\frac{1}{2}$ teaspoon rosemary essential oil
$\frac{1}{2}$ teaspoon lemon essential oil
20 drops pine essential oil
20 drops lemon grass essential oil

Place all the ingredients in a labeled dropper bottle. Shake to blend.
    If possible leave for four days to synergize. Store in a dark, cool place.

Pre-soak

If there is contagious or infectious illness in the house, pre-soak bed linen, nightwear, and any other appropriate garments in water to which you have added 10 drops of the Laundry Blend and 10 drops of eucalyptus essential oil.

Washing

Add 4–5 drops of Laundry Blend to the final rinse water in the washing machine.
    Add 2 drops of this blend to rinse water if hand washing.

Tumble dryer

Put two to three drops Laundry Blend on a small piece of cloth and throw into the dryer with the damp clothes.

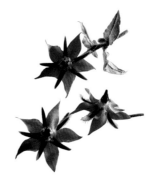

Laundry trouble spots

Floors, cupboards, and sinks	Use All-Purpose Disinfectant Cleaner.
Air spray	Spray the air, the inside of cupboards, and baskets with Anti-Plague Blend, page 352. This ensures a sweet and safe environment.
Ironing	Add 2 drops Laundry Blend to a spray bottle containing 10 fl oz (300 ml) purified water. Shake well before spraying. If in doubt, test in an inconspicuous place. Don't put essential oils directly into the iron.

Furniture polish

This furniture polish gives a lovely gloss to furniture and nourishes the wood as well. Just take very little onto a soft cloth and apply with gusto to the woodwork! Use only about once every two weeks.

LEMON FURNITURE POLISH

$^{1}/_{4}$ cup (60 ml) olive oil

$^{1}/_{4}$ cup (60 ml) lemon juice, strained

1 teaspoon lemon essential oil

To make and use

Mix the ingredients together in a labeled bottle. Shake until the mixture is blended.

Use to polish wooden furniture

Lemon Furniture Polish needs firm application with a soft cloth.

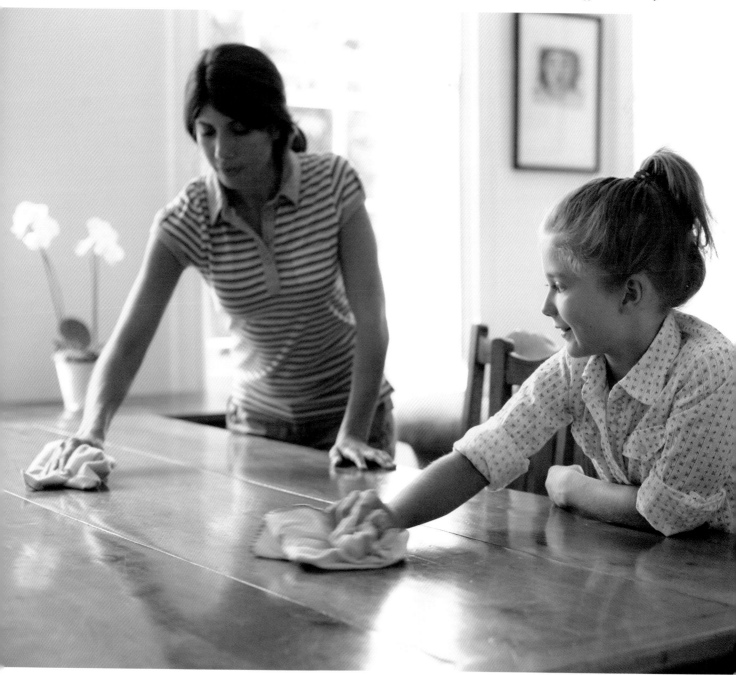

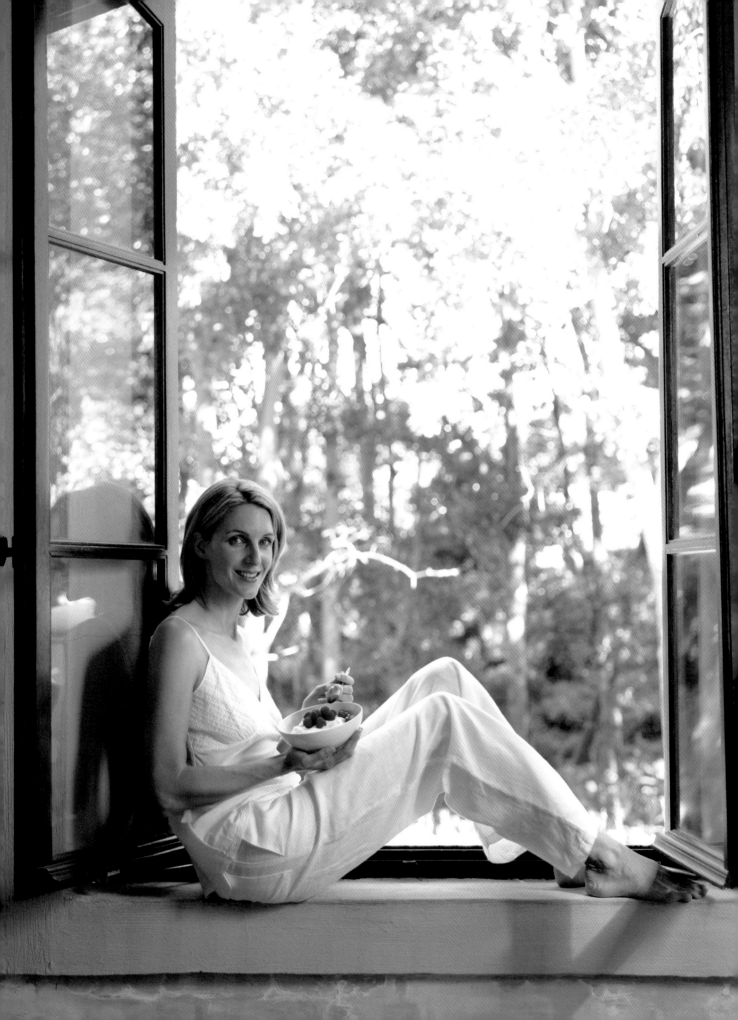

Home remedies

When we were living on our herb farm, we used the plants and their oils in skin- and hair-care products, healing creams, and as remedies for ourselves, our pets, and our gardens. My heart-shaped first-aid box seemed to contain a panacea for one and all—a visitor with a headache, a friend feeling stressed, a child with a cut or bruise. In fact, sometimes the mere sight and smell of the box seemed to bring about an almost magical improvement!

The art of home herbalism is simple and effective, and more and more people are turning to this age-old and well-proven skill to empower themselves and heal their families. I believe that it is empowering and comforting to know that you can deal with simple complaints, common ailments, and first-aid situations promptly at home. I hope you will feel enriched when you, your family, and friends are using the gifts of the earth to improve your health and well-being.

These remedies are not intended to take the place of advice from your health practitioner, and you need to remember that even seemingly simple symptoms can mask serious complaints. If symptoms are severe or of long duration, the condition needs to be assessed professionally. What herbs and essential oils can do is assist the body to heal itself. They can help you:

* Treat everyday ailments.
* Strengthen your immune system, organs, and glands to fight invading bacteria, fungi, and viruses.
* Lower your stress levels.
* Tone, relax, and strengthen your muscles.

Anyone with more serious complaints can also benefit from using herbs and essential oils. Where appropriate you can use them as an adjunct to the treatment you are receiving. Of course it is important to discuss this with your health practitioner.

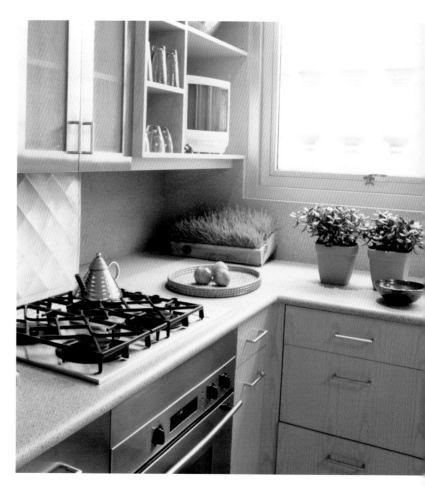

A sunny kitchen window is the perfect place for herbs to thrive. It also keeps them free from bugs.

It is important to take careful note of the cautions for using particular essential oils and the suggestions for quantities to use. The difference in action between one and two drops is very great. Always use the appropriate proportions of the essential oils and the carrier oil. The total amount of essential oils should rarely exceed three to four percent of the total amount, and some oils should be used in far smaller amounts.

Many of my recipes suggest that you leave the blends for four days to synergize or combine well. This isn't absolutely essential, but leaving the blends to synergize in this way increases their potency and enhances their therapeutic action.

When you make and use your own preparations, there are a few cautions to be observed:

* Ensure that the herb you are about to use is the correct one. Check and check again using the botanical name for reference. The common names for herbs have been used in this section. The botanical names may be found in the A-Z chapter.

* If you intend to make a tincture for internal use, be sure to use alcohol that is safe for consumption. Rubbing alcohol is NOT suitable.

* Adhere to dose recommendations and take no medicines for more than six days of the week, the seventh day being a rest day for the system.

* If a problem is severe or of long duration, seek the help of a qualified professional. After he or she establishes the nature of the problem, you can then suggest that you would like to use herbs as part of your healing process.

Many people who are ignorant of the properties of herbs consider them to be harmless. This is a dangerous

It's great to get the whole family involved in the preparation of home remedies. They seem to work better that way.

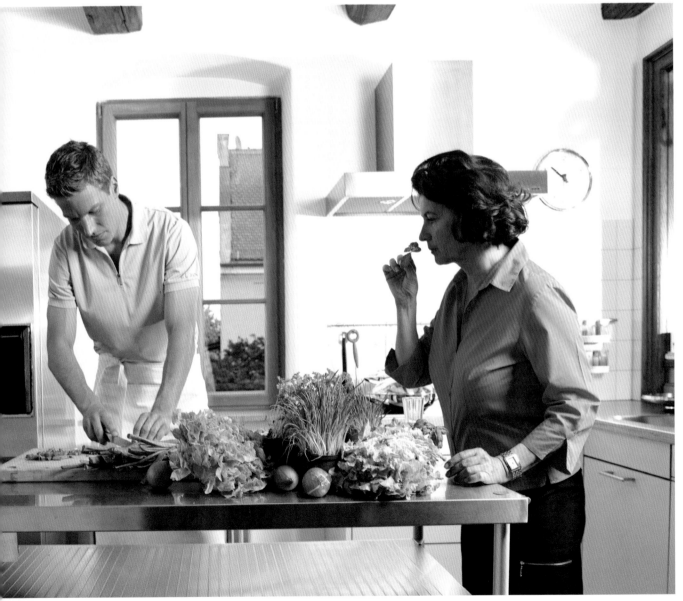

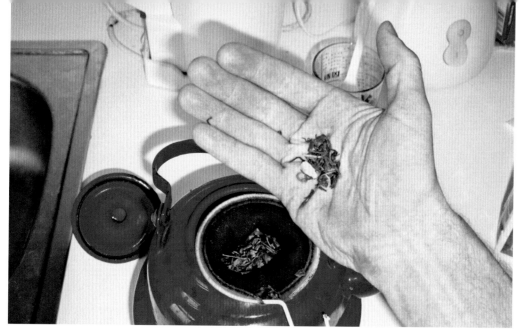

Always use a teapot that has a good infusion insert or use paper coffee filters.

misconception. To be of use, any herb needs pharmacological activity. This is the property which can alter the state of the body and which, if used correctly, can promote healing.

There are several ways to use your chosen herbs. The easiest is called a "simple," meaning that only one herb is used. An example of a simple is a cup of chamomile tea taken at bedtime to help you to achieve a good night's sleep.

The more usual and possibly safer way to use herbs is as a "compound," using several in a mixture. The reasons for the great use of compounds are:

1. **Active botanicals.** Some problems need a variety of actions for relief to be gained, as a disorder in one organ can result in other organs becoming involved and needing treatment. For instance, the symptoms of an overloaded and sluggish liver could be headache, constipation, upset stomach, and bad breath, and would require the use of hepatic and possible digestive, antispasmodic, and aperient herbs. A herb used in such a way to address a problem directly is known as an "active botanical."

2. **Adaptogens.** These gradually produce a beneficial change in bodily functions. They improve detoxification of the body by improving digestion and the function of elimination. Once known as "blood cleansers."

3. **Demulcents**. If there is inflammation or irritation present it is necessary to use demulcent herbs to buffer the action of the other ingredients and to soothe membranes.

4. **Aromatics.** These help to make terrible tasting herbal mixtures more acceptable.

5. **Aperients**. These are laxatives and, unless diarrhea is a problem, are always helpful; having the bowels functioning well helps the system rid itself of toxins.

FORMULA FOR A HERBAL COMPOUND

4 parts active botanical (or as few or many as needed) (see 1)
1 part adaptogen (see 2)
1 part demulcent (see 3)
1 part aromatic (see 4)
1 part aperient unless diarrhea is present (see 5)

This formula can be used to make tinctures, pills, capsules, teas, and decoctions, and any other method where a compound formula is more effective than a single herb.

You may find that one or more of the herbs you have chosen fulfils more than one function and you can adjust the formula accordingly.

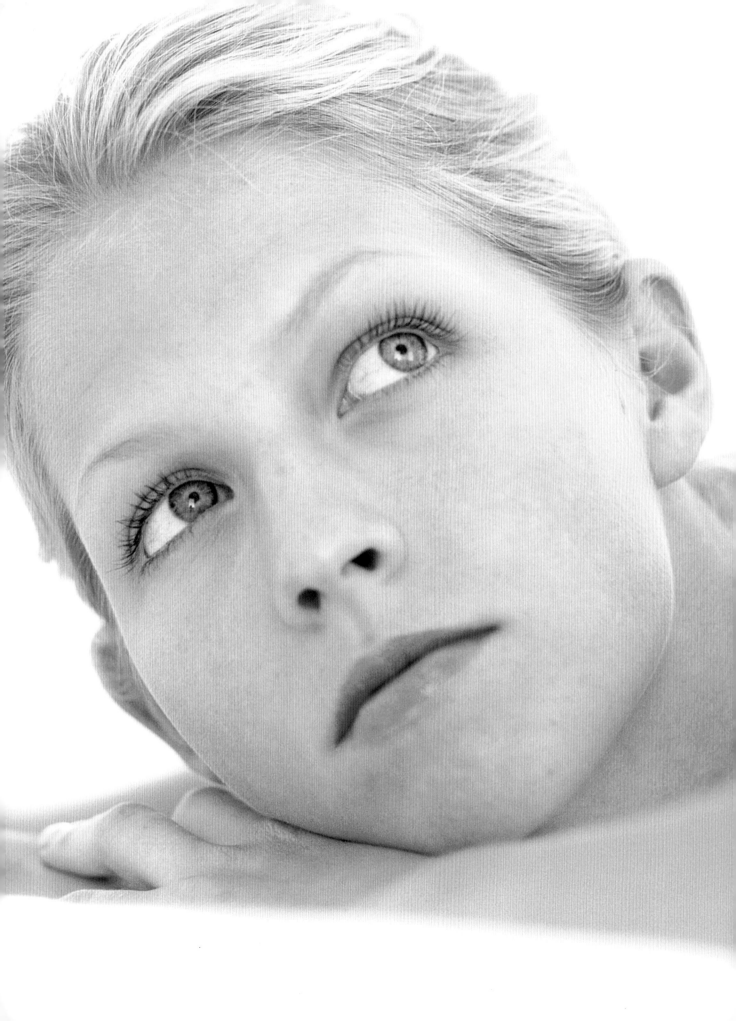

Women's health

The subject of health for the different sexes has become a major feature of healthcare in the twenty-first century and special centers and groups have been set up to deal with the specific problems encountered by the modern woman and man. These centers have enabled women, in particular, to get specialist care for many of their day-to-day health concerns. Although modern medicine is making radical improvements in the treatment of individual complaints, the use of herbal and natural treatments can often alleviate many of the symptoms and enhance the effect of regular medicines.

Always consult a health professional if the symptoms you have are chronic or long term and always inform your health worker of any natural remedies that you are using. It is important that all the information about your condition is available so that your treatment is refined accordingly. The following treatments are designed to assist you through the trials and tribulations of being a woman.

Menstruation

Women begin their 28-day cycle at about twelve years of age and continue (except during pregnancy or some illnesses) until they are around 50. The cycle contains many hormonal changes that culminate in the shedding of the lining of the uterus and the egg; this shedding is referred to as menstruation or "having a period."

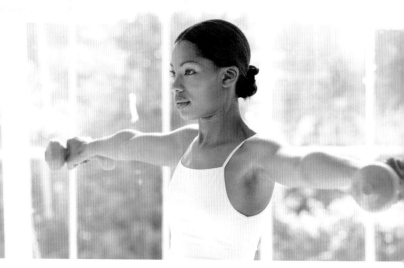

Simple exercise can be done at home without the need to attend a gym.

This cycle affects women very differently. Some scarcely notice any changes, have no pain, and no emotional problems. Many suffer from menstrual problems such as bloating, uterine cramps, pelvic pain, constipation, backache, headaches, fatigue, and other unpleasant and incapacitating symptoms for almost the whole 20 days and refer (understandably) to menstruation as "the curse."

The four complaints I will deal with here are amenorrhea (absence of, or scanty periods), dysmenorrhea (painful periods), menorrhagia (heavy bleeding), and premenstrual syndrome (PMS). Essential oils are a useful part of the total treatment that should consist of herbal and homeopathic remedies, relaxation, and, where necessary, consultation with a health practitioner.

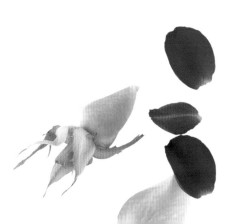

Amenorrhea

Amenorrhea means irregular or absent periods. There are many reasons for scanty periods including pregnancy, menopause, severe weight loss, overexercising, stress, and illness. Before using essential oil remedies (they all encourage menstruation), make sure that you are not pregnant. Consult your doctor if you stop menstruating suddenly. If no serious medical condition exists, the following tincture can be helpful for this problem.

ESSENTIAL OILS

Basil, chamomile, cinnamon, clary sage, jasmine, lavender, marjoram.

AMENORRHEA TINCTURE

2 parts angelica root
2 parts chaste tree (*Vitex agnus-castus*) berries
1 part calendula petals
1 part yarrow leaf

To make and use

Make up a tincture using the above ingredients and take 15 drops in water three times a day.

MASSAGE OIL BLEND FOR MENSTRUATION

3 tablespoons (45 ml) sweet almond oil
15 drops basil essential oil
10 drops marjoram essential oil
10 drops clary sage essential oil

To make and use

Mix all the oils together in a small bottle and shake to blend.

Leave for four days before using so the oils have time to synergize or combine well.

Massage the lower back and abdomen twice a day with the blend, then massage your feet and ankles very firmly.

Add two teaspoons of the blend to a warm bath, massaging floating drops of oil into the abdomen.

Pour a little of the blend into the palm of your hand and massage over your body after showering, while the skin is still damp. Pay particular attention to the lower back and abdomen.

Use the appropriate number of essential oils for a soothing fomentation over the pelvic area.

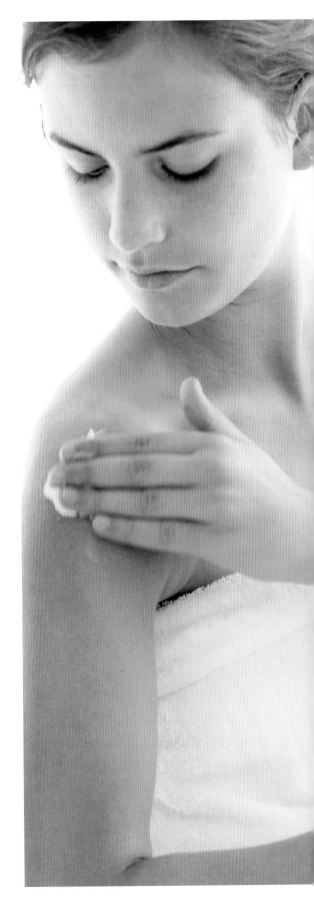

Remember to pamper your whole body even when it feels well.

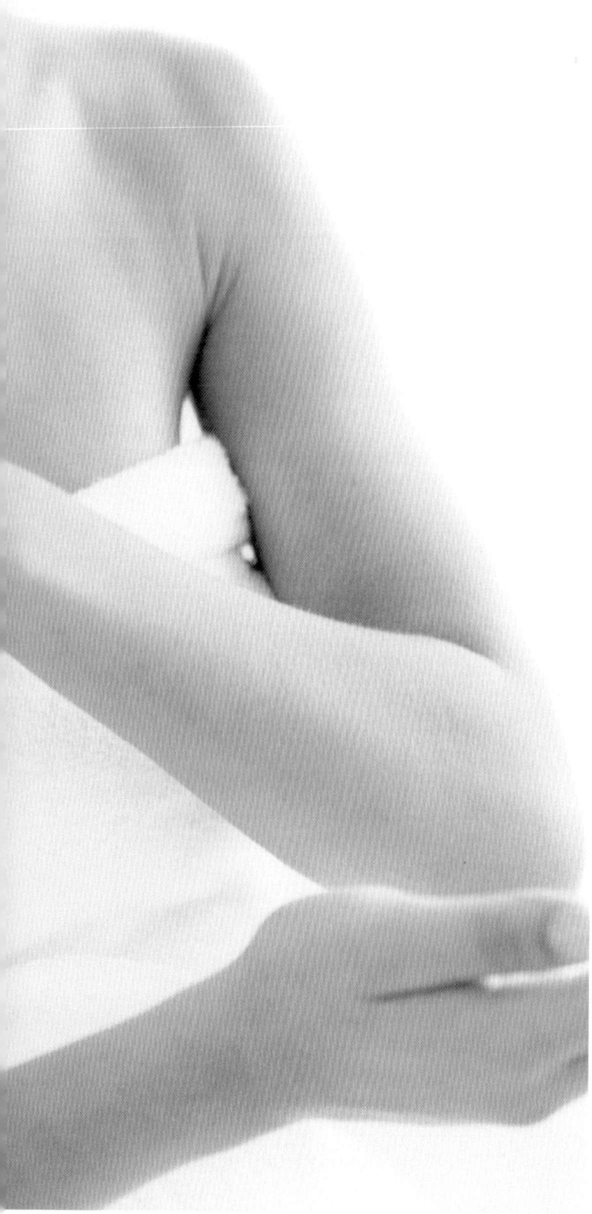

Dysmenorrhea (cramps and pain)

This is another word for painful periods. Taking 2,000–4,000 mg of borage (starflower) oil or evening primrose oil can ease the pain.

The herbs black cohosh, cramp bark, chaste tree, wild yam, and don quai are most helpful, particularly when taken in combination. They may be found singly or as a combination in tablet or extract form at health food stores. Be sure to follow the directions on the bottle.

ESSENTIAL OILS

Lavender, clary sage, cypress, geranium, marjoram.

PAIN-EASE TEA

2 parts willow bark, finely crushed
1 part vervain leaf
2 parts yarrow leaf and flower

To make and use

Mix the herbs together and use one teaspoon of dried or one teaspoon of fresh herbs in one cup of boiling water. Steep, covered, for 15 minutes. Drink one cup of the tea three times daily.

"OUCH DURING THE PERIOD" BLEND FOR CRAMP

3 tablespoons (45 ml) sweet almond oil
15 drops lavender essential oil
10 drops cypress essential oil
5 drops geranium essential oil

To make and use

Mix all the oils together in a small bottle and shake to blend. Leave for four days before using so the oils have time to synergize or combine well.

Massage the lower back and abdomen twice a day with the blend then massage your feet and ankles very firmly.

Add two teaspoons of the blend to a warm bath, massaging floating drops of oil into the abdomen.

Pour a little of the blend into the palm of your hand and massage over your body after showering while the skin is still damp. Pay particular attention to the lower back and abdomen.

Menorrhagia

The term "menorrhagia" covers any abnormally heavy bleeding or clotting, or irregular bleeding (between periods), and merits a trip to your health practitioner, as it can be caused by a pelvic infection, endometrial polyps, endometriosis, uterine fibroids, or thyroid abnormalities. It can also occur for no apparent reason.

Half a teaspoon (2.5 ml) of tincture of shepherd's purse in water, four times daily makes a first-rate remedy for easing internal bleeding. So do three cups of cinnamon tea daily, or chaste tree capsules or extract, as directed. If the problem persists, professional help must be sought, as it could be caused by any of the conditions listed above.

ESSENTIAL OILS

Use only these three essential oils: Cypress, geranium, lemon.

Caution: Avoid antispasmodic essential oils: Basil, aniseed, chamomile, clary sage, dill, fennel, ginger, juniper, lavender, marjoram, melissa, myrrh, orange, oregano, peppermint, rosemary, spearmint.

MASSAGE OIL BLEND FOR HEAVY BLEEDING

3 tablespoons (45 ml) sweet almond oil
15 drops cypress essential oil
10 drops geranium essential oil
8 drops lemon essential oil

To make and use

Mix all the oils together in a small bottle and shake to blend.

Leave for four days before using so the oils have time to synergize or combine well.

Use the massage blend once or twice daily throughout the month to massage the abdomen and lower back.

Mix five drops cypress and five drops lemon essential oils in one teaspoon of sweet almond oil. Add to a warm bath, agitate to disperse, soak for 10 minutes, massaging the floating droplets of oil into your lower abdomen.

Pour a little of the bath blend into the palm of the hand and massage over the lower back and abdomen after showering, while the skin is still damp.

Use clean utensils for harvesting your herbs and keep them aside only for that job.

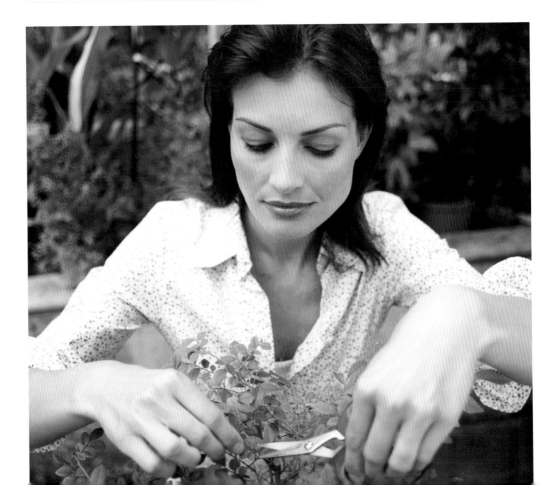

Premenstrual syndrome (PMS)

The following can help in treating premenstrual syndrome.

* Take 2,000–3,000 mg of borage (starflower) oil or evening primrose oil.
* Take two capsules of dong quai three times a day. Discontinue a few days prior to menstruation and recommence when menstruation has finished.
* Take 2,000 mg garlic oil capsules three times daily.
* Drink dandelion leaf tea to help disperse excess fluid.
* Drink chamomile tea in place of regular tea or coffee for its calming effect.
* Take chaste tree tea, tincture or tablets.
* Take 500–1,000 mg of skullcap, passionflower, or valerian at night, or 20 drops of mixed tinctures in water.

ESSENTIAL OILS

Bergamot, chamomile, clary sage, grapefruit, geranium, petitgrain, rosemary.

PRE-PERIOD CRAMPING BLEND

3 tablespoons (45 ml) sweet almond oil
15 drops marjoram essential oil
5 drops clary sage essential oil
10 drops lavender essential oil

To make and use

Mix all the oils together in a small bottle and shake to blend.

Leave for four days before using so the oils have time to synergize or combine well.

Massage the lower back and abdomen twice a day with the blend, then massage your feet and ankles very firmly.

Add two teaspoons of the blend to a warm bath, massaging floating drops of oil into the abdomen.

Pour a little of the blend into the palm of your hand and massage over your body after showering, while the skin is still damp. Pay particular attention to the lower back and abdomen.

Essential oils are only part of a total strategy for this condition, but you may be agreeably surprised by the benefits you will receive from using a combination of these essential oils, along with appropriate herbal remedies and stress management techniques.

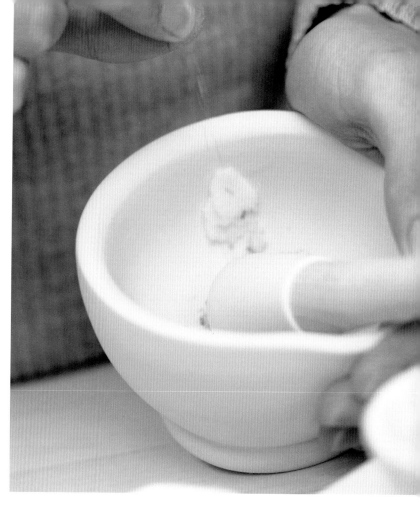

A mortar and pestle are the perfect tools for crushing or blending herbs.

PMS CHASER

2 teaspoons bergamot essential oil
$\frac{1}{2}$ teaspoon chamomile essential oil
$\frac{1}{2}$ teaspoon clary sage essential oil
$1\frac{1}{2}$ teaspoons geranium essential oil
$\frac{1}{2}$ teaspoon grapefruit essential oil

To make and use

Mix all the oils together in a small bottle and shake to blend. Leave for four days before using so the oils have time to synergize to combine well.

Stimulate the lymphatic system with a skin-brush before showering. Begin at the feet and, using a circular motion, work up the legs, body, and arms. Don't wait until you are feeling really bad. Use the essential oils every day.

Include this PMS Chaser blend in baths, after-shower treatments, and massage oils, and in air sprays and oil burners.

Use PMS Chaser as a pulse point oil and toilet water splash, or during meditation.

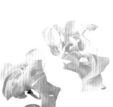

Fluid retention

To reduce fluid retention, drink one cup of dandelion leaf tea three times daily for one week, then drink one cup daily for two weeks. Discontinue for one week. This regimen may be followed as long as needed.

It is also helpful to take a 1,000 mg garlic oil capsule twice daily. Celery seed extract as recommended on the container is also beneficial.

BEAT WATER RETENTION BLEND

3 tablespoons (45 ml) sweet almond oil
15 drops fennel essential oil
10 drops juniper essential oil
8 drops rosemary essential oil

To make and use

Mix all the oils together in a small bottle and shake to blend.

Leave for four days before using so the oils have time to synergize to combine well.

Begin to use the blend on day 21 of your cycle, counting from the first day of the last period. This blend will help to rid the body of excess fluid and ease the "bloated" feeling. Use one teaspoon in a warm bath. Massage floating droplets of oil into the skin.

Pour a little into the palm of your hand and massage into the body after showering.

Use $\frac{1}{4}$ teaspoon of the blend for a foot massage every evening. Try to use the oil at least twice a day.

DEPRESSION AND IRRITABILITY BLEND

2 tablespoons grape seed oil
15 drops chamomile essential oil
10 drops bergamot essential oil
10 drops petitgrain essential oil

To make and use

Mix all the oils together in a small bottle and shake to blend.

Leave for four days before using so the oils have time to synergize or combine well.

Begin to use the blend on day 21 of your cycle, counting from the first day of the last period. This blend will help to rid the body of excess fluid and ease the "bloated" feeling. Use one teaspoon in a warm bath. Massage floating droplets of oil into the skin.

Pour a little into the palm of your hand and massage into the body after showering.

Use $\frac{1}{4}$ teaspoon of the blend for a foot massage every evening. Try to use the oil at least twice a day.

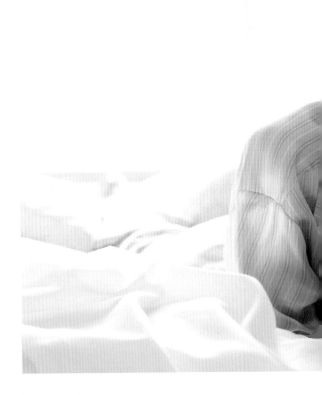

Endometriosis

Endometriosis is an acutely painful condition including heavy and painful periods, internal bleeding, painful sexual intercourse, painful bowel movement, constipation and diarrhea, infertility, and more. It affects about 10 percent of all women.

Aromatherapy treatments often ease the pain and discomfort being experienced, but lifestyle changes—diet, more exercise, and vitamin and mineral supplements are advised.

ESSENTIAL OILS

Geranium, chamomile, clary sage, cypress, lavender.

SITZ BATH

A daily sitz bath (sitting alternately in hot and cold baths) will stimulate the pelvic region. You need enough hot water to cover the lower abdomen. Run hot water into your bath and have a baby bath or similar filled with cold water on the floor alongside.

Make a blend of two drops of each of the recommended essential oils in one teaspoon vegetable oil and add to the hot bath, stirring well to distribute evenly. Sit for 10 minutes in the hot bath, massaging the oil droplets into the abdomen and pelvic area.

Now sit for five minutes in the cold bath (no essential oils added). Repeat.

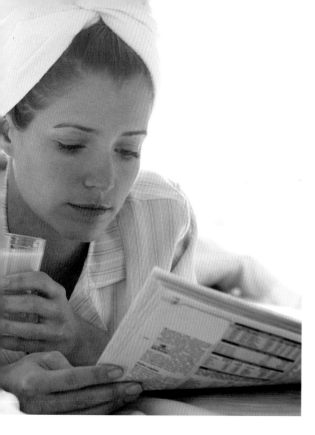

MASSAGE BLEND FOR ENDOMETRIOSIS

3 tablespoons (45 ml) sweet almond oil
20 drops cypress essential oil
5 drops clary sage essential oil
5 drops nutmeg essential oil

To make and use

Mix all the oils together in a small bottle and shake to blend.

Leave for four days before using so the oils have time to synergize or combine well.

Massage the abdomen and lower back once or twice a day.

Fibrocystic breast disease (lumpy breasts)

The symptoms of fibrocystic disease are nodules or lumps in the breasts that can change in size and location. Sometimes there is soreness, swelling, pain, and tenderness. Lumpy breasts are often a part of the symptoms of PMS as they appear to be caused by hormonal changes in the body. The lumps usually disappear at menopause unless you are on a hormone replacement program. See your doctor for a breast examination.

Check with a health professional before using home treatments.

* Take a 1,000 mg garlic oil capsule three times daily.

* Take 3,000 mg borage (starflower) oil or evening primrose oil once daily.
* Sore or swollen breasts may be eased by the application of the cabbage leaves that have been ironed or steamed to soften, then chilled in the refrigerator. Place over breasts, cover with a piece of plastic wrap, and hold in place with a bra.
* Apply warm fomentations using a triple-strength chamomile and lavender tea three times daily.

ESSENTIAL OILS

Chamomile, cypress, geranium, lavender.

BREAST MASSAGE CREAM

4 tablespoons (60 ml) coconut oil
2 teaspoons grape seed oil
30 drops chamomile essential oil
10 drops lavender essential oil
10 drops geranium essential oil

To make and use

Melt the coconut oil together with the grape seed oil.

When cool but still liquid, mix together with the essential oils.

Pot in a small labeled jar. Shake occasionally until set.

Store in the refrigerator in warm weather.

Massage both breasts twice daily using the above blend. Apply warm fomentations using six to eight drops of mixed chamomile and lavender essential oils.

Leucorrhea

This is a thick white or colorless, non-infectious vaginal discharge.

ESSENTIAL OILS

Lavender, myrrh.

DOUCHE BLEND

1 teaspoon cider vinegar
1 drop lavender essential oil
1 drop myrrh essential oil
2 cups warm water

To make and use

Mix the oils with the vinegar and leave for a few minutes to dissolve a little.

Add the mixture to the warm water just prior to pouring into a douche bag (available from pharmacies). Shake well just prior to using.

Take "Me Time" when you are feeling low. An hour alone can do wonders.

TIP THE BAG CONTAINING THE DOUCHE MIX SHOULD BE AGITATED IMMEDIATELY BEFORE USING TO PREVENT HOT SPOTS OF OILS.

Menopause

Menopause is the time when periods and ovulation cease, but the symptoms may begin one, two, or three years before this happens. Many authorities assure us that there is no reason why women should suffer from unpleasant menopausal symptoms, but the depressing fact is that many, many women have an unhappy and uncomfortable time.

If your life is being ruined or dominated by mood swings, depression, hot flashes, sweating, anxiety, insomnia, loss of libido, and dryness of the skin, mucous, and vagina, some or all the following suggestions may bring relief.

Careful use of essential oils in your daily life can alleviate many of the symptoms of menopause.

* Walk daily alone or with your partner or walking buddy. It will not only help to increase bone density and prevent osteoporosis, but being active every day is good for your long-term health and well-being and being outdoors can often bring a new perspective to life.
* Eat foods containing the anti-ageing essential fatty acids to promote hormonal balance. These are found in olive oil, light olive oil, avocados, sunflower and sesame seeds, wheat germ (must be fresh and stored in the freezer), mackerel, herrings, sardines, salmon, and tuna.
* Taking borage (starflower) oil or evening primrose oil capsules can also be of benefit.

* Drink a cup of sage tea twice daily to help in the reduction of hot flashes. Two capsules of passionflower (or 1 dropperful of tincture) up to four times a day can help calm the nerves.

MENOPAUSE TEA OR TINCTURE

Licorice root
Alfalfa herb
Red clover herb
Burdock root
Motherwort
Fennel
Vervain

To make and use

Combine as many as possible of these dried herbs in equal parts and make into a tincture of your choice (see Practicalities).

Take 40 drops in water three times daily.

HORMONAL BALANCE MASSAGE AND BATH OIL

$^{1}/_{3}$ cup (80 ml) sweet almond oil
20 drops borage seed oil
20 drops clary sage essential oil
20 drops geranium essential oil
15 drops bergamot essential oil

To make and use

Mix all the oils together in a small bottle and shake to blend.

Leave for four days before using so the oils have time to synergize or combine well.

Float one teaspoon of the blend on warm water in a small bowl and use for a massage of the abdomen and lower back.

Pour two teaspoons of the blend into a bath or footbath, agitate to disperse and soak in the bath for 30 minutes, massaging any floating oil droplets into the skin.

Pour a little into the palm of your hand and massage over your body after showering while your skin is still damp.

Use the essential oils (without the sweet almond oil) in an air spray or oil burner.

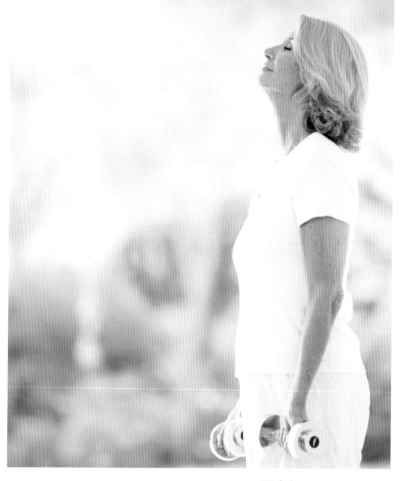

Weight-bearing exercise is important for strong bones and a healthy heart.

Hot flashes

ESSENTIAL OILS

Clary sage, cypress, geranium, lime.

BATH AND MASSAGE BLEND TO BEAT HOT FLASHES

$^{1}/_{3}$ cup (80 ml) sweet almond oil
20 drops borage seed oil
20 drops clary sage essential oil
20 drops geranium essential oil
15 drops cypress essential oil

To make and use

Mix all the oils together in a small bottle and shake to blend.

Leave for four days before using so the oils have time to synergize or combine well.

Float one teaspoon of the blend on warm water in a small bowl and use for a massage of the abdomen and lower back.

Pour two teaspoons of the blend into a bath or footbath, agitate to disperse and soak in the bath for 30 minutes, massaging any floating oil droplets into the skin.

Pour a little into the palm of your hand and massage over your body after showering while your skin is still damp.

Use the essential oils (without the sweet almond oil) in an air spray or oil burner.

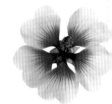

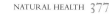

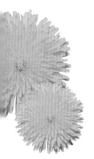

Depression

ESSENTIAL OILS
Ylang-ylang, clary sage, bergamot.

"BEAT THE BLUES" MASSAGE BLEND
$1/_3$ cup (80 ml) sweet almond oil
20 drops borage seed oil
20 drops clary sage essential oil
20 drops ylang-ylang essential oil
15 drops bergamot essential oil

To make and use
Mix all the oils together in a small bottle and shake to blend.

Leave for four days before using so the oils have time to synergize or combine well.

Float one teaspoon of the blend on warm water in a small bowl and use for a massage of the abdomen and lower back.

Pour two teaspoons of the blend into a bath or footbath, agitate to disperse, and soak in the bath for 30 minutes, massaging any floating oil droplets into the skin.

Pour a little into the palm of your hand and massage over your body after showering while your skin is still damp.

Use the essential oils (without the sweet almond oil) in an air spray or oil burner.

Nerves and mood swings

ESSENTIAL OILS
Chamomile, geranium, marjoram.

CALMING BLEND FOR NERVES
$1/_3$ cup (80 ml) sweet almond oil
20 drops borage seed oil
20 drops chamomile essential oil
20 drops geranium essential oil
15 drops marjoram essential oil

To make and use
Mix all the oils together in a small bottle and shake to blend.

Leave for four days before using so the oils have time to synergize or combine well.

Float one teaspoon of the blend on warm water in a small bowl and use for a massage of the abdomen and lower back.

Pour two teaspoons of the blend into a bath or footbath, agitate to disperse and soak in the bath for 30 minutes, massaging any floating oil droplets into the skin.

Pour a little into the palm of your hand and massage over your body after showering while your skin is still damp.

Use the essential oils (without the sweet almond oil) in an air spray or oil burner.

Cystitis

Cystitis is an inflammation of the bladder caused by bacterial infection of the urinary tract. The symptoms are burning and scalding when passing urine, wanting to pass urine frequently, a persistent dull ache above the pubic bone, urine which smells or contains blood or pus. If the attack is accompanied by fever and low back pain, the infection may be in the kidneys as well as the bladder and urethra, so professional help is needed.

Make a special time each month to blend your own massage oil.

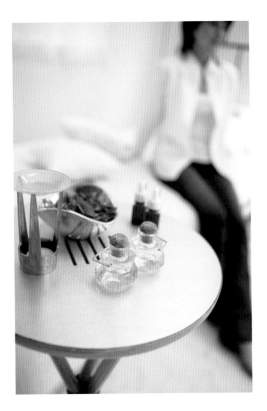

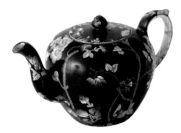

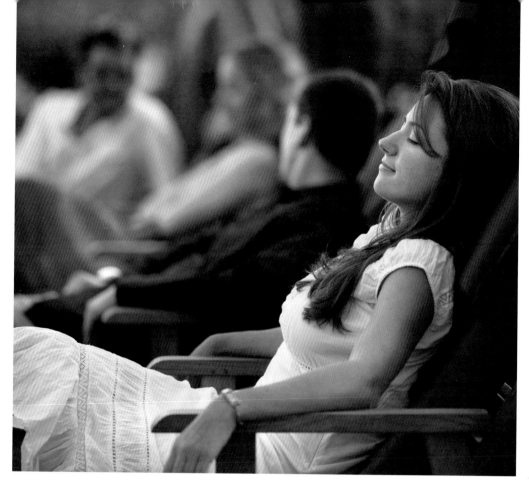

Sometimes it's necessary to take time alone even in the midst of a crowd. Keep a tissue infused with your favorite oil in your purse for just such occasions.

ESSENTIAL OILS

Bergamot, chamomile, eucalyptus, sandalwood.

CYSTITIS MASSAGE AND FOMENTATION BLEND

4 teaspoons grape seed oil
6 drops bergamot essential oil
3 drops chamomile essential oil
3 drops eucalyptus essential oil
4 drops sandalwood or parsley essential oil

To make and use

Mix all the oils together in a small bottle.

Shake to blend thoroughly.

Warm $^1/_2$ teaspoon of the blend in a hot spoon and use to massage over the bladder area.

Use 10 drops of mixed essential oils in a fomentation over the bladder area

Add two teaspoons of the blend to a hot bath. Soak for 10 minutes.

During an attack, drink at least eight glasses of fluid a day, and take 20,000 mg cranberry capsules, or unsweetened cranberry juice may be drunk instead.

Other treatments are:

- Take 1,000 mg garlic oil capsule three items daily.
- Take goldenseal capsules or tincture dosage as prescribed on the package.
- Take $^1/_2$ teaspoon (2.5 ml) of fluid extract of echinacea in 2 tablespoons (40 ml) of water every two hours during an attack and twice daily for two months after an attack to help prevent a recurrence.

CYSTITIS TEA

2 parts yarrow
1 part dandelion leaf
1 part chamomile flowers

To make and use

Combine the ingredients and drink $^1/_2$ cup (125 ml) of hot tea every hour until relief is obtained.

CYSTITIS FOMENTATION

Make a hot fomentation using as many of the following herbs as possible: Cayenne (use one part cayenne to eight parts other herbs), chamomile, plantain, wormwood, yellow dock. Place over the bladder and repeat every two hours until relief is obtained.

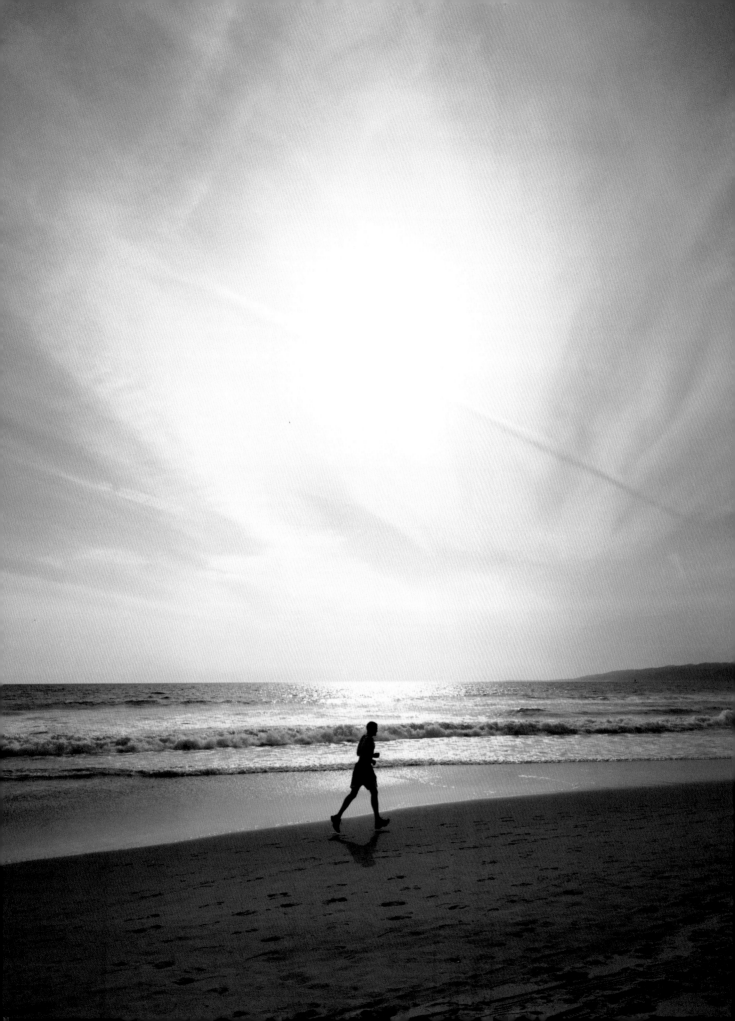

Men's health

Men aren't usually as in tune with their bodies as are women. In the past it was considered "not manly" to worry about physical problems—men were supposed to tough it out and not complain. However, attention to the particular problems that men encounter has become accepted and important, and there are many clinics specifically set up to help with men's problems.

The following treatments should be used as a starter, and your health professional should be informed of any natural or alternative treatment that you are using. Always consult a professional if symptoms persist or become aggravated.

ASK YOURSELF

Did anyone in my family die of a heart attack?

Is my blood pressure high?

Can I reduce the stress at work or home?

Am I smoking or drinking too much?

Am I physically fit?

Do I need to exercise more?

Am I overweight?

Do I eat too much junk and not enough fish, grain, fruit, and vegetables?

If the answer is "Yes" to any or many of the above questions, you need to make a change.

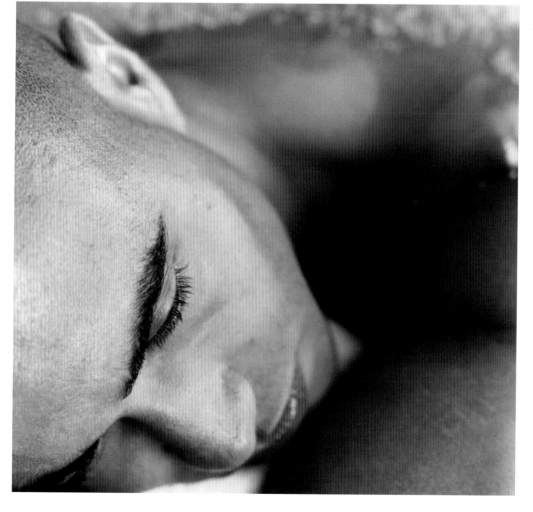

For good health adequate rest is just as important as exercise.

Heart health

The biggest problems that men have to address are diet and stress, and their dire consequences. Heart attacks strike men during their middle years, and many could have been avoided if the warning signs had been heeded. There is so much help out there these days—the Heart Association (Heart Foundation) is only a phone call away. The following recipes will improve the circulation, reduce stress, and aid in lowering blood pressure.

ESSENTIAL OILS TO STIMULATE CIRCULATION

Black pepper, clary sage, eucalyptus, geranium, ginger, hyssop, marjoram, rose, rosemary.

ESSENTIAL OILS TO REDUCE STRESS

Basil, bergamot, chamomile, clary sage, cypress, frankincense, marjoram, sandalwood

HEART'S EASE BLEND

$^1/_3$ cup (80 ml) grape seed oil
20 drops geranium essential oil
20 drops clary sage essential oil
10 drops bergamot essential oil
10 drops rosemary oil
5 drops marjoram oil

To make and use

Mix all the oils together in a small bottle and shake to blend.

If there's time, leave for four days before using so the oils have time to synergize or combine well.

Float one teaspoon of the blend onto warm water in a small bowl, and use for massage. Pour two teaspoons of the blend into a bath or footbath, agitate to disperse, and soak in the bath for 20–30 minutes, massaging any floating oil droplets into the skin.

Pour a little of the blend into the palm of the hand, and massage over the body after showering, while the skin is still damp.

Alternatively, just blend the essential oils together to use as an air spray or in an oil burner.

Group exercise is often a popular choice for men.

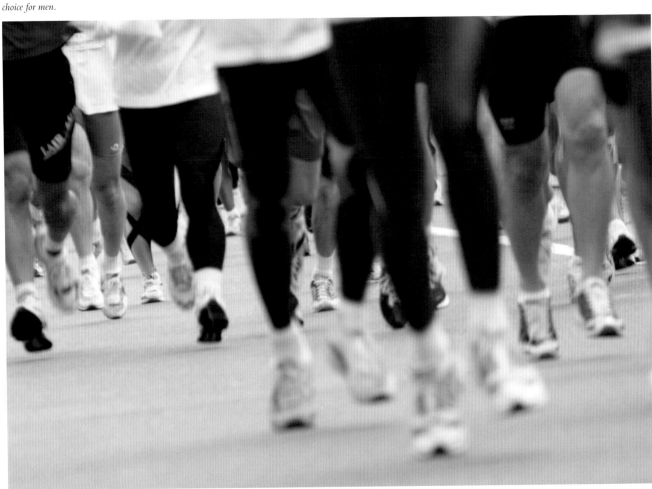

Prostate gland, enlarged

If the prostate becomes enlarges, urination is difficult or impossible, and there is a risk of urinary and kidney damage. All the following treatments can help.

* Take 4 teaspoons (20 ml) of flaxseed oil a day (must be fresh and stored in the refrigerator).
* Take 160 mg saw palmetto extract capsule twice daily, to reduce night time urination, and improve urinary flow rate.
* Take $\frac{1}{2}$-$\frac{3}{4}$ teaspoon tincture of nettle root in 3 tablespoons (45 ml) water, three times a day. This may increase urinary volume and the maximum flow rate of urine.
* Take 160 mg pumpkin seed oil capsule three times a day, with meals. When taken with the saw palmetto and nettle remedies above, this seems to effectively reduce symptoms.
* Take panax ginseng as recommended on the container.
* Take two 10,000 mg cranberry capsules, or drink lots of unsweetened cranberry juice.

There are formulae available in health food stores and through naturopaths that contain all the most important supplements needed to treat problems of the prostate gland. The formula you choose should ideally contain zinc (picolinate) and essential fatty acids among the other ingredients.

You and your partner can make a pact that for as long as it takes—maybe weeks, maybe months—you will give each other lots of TLC and this includes body massages without any expectation of intercourse—take time to enjoy shared and sensual experience without the stress of "performing."

Try to keep your coffee levels low, even when busy. Stick to herbal tea.

Impotence

Women these days have such high expectations of sex that men are often completely intimidated, and can become impotent due to "performance anxiety." There is demand for long exciting foreplay, "multiple" orgasms and the discovery of new and thrilling erogenous zones. Work stresses and money worries add to the load, until the whole thing becomes too much of a problem, and the poor penis remains sullen and unresponsive. Let's see what a little tenderness and sharing can achieve.

Some problems require understanding and support. An essential oil massage can be shared.

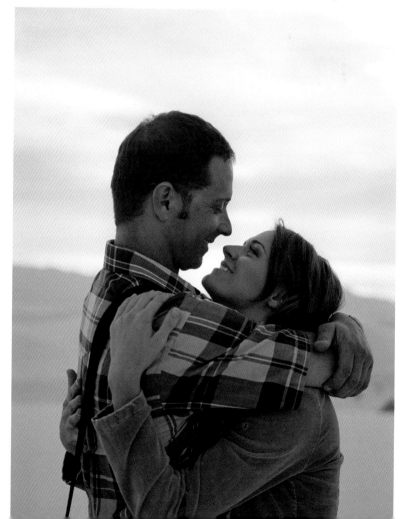

ESSENTIAL OILS

Cedarwood, clary sage, black pepper, jasmine, neroli, rose, sandalwood, vetiver, ylang-ylang.

LOVING TOUCH BLEND

$^{1}/_{3}$ cup (80 ml) grape seed oil
20 drops sandalwood essential oil
20 drops cedarwood essential oil
15 drops clary sage essential oil (not if you have
   been drinking alcohol)
10 drops rosewood essential oil

To make and use

Mix all the oils together in a small bottle and shake to blend. If there's time, leave for four days before using the blend, so the oils have time to synergize or combine well.

Float one teaspoon of the blend onto warm water in a small bowl and use for the massage.

Pour two teaspoons of the blend into a bath (a shared bath maybe) agitate and disperse, and soak in the bath for 30 minutes, massaging any floating oil droplets into the skin. If you prefer to shower (shared showers are fun as well and help the ecology by saving water!), pour a little of the blend onto the palm of the hand and massage each other over the whole body after showering, while the skin is still damp.

Alternatively, just blend the essential oils together to use as an air spray or in an oil burner.

Prostatis

Prostatis is an infection that causes a burning sensation when passing urine, pain and tenderness in the area of the prostate, pelvic area and lower back, fever, and exhaustion. The suggestions in this section must only be followed after an examination by a doctor has ruled out anything more serious.

ESSENTIAL OILS

Chamomile, cypress, eucalyptus, lavender, myrrh.

PROSTATIS BATH AND MASSAGE BLEND

3 tablespoons grape seed oil
15 drops cypress essential oil
15 drops eucalyptus essential oil
10 drops lavender essential oil
10 drops myrrh essential oil

To make and use

Mix all the oils together in a small bottle and shake to blend.

If there's time, leave for four days before using, so the oils have time to synergize or combine well.

Float one teaspoon of the blend onto warm water in a small bowl, and use for a massage of the abdomen and lower back.

Pour two teaspoons of the blend onto a bath or foot bath, agitate to disperse, and soak in the bath for 30 minutes, massaging any floating oil droplets into the skin.

Pour a little of the blend into the palm of the hand and massage over the body after showering, paying special attention to the lower back, and sacrum area.

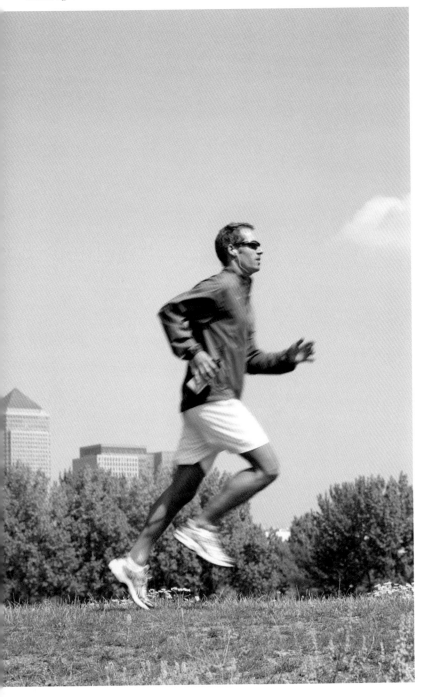

Ensure you do not neglect your exercise regime.

"Jock itch"

This is a fungal infection of the groin area often caused by wearing underwear and/or pants that are too tight, and which are made of synthetic material. The perspiration can't evaporate, and the area becomes a perfect breeding ground for the fungus. The condition is typified by small red itchy spots that can become very sore.

ESSENTIAL OILS
Tea tree, lavender.

Treatment
Wash the area carefully twice a day with two drops of lavender oil in a small bowl of water. Dry gently but thoroughly.

Add five drops of each essential oil to four teaspoons (20 ml) of olive oil. Massage into itchy area two or three times a day.

Gout

Gout is caused by an excessive build-up of uric acid in the body that turns into crystals around joints, most commonly the base of the big toe. Attacks are accompanied by extremely painful swelling, and inflammation.

Internal remedies are of paramount importance in the treatment of gout. The absolute number one remedy for gout is to eat cherries – canned, frozen, or fresh. If you keep including them in your diet the gout won't occur. Another remedy is the following tea. It's easiest to make a few days supply at one time, (12 cups/3 liters would be a four-day supply).

Use one teaspoon of the dried (two teaspoons fresh) herb to 1 cup (250 ml) of water, or 12 teaspoons of dried (24 teaspoons fresh) herb to 12 cups (3 liters) of water.

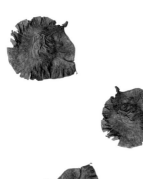

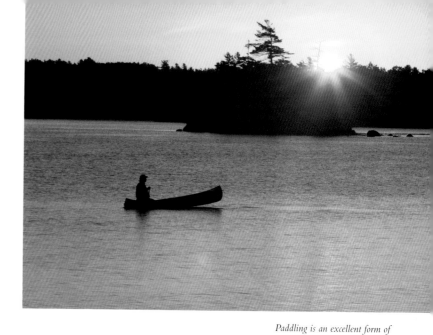

Paddling is an excellent form of sustained exercise and it has the benefit of relieving stress as well.

GOUT DECOCTION OR TINCTURE
1 part meadowsweet
1 part burdock root
1 part yellow dock toot
1 part celery seed
1 part nettle

To make and use
Take one cup three times daily, or 20 drops of tincture in water three times daily.

For external treatment, apply poultices of meadowsweet to the inflamed area.

Cool footbaths, containing triple strength teas of fennel and juniper, are also helpful.

ESSENTIAL OILS
Chamomile, rosewood, peppermint, fennel, juniper, cypress.

GOUT MASSAGE OIL
3 tablespoons (45 ml) grape seed oil
15 drops chamomile essential oil
15 drops rosewood essential oil
5 drops peppermint essential oil

To make and use
Mix all the oils together in a small bottle and shake to blend.

If there's time, leave for four days before using, so the oils have time to synergize or combine well.

Float one teaspoon of the blend in a small bowl of warm water.

Massage the affected parts very gently three times a day.

If massage is too painful at first, soak the feet in warm water, and then in a cool footbath, containing two drops each fennel, juniper, and cypress essential oils.

TIP WEAR COTTON BOXER SHORTS AND IF POSSIBLE, LOOSE FITTING COTTON TROUSERS.

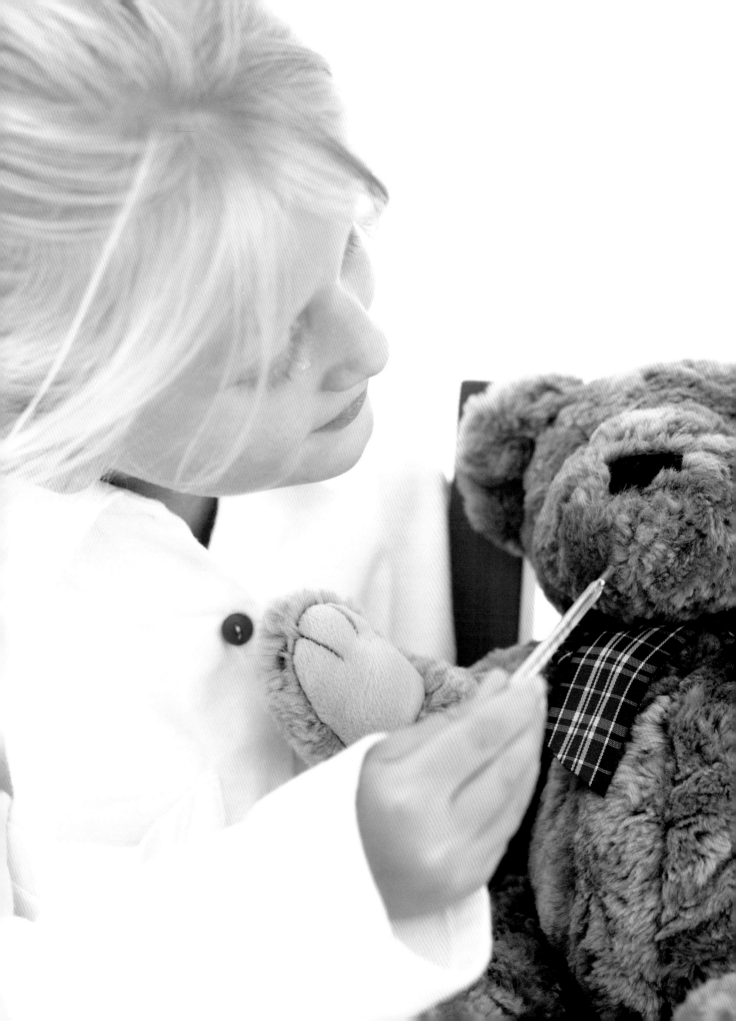

Children and babies

When treating children we need to be very careful. The herbs suggested here have all been shown over centuries to be suitable for children but, even so, we must never forget that everything on this planet will be an allergen to someone. If your child suffers from allergies, a "patch" test can be helpful.

To do this, make a very strong tea of the suspected herb, dab it thoroughly on the inside skin of the elbow, cover, and leave for 24 hours. If there is any redness or soreness at the end of this time the herb should be avoided.

Babies need special treatments—their tender and sensitive little bodies can't tolerate any but the most gentle of remedies. They can become very ill very quickly, but can also recover just as dramatically. Never take chances with your baby. If in doubt, get professional help.

In this section we cover some of the more common complaints that can afflict babies and children, with recommendations for herbal treatments and essential oils.

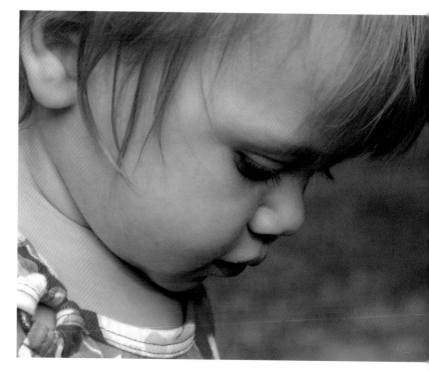

Extreme care must be taken before administering herbs or essential oils to babies and young children.

Herb teas for children

It's good to encourage children to drink mild herbal teas mixed with fresh fruit juices from an early age. If they develop a taste for these drinks it will have a twofold benefit; drinking the teas is a preventative act, and the children won't be resistant to the teas if they become sick and need them.

Herbs which are good to use for these drinks are lemon grass, spearmint, and red raspberry leaf or fruit, mixed with apple, orange or lemon juice, water and honey. Fruit juices should always be diluted with water or herb tea before being given to children; the undiluted juice is too strong for immature digestive systems to cope with. Avoid giving the same herb over long periods. Vary them from day to day.

Discontinue treatment with the chosen herb after three weeks.

Resume after a further week if the treatment is working, or change to another herb if no improvement is seen.

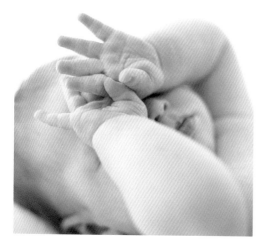

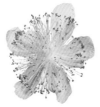

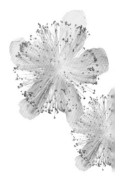

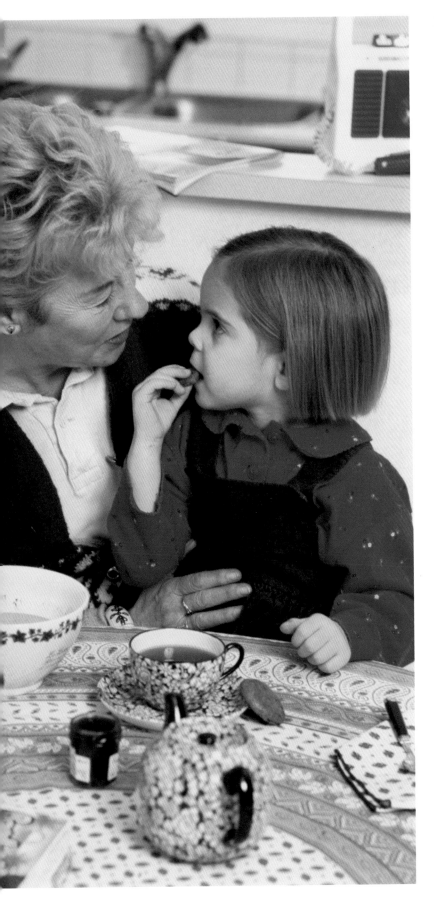

DOSAGE

Over 65 lb (30 kg): $^{1}/_{2}$ cup (125 ml)—three times daily, half an hour before food.

33-63 lb (15–29 kg): 2 tablespoons (30 ml)—three times daily, half an hour before food.

15-30 lb (7–14 kg): 4 teaspoons (20 ml)—three times daily, half an hour before food.

Children and essential oils

Most of the recipes in this book are calculated in adult doses. All will need to be adapted before using on babies, toddlers and children.

Most essential oils are too powerful to use on the skin of newborn babies and there are few that are safe to use until the baby is two to three months old.

Caution: Essential oils must never be used internally and must always be correctly diluted before use. This is particularly important for babies and children as undiluted essential oils rubbed from the hands into the eyes could cause permanent damage.

The following chart gives the amounts of oils to use in preparations for babies and children.

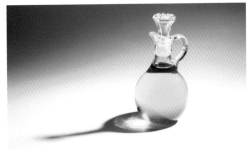

Above: *Olive oil should be added to essential oils in all children's baths.*
Left: *Introduce children to herbal teas at a very young age. Add them to fruit juice to enhance the taste.*

Which essential oils to use when

Age	Essential Oils
2–3 months	Chamomile and lavender (after the first 48 hours)
3–2 months	Add calendula, grapefruit, tea tree
1–5 years	Add geranium, lemon palmarosa, spearmint, rose
5 years–puberty	All the oils considered safe for adults may be used but in smaller amounts

Bath time

Use age	Appropriate oils
2–3 months	1 drop of either chamomile or lavender essential oil mixed thoroughly with 4 teaspoons (20 ml) olive oil and dispersed thoroughly into the bath water
3–12 months	2 drops of appropriate essential oil with 4 teaspoons (20 ml) olive oil and dispersed thoroughly into the bath water
1–5 years	3–5 drops of appropriate essential oils with 4 teaspoons (20 ml) olive oil and dispersed thoroughly into the bath water
5 years–puberty	5–8 drops of appropriate essential oil with 4 teaspoons (20 ml) olive oil and dispersed thoroughly into the bath water

Massage

Use age	Appropriate oils
2–3 months	10 drops (total) mixed or single essential oils in $\frac{1}{2}$ cup (125 ml) mixed olive oil and almond oils. Shake well before use
3–12 months	10–16 drops (total) mixed or single essential oils in $\frac{1}{2}$ cup (125 ml) mixed olive and almond oils. Shake well before use
1–5 years	10–16 drops (total) mixed or single essential oils in $\frac{1}{2}$ cup (125 ml) mixed olive and almond oils. Shake well before use
5 years–puberty	16–20 drops (total) mixed or single essential oils in $\frac{1}{2}$ cup (125 ml) mixed olive and almond oils. Shake well before use

Air Sprays

Use age	Appropriate oils
2–3 months	Not recommended
3–12 months	Not recommended
1–5 years	Use one-quarter the adult amount
5 years–puberty	As 1–5 years gradually increasing (drop by drop) with child's age

Babies

Babies deserve the best. By using pure, natural oils on their bodies we are giving them just that. Massage your baby every day—you will both love it and to will help to strengthen that special bond. It also helps to ease the pain of colic.

The first 48 hours

The best oils for newborn babies are extra virgin olive oil and sweet almond oil; these can be combined or used alone for the first two days.

Newborn babies can be massaged with sweet almond oil or virgin olive oil.

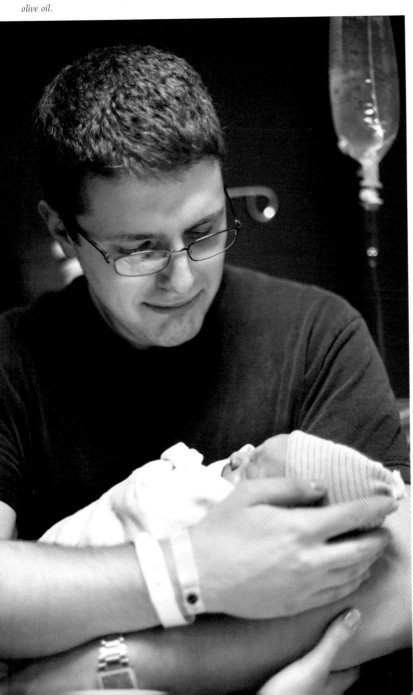

Three days to two months

Chamomile and lavender oils may be introduced and used for babies after the first 48 hours. These oils both calm the nervous system, boost the immune system and are antibacterial and mildly antiviral.

You can use these oils in the bedroom to soothe babies who are restless, "scratchy," or suffering from colds.

A drop of either of these oils in a diffuser, or floating in a bowl of warm water near the cot, should help to ensure restful sleep.

Two months to twelve months

This is a time when you can extend the range of essential oils you use for baby and carefully increase the amount. However, do not exceed the quantity of essential oils given in the ingredients list of recipes.

GENTLE BABY OIL

All babies love to be massaged. It's good for bonding and has a calming effect on a baby who is suffering from colic, restlessness, or just "the miseries." Gentle Baby Oil can be used for any of these problems and for general skin care, to loosen cradle cap, or as an after-bath oil.

1/3 cup (80 ml) sweet almond oil
4 teaspoons (20 ml) olive oil
5 drops chamomile essential oil
8 drops lavender essential oil

To make and use

Mix all the oils together in a small, labeled bottle and shake to blend.

Leave for four days before using so that the oils have time to synergize or combine well.

Sprinkle Gentle Baby Oil on absorbent cotton (cottonwool) and use to clean baby during a diaper change.

Massage baby after bathing with Gentle Baby Oil or if baby is restless and "scratchy." Avoid the genitals and eyes when massaging and pay particular attention to the feet.

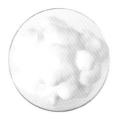

Cradle cap

Use Gentle Baby Oil to lift cradle cap.

The oil may be massaged gently on the scalp, left on overnight, and washed off in the morning.

Repeat for as long as necessary.

CRADLE CAP INFUSED OIL

Chamomile flowers, dried elder flowers, dried calendula petals, dried nettle.

To make and use

Make an infused oil using sweet almond oil as the base oil and as many of the herbs as possible.

Massage gently into the scalp. This is also a lovely massage oil to use all over your baby's body.

Diaper rash

Babies should be allowed to crawl around with their bare bottoms exposed to the fresh air for some part of every day as a good preventive measure against diaper rash. Be sure to keep them out of the sun at the hottest part of a summer's day, though, to protect their skin. Small babies love being in a pram under a tree—no diaper, legs waving in the air, watching the leaves and the clouds moving. It keeps them, and you, happy for hours. A strong net (cat- and insect-proof) fastened firmly over the pram is a safety precaution.

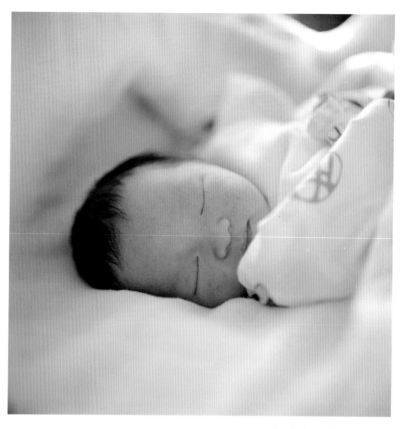

INFUSED OIL

Make an infused oil using chamomile, elderflower and mallow root and use this to make an ointment. This makes a really effective, soothing, and healing treatment that acts as a barrier cream as well.

ESSENTIAL OILS

Lavender, chamomile, tea tree

Treatment

Wash baby's bottom, using warm water to which you have added two drops of tea tree oil for every two cups of warm water.

Agitate the water well before using.

Dry skin gently and use either Diaper Rash Powder or Healing Bottom Cream.

Although the use of disposable diapers has greatly reduced diaper rash, it still occurs and needs immediate treatment with oils.

Cradle cap is very common in babies. A gentle infused oil will reduce it.

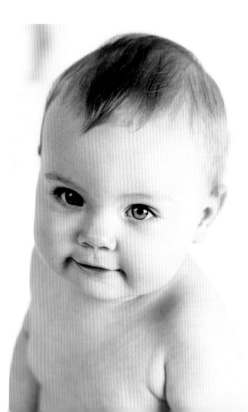

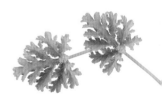

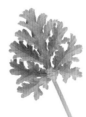

HEALING BOTTOM CREAM

1 cube (12–14 g) beeswax
2 $\frac{3}{4}$ oz (80 g) anhydrous lanolin
$\frac{1}{4}$ cup (60 ml) calendula or sweet almond oil
$\frac{1}{4}$ cup (60 ml) olive oil
8 drops lavender essential oil
5 drops chamomile essential oil

To make and use

Gently melt the beeswax in a double boiler. Add the lanolin and melt.

Combine the olive and calendula (or sweet almond) oils and add slowly to the pan. Do not overheat. Set aside.

Add the lavender essential oil when the temperature falls below 110° F (45°C) and combine until thoroughly incorporated but not set.

Spoon into a clean, labeled pot

DIAPER RASH POWDER

Zinc oxide powder and lavender essential oil combined, are wonderful for healing or preventing diaper rash.

2 cups cornstarch (cornflour)
3 tablespoons (45 ml) zinc oxide powder
  (from pharmacies)
20 drops lavender essential oil

Often, diaper rash is worse as babies begin solid food.

To make and use

Thoroughly combine the cornstarch and zinc oxide powder.

Add the lavender oil one drop at a time, stirring constantly to prevent lumps forming.

Allow to stand for four days to blend then store in an air tight container.

Shake occasionally to mix.

Overuse of powders is not recommended but a light dusting helps keep little creases sweet and dry.

Colic

For convenience, make tea mixtures, store them in glass jars and mark with the mixture name. You might find that one blend is more effective for your baby than another. If the problem persists, seek professional help.

COLIC MIXTURE 1
Anise seed, fennel seed, dill seed

COLIC MIXTURE 2
Catnep, dried spearmint, dried dill seed

COLIC MIXTURE 3
Chamomile, dried lemongrass, dried fennel seed

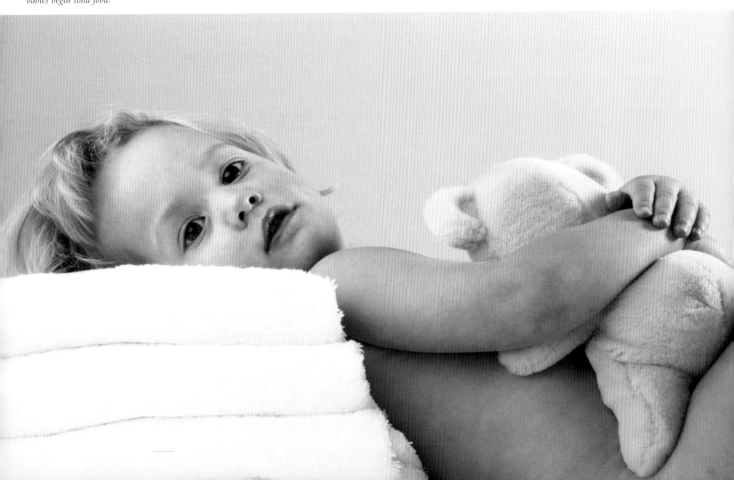

To make and use

Make tea mixtures, store them in glass jars and mark with the mixture name.

Pour 1 cup (250 ml) boiling water over one heaped teaspoon of the crumbled dried herb and seed mix, in a warmed teapot.

Cover and stand for 5–10 minutes,

Strain and sweeten with honey if you wish. Give in doses of one to two teaspoons as needed.

Store unused tea in the refrigerator in a covered container.

Make fresh every third day, or make a larger quantity and freeze in ice-cube trays.

Massage baby's abdomen in a clockwise direction with Gentle Baby Oil. Avoid the genitals.

Teething pain

Acupressure often gives relief. On the outside of the baby's face, use your second finger to press gently along the jaw line. If the baby flinches or cries, keep very gentle pressure on that point for up to 10 seconds. Release the pressure and continue along the jaw line.

Combine one drop chamomile essential oil with one teaspoon sweet almond oil. Massage baby's cheeks and jaw gently, carefully avoiding the eye area.

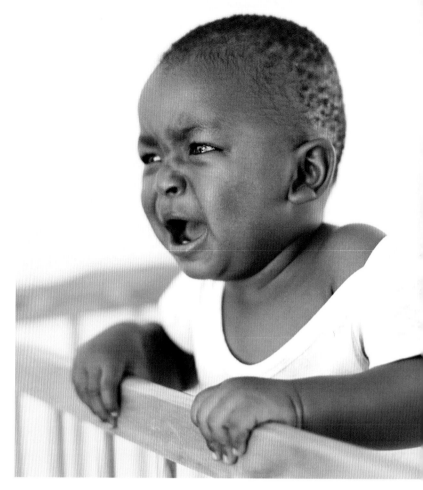

Teething pain can make baby miserable. It helps to rub the gums with chamomile tea.

Even if your baby has just graduated to the great age of one, he or she still needs smaller amounts of essential oils than an older child. If in doubt, use the dosages suggested for babies aged two to twelve months.

Chill an eggcupful of chamomile tea in the refrigerator and, when really cold, dip your finger (well scrubbed, of course, and with a very short nail!) into the tea and use to gently massage the sore gums. Use fresh tea each time.

Caution *Babies sometimes develop diarrhea and fever when teething, but it's dangerous to assume that teething is the cause. The help of a professional is needed if the symptoms persist.*

Over-excitement

Bath baby with a mix of mandarin and lavender essential oils. Use the number of drops of oil appropriate for baby's age.

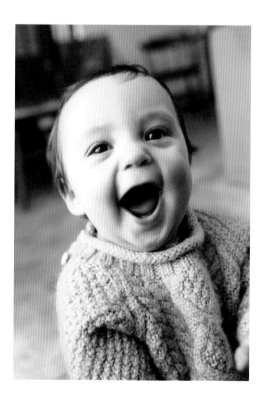

Essential oils can really assist in calming down excited toddlers.

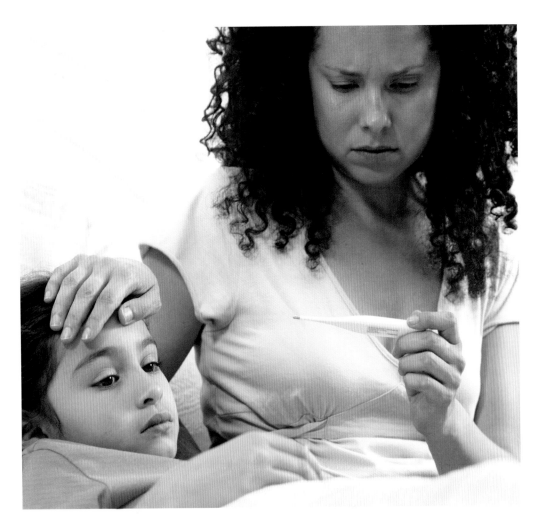

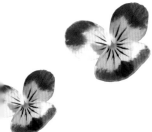

Common childhood complaints

Coughs and colds

Most of the same herbs used to treat colds in adults can also treat colds in children. You will want to reduce the dosages, however, or make the infusion half or a quarter of the normal strength, depending on the age of the child.

Steam or inhalations can also help, using handfuls of lavender, tea tree, eucalyptus, and/or peppermint in the boiling water. Be very cautious when using inhalations for children. Pour boiling water into a basin, have the child sit on your knee and use a large bath or beach towel to cover both of you and enclose the steam.

Make sure the child is getting plenty of vitamin C in his/her daily diet for the duration of the cold.

ESSENTIAL OILS
Tea tree, lavender and rosemary

To make and use
Float three drops of tea tree or lavender essential oil on a bowl of warm water and place the bowl under the baby's cot or bed.

Combine one drop each of tea tree, lavender and rosemary essential oils with four teaspoons grape seed oil. Float on a small bowl of warm water. Massage onto the chest and back.

Combine one to two drops (depending on age) each of tea tree, lavender and rosemary essential oils to one teaspoon grape seed oil or full cream milk. Add to a warm bath. Agitate the water to disperse.

Catarrh

To reduce inflammation of mucus membranes, give the child fresh alfalfa and red clover sprouts to eat twice daily.

Make a tea of as many as possible of the following: Anise, chamomile, fennel, hyssop, lemon balm, and mullein; sweeten with honey or oxymel and give three times daily. (See page 396 for dosages).

Coughs

The following treatment aims at loosening, lessening and expelling mucus and strengthening the lungs. If a cough is persistent, it would be advisable to consult a health professional.

COUGH SYRUP
Not suitable for children under 18 months.

1 part dried angelica root
1 part dried mallow root
1 part dried mullein
1 part anise
1 part dried sage
1 part dried thyme
1 part dried violet leaf

To make and use
Make an extract of the herbs and then follow the instructions for making a syrup (see page 522).

Add two drops of cider vinegar to each teaspoon of the mixture.

Give $\frac{1}{2}$-1 teaspoon (2.5-5 ml) as needed, according to age.

Earache

Never ignore earache. It can be a warning of more severe problems and lead to infections resulting in permanent deafness or other major traumas. The infection may even reach the brain. If earache persists for more than an hour or two, seek medical help. The following treatment is for first aid for earaches and if the condition is mild (such as that caused by a cold) may clear it up very quickly.

ESSENTIAL OILS
Chamomile, tea tree

CUTS, ABRASIONS AND BITES

If your child is entering a phase when his or her legs and arms are usually covered in abrasions, cuts and bruises—worn like medal earned on a battlefield—wash with Antiseptic Wound Wash (see Practicalities) and leave open to the air if possible. Use Antiseptic Wound Wash to swab the wound clean and give instant relief in emergencies. Basic Healing Ointment may be used after Antiseptic Wound Wash or at any time an ointment is needed.

For insect bites, add one drop lavender essential oil to one teaspoon bicarbonate of soda. Mix to a soft paste with a little water. Dab frequently on bites.

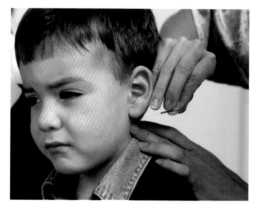

Only use essential oils for a mild earache.

Treatments
Put one teaspoon olive oil into a hot tablespoon (this will heat the oil slightly).

Add one drop of either of the recommended essential oils.

Using a dropper, squeeze a few drops into the ear and plug the external opening of the ear with a cotton ball.

Squeeze the contents of a garlic capsule into a warm, sterile teaspoon and add half a teaspoon of vegetable oil.

Draw up into an ear dropper and squeeze gently into the ear.

Plug the outside of the ear with a cotton ball.

Infused mullein flower oil is also a wonderful treatment for earache.

Caution *The pure oil from garlic oil capsules must never be used undiluted in the ears of children. It is far too strong and could cause intense pain and damage to the eardrum. If the earache is intense and/or prolonged, seek professional help. Earache can be an indication of severe problems.*

Stomachache

Stomachache in children can be indicative of many different problems, such as overeating, constipation, nerves or tiredness, or a more serious problem such as appendicitis. If a stomachache is severe or prolonged it requires medical attention.

STOMACHACHE FROM OVEREATING AND/OR CONSTIPATION

Give a tea of spearmint, dill, and ginger, sweetened with honey.

STOMACHACHE FROM NERVES AND TIREDNESS

Give a tea of catnep and chamomile sweetened with honey.

Dosages

Over 65 lb (30 kg): $1/2$ cup (125 ml)—three times daily, half an hour before food

33-63 lb (15–29 kg): 2 tablespoons (30 ml)—three times daily, half an hour before food

15-30 lb (7–14 kg): 4 teaspoons (20 ml)—three times daily, half an hour before food

Vomiting

Vomiting can lead to dehydration, so an adequate fluid intake needs to be maintained. Never give flat lemonade to children suffering from vomiting, as the sugar content causes further dehydration. See professional help if the vomiting persists. See the suggestions for stomachache above.

ANTI-NAUSEA TEA

$1/2$ teaspoon fresh spearmint leaves, crushed
$1/4$ teaspoon anise seeds, crushed
$1/8$ teaspoon finely grated fresh ginger

To make and use

Add the herbs to $1 1/2$ cups of boiling water, cover and steep for five minutes.

Sweeten with honey.

Give two-teaspoon sips of the tea as often as needed.

Over-excitement and insomnia

Children suffer from insomnia if they are over-tired, scared of the dark, worried about an event, or, sometimes, for no apparent reason. Try to work out why and follow one of the suggestions below.

Run a warm bath. Add the appropriate number of drops of both mandarin and lavender essential oils to one teaspoon grape seed oil. Add to the bath agitating well to disperse. Let the child remain quietly in the water (under supervision of course and no playing games) while you massage his or her limbs. Try to keep your child calm.

Give a tea of one or all of the following herbs; catnep, chamomile, lemon balm. Sweeten with honey and give after a warm (not hot) bath. Keep bedtime very calm and low-key.

Put a few drops of calming lavender oil on a curtain where the breeze through the open window will waft it into the room.

If stomachache is accompanied by fever, seek medical advice.

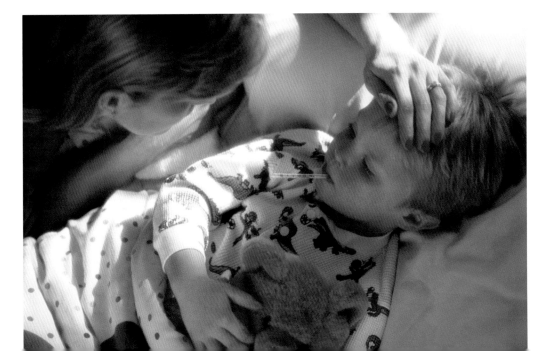

Insomnia

ESSENTIAL OILS
Chamomile, geranium, lavender, mandarin

OVER-TIRED AND STRUNG-OUT BLEND
2 teaspoons grape seed oil
2 drops lavender essential oil
2 drops chamomile essential oil

To make and use
Mix all the oils together in a small, labeled bottle and shake to blend.

Add half the blend to a warm bath and agitate thoroughly to disperse to oils.

After the bath, put the little one to bed in a dimly lit room and massage the remainder of the oil into the child's feet.

BANISH-THE-BOGEYMAN-BLEND
Add one drop each of lavender and mandarin essential oils to 7 fl oz (200 ml) water in a spray bottle. Shake really well then lightly spray the floor around the child's bed. While you are spraying, tell the child that this spray gets rid of bogeymen. The oils in the spray will help to allay fears and give sound sleep.

Achy and Grumpy

This blend is for children over five years of age who have been to a sports day, energetic parties or have over-extended themselves emotionally and physically.

ESSENTIAL OILS
Geranium, lavender, peppermint

ACHY AND GRUMPY BATH AND MASSAGE BLEND
4 teaspoons (20 ml) grape seed oil
5 drops lavender essential oil
3 drops geranium essential oil
2 drops peppermint essential oil

To make and use
Mix all the oils together in a small, labeled bottle, and shake to blend.

Pour two teaspoons of the blend into a bath or foot bath, agitate to disperse then pop the child into the bath to soak (under supervision) for 10-15 minutes, massaging any floating oil droplets into the skin.

Pour a little of the blend into the palm of your hand and massage over your child's body after showering.

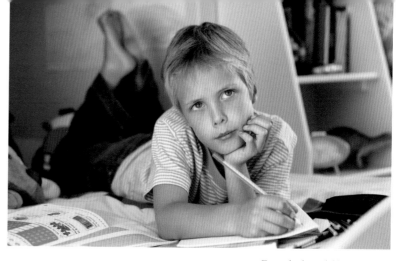

Float one to two teaspoons of the blend on a little warm water in a bowl and massage the child's back, legs or wherever aches the most!

Even school-age children can suffer stress and can be treated with calming teas.

Hyperactivity

A treatment plan should consist of chamomile, gotu kola, skullcap, red clover, milk thistle and ginkgo biloba taken as tea, tincture, or capsules.

A daily supplement of evening primrose oil has also shown to be beneficial for children suffering from hyperactivity.

Try giving your child a herbal bath using crushed lavender, catnep, and lemon balm tied in handkerchief or a piece of cloth and hung on the faucet where the water can run over it. The little bundle can then be squeezed into the bathwater and used as a washcloth.

Keep the home scented with calming essential oils such as lavender and geranium.

A natural diet is best. Eliminate foods that could cause an allergic reaction and return them to the diet one at a time, watching for any changes in the child's behavior. Be sure the child gets adequate amounts of zinc and B-complex vitamins.

Catnep tea is an ideal tranquilizer for children. Give one to two cups a day in half-cup doses sweetened with honey. Children often prefer to drink this tea cold.

After a busy day out, it's best to calm everyone with essential oils.

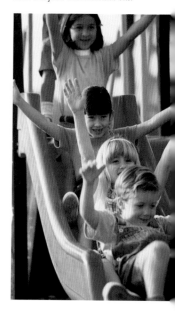

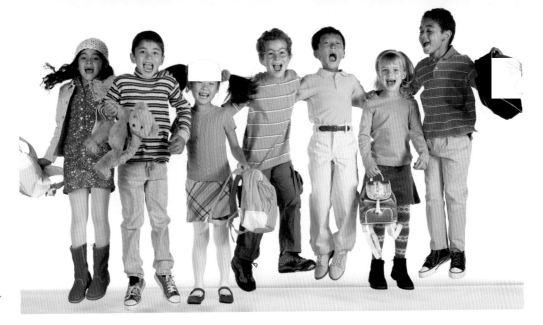

Kids can share more germs in a single day at school than they ever will again in their lives.

School infections

Head lice

Lice can also be treated by placing drops of tea tree oil on a fine-toothed comb and combing the hair thoroughly every day for two weeks.

LICE TREATMENT

3¹/₂ fl oz (100 ml) any inexpensive hair conditioner
20 drops tea tree oil
10 drops each of rosemary, lavender and lemon oil

To make and use

Combine the ingredients.

Apply to dry hair and cover with a plastic bag or shower cap. Wrap the head in a towel. Leave on for one hour. Rinse, shampoo, and rinse again.

When the hair is dry, comb with a very fine comb designed for the removal of lice eggs.

Repeat in one week if necessary.

Another treatment is to wash the hair nightly with a mild shampoo that has oil of thyme and tea tree oil added. Add 10 drops on thyme oil and 10 drops of tea tree oil to each 1 cup (250 ml) of shampoo, stir well to mix and gently invert the bottle a few times before using to make sure there is no essential oil floating on the top of the shampoo.

Impetigo

This contagious skin disease is marked by superficial pustular eruptions, particularly on the face. To help, give children over the age of five, 1,000 mg garlic oil capsules once daily with food, or echinacea extract as recommended on the bottle.

Half a cup of chickweed tea drunk three or four times per day is also beneficial.

Wash the sores carefully with a strong infusion of calendula several times per day.

Goldenseal, echinacea, and myrrh ointment is effective used as an adjunct to orthodox treatment.

NOSEBLEED

Pack the nose with an absorbent cotton (cottonwool) plug soaked in a cold, triple-strength infusion of mullein, plantain, and yarrow. Leave the plug in place for as long as possible and take care to withdraw it very gently, or the bleeding may start again.

Pinch the nose firmly but gently with the thumb and first finger, below the point where the bone begins. Keep the patient sitting upright and maintain the pinching for at least 10 minutes.

Putting the hands of the patient in cold water is often very effective.

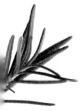

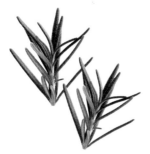

Childhood diseases

Fevers

Children can run alarmingly high fevers very quickly. Usually the temperature drops just as fast. But it is important to reduce fevers promptly to lessen the chance of complications.

ESSENTIAL OILS

Eucalyptus, lavender, tea tree

Treatment

Place cool (not icy cold) compresses on the child's forehead using eucalyptus, lavender, or tea tree essential oils; replace often. Then proceed with one of the following:

• Run a deep, cool to lukewarm bath (have as much as possible of the child's body under the water). Add one to two drops (depending on age) of each of the recommended essential oils, to one teaspoon grape seed oil. Add to the bath, agitating well to disperse. Massage any floating oils into the child's body.

• Add two drops each of tea tree, lavender, and eucalyptus essentials oils to a bowl of cool to lukewarm water, and agitate well to mix. Soak pieces of cloth in the water, wring out, and lay over the body of the child, avoiding the genitals. Change as soon as the sheeting warms up.

Feverish, fretful children will benefit from chamomile and/or catnep tea. Give 1 teaspoon (5 ml) doses to children under four; and 4 teaspoon (20 ml) doses to children over four. Repeat at three hourly intervals.

SOOTHING TEA

1 teaspoon dried catnep leaves
1 teaspoon dried raspberry leaves
1 teaspoon dried spearmint leaves

To make and use

Crumble the herbs, mix together and use half a teaspoon to $^1/_2$ cup (125 ml) of boiling water.

Allow to steep, covered, for five minutes. Sweeten with honey and give up to $^1/_2$ cup (125 ml) three times daily.

Dosages

Over 65 lb (30 kg): $^1/_2$ cup (125 ml)—three times daily, half an hour before food.

33-63 lb (15–29 kg): 2 tablespoons (30 ml)—three times daily, half an hour before food

15-30 lb (7–14 kg): 4 teaspoons (20 ml)—three times daily, half an hour before food

Chickenpox

Chickenpox is a highly infectious viral disease with an incubation period of 10–21 days. It starts off as a feverish cold before a red, spotty rash appears, and then develops into blisters that are often intensely itchy.

Treatments

Trim the child's nails very short or put gloves or mittens on their hands, as there is a risk of infection and/or scarring if the blisters are broken.

Encourage the child to drink copious amounts of fluid (filtered or bottled water, or diluted fruit juice).

Frequent baths using oats and lavender bath bags are soothing. Tie a handful of rolled oats and crushed lavender flowers in muslin or thin cloth, drop in the bath and squeeze to release the milky liquid. Use the bag to dab spots, but be gentle—it's important not to break the blisters.

Compresses and washes, or sprays of chamomile tea, will help to cool and reduce itching.

ANTI-ITCH LOTION

Fill a 2-cup (500 ml) jug with a mixture of chopped, fresh, lavender flowers, chamomile flowers, plantain leaves, and chickweed, and cover with boiling water.

Cover and leave to go cold.

Strain, squeeze the herbs thoroughly, and repeat the process using the reheated strained liquid and fresh chopped herbs.

Strain through coffee filter paper, then add 1 cup (250 ml) of witch hazel.

Pour into a labeled spray bottle.

Keep refrigerated, and spray the spots lightly, or use as a lotion to dab on and cool the blisters.

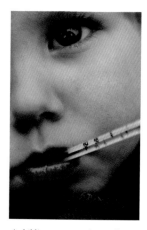

A child's temperature is usually an accurate guage to their health.

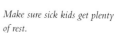

Make sure sick kids get plenty of rest.

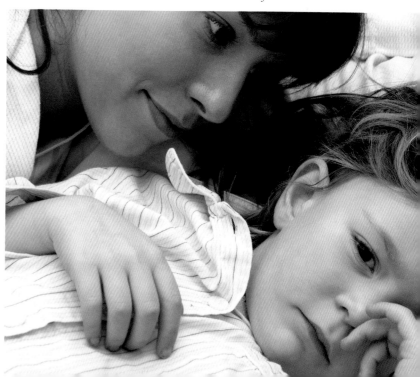

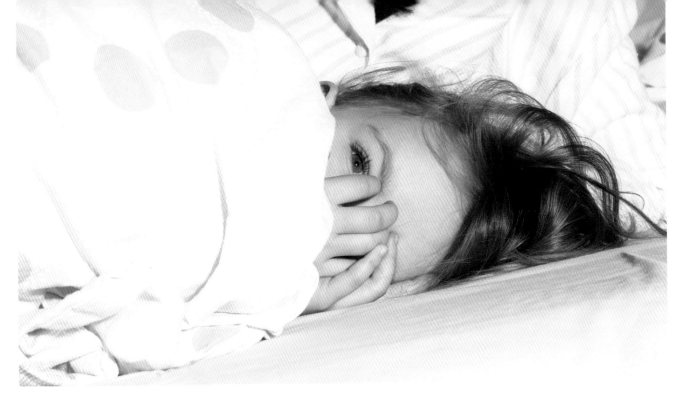

Although mild in children, rubella is serious during pregnancy.

Rubella (German measles)

German measles, or rubella, is a highly infectious viral disease. The symptoms are fairly mild in children, but if caught in pregnancy the effect can be very serious. Professional advice must always be sought to deal with this complaint.

Treatments

Trim the child's nails very short or put gloves or mittens on their hands, as there is a risk of infection and/or scarring if the blisters are broken.

Encourage the child to drink copious amounts of fluid (filtered or bottled water, or diluted fruit juice).

Give frequent baths using oat bath bags; tie a handful of rolled oats in a muslin or thin cloth, drop the bag in the bath, and squeeze it to release the milky liquid. Use the bag to gently dab the spots.

Compresses and washes, or sprays of chamomile tea, will help to cool and reduce itching.

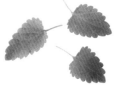

Measles

Measles is a potentially dangerous disease. Professional advice must always be sought to deal with this complaint, but there are also measures that can be taken at home to reduce the discomfort of the symptoms.

Treatments

Trim the child's nails very short or put gloves or mittens on their hands, as there is a risk of infection and/or scarring.

Encourage the child to drink copious amounts of fluid (filtered or bottled water, or diluted fruit juice).

Give frequent baths using oat bath bags; tie a handful of rolled oats in a muslin or thin cloth, drop the bag in the bath, and squeeze it to release the milky liquid. Use the bag to gently dab the spots.

Compresses and washes, or sprays of chamomile tea, will help to cool and reduce itching.

Mumps and swollen glands

Mumps is a viral infection characterized by swollen glands on one or both sides of the jaw, and possibly earache, mild fever, and headache. The very uncomfortable stage lasts for only a few days, but during this time bed rest is essential to avoid complications. The swollen glands under the ears may make the child very miserable, as it becomes painful to eat or swallow. Adults contracting mumps can suffer from swelling and inflammations of the testicles.

SOOTHING AND CLEANSING TEA

1 teaspoon dried catnep leaves
1 teaspoon dried raspberry leaves
1 teaspoon dried chamomile flowers

To make and use

Crumble the herbs to the consistency of tea leaves, and use one teaspoon of the blend for each cup of boiling water.

Dosages

Over 65 lb (30 kg): $^1/_2$ cup (125 ml)—three times daily, half an hour before food.

33-63 lb (15–29 kg): 2 tablespoons (30 ml)—three times daily, half an hour before food

15-30 lb (7–14 kg): 4 teaspoons (20 ml)—three times daily, half an hour before food

Use chamomile, mullein, violet, as a fomentation on swollen glands.

Tonsillitis

Use echinacea extract as recommended for the child's age on the container.

Give a tea of catnep, chamomile, lemon balm, and yarrow, sweetened with honey, three times daily.

Dosages

Over 65 lb (30 kg): $^1/_2$ cup (125 ml)—three times daily, half an hour before food.

33-63 lb (15–29 kg): 2 tablespoons (30 ml)—three times daily, half an hour before food

15-30 lb (7–14 kg): 4 teaspoons (20 ml)—three times daily, half an hour before food.

If the child is old enough, encourage him/her to gargle with a tea of hyssop, sage, and a pinch of salt.

Whooping cough

This highly infectious, and serious bacterial disease, usually affects the very young, and professional help is always needed. The following treatment may be of some benefit.

* Give echinacea fluid extract for children as directed on the bottle.
* Keep a bowl of steaming water and/or an oil burner in a safe place in the room at all times. Eucalyptus leaves, lavender flowers, and thyme leaves may be crushed and used as an inhalation, and also used in steam kettles.
* Massage the chest and back with infused oil of lavender.
* Give half a cup of chamomile tea three to six times a day.
* Very finely chop half an onion and one clove of garlic, put in a jar, add the juice

of one lemon and cover to twice the depth with honey. Leave overnight. Give children $^1/_2$–1 teaspoon (2.5–5 ml) of the liquid three times a day, depending on age (not to be given to children under two years of age).

WHOOPING COUGH INHALATION BLEND

1 drop tea tree essential oil
1 drop lavender essential oil
1 drop thyme essential oil

Mix oils together well, and use as an inhalation for children over three years of age.

WHOOPING COUGH MASSAGE BLEND

This treatment should only be used on children over two years of age.

4 teaspoons (20 ml) grape seed oil
8 drops cypress essential oil
4 drops tea tree essential oil
4 drops lavender essential oil

To make and use

Mix all the oils together in a small, labeled bottle, and shake to blend.

Leave for four days before using, so the oils have time synergize or combine well.

Add one teaspoon (for children over 12 years) or $^1/_2$ teaspoon (for children from 2–12 years) to a warm bath. Use the floating droplets of oil to massage chest, back and throat.

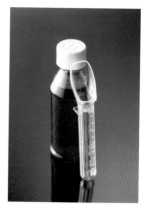

Buy a special medicine measure for children from a pharmacy.

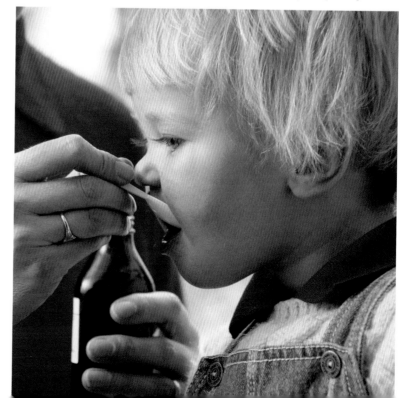

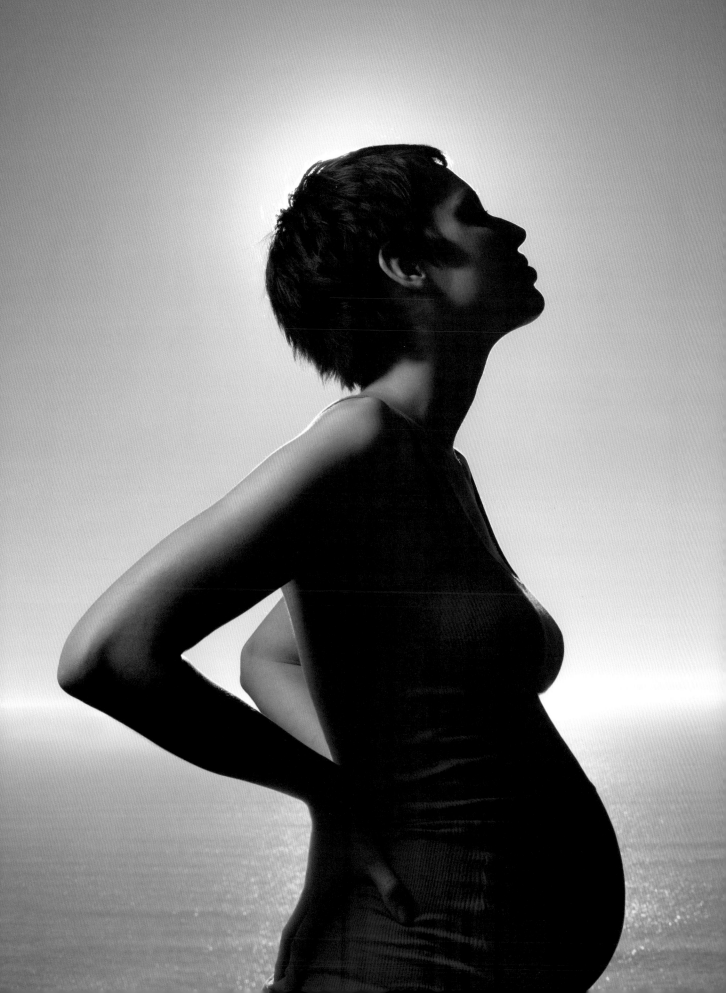

Pregnancy and birth

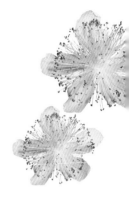

There should be no more satisfying and special time in a woman's life than the nine months of pregnancy, but women are often beset by anxiety and discomfort. This is a time to take the ultimate care of yourself to help to ensure that you and your baby are as healthy as it is possible to be.

The use of essential oils during pregnancy, labor, and after delivery can help immeasurably, both physically and emotionally. The essential oils will pass through the skin and be experienced by your baby, so don't be tempted to either increase or change the recommended oils.

There are some oils which should never be used during pregnancy; and some that should be avoided for the first three months.

The recipes here are for external use.

Pregnancy

Essential oils for use during pregnancy
Benzoin, chamomile (but not during the first four months), cypress, geranium, (see caution following), ginger, grapefruit, lavender (see caution following), lemon, mandarin, palmarosa, patchouli, rose (see caution following), ylang-ylang.

Essential oils for postnatal care
Chamomile, clary sage, fennel, frankincense, geranium, grapefruit, lavender, patchouli.

Caution: Oils which may be unsafe to use during pregnancy
Basil, cedarwood, celery seed, cinnamon, clary sage, fennel, galbanum, hyssop, jasmine, juniper, marjoram, melissa, myrrh, nutmeg, parsley, pennyroyal, peppermint, rosemary, thyme.

PREGNANCY TEA

Dandelion root and leaf are rich sources of vitamins and minerals, including beta-carotene, calcium, potassium, and iron. Dandelion leaf is mildly diuretic; it also stimulates bile flow and helps with the common digestive complaints of pregnancy. Dandelion root tones the liver.

Raspberry leaf is rich in vitamins and minerals (especially iron). It tones the uterus, increases milk flow and restores the mother's system after childbirth.

Nettle leaf provides the minerals calcium and iron, is mildly diuretic, and aids in the elimination of excess water from tissues. Nettle enriches and increases the flow of breast milk and restores the mother's energy following childbirth.

To be used only after the first trimester.

1 part dried dandelion root, very finely crushed
1 part dried dandelion leaf
1 part dried raspberry leaf
1 part dried nettle leaf

To make and use
Crumble the leaves to the texture of tea leaves. Mix them together. Drink one cup of the tea three times daily.

Morning sickness
Morning sickness has been associated with low blood sugar. A ginger capsule or a cup of ginger tea and a couple of dry water biscuits before raising the head from the pillow in the morning (eat on your side, not your back, to prevent choking) may help to avoid nausea.

Ginger or spearmint tea (no more than two small cups a day), or crystallized ginger, can be taken for nausea. No more than one gram of ginger should be taken in a 24-hour period.

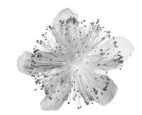

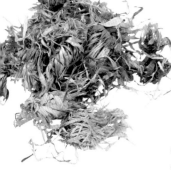

If the sickness is prolonged or frequent and causing distress, a health-care professional needs to be consulted, as the vomiting may be indicative of a more serious problem.

The following suggestions should work very quickly to dispel morning sickness.

The scent of the spearmint or ginger oil will calm your tummy during the night and you should wake up with no nasty queasiness. Use any or all of the following ideas.

Put one drop of spearmint or ginger essential oil on the light globe before switching on the bedside light at night.

Put another two drops on absorbent cotton (cottonwool) and tuck under your pillow.

Place a small bowl of lukewarm water in the bedroom before going to bed and sprinkle with one drop of spearmint and two drops of lavender essential oils.

Also, keep a bottle of spearmint or ginger oil next to the bed and sniff the aroma on waking.

TIP OILS TO AVOID DURING THE FIRST FOUR MONTHS OF PREGNANCY: GERMAN AND ROMAN CHAMOMILE, GERANIUM, LAVENDER, ROSE.

Stretch marks

As soon as pregnancy is confirmed, it's time to start taking extra care of the skin on the tummy, thighs, bottom, and breasts. Stretch marks can be largely avoided but not easily cured and the use of these oils morning and night will certainly help to keep the constantly and rapidly stretching skin supple and pliable.

TUMMY OIL

4 x 250iu vitamin E capsules
5 fl oz (150 ml) sweet almond oil
3 teaspoons olive oil
2 teaspoons avocado oil
1 teaspoon wheat germ oil
10 drops mandarin essential oil
10 drops palmarosa essential oil
20 drops lavender essential oil

To make and use

Pierce the vitamin E capsules and squeeze the oil into a 7 fl oz (200 m) labeled bottle.

Add the remaining oils and shake to blend. If possible, leave for four days to synergize.

Shake the bottle well before use.

Massage the oil thoroughly into the skin of the breasts and from the waist down to the knees. Use twice daily if possible.

As your pregnancy progresses, nausea usually subsides. But continue with your herbal teas and essential oils to keep it away.

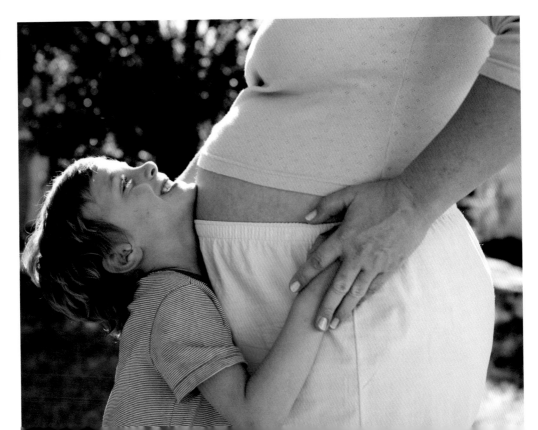

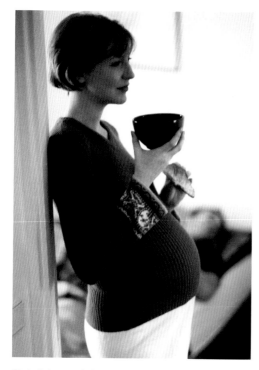

Sip herbal tea regularly throughout your pregnancy.

Nipples

It's a good idea to begin to massage the nipples for a couple of months before the birth. Massaging will help to avoid the painfully cracked nipples from which so many mothers suffer, and which change the joyful time of breastfeeding into a miserable experience.

Make the following oil and begin to use several weeks before the baby is due.

If you prefer, calendula ointment and calendula infused oil are available in health food stores.

NIPPLE OIL

3 tablespoons (45 ml) calendula infused oil or sweet almond oil

1 teaspoon wheat germ oil

10 drops carrot essential oil

15 drops chamomile essential oil

To make and use

Mix all the oils together in a small bottle. Shake well to blend. Label the bottle and secure with a well-fitting lid.

Leave for four days before using so the oils have time to synergize or combine well.

Essential oils are absorbed through the skin, and will have a soothing effect on your baby.

Massage the oil well into the nipples and surrounding area in a firm but gentle squeezing motion. This should be done three times a day up to the birth.

Do not leave any residue oil on the nipples when breastfeeding, as they will be absorbed by the baby.

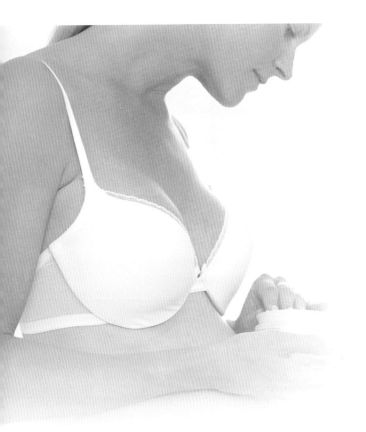

*Massage your tummy twice a day
to try and avoid stretch marks.*

Perineum massage

Massaging the perineum (the area between the vagina and the anus) has been shown to lessen the risk of tearing. Massage twice daily with a mixture of olive and wheat germ oils for the last two months before the birth.

Varicose veins

Varicose veins are largely hereditary so if any members of your family suffer from them, take precautionary measure as early as possible.

Caution: *If you already have varicose veins, avoid massaging over the veins.*

VARICOSE MASSAGE BLEND
4 teaspoons grape seed oil
4 teaspoons sweet almond oil
10 drops geranium essential oil
10 drops lemon essential oil
5 drops cypress essential oil

To make and use
Mix all the oils together in a small, labeled bottle and shake to blend.

Leave for four days before using, so the oils have time to synergize or combine well.

Stroke the oil on your legs twice daily starting at the ankle, stroking firmly but gently upwards. In the later stages of pregnancy it will be difficult and you may need a partner or friend to do this for you.

The "blues"

It's very natural for you to feel conflicting emotions during pregnancy. Your body is undergoing immense changes and this, combined with tiredness, can result in tearfulness and the miseries. When this happens, stop what you are doing and have a bath! During my five pregnancies I often relied on a bath to see me through the day. The water supports your tummy and removes the heavy feeling, while the warm water (not hot) with essential oil takes away the gloominess.

Aching backs

Towards the end of pregnancy can be a trying time as the body gets heavier and backaches more frequent. This oil is very gentle and will help to alleviate the depressing, dragging feeling. If used regularly it may help to prevent the backache.

Caution: *Use only after the first four months.*

ACHING BACK MASSAGE BLEND
3 tablespoons (45 ml) grape seed oil
4 teaspoons sweet almond oil
20 drops chamomile essential oil
20 drops lavender essential oil

To make and use
Mix all the oils together in a small, labeled bottle and shake to blend.

Leave for four days before using, so the oils have time to synergize or combine well.

Ask a friend or partner to massage your lower back very gently with the blend after you have had a bath or shower.

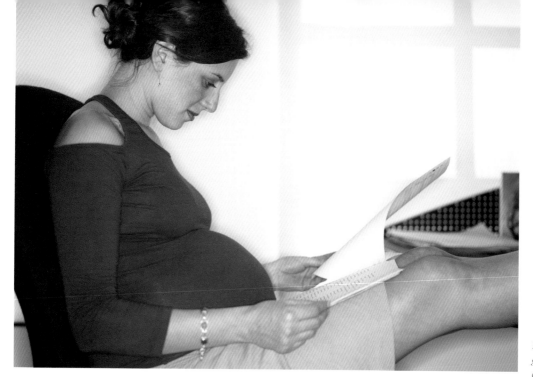

Elevate your legs every chance you get while pregnant. Essential oils can't do everything.

BABY BLUES BATH BLEND

1 teaspoon grape seed oil
2 drops mandarin or lavender essential oil
2 drops grapefruit or geranium essential oil
1 drop sandalwood or ylang-ylang essential oil

To make and use

Mix the oils together in a small bowl.

Choose a time when the other children are at school, or ask a friend or relative to mind young children for half an hour or so.

If you don't own a bath pillow, fill a hot water bottle with warm water and tuck under your neck; the warmth will help you to relax. Add the oils after running the bath and swoosh the water to disperse the drops. Massage the floating drops of oil into your tummy and breasts, relax, talk to your baby and enjoy!

Caution: *This bath only to be taken after the fourth month.*

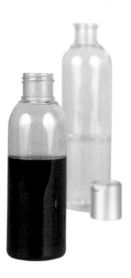

The birth

This is it! Soon you will see the baby who has been your constant companion for nine months. There are a few oils that are going to help you welcome your baby into the world. You're going to be working very hard for the time the journey takes from the womb to the world. Your needs and desires are paramount at this time so make the most of it! Don't hesitate to say what you want.

The first stages of labor can really drag on if you sit around waiting for the next contraction. It's a good idea to go for a walk (near to home and accompanied of course) as this will help to speed things up. If you feel nervous about leaving the house you can occupy yourself with household chores.

When the contractions begin to get stronger and closer together you may enjoy a warm bath to which you have added six drops of lavender essential oil. A few comforting things may be soft music, a hot water bottle for a sore lower back, lip salve for dry lips, frozen fruit juice, or water cubes to suck, and diluted apple juice to keep the blood sugar level up.

The following massage blend will help to lesson the discomfort of contractions, gently speed up contractions, create a calm and tranquil atmosphere, and help to keep you and the surrounding air free of bacteria.

"WAITING FOR BABY" MASSAGE BLEND

Do invest in jasmine or rose oils for this very special occasion if you possibly can!

2 teaspoons grape seed oil
2 teaspoons sweet almond oil
5 drops clary sage essential oil
5 drops lavender essential oil
3 drops geranium essential oil
3 drops jasmine or rose essential oil

To make and use

Mix all the oils together in a small, labeled bottle, and shake to blend.

Leave for four days before using, so the oils have time to synergize or combine well.

Massage the lower back with the blend, as often and as firmly as liked during the labor. If it can be tolerated, the abdomen can be massaged once during the first stage using only the lightest strokes. Guide the person conducting the massage as to the movements and areas that are most comfortable and helpful.

Wow! Now is the time to begin using teas and oils to keep up your milk production.

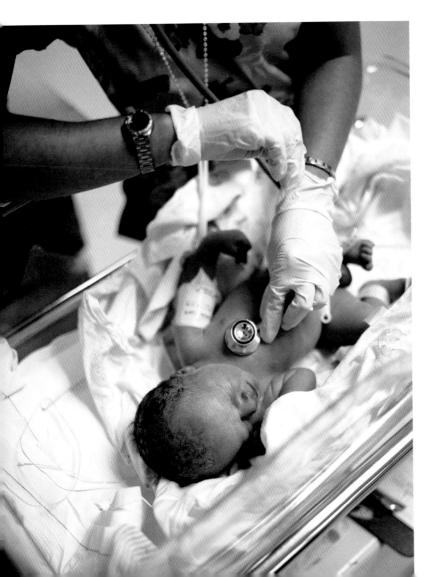

After the birth

Now you have your baby and will be having a wonderful time getting to know each other. This time can be stressful and demanding however, and the essential oils can help you to avoid or banish some of the annoying problems which occasionally arise. The choice of oils is still limited as breast-fed babies will receive these oils in the breast milk.

Breast-feeding

It's beyond the scope of this book to talk in depth about this subject but I would urge you, even if you have decided not to breast-feed, to consider feeding for the first vital days when the baby will receive colostrum. This is a think, creamy-coloured fluid which contains constituents important for the baby's immunity to disease.

BREAST MILK TEA

It's a good idea to triple this recipe (enough for three days) and store in a covered container in the refrigerator.

4 teaspoons fennel seed
1 teaspoon anise seed
2 teaspoons caraway seed
1 teaspoon fenugreek seed

To make and use

Lightly crush the seeds and place in a small saucepan.

Pour three cups of cold water over, place a lid on the pan and slowly bring to the boil.

Turn the heat off immediately and leave the tea to stand for 10–15 minutes. Stand and store in the refrigerator in a covered container.

Drink three cups a day, sweetened with honey if desired.

BLEND TO INCREASE MILK FLOW

3 tablespoons (45 ml) grape seed oil
20 drops fennel essential oil
10 drops clary sage essential oil

To make and use

Mix all the oils together in a small, labeled bottle, and shake to blend.

Leave for four days before using, so the oils have time to synergize or combine well.

Massage the oil blend gently into the breasts two to three times a day using a circular movement. Wash off thoroughly before breast-feeding.

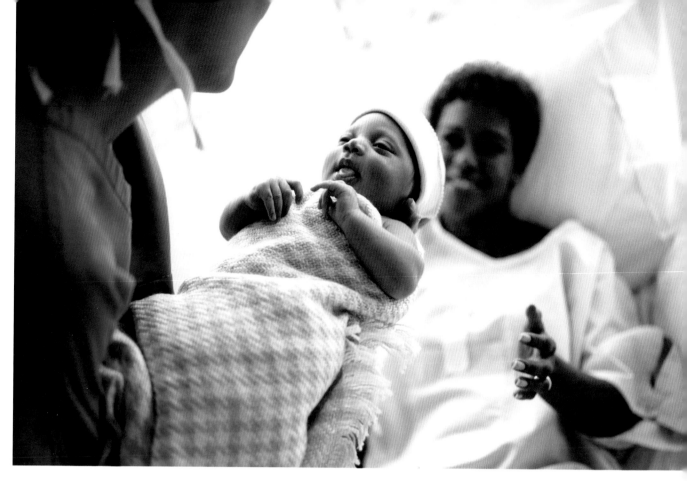

By day three, your milk is fully in. Watch for sore areas in the breast and treat them immediately.

Breast abscess

A breast infection at this time can be very painful and distressing. Consult your health practitioner if there's a fever.

BREAST ABSCESS FOMENTATION BLEND
5 drops geranium essential oil
5 drops chamomile essential oil
small bowl of hot water

To make and use
Add the oils to the water.
   Fold a piece of soft cloth in four and soak in the water.
   Apply fomentation to the breast every 4 hours.
   Cover cloth with a piece of plastic and keep in place with a bra.
   Iron a cabbage leaf until very soft. When cool enough, slip the leaf over the breast under your bra. Alternate this treatment with the fomentation method.

BREAST ABSCESS OIL
3 tablespoons (45 ml) grape seed oil
10 drops geranium essential oil
15 drops chamomile essential oil

To make and use
Mix all the oils together in a small, labeled bottle, and shake to blend.
   Leave for four days before using, so the oils have time to synergize or combine well.
   Massage breasts very gently 4 times daily.

Perineum

The perineum may be very sore after the birth. Even though you may not have had stitches, there are often tiny little tears or sore areas that can be very uncomfortable.

PERINEUM MASSAGE OIL
4 teaspoons olive oil
4 teaspoons wheat germ oil
6 drops lavender essential oil

To make and use
Mix together in a small, labeled bottle.
   Shake to blend.
   Massage the perineum for two minutes twice daily.
   If the area is too sore for massage, try a cool compress containing five drops lavender essential oil instead.

TIP TO STOP MILK PRODUCTION, DRINK HALF A CUP OF SAGE TEA (EITHER RED OR GARDEN SAGE) EVERY TWO HOURS.

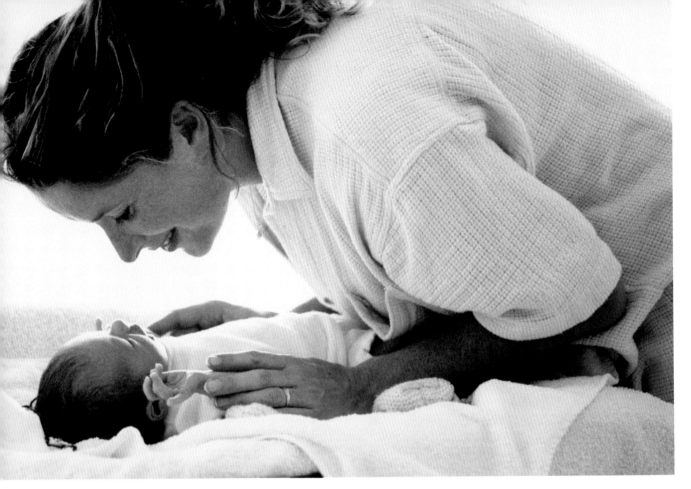

Home time is the busiest of all. Try to get help occasionally so that you can pamper youself with a bath.

SITZ BATH

1 teaspoon vegetable oil

2 drops lavender essential oil

2 drops tea tree essential oil

2 tablespoons salt

To make and use

Mix the oils together in a small bowl. Stir well to blend and add the salt.

Add to the bath and stir to dissolve.

Run enough warm water in the bath to cover the lower hips. Add the above mixture, agitate the water to dissolve the sale and soak in the bath for 10 minutes.

Postnatal depression

Few people can understand or sympathize with postnatal depression unless they have suffered themselves. The depression can range from mild (experienced by most women on the second or third day after the birth), to very severe. Plenty of rest and pampering yourself will help you feel relaxed. And you will have more energy and enthusiasm to cope with the baby and household chores. Use the following oils

Breast-feeding is the ultimate experience for you and baby. Massage your nipples and breasts regularly to keep them supple.

to lift your spirits and give confidence. Consult a health professional if the symptoms persist as this condition is very serious if left untreated.

ESSENTIAL OILS

Bergamot, frankincense, geranium, grapefruit, lavender, lemon, mandarin, jasmine.

POSTNATAL BLUES BEATER

60 drops bergamot essential oil

60 drops lavender essential oil

40 drops geranium or frankincense essential oil

40 drops grapefruit or mandarin essential oil

To make and use

Mix all the oils together in a small, labeled bottle, and shake to blend.

Add 10 drops to one teaspoon grape seed oil for a bath, agitate the water well to disperse.

Sprinkle two to three drops on a wet wash cloth and use as a final rub after showering.

Add 15 drops to four teaspoons grape seed oil for a massage.

Alternatively just blend the essential oils together to use an as air spray or in an oil burner.

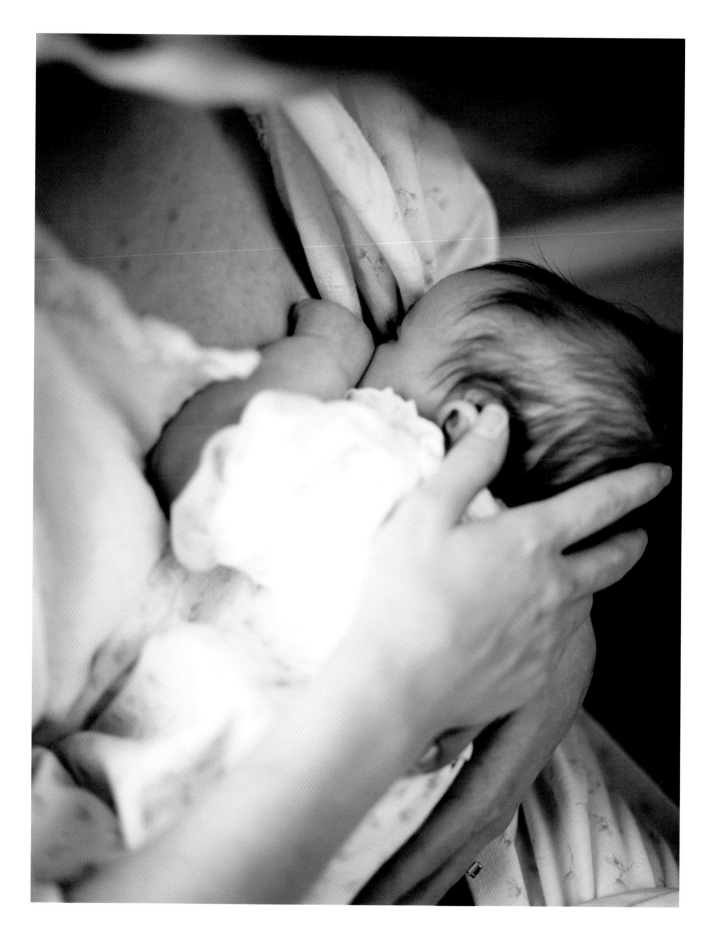

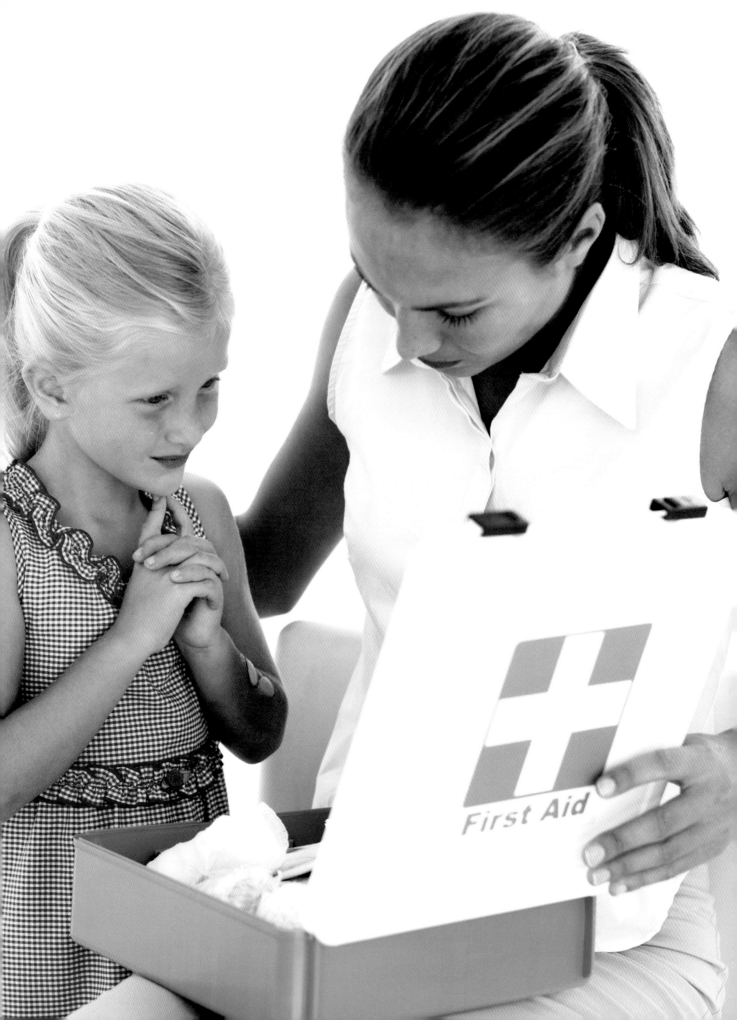

First aid for families

Everyone at some time has been, or will be faced with a minor or major injury to themselves or others: Cuts, burns, and stings and more serious things such as heart attacks and broken bones.

Knowing what to do in theses situations can prevent excessive trauma or pain, and in some cases can save a life.

It should be noted that this section deals with first aid only. Many injuries need professional help as soon as possible: The dirt in a seemingly innocent cut can carry infections such as tetanus; the pain of earache may be a symptom of middle ear infection, a potentially serious condition.

There are three things needed in order to be an effective helper.

First, take a short first-aid course with a reputable organisation such as American Red Cross or St John Ambulance. Buy a good reference book on first aid and keep it handy. If possible, familiarize yourself with the most common procedures before something happens: The middle of a crisis is not a good time to have to learn a new skill.

Second, provide the car and house with well-equipped first-aid boxes. Check them regularly and re-stock as supplies run low. Ideally, the containers should be robust, weatherproof, and, if you have children, lockable. I use a small, bright red, metal toolbox.

Keep a list of emergency numbers (ambulance, doctor, hospitals, poisons information center) both in the first-aid boxes and next to the telephone.

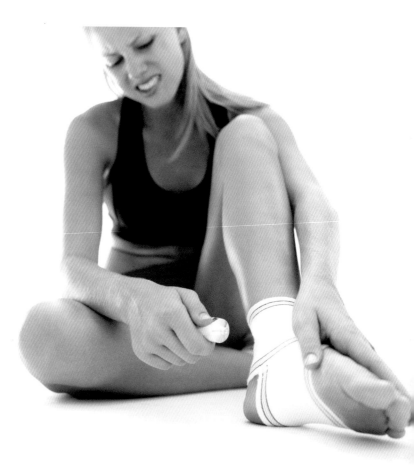

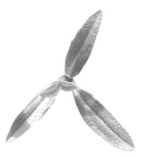

A first-aid box should contain immediate remedies for all sorts of injuries, including sport.

The first-aid box

Every home and car should have a well-equipped first-aid box. The ability to give prompt assistance can often prevent excessive pain and trauma and, in some cases, save a life.

The following first-aid box contents are in addition to the usual bandages, sticking plasters, tweezers, and scissors. If you are a frequent traveller (particularly overseas), you may find it easier to carry an essential oil first-aid kit rather than the more conventional one.

You can make some items for your first-aid box from your home-grown herbs, while others are best bought ready-made from the health food shop or pharmacy.

You may, of course, wish to vary these suggestions for your first-aid supplies to suit your own family needs.

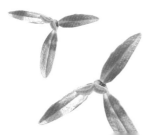

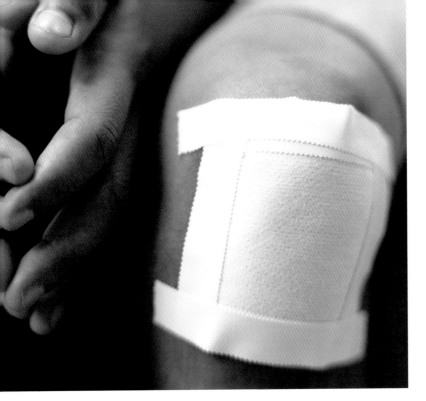
Keep the contents of the first-aid box clean to avoid cross infection.

Aloe vera gel
Buy a reputable brand of pure aloe vera gel and use it on minor burns and scalds.

Arnica cream
This is a wonderful remedy for bruising but must never be used on broken skin.

Castor oil
Castor oil comes from the seed of the castor oil plant and was once used as a laxative, but is no longer considered safe treatment. As an external remedy, it has amazing drawing power, soothing as it draws splinters or foreign bodies from the flesh.

Chamomile tea bags
Idea to calm tension, depression and anxiety, insomnia, internal inflammation such as gastritis, diarrhea, cystitis, menstrual pain, PMS.

Charcoal tablets
This antacid remedy is a powerful absorbent in the stomach and intestinal tract, acting like a sponge. Modern charcoal is "activated," treated with steam to make it even more absorbent. It disinfects and deodorizes, picks up harmful bacteria and passes them from the body. Some say it can cure a hangover. Use it with care as it can cause constipation if overused, but it is useful to treat simple diarrhea.

Dr Bach's Rescue Remedy
This is a ready-made mixture of the homeopathic flower tinctures of cherry plum, clematis, impatiens, rock rose, and star of Bethlehem. The tincture is useful in many minor or major situations where there is shock and nerves need to be calmed. Take four drops at a time under the tongue. Use as often as every 15 minutes if the situation warrants it. It can be rubbed on the pulse points if the patient is unconscious.

Essential oils
* Chamomile essential oil to calm tension, depression and anxiety, insomnia, internal inflammation such as gastritis, diarrhea, cystitis, menstrual pain, PMS (external treatments), and also to ease dull pain.
* Eucalyptus essential oil—it is anti-inflammatory, antiseptic, antiviral and pain relieving
* Geranium essential oil to use with lemon essential oil and witch hazel to stop bleeding. Nerve tonic when stressed. Use with lavender essential oil to repel insects.
* Ginger essential oil for nausea, muscular pain, and fatigue.
* Grapefruit essential oil to combat fatigue, depression, and nervous exhaustion. Blend with geranium to counteract muscle stiffness.
* Lavender essential oil may be used undiluted over small areas. Antibacterial, antiviral, antidepressant. Mix with witch hazel for insect bites, insect repellent, bruises, minor burns, and sunburn. Also for headaches, depression.
* Lemon essential oil—use with geranium essential oil and witch hazel to stop bleeding and prevent bacterial infection of wounds. One drop of oil in a cup of water is reputed to make the water safe to drink but I would hesitate to recommend this in

Third World countries or whenever you are off the beaten track and unsure of the water supply.

* Peppermint and/or ginger essential oils—ease stomach cramps, travel sickness, and nausea. Caution—use 0.5 percent only of ginger and peppermint essential oils.
* Rosemary essential oil stimulates the central nervous system (and therefore the brain), gives clarity to the brain, and inhalations ease the symptoms of colds, coughs, catarrh. Eases the pain of muscles that are tired and stiff from sitting for long periods. Caution—not to be used by epileptics or during pregnancy.
* Tea tree essential oil—antibacterial, antiviral, antiseptic, antifungal. Maybe used undiluted over small areas. Use to treat abscesses, athlete's foot, cold sores, cuts, grazes, bites, ringworm, and sunburn.
* Witch hazel extract to reduce the pain of bites and stings as well as inflammation.

Garlic oil capsules

Garlic oil contains a very powerful antibacterial agent called allicin, which prevents the growth of bacteria and also promotes the healing of infections. This makes it an ideal preventative herb.

Ipecac (ipecacuanha) syrup

This Brazilian herb, used in small doses, is an expectorant and in large doses becomes an emetic. Its main use in the first-aid box is in cases of poisoning. It must never be used if a strong corrosive liquid or a substance with strong fumes has been swallowed, or if the patient is an infant under one year old. Always follow the instructions on the manufacturer's label.

In cases of child poisoning, it is always best to obtain urgent medical advice before you administer any remedy. Your doctor, ambulance service, health service or, if you have one, poisons information center or equivalent service, will usually give advice over the phone on what to take, according to what has been swallowed.

Caution: Keep emergency telephone numbers next to the telephone and stored in all your cell phones.

Menthol crystals

Menthol is crystallized out of peppermint oil. In the first-aid box it is used for an inhalation.

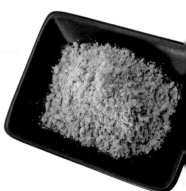

Ointments
Basic healing ointment

Make and choose the ointments for your first-aid box from the recipes in this book by following the methods described in Section 4, Practicalities.

Slippery elm

The powdered bark of this tree from North America is a specific treatment for soothing inflamed membranes, both internally and externally. Follow the instructions on the container.

Tinctures

Some of the tinctures you will find useful are calendula, chamomile, cayenne, ginger, and shepherd's purse. Distilled witch hazel is a must, as this tincture is one of the finest and gentlest astringents there is. It is available from pharmacies.

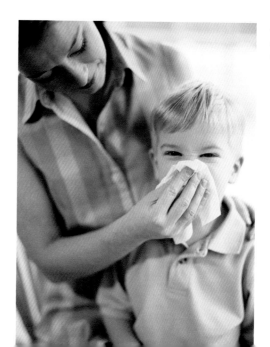

Nosebleeds are common in some kids and you should be ready at any time to deal with them.

You also need:

* Bandages, slings, clean cloth
* Plasters, eye patches
* Scissors, tweezers
* Steel or enamel dish
* Small funnel
* Thermometer
* Two or three eye-droppers
* Glass or plastic 25 ml medicine measure
* Cotton buds and absorbent cotton (cottonwool)
* Two empty dropper bottles for mixing
* Two eye droppers for measuring essential oils
* Paddle pop sticks for taking ointment out of jar
* 15 ml bottle sweet almond oil for making blends

Playgrounds are the most common situation for minor injuries.

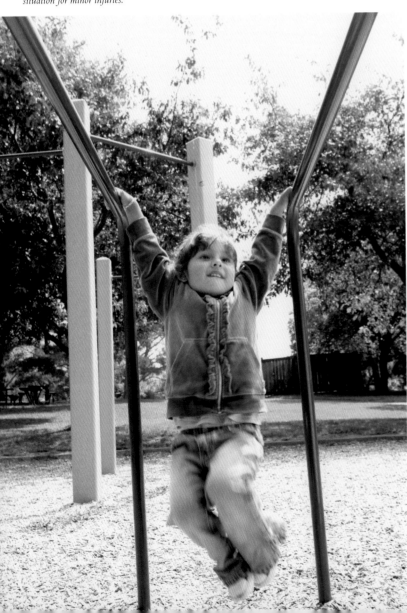

FIRST AID A–Z
BITES AND STINGS

Bee
Scrape the sting out sideways, never remove with tweezers. Massage with a paste of bicarbonate of soda and water. Repeat often. If an allergy is suspected, use the treatment on the way to the hospital or emergency center.

Dog
Wash the area immediately and thoroughly with tea tree or manuka oil in water. Apply neat tea tree oil and a dressing. Go to the nearest doctor or hospital for treatment.

Insects
(mosquitoes, gnats, or flies)
Apply neat lavender oil directly on the bite until relief is obtained.

Spiders
Spray the area with vinegar and then cover with neat lavender oil. Try to identify the spider. If you suspect that it is the venomous variety, go straight to hospital, dripping the puncture with lavender essential oil until medical treatment begins.

Wasps
Add four drops of lavender oil to one teaspoon of vinegar. Dab on the wound to counteract the alkaline poison of the sting and reduce pain and swelling. Repeat hourly.

BLEEDING, EXTERNAL
Apply a cold compress of either tincture of calendula or distilled witch hazel. Bandage firmly if possible. Apply plantain ointment when bleeding has lessened, and cover with a dressing if necessary.

BRUISES
Use a witch hazel compress, then massage arnica ointment or aloe vera gel gently into the bruised area.

BURNS, MINOR

Hold under cold water for 10 minutes. Smear aloe vera gel or lavender oil into the burn. Repeat every 15–20 minutes until the pain is gone. Don't cover—leave open to the air.

COLD SORES

Dab cold sore with tea tree oil or tincture of myrrh.

CUTS AND GRAZES

Add one teaspoon of calendula tincture and three drops of tea tree or manuka oil to one cup (250 ml) of boiled water. Use to cleanse the wound. Leave wound open to air unless severe. If a dressing is needed, place two drops of tea tree oil on the dressing before applying.

EARACHE

Squeeze the contents of a garlic oil capsule into a warm teaspoon. Add half a teaspoon of vegetable oil, mix, and drip into the ear. Plug the opening of the ear with absorbent cotton (cottonwool).

Alternatively, warm one teaspoon of vegetable oil and add three drops of tea tree oil. Drip into the ear and plug the opening with a cotton ball.

EYES, GRIT AND DUST

Don't attempt first-aid treatment if the foreign body has penetrated the eye, Cover loosely with an eye patch and seek medical assistance.

If the foreign body is loose, put one linseed under the lower eyelid. Within half an hour or so it will appear as a jelly (containing the grit) in the corner of the eye. Remove with a cotton bud or tissue.

An alternative treatment is to put three drops of castor oil in the eye and cover with an eye patch.

FAINTING

Loosen tight clothing and encourage the patient to put his/her head between the knees. Massage a few drops of lavender oil on the pulse points of the wrist and temple. Hold the bottle of oil under the nose of the patient so that he/she breathes directly from the bottle.

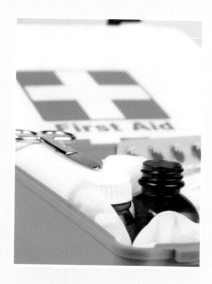

FLATULENCE

Take the appropriate number of charcoal tablets as directed on the container.

Alternatively, add one teaspoon of tincture of ginger to a glass of warm water, sweeten with honey if liked, and sip very slowly.

HEADACHES

Inhale menthol crystals as instructed on the container.

Alternatively, massage the back of the neck and the temples (avoiding the eyes) with lavender or rosemary oil.

HEARTBURN

Mix one drop of peppermint oil in one teaspoon of honey in a glass. Fill with warm water and sip slowly.

NAUSEA AND VOMITING

Mix one teaspoon of tincture of ginger into one teaspoon of honey in a glass. Fill the glass with warm water and sip very slowly.

If the vomiting has made the stomach sore, slippery elm tablets will soothe the lining of the stomach. Take as directed on the container.

SHOCK

Use Dr Bach's Rescue Remedy (see page 414). Put directly onto the tongue as directed on the bottle. If the patient is unconscious, rub the remedy onto the pulse points every 5–10 minutes.

Alternatively, hold a bottle of lavender oil under the nose for the patient to sniff.

SPLINTERS, DEEPLY EMBEDDED

Soak lint or gauze in castor oil. Apply as a compress. Bandage loosely in place and change two hourly until the splinter is drawn to the surface.

SPRAINS AND STRAINS

Thoroughly dampen a piece of absorbent cloth with witch hazel extract, sprinkle with five drops of rosemary oil, wring out and bandage onto the sprained area. Repeat every two hours.

Alternatively (or as well), the oil may be mixed with one tablespoon of vegetable oil and massaged into the sprained area.

SUNBURN

Run a lukewarm bath into which is sprinkled 10 drops of lavender oil. Soak for 20–30 minutes, splashing the burned areas with the water.

After the bath, apply aloe vera gel mixed with witch hazel onto sore area.

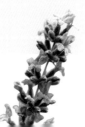

Essential oil first-aid treatments

Ailment	Essential oil	Treatment
Bites, animal	Lavender, tea tree	Neat
Bleeding	Lemon, geranium, which hazel	Compress
Blisters	Geranium, tea tree	Neat
Bruises	Witch hazel, lavender	Compress
Burns	Lavender	Neat
Chills and fevers	Ginger, geranium	Bath, shower, massage
Colds	Eucalyptus, ginger	Bath, massage
Cramp	Geranium, ginger	Massage
Cuts and grazes	Lavender, tea tree	Wash
Exhaustion, physical	Lavender, peppermint	Bath, shower, massage
Hay fever	Chamomile, eucalyptus	Inhalation
Headaches	Lavender, peppermint	Inhalation, neck massage
Heatstroke	Lavender, eucalyptus, lemon	Cold water sheet wrap
Indigestion	Peppermint or ginger	Drink
Insect bites	Lavender, tea tree	Neat
Insect repellent	Lavender, peppermint	Lotion
Insomnia	Chamomile, lavender	Bath, massage
Itching	Lavender, eucalyptus	Lotion
Jelly fish sting	Lavender, vinegar	Flood with vinegar and neat oil
Jet lag	Lavender, rosemary, grapefruit	Bath, shower, massage
Muscles, aching	Lavender, rosemary, ginger	Bath, massage
Prickly heat or rashes	Geranium, lavender, witch hazel	Lotion
Sprains, strains	Lavender, chamomile, witch hazel	Compress for four days
Sunburn	Lavender	Bath, neat
Sunstroke	Lavender, eucalyptus, lemon	Cold water sheet wrap
Toothache	Chamomile lotion	Massage on gum, spit out
Travel sickness	Peppermint or ginger	Inhalation, drink
Tummy troubles	Ginger, peppermint	Inhalation, stomach massage
Vomiting	Peppermint or ginger	Inhalation, drink
Wounds	Lavender, tea tree, witch hazel	Lotion

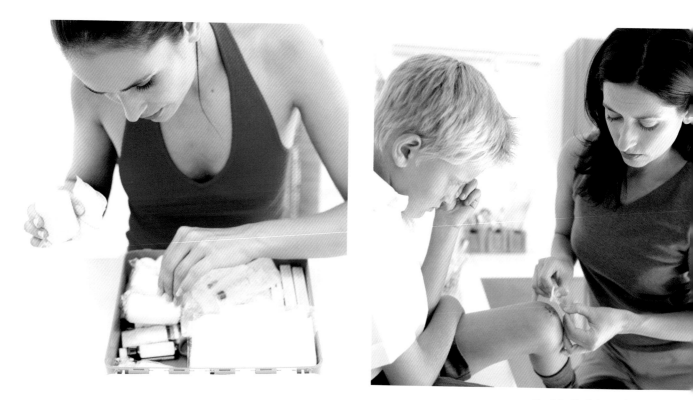

Top left: *Don't just stock the first-aid box for kids. Adults hurt themselves too.*

Top right: *Try giving injured children a tissue infused with a suitable essential oil to calm them while you deal with the wound.*

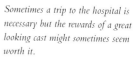

Sometimes a trip to the hospital is necessary but the rewards of a great looking cast might sometimes seem worth it.

Key to first-aid treatments

Massage	Four drops total of oils in one teaspoon almond oil
Inhalation	Sniff straight from the bottle
Compress	Four drops total of oils on cold, wet cloth, wring cloth to distribute oils
Wash	Three drops total of oils to one cup warm water
Bath	5-10 drops total of oils in one teaspoon almond oil. Add to bath
Drink	One drop oil in one cup warm water, stir vigorously before drinking
Neat	Oil may be applied neat
Lotion	Mix four drops total of oils with one teaspoon with hazel
Shower	Sprinkle three drops total of oils on wet wash cloth. Rub briskly over body.

Neck injuries can be very serious. Always see a health professional if neck pain persists.

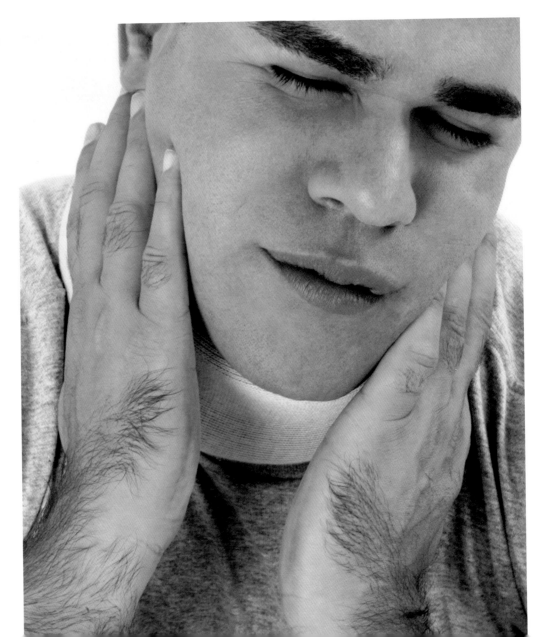

What to do about

Fever

Fever is the way the body reacts to defend itself against infection. Left to run its natural course, fever can heal the body—a temperature of 102–104°F (39–40°C) can help shorten the duration of the complaint. If the temperature soars or continues for more than two days you may need to reduce it by encouraging sweating, or giving the patient cool baths or sponge baths and this is where aromatherapy helps.

ESSENTIAL OILS
Lavender, tea tree, eucalyptus, peppermint

Treatment to promote sweating
Add 5–10 drops of mixed lavender and tea tree essential oils (depending on the patient's age) to a warm bath. For a sponge bath, add three to four drops of mixed lavender and tea tree essential oils to a bowl of warm water.

Treatment to soothe a fever or headache
Use three to four drops of mixed lavender and tea tree essential oil as a cool compress on the forehead and temple.

Treatment to reduce a temperature
Add two drops of lavender, one drop of peppermint, and one drop eucalyptus essential oils to a small bowl of cool (not cold) water, and sponge the body and head at hourly intervals.

Soak the feet in a warm eucalyptus foot bath for 10–15 minutes with six drops of eucalyptus essential oil mixed thoroughly into the water.

Nausea and vomiting

Nausea and that awful feeling of wanting to vomit can be the result of smelling something putrid, seeing something really distressing, overeating or drinking, fever, migraine, early pregnancy, or simple motion sickness.

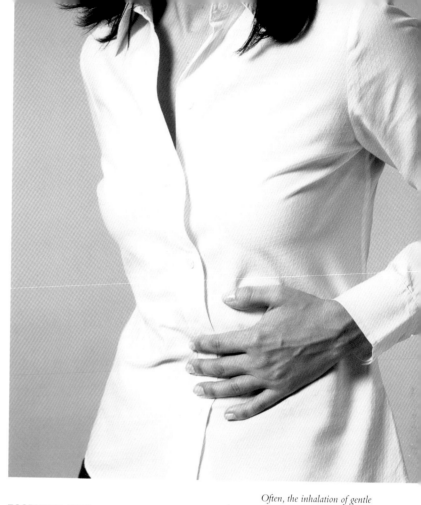

ESSENTIAL OILS
Peppermint, lavender.

Treatment
Put two drops peppermint or lavender oil in a paper bag. Place the open bag over the nose and mouth and inhale deeply. If you don't have a paper bag, put one drop of the oil on the palm of your hand and rub your hands together. Cup the palms over your nose and mouth and inhale deeply.

Mix one drop of peppermint essential oil with one teaspoon honey in a glass. Fill the glass with warm water, mixing the contents well. Sip slowly.

Often, the inhalation of gentle essential oils can remove that awful sensation of nausea.

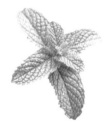

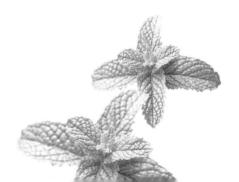

ESSENTIAL OIL POISONING

Always bear in mind that the essential oils are potentially lethal if swallowed—even $\frac{1}{4}$ teaspoon could kill a child. There is no such thing as a "child proof," merely a child-resistant cap. Children are persistent and patient and will spend an extraordinary length of time to solve a problem that interests them. Children are also curious and impatient, they rarely smell the contents of a bottle, and rarely sip; the bottle is up-ended and the contents gulped. This has led to several recorded fatalities.

The following suggestions are appropriate if essential oils are swallowed, spilt undiluted on the skin, or rubbed into the eyes of a child or adult.

FIRST-AID PROCEDURES

Try to find someone (a neighbor or other person) to begin the treatment below while you telephone the Poison Control or Information Center in your area.

Keep the number handy to the telephone and in all first-aid kits.

Have the particular bottle of essential oil with you when you telephone. You will be asked a list of questions that may include some of the following:

- Age and weight of patient?
- What oil has been swallowed?
- Was the oil undiluted or diluted with another liquid? If diluted, what percentage dilution?
- How much oil has been swallowed?
- How long ago did the accident happen?
- What has been done so far in the way of treatment?
- Are there any symptoms?

Do not wait to find out this information before calling the center. It's best to get someone else to gain the information while you call or handle each question as it arises.

Do not induce vomiting.

Don't give milk or oil to drink as the fat contents may accelerate the rate of absorption of the oils.

Wash the mouth out with lots of cool water, spit the water out.

If undiluted essential oil has been spilt on the skin, wash the area with soap and constantly running warm water until all traces of the oil have disappeared from the skin.

If essential oil has been rubbed into the eyes, run cool running water over the eyes for 10–15 minutes.

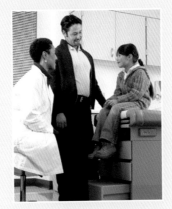

Fainting

A cup of peppermint tea is a good restorative for someone who has awoken from a faint.

Alternatively, hold a bottle of any of the following oils under the nose, or sprinkle a few drops on a tissue or handkerchief for the patient to sniff regularly: Lavender, marjoram, or rosemary.

To aid recovery, massage two to three drops of lavender oil on the temples (keep away from the eyes).

If the patient is unconscious, rub Dr Bach's Rescue Remedy (see page 414) on the inner side of the wrist. Repeat at 10 minute intervals until the patient is recovered. If the patient is conscious, place four drops of the remedy under the tongue.

ESSENTIAL OILS

Lavender, marjoram, peppermint.

Treatment

Put a few drops of one of the recommended essential oils on a tissue and hold just under the nose of the person who is feeling faint (or has fainted), or encourage them to gently sniff the aroma from the oil bottle.

Massage two to three drops of lavender essential oil on their temples, keeping the oil well away from their eyes.

SMELLING SALTS

20 drops marjoram essential oil
10 drops peppermint essential oil
20 drops lavender essential oil
4 tablespoons coarse sea salt crystals

To make and use

Mix the oils together and sprinkle over the sea salt crystals.

Pack mixture into a small jar and seal tightly.

Sniff the contents to restore equilibrium when feeling faint.

Smelling salts are also useful for relieving tension headaches.

Shock

In addition to essential oils, every first-aid box should have a bottle of Dr Bach's Rescue Remedy (see page 414).

ESSENTIAL OILS
Chamomile, peppermint, lavender.

Treatment
Drip a few drops of Rescue Remedy under the tongue and massage two or three drops on the inside of the wrists.

Sprinkle a couple of drops of peppermint essential oil onto a tissue and inhale deeply.

If possible, run a deep warm bath and add five drops of chamomile essential oil and five drops lavender essential oil dissolved in 1 teaspoon grape seed oil. Agitate the water to disperse. Allow the patient to soak for at least 30 minutes.

Convalescence

Convalescence can range from a few days of feeling weak after a bad cold to weeks of recovery from serious illness, an accident, or an operation. Aromatherapy can help speed up the recovery process by increasing the body's own defenses. The oils will increase appetite, strengthen nerves, and generally regenerate the bodily system. The Pick-Me-Up Blend is a tonic, gently stimulating and raising energy.

ESSENTIAL OILS
Geranium, ginger, grapefruit, lavender, lemon, rosemary, thyme.

PICK-ME-UP BLEND
$^1/_4$ cup (60 ml) sweet almond oil
20 drops grapefruit essential oil
10 drops lavender or geranium essential oil
10 drops rosemary essential oil
5 drops lemon essential oil
5 drops thyme or ginger essential oil

To make and use
Mix all the oils together in a small, labeled bottle, and shake to blend.

Leave for four days before using, so that the oils have time to synergize or combine well.

Float one teaspoon of the blend on a little warm water in a bowl and use for a gentle massage. The patient may feel too weak for a full massage in which case a hand, foot, and/or back massage may be the best treatment.

Pour two teaspoons of the blend into a bath or foot bath, agitate to disperse and soak in the bath for 30 minutes, massaging any floating oil droplets into the skin. Pour a little of the blend into the palm of your hand and massage over your body after showering, while the skin is still damp.

Alternatively, you can simply blend the essential oils together to use as an air spray or in an oil burner.

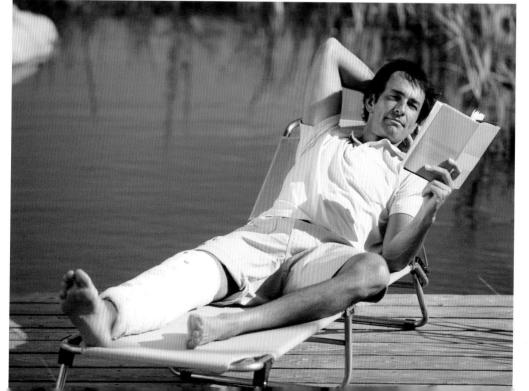

Speed your convalescence with the use of good home-made massage oils and the inhalation of essential oils.

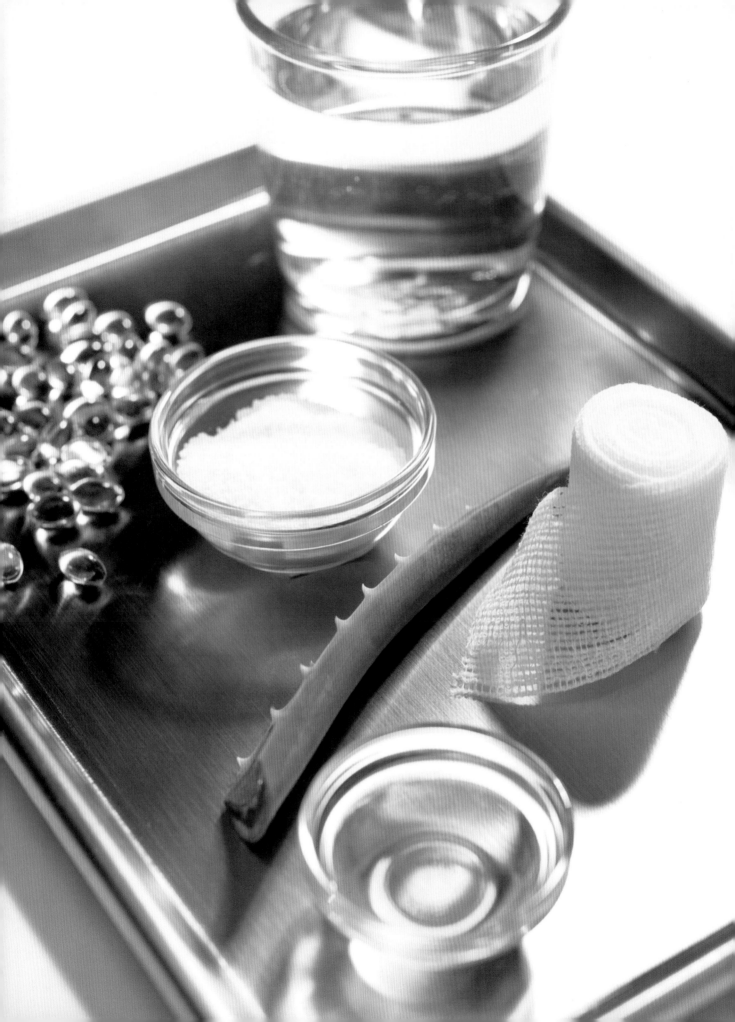

Ailments and remedies

Along with the joy of daily living, unfortunately our lives are also filled with ailments, from minor…to serious. Although we have excellent medical practitioners to assist and heal these complaints, sometimes they need a little help from nature. The remedies here are designed to take the edge off aches and pains and, in the case of minor ailments, they may even alleviate the problem completely.

Always consult a medical professional if the complaint is severe or persists past a day or so. Inform your doctor what remedies you have been using so that they can be combined with the regular medicines you receive and not inhibit their curative powers.

Skin deep

Abrasions and cuts

Abrasions are not usually serious but they can be very painful, as nerve endings have been abraded. They usually heal quickly and just need careful cleansing.

ESSENTIAL OILS

Lavender, tea tree, manuka

TREATMENT

Thoroughly clean the abrasion with Antiseptic Wound Wash (see page 426) using single or mixed oils or use Antiseptic Vinegar. Repeat every two hours. Unless the wound is bleeding profusely, or is an area that will get dirty, it's best to leave the wound uncovered. If a plaster is needed use one drop of lavender, tea tree, or manuka essential oil on the plaster.

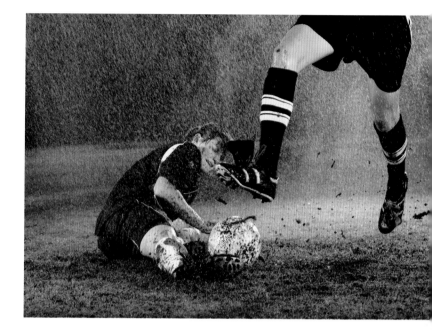

Contact sports are a major source of cuts and abrasions.

HERBAL ICE CUBES

It's useful to make herbal ice cubes so that a treatment is readily available when needed. For abrasions and cuts, drop a cube in a little boiled water and when dissolved swab the wound clean.

These provide an instant method of easing the pain of cuts, abrasions, minor burns, and sprains, and for reducing inflammation. The recipe which follows contains antibacterial and antiviral herbs, to help prevent infection.

To make, fill a pitcher (jug) with a mixture of as many as possible of the following chopped fresh herbs, or half-fill with dried, crumbled herbs. Use calendula, chamomile, comfrey leaf, lavender, mallow, plantain, rosemary, sage, thyme, and yarrow. (If you don't have all the herbs it doesn't matter.) Fill the pitcher with boiling water, cover and leave to go cold.

Strain the herbs through a sieve, squeezing them to extract as much liquid as possible, then strain again through coffee filter paper.

Freeze the liquid in ice-cube trays and when frozen decant into a freezer bag clearly labeled with the name of the remedy and the date frozen. The cubes can be kept frozen for up to 12 months.

To use on cuts, abrasions, minor burns, and inflammations, wrap as many cubes as needed in a handkerchief or similar piece of clean cloth, and apply to the wound. To use in compresses, drop three or four cubes in enough water to dissolve them. To use in fomentations, drop three or four cubes in enough boiling water to dissolve them.

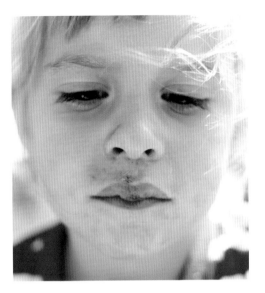

Dab grazes and weeping wounds with Antiseptic Vinegar to dry them out.

ANTISEPTIC VINEGAR

This is a useful addition to the medicine and first-aid cupboard; it is used to wash and disinfect wounds of all types and can also help to ease itching.

$\frac{1}{2}$ cup (125 ml) cider vinegar
$\frac{1}{2}$ cup (125 ml) distilled or purified water
30 drops tea tree essential oil
30 drops lavender essential oil

To make and use

Mix together in a dark-colored bottle. Shake well to blend.

Pour a little onto a absorbant cotton (cotton-wool) ball and use it to swab the affected area.

Always bandage a deep wound before taking the patient to the hospital or surgery.

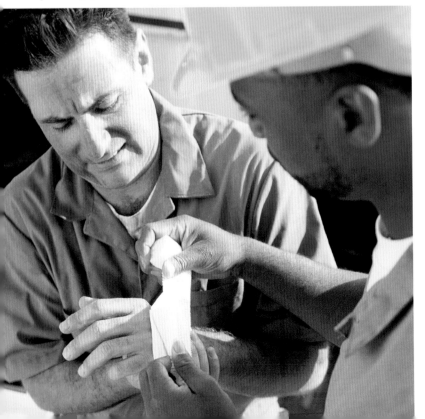

ANTISEPTIC WOUND WASH

Wound washes are used to cleanse wounds which are contaminated with dirt. They are made by adding 5–10 drops (depending on the age of the patient) of essential oil (such as lavender, tea tree, or manuka) to $\frac{1}{2}$ cup (125 ml) of warm or cold pre-boiled water. The water should be agitated before being used, to avoid the possibility of "hot spots" of oil.

HEALING BLEND

4 teaspoons (20 ml) distilled witch hazel
1 cup (250 ml) cooled strong calendula tea
OR
1 teaspoon (5 ml) calendula tincture in 1 cup (250 ml) cooled boiled water.

To make and use

Mix the ingredients together and use the blend to wash dirt from the abrasion.

Smooth aloe vera or calendula ointment over the area, and cover with a non-stick dry dressing.

Wounds

If a cut is very deep and needs stitches, cover the wound with a firm dressing onto which you have dripped distilled witch hazel and two drops of tea tree oil. Bandage in place and get to the nearest hospital or surgery.

If the wound is dirty, it should be gently washed using a herbal ice cube dissolved in boiled water, or one drop each of lemon, lavender, and geranium oil to $\frac{1}{2}$ cup (125 ml) of boiled water and $\frac{1}{2}$ cup (125 ml) of distilled witch hazel.

Use as many as possible of the following herbs made into a poultice, wash, fomentation, compress, or an ointment: Calendula, mallow, oregano, mullein, plantain, rosemary, yarrow.

ESSENTIAL OILS

Geranium, lavender, lemon, tea tree

TREATMENT

Add one drop each of geranium, lavender, lemon, and tea tree essential oils to $\frac{1}{2}$ cup (125 ml) boiled water and bathe the wound with this blend.

Drip two drops of tea tree essential oil on a firm sterile pad of gauze, and apply to the wound if bleeding persists. Bandage in place.

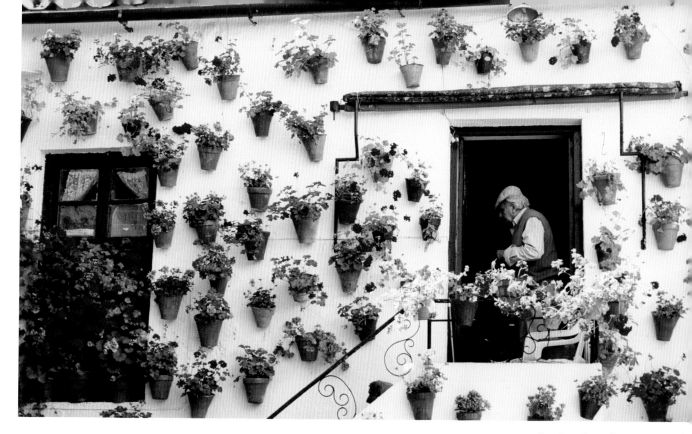

To stop bleeding

ESSENTIAL OILS
Geranium, lemon, cypress

TREATMENT
Fold a piece of cloth into a pad a little bigger than the wound. Apply as a cold compress containing any of the above essential oils. Bandage the pad firmly, but not too tightly, in place. If bleeding doesn't stop, reapply the compress and seek professional help.

Scar tissue

ESSENTIAL OILS
Frankincense, lavender, helichrysum, sandalwood

SCAR TISSUE OIL
Patience will be rewarded with this treatment.

4 teaspoons (20 ml) wheat germ oil
2 x 500iu vitamin E oil capsules
3 drops each frankincense, lavender, helichrysum, and sandalwood essential oils

To make and use
Pierce and squeeze the vitamin E capsules into the wheat germ oil in a small, labeled bottle.

Add the essential oils. Mix well. If possible, leave for four days to synergize.

Massage a little of the blend into the scar twice daily, as long as is needed.

Blisters

ESSENTIAL OILS
Lavender, tea tree

TREATMENT
Apply two drops neat of either lavender or tea tree essential oil. Pat in gently.

Don't break the blister unless it's very big. If you have the break the blister, use a needle that has been sterilized in a flame, then press the skin flat and apply a drop of lavender essential oil and a plaster.

Black eyes

TREATMENT
In a small bowl, drop one ice cube in two teaspoons witch hazel. Stir until the ice is melted and the mixture well blended. Cut lint into a suitable shape to cover the blackened area and soak in the mixture. Squeeze until it is no longer dripping, and gently lay over the closed eye. Repeat when the pad gets warm.

Geranium oil is used in many wound treatments. Here geraniums grow all over a wall in Cordoba, Andalucia, Spain.

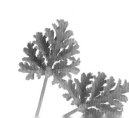

Bruises

Any of the following treatments can ease the pain and speed the healing of bruises.

* Apply an ice-cold compress of distilled witch hazel. Reapply for 8–10 hours.
* Apply a poultice made with crushed comfrey root.
* Gently massage the bruise with calendula ointment. Or, gently massage with arnica ointment (though not if the skin is broken).

ESSENTIAL OILS
Geranium, lavender

TREATMENT
Hold a bag of frozen peas or ice cubes wrapped in cloth on the area for a few minutes. Massage the area gently with a blend of four drops of either geranium or lavender oil in one teaspoon grape seed oil.

Bites and stings

Carry a bottle of lavender and tea tree oil with you if hiking. If swimming, add a spray bottle of vinegar to the kit, because essential oils are a quick way of dealing with insect bites and stings.

Bee stings

ESSENTIAL OILS
Chamomile, lavender

TREATMENT
Carefully scrape the sting out sideways, don't pull it out. If allergy is suspected go immediately to a hospital casualty department.

Mix one drop chamomile essential oil and one drop lavender essential oil with one teaspoon bicarbonate of soda (counteracts the acidity of the sting) with enough water to make a soft paste.

Apply the paste to the painful area hourly (or on the way to hospital).

The following suggestions can be used for gnat and sandfly bites too.

ESSENTIAL OIL
Lavender

TREATMENT
If bitten, apply neat lavender essential oil frequently to the bite until the pain is relieved.

INSECT AND MOSQUITO BITES

* Protect yourself from mosquito bites by wearing loose-fitting, long-sleeved clothes when outside in known mosquito areas or in the evening during summer—avoid dark clothes and perfume.
* Avoid being out of doors at dusk and dawn.
* Use a personal insect repellent lotion at all times when out of doors.
* Use mosquito nets around beds at night and screen windows.

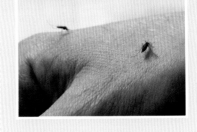

Insect repellents

ESSENTIAL OILS
Lavender, citronella, lemon, tea tree, peppermint

MOSQUITO AND SANDFLY REPELLENT
This is probably the only time that I would recommend using paraffin oil on the skin, the reason being that it remains effective, holding the essential oils on the skin for a longer time than grape seed oil, which is absorbed more quickly.

40 drops lavender essential oil
40 drops citronella essential oil
30 drops peppermint essential oil
$1/_4$ cup (60 ml) cider vinegar or distilled witch hazel
$1/_4$ cup (60 ml) paraffin oil

To make and use
Mix all the oils together in a small, labeled bottle and shake to blend.

Leave for four days before using so that the oils have time to synergize or combine well.

Smooth the repellent over all exposed areas. Keep well clear of eyes.

Re-apply every two to three hours.

Wasp stings

ESSENTIAL OIL
Lavender

TREATMENT
Add eight drops lavender essential oil to one teaspoon vinegar. Dab on sting to counteract the alkaline poison of the sting and reduce pain and swelling. Repeat hourly.

Spider bites

If you suspect the spider was of the poisonous variety, go straight to hospital, dabbing wound constantly with neat lavender essential oil until hospital treatment begins. It is important to identify the spider. Take the spider along in a jar, if possible.

ESSENTIAL OIL
Lavender

TREATMENT
Add five drops lavender essential oil to one teaspoon vinegar. Dab on bite hourly.

Dog bites

ESSENTIAL OILS
Tea tree, lavender

TREATMENT
Wash the area of the bite immediately and thoroughly (even if the skin isn't broken), with four drops of tea tree and/or lavender oil in water, then dab on a little neat tea tree essential oil and a dressing if necessary. If the skin is broken, go to the nearest doctor or hospital casualty department for further treatment.

Ticks and leeches

Ticks and leeches are disgusting when they choose your body on which to lunch. We spend quite a lot of our time in the tropics and both my husband and our dogs have played host to these creatures! Prevention is obviously better than cure, but in the case of ticks and leeches it's fairly difficult to deter them. The following recipe may help, but dressing sensibly is best. Wear long pants with socks pulled up over the bottom of the legs. Wear long sleeves with elastic bands around the wrists (not tight enough to restrict blood supply).

TREATMENT
No matter how anxious you are to get rid of them, don't just pull them off, as the head or teeth may remain embedded in your flesh and set up infections and irritations for a long time.

There are many ways for removing leeches and ticks, but we found that it works well if you sprinkle plenty of salt on the creature, leave for a minute and then follow with plenty of tea tree essential oil dripped onto the head and body. Hold the body gently with a pair of tweezers and slowly twist until the whole animal releases its grip.

Apply more neat tea tree or lavender essential oil to prevent infection and treat with the oil for several days.

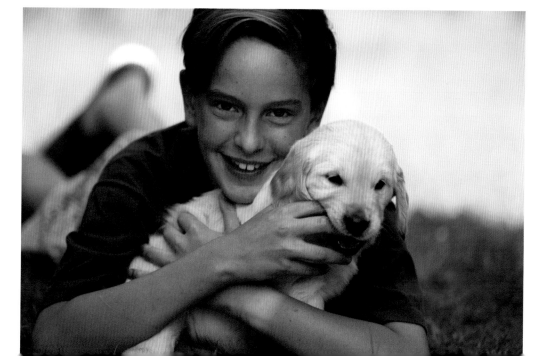

Dog bites should be treated immediately by washing thoroughly.

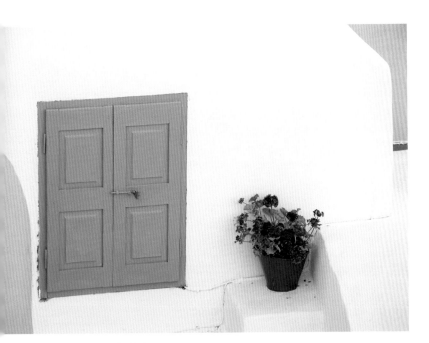

Geraniums make a colorful display on a wall in Santorini, Greece. Their decorative value is equaled by the value of the essential oil obtained from them.

TICK REPELLENT OIL BLEND

40 drops lavender essential oil
40 drops lemon tea tree essential oil
20 drops peppermint essential oil
10 drops marjoram essential oil
$\frac{1}{4}$ cup (60 ml) cider vinegar or distilled witch hazel
$\frac{1}{4}$ cup (60 ml) paraffin oil

To make and use

Mix all the oil together in a labeled bottle. Shake well before use.

Rub on all exposed areas of the body.

Reapply every two to three hours.

Minor burns and scalds

Moderate to severe burns need urgent medical attention. If there is clothing stuck to the burn, make no attempt to remove it. Hold the burned area under cold water or apply cold compresses for at least 10 minutes to reduce the heat in the area.

For minor burns and scalds over a small area, reduce the heat by holding the burned area under cold water or ice cold compresses for 10 minutes. Then apply neat aloe gel (split open the leaf and apply the gel directly to the burn) and honey, which should be dabbed on gently. Repeat at 10–15 minute intervals if needed.

Drink six to eight glasses of water a day to maintain good health.

DR CHRISTOPHER'S BURN REMEDY

4 teaspoons (20 ml) comfrey root powder
4 teaspoons (20 ml) wheat germ oil
4 teaspoons (20 ml) honey

To make and use

Stir the comfrey, oil, and honey together and apply gently but liberally to the burn.

Wrap in gauze to hold it on. Replenish as necessary.

Carry on with the treatment until the burn is completely healed and it will prevent scarring.

If you get tired of wearing a bandage, you can start applying wheat germ oil or vitamin E alone on the burn after most of the healing work has been accomplished by the ointment. This period is identified by absence of pain and general tissue healing to the point that the skin has reformed and closed, with a scab or pinkish red skin. Keep applying the oil on a daily basis until you cannot identify where the burn was.

ESSENTIAL OILS

Lavender, niaouli

TREATMENT

For minor burns, cool then dab lavender or niaouli essential oil or honey gently on the burn area. Repeat at 10–15 minute intervals.

Rashes

Urticaria

Also known as nettle rash or hives, urticaria is characterized by angry, red, raised welts on the skin that are very itchy, and is triggered by an allergic reaction that releases histamines. The amount of essential oil used in treatment is less than for many complaints as the skin is very sensitive and a high percentage of oil could irritate.

ESSENTIAL OILS

Bergamot, lavender, chamomile

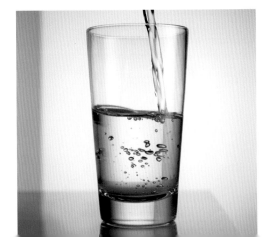

TREATMENT

Mix two drops of each of the recommended essential oils with one teaspoon grape seed oil and add to a bath. Massage floating drops of oil on the affected areas. Mix two drops of each essential oil in two teaspoons grape seed oil for topical application.

Mix four drops lavender essential oil in two teaspoons cider vinegar and apply topically to ease itching. Apply a compress using chamomile essential oil. Repeat every few hours.

If the rash covers a large area, it may be more appropriate to soak in a lukewarm bath to which is added $\frac{1}{2}$ cup bicarbonate of soda and six drops chamomile essential oil.

Make a tea of chamomile, cool to lukewarm, and use as a compress on the area. If the rash covers a large area, soak in a lukewarm bath to which you have added 1 quart (1 liter) of very strong chamomile tea mixture with half a cup of bicarbonate of soda.

Heat rash

Heat rash is an itchy, uncomfortable rash that occurs during hot weather when skin hasn't been able to "breathe" and sweat to evaporate. Wear natural fibers such as cotton and loose or as little clothing as possible.

ESSENTIAL OILS

Eucalyptus, lavender

TREATMENT

Add eight drops lavender essential oil to one cup bicarbonate of soda, mix well and add to a warm bath. Agitate the water to dissolve the powder. Soak for as long as you like, keeping the itchy rash under water. After bathing, pat rather than rub the skin dry. If the sufferer is a child, see Children and Babies, page 386, for the amount of essential oil to use and adjust the amount of bicarbonate of soda.

HEAT RASH ANTI-ITCH SPRAY

3 tablespoons (45 ml) distilled witch hazel
6 drops essential oil
6 drops eucalyptus essential oil
1 cup (250 ml) water

To make and use

Mix the witch hazel and essential oils in a labeled, spray bottle. Shake well to blend. Add the water and shake once more.

The spray needs shaking every time before use. Spray the affected areas with the blend and allow to air dry.

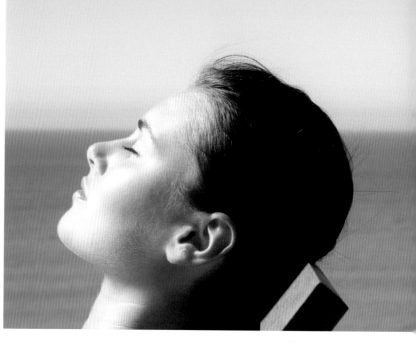

We should only expose our skin to sunlight for 10 minutes early morning and late afternoon.

Sunburn

We should all now be completely aware of the dangers of overexposure to sunlight. We only need to expose our skin to sunshine for 10 minutes a day in the early morning or late afternoon to achieve the necessary manufacture of vitamin D in our skin.

ESSENTIAL OILS

Lavender, chamomile

TREATMENT

If the face and head are burned, apply cool compresses using the essential oils. Run a cool bath deep enough to submerge the body up to the neck. Add 10 drops of either chamomile or lavender essential oil (depending on age) to one teaspoon vegetable oil, and disperse into the water. Stay in the bath 15–30 minutes. Pat dry. Smooth Sunburn Blend all over the burned skin. Be very gentle when applying it, or the skin will be even more painful! Apply neat lavender essential oil to any sunburned blistered areas.

SUNBURN BLEND

4 teaspoons (20 ml) aloe vera gel or juice
1 teaspoon grape seed oil
20 drops lavender essential oil

To make and use

Mix oils in a bowl and beat together well with aloe vera. Beat "left-overs" before reapplying.

TIP SQUEEZING THE OIL FROM VITAMIN E CAPSULES ON THE BURN AREA THE DAY AFTER THE FIRST-AID TREATMENT DESCRIBED WILL FACILITATE SWIFT AND SCAR-FREE HEALING.

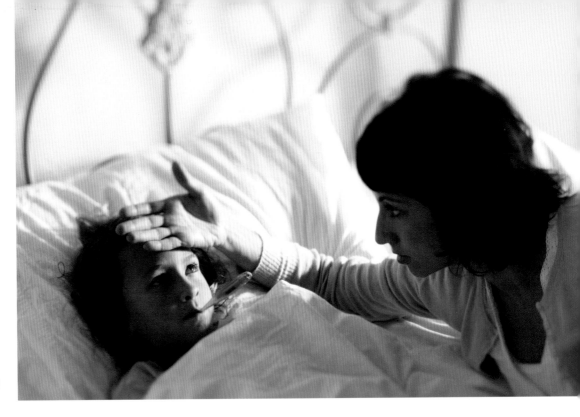

Children are very prone to high temperatures and should be treated quickly to avoid complications.

Viruses

Warts and verrucas

Warts and verrucas (plantar warts on the soles of the feet) are caused by a virus. If you suffer from either recurrent or a large number of warts or verrucas, your immune system may need help.

The best treatment for warts is to make the body pay attention to them by applying either of the following treatments. The body will be alerted and will begin to fight the virus and the warts.

Use the white latex that oozes out when the stalk of the dandelion flower or fig is snapped. Apply one drop only onto the wart, taking care not to get any on the surrounding skin. Cover with a sticking plaster. Repeat twice daily until the wart has completely gone.

If the skin is dry where the wart dropped off, the contents of a vitamin E capsule may be squeezed onto the area and gently massaged into the area.

ESSENTIAL OILS
Tea tree, lemon, calendula infused oil

TREATMENT
Paint one drop of tea tree or lemon essential oil directly onto the wart and cover with a sticking plaster. Repeat treatment twice daily until the wart has gone. If the skin is very dry afterwards, massage the skin with a little calendula infused oil.

Herpes

There are numerous viruses in the herpes family. *Herpes simplex* is the one responsible for those painful blisters that turn into sores on the lips (called cold sores), vulva, anus, or buttocks. This virus tends to recur and can be triggered by stress, too much sun, and minor infections.

ESSENTIAL OILS
Lavender, manuka, melissa, myrrh, tea tree

TREATMENT
Dab blisters and sores with one drop of neat essential oil chosen from the recommended list. If the blisters are on the vulva or anus, add three drops tea tree essential oil to one teaspoon unscented gel, mix very well and gently apply to external lesions with a cotton bud.

In the case of outbreaks, use aloe vera gel or hypericum ointment if the area is very sensitive. Repeat three times daily.

Dab tincture of myrrh frequently on lip lesions.

Recent tests show that lemon balm is useful in helping to heal the blisters and sores of genital herpes. Use it in an ointment or an infused oil.

Bacterial and fungal infections

Abcesses

An abscess is a localized, pus-filled cavity created by bacterial invasion.

ESSENTIAL OILS

Chamomile, lavender, tea tree

ABSCESS FOMENTATION

$\frac{1}{2}$ cup (125 ml) hot water
4 drops tea tree essential oil
3 drops lavender essential oil
3 drops chamomile essential oil

To make and use

Pour the water into a bowl and add the oils. Apply fomentation every two hours.

SLIPPERY ELM POULTICE

Make a hot poultice from slippery elm powder, mashed potato or bread, and any of the following herbs you have available: Garlic, hyssop, marjoram, oregano, sage, yarrow.

Apply as hot as can be borne. Reapply every two to three hours.

Boils and carbuncles

Boils are a staphylococcal infection. Treatment aims to bring the boil to a head, allow the pus to escape and the area to heal. If a fever develops or red lines radiate out from the boil, professional help is needed. Boils are very contagious.

* The patient should avoid handling and preparing food while infection is present.
* Any clothes in contact with the area should be washed separately. Add a few drops of tea tree or lavender essential oil to the washing and rinsing water.

ESSENTIAL OILS

Bergamot, lavender, tea tree

TREATMENT

Wash three times daily with two drops bergamot essential oil and three drops lavender essential oil in $\frac{1}{4}$ cup (60 ml) warm, boiled water. Dip absorbent cotton (cottonwool) into the mixture and use to wash the boil and surrounding area. Apply a fomentation twice a day using the above oils. Keep the boil covered with a non-stick dressing, on which two drops of tea tree essential oil have been sprinkled.

Take 1,000 mg garlic oil capsule three times daily.

Take $\frac{1}{2}$ teaspoon (2.5 ml) fluid extract of echinacea three times daily.

Mix slippery elm powder or potato mashed with calendula tea and apply as a hot poultice twice a day until the boil bursts.

OR

Apply a fomentation of 3 tablespoons (45 ml) of Epsom salts in 1 cup (250 ml) of hot water. Repeat every three to four hours until the boil comes to a head and bursts, then apply calendula ointment and a non-stick dressing.

Make triple-strength calendula tea or add 2 teaspoons (10 ml) of calendula tincture to $\frac{1}{2}$ cup (125 ml) of warm water. Add 4 drops of tea tree oil and wash the area using absorbent cotton (cottonwool). Dispose of the cotton down the toilet. Add five drops of tea tree oil to one teaspoon of vegetable oil and smooth on after the wash. Wash the hands well after finishing the treatment.

Add 10 drops of tea tree oil to water to soak clothing that has been in contact with the infected area. Wash separately.

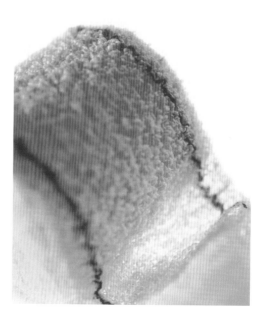

Open infections should be kept covered with a sterile dressing, into which a few drops of appropriate essential oil have been added.

Whitlow

A whitlow is a very painful infection that develops down the side, and sometimes under, the nails. Pus collects, and the pressure sometimes necessitates removal of the nail. Early treatment can often cure the problem before such drastic action is needed.

ESSENTIAL OILS

Lavender, tea tree, thyme

TREATMENT

Put one cup of hot boiled water into a small bowl. When the water is cool enough to be tolerated, add two drops tea tree essential oil and two drops thyme essential oil and stir vigorously. Immerse the finger for a few minutes in the mixture, then dry gently and drip neat lavender essential oil on the affected part. Cover the area of the whitlow with a non-stick "breathable" dressing. Repeat the treatment three times a day.

Impetigo

Impetigo is very contagious. The weeping blisters which crust over are sometimes known as school sores. The infection is produced by the *Streptococcus* bacterium. Swift intervention is absolutely essential to prevent the condition spreading to other parts of the body and other people. Often the sores won't clear without orthodox treatment. Essential oils can be an effective adjunct to orthodox treatment.

ESSENTIAL OILS

Myrrh, goldenseal infused oil, echinacea infused oil

TREATMENT

Add these essential and infused oils to the Orange Moisture Lotion recipe (see page 266) and apply the ointment regularly.

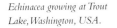

Echinacea growing at Trout Lake, Washington, USA.

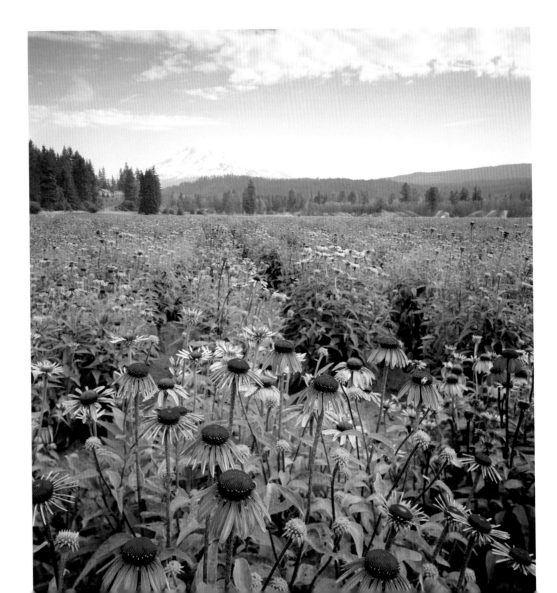

Ringworm

Ringworm is not actually a worm but a highly contagious fungal skin condition. It is an itchy rash that appears in the shape of a red ring. It often affects the scalp and can cause hair to fall out. Very strict hygiene needs to be observed in order to prevent the spread of the problem.

To help combat ringworm, try any of the following remedies.

Take a 1,000 mg garlic oil capsule three times a day.

Take $^1/_2$ teaspoon (2.5 ml) of echinacea liquid extract three times a day.

Take a daily dose of 500 mg of vitamin C with bioflavoids.

In the early stages, drip calendula tincture alternately with myrrh tincture directly onto the ringworm. Leave the tincture to dry on the skin. As the infection dries out, use calendula, echinacea, and goldenseal ointment.

ESSENTIAL OILS

Tea tree, myrrh, lavender

TREATMENT

Dab the ringworm with neat tea tree, lavender, and myrrh essential oils several times daily for a few days. Alternate which oils you use. When the moist stage has passed, massage the area with equal parts of tea tree, lavender, and olive oil. The olive oil will help to prevent excessive drying out of the skin.

Itching (pruritis)

The most embarrassing and awkward itch is pruritus ani or itching of the anus or vulva as you can't scratch it in public! Causes can range from inadequate washing or inadequate rinsing away of soap, antibiotics, allergic reaction to chemicals in toilet paper and toiletries, or from wearing synthetic fabrics.

Because the area is warm, dark, and moist, it is the perfect breeding ground for fungi and bacteria.

Fill a bath with enough warm water to cover the lower hips. Add one cup of bicarbonate of soda and one quart (one liter)

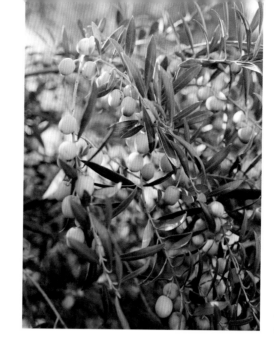

Olive tree bearing fruit. Olive oil helps to prevent skin drying out during treatment for ringworm.

of very strong chamomile tea. Sit in the bath for up to 10 minutes. Dry gently and apply the powder recommended below.

ANTI-ITCH POWDER

4 teaspoons (20 ml) dried lavender flowers
4 teaspoons (20 ml) dried chickweed leaves
4 teaspoons (20 ml) dried calendula petals
4 teaspoons (20 ml) dried chamomile flowers
4 teaspoons (20 ml) dried plantain leaves
$1^1/_2$ cups cornstarch (cornflour)
tea tree oil

To make and use

Grind the herbs to a powder, add the cornstarch and pass through a very fine sieve.

Add 10 drops of tea tree oil a few drops at a time, stirring constantly to prevent lumping.

Store in a labeled, airtight container.

Use absorbent cotton (cottonwool) dipped into the powder to dust the area after bathing, showering, or washing. Discard and use fresh cotton each time.

Another remedy is to make a chickweed ointment and apply gently to the itchy parts.

ESSENTIAL OILS

Bergamot, chamomile, lavender, myrrh, tea tree

ANTI-ITCH WASHING BLEND

1 cup (250 ml) water
1 drop lavender essential oil
1 drop tea tree essential oil

To make

Add the oils to the water and agitate just prior to using.

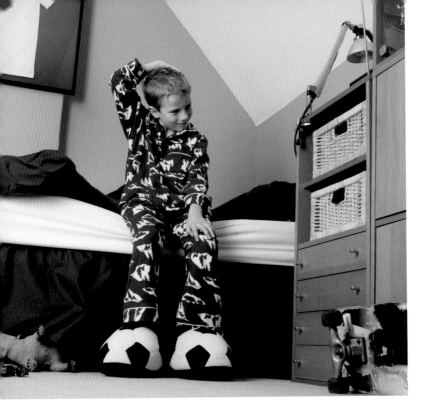

Unfortunately children get head lice, even when everything seems clean. The remedies here will help, without the use of strong chemicals.

TIP WEAR UNDER-CLOTHES MADE FROM NATURAL FIBERS AND AVOID WEARING PANTS OR JEANS THAT ARE TIGHT IN THE CROTCH.

ANTI-ITCH MASSAGE BLEND

4 teaspoons (20 ml) grape seed oil or unscented gel
6 drops lavender essential oil
6 drops chamomile or bergamot essential oil

To make and use

Mix the ingredients together in a small, labeled bottle or jar, shaking or stirring well to blend.

Dip absorbent cotton (cottonwool) in the Anti-Itch Washing Blend (see page 435) and clean the affected area after going to the toilet.

Apply Anti-Itch Massage Blend after bathing, showering, or washing. Stir well before use

Insects

Scabies

Scabies is an intensively itchy skin condition caused by a tiny insect that burrows beneath the skin and lays its eggs. It is difficult to treat and you may need medical help. It is essential to wash all clothing, towels, and bedding in very hot water. Add eucalyptus essential oil to the washing and rinse water and dry in the sun. Wipe mattresses and pillows with a mixture of tea tree, clove, and lavender essential oils, and dry in sun.

ESSENTIAL OILS

Bergamot, clove, lavender, lemon grass, peppermint

SCABIES OINTMENT

1 cube (12–14 g) beeswax
1$^1/_2$ oz (40 g) anhydrous lanolin
3 tablespoons (45 ml) olive oil or (even better)
 calendula infused oil
$^1/_2$ teaspoon tincture of calendula
20 drops bergamot essential oil
40 drops lavender essential oil
20 drops peppermint essential oil
10 drops rosemary essential oil
10 drops clove essential oil

To make and use

Melt the beeswax gently, taking care that it does not overheat.

Add the lanolin and stir until melted. Slowly add the olive or calendula infused oil; don't re-harden the wax. Take off heat, cool slightly.

Mix together the calendula tincture and essential oils and add slowly while stirring thoroughly to incorporate until the mixture is just beginning to thicken. Pour into labeled jars.

This ointment has a much higher proportion of essential oil than is usual. Apply very frequently but take care to use only on the affected areas of skin.

Head lice

Lice have always been, and will continue to be, a problem among school-age children. Young children are cosy creatures, they get their heads together to share secrets, caps, combs, and head lice. Broad spectrum treatment is needed, because if the nits (eggs) of head lice aren't destroyed then the problem will recur.

Essential oils are an excellent way of dealing with the problem, and you may notice that the percentage of oils is higher than that normally used. If there is any burning or discomfort to their skin, increase the amount of grape seed oil in the mixture from 3$^1/_2$ fl oz (100 ml) to $^1/_2$ cup (125 ml).

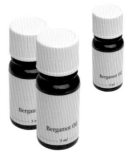

ESSENTIAL OILS

Bergamot, eucalyptus, geranium, lavender, rosemary

TREATMENT

Wash all bedding and personal clothes in very hot water. Add two teaspoons eucalyptus oil to the rinsing water. Hang in the sun for a whole day, turning inside out at intervals, so that every part of the material (particularly seams and hems) receive air and sun. Head lice hatch out at 48 hour intervals so the treatment of clothes and bedding will need to be carried out every two days until the problem no longer exists.

HEAD LICE OIL TREATMENT

3$\frac{1}{2}$ fl oz (100 ml) grape seed oil
30 drops eucalyptus essential oil
30 drops geranium essential oil
30 drops lavender essential oil

To make and use

Mix the oils together in a small, labeled bottle and shake to blend. Leave for four days before using so the oils have time to synergize or combine well.

Massage thoroughly into the hair and scalp; cover with a shower cap and leave on either all day or all night.

The following morning, shampoo the hair, and comb through with a fine tooth comb paying particular attention behind the ears and the back of the neck—this will help to get rid of head lice.

Add two drops of rosemary essential oil in the final rinse water.

When hair is dry, comb it with the cleaned fine tooth comb.

Repeat the process every two days for a week, but don't continue on a regular basis after that. Instead, to prevent re-infestation, use one of the shampoo recipes in the "Hair" section adding appropriate oil or oils from the list above.

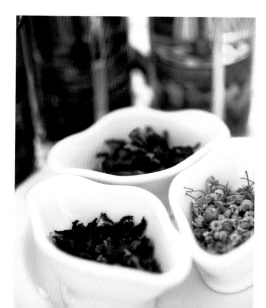

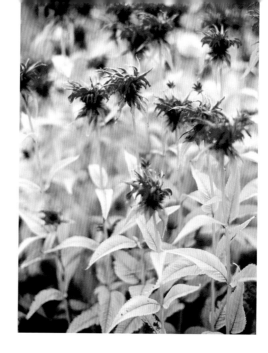

Red bergamot in flower. The flowers are crushed to make essential oil.

Headaches and migraine

Headaches

There are many reasons why headaches develop, some of these being indigestion, stress, muscle tension in the neck and back, eye strain, tiredness, and nasal congestion.

If a headache is persistent and a cause isn't obvious, it would be advisable to seek professional help (an optician if you suspect eyestrain, or a chiropractor if you feel that a spinal adjustment may be needed).

Foods that contain tyramine, an amino acid found in many foods, are often implicated in throbbing headaches or migraine and should be avoided. These foods are: Most alcoholic drinks, preserved meats (salamis, smoked meats, bacon, and ham), all cheeses (except cottage and ricotta cheese), chocolate, soy sauce, sour cream, and yeast concentrates.

Other foods that may cause headaches are those containing monosodium glutamate (often found in Chinese food and many very salty foods), pickles, and preservatives.

To ward off headaches:

* Drink eight glasses of filtered or bottled water daily. Taking a garlic oil capsule according to packet directions can also help.
* Drink chamomile or peppermint tea for headaches caused by digestive disorders.

Left: *Cloves, bergamot, and calendula flowers are all distilled to make essential oils for Scabies Ointment.*

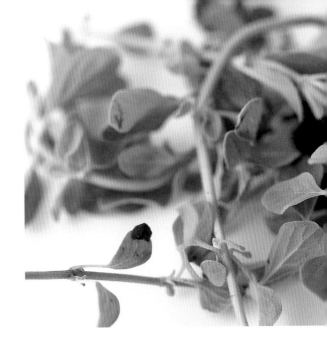

- Drink rosemary tea for headaches caused by mental or physical exhaustion.
- Make a very cold compress using a strong lavender and rosemary tea or vinegar. Lie down and place the compress over the forehead. Replace as it gets warm.
- Alternate hot and cold footbaths can also ease an aching head. Add two drops each of lavender, basil, and marjoram oil to the cold water, agitating well to disperse. Soak the feet for five minutes in each bath and repeat two or three times.
- A simple but often effective treatment for headache is a vinegar inhalation. Heat a tablespoon or so of vinegar and inhale the steam as it rises.

TIPS: ALTERNATE HOT AND COLD FOOTBATHS WILL OFTEN EASE A HEADACHE. MAKE AN INHALATION, USING TWO DROPS OF LAVENDER OR MARJORAM OIL IN 3 TABLESPOONS (45 ML) HOT VINEGAR. DECANT SOME "SMELLING BOTTLE FOR NERVOUS HEADACHES" OIL INTO A TINY BOTTLE YOU CAN CARRY WITH YOU; INHALE TO EASE HEADACHES, CLEAR THE BRAIN, AND LESSEN TENSION.

DECOCTION OR TINCTURE FOR HEADACHE

2 parts dandelion root and leaf
1 part milk thistle
1 part willow bark

To make and use

Make as a decoction or tincture.

Drink three cups daily of the decoction, or take 20 drops of tincture in water three times daily.

ESSENTIAL OILS

Nervous headaches: Lavender, marjoram, peppermint

Gastric headaches: Peppermint

HEADACHE MASSAGE AND BATH BLEND

4 teaspoons grape seed oil
8 drops lavender essential oil
5 drops marjoram essential oil
3 drops peppermint essential oil

To make and use

Mix all the oils together in a small bottle and shake to blend.

Leave for four days before using so that the oils have time to synergize or combine well.

Alternatively, blend the essential oils together to use as an air spray or in an oil burner.

SMELLING BOTTLE FOR NERVOUS HEADACHES

3 tablespoons cider vinegar
30 drops lavender essential oil
20 drops rosemary essential oil
15 drops peppermint essential oil
15 drops marjoram essential oil

To make and use

Mix all ingredients in a dark-colored, labeled glass bottle. Shake well. Leave for one week, shaking daily.

Strain the mixture through coffee filter paper. Add 3 tablespoons (45 ml) purified water.

Store in a cool, dark place.

TREATMENT

- Massage a few drops of Headache Massage and Bath Blend on the temples and the nape of the neck. Be careful not to get any in the eyes.
- Add two teaspoons of the Headache Massage and Bath Blend to a warm bath, and agitate the water. Soak for 30 minutes, inhaling the vapors and massaging the floating oil drops onto the back of the neck

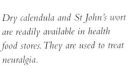

Dry calendula and St John's wort are readily available in health food stores. They are used to treat neuralgia.

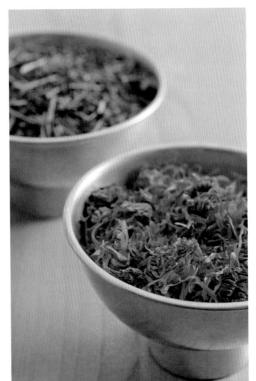

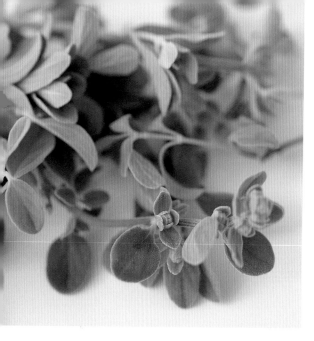

GASTRIC HEADACHES

- Massage the stomach and abdomen with two drops of peppermint essential oil in one teaspoon grape seed oil.
- Make an inhalation using peppermint essential oil.
- Add eight drops peppermint essential oil to one teaspoon vegetable oil. Pour into a warm bath, agitate the water to disperse. Soak for 30 minutes, massaging floating oil droplets into the back of the neck, the stomach, and abdomen.

Migraine

Migraine is not just a bad headache! There seems to be a range of causes including food allergy and stress.

ESSENTIAL OILS

Lavender, marjoram, peppermint

TREATMENT

Essential oil treatments are useful especially as preservative measures—usually by the time a migraine begins, migraine sufferers can't bear to be touched or tolerate smells.

Hot fomentations to the back of the neck using marjoram essential oil can help in the very early stages when the blood vessels are constricting, but only if the sufferer can bear it at this point.

Cold compresses of lavender and/or peppermint essential oil on the forehead may help when the blood vessels are dilating. Mix one teaspoon grape seed oil with five drops lavender and five drops peppermint essential oils. Pour the blend into a footbath of cold water; stir to disperse.

Soak the feet for 15 minutes while doing some stress-relieving deep breathing.

HERBS

Taking 2,000 mg of borage (starflower) oil or evening primrose oil daily has proved useful to many who suffer from migraines.

If the patient is open to the treatment, hot fomentation to the back of the neck using a strong, hot tea of marjoram and lavender will help in the very early stages when the blood vessels are constricting.

Cold compresses of lavender on the forehead may help when the blood vessels are dilating.

Passionflower and valerian are antispasmodic and sedative herbs that often reduce the severity of a migraine attack. Take as either capsules or a tincture, as the unpleasant taste of valerian tea might provoke nausea.

Feverfew is now being used extensively in the treatment of migraine. The effects may not be felt for a month or so, so it's important to persevere. Chew one fresh leaf one to three times a day or drink 15 drops of tincture in one tablespoon of water three times daily. In rare cases, chewing the leaf can cause mouth ulcers, so if this occurs discontinue use, and try taking the tincture instead.

Caution: *The leaves of fresh feverfew occasionally cause soreness of the mouth. Feverfew must not be used during pregnancy.*

TIP CONSULT A DIETITIAN REGARDING FOOD INTOLERANCE. LEARN STRESS MANAGEMENT TECHNIQUES.

Marjoram is a common herb in the treatment of headaches.

Migrane headaches are debilitating and should be treated seriously.

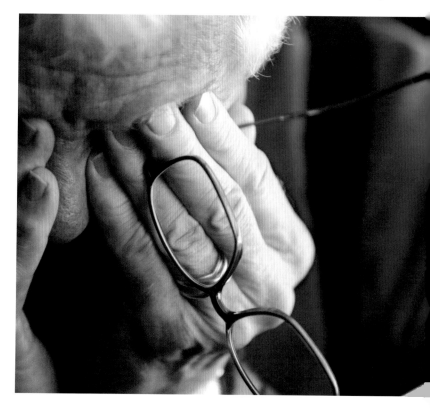

Neuralgia

Neuralgia is a pain originating in a nerve that radiates from the central nervous system. The pain, especially when in the face, can sometimes be intense. Any of the following treatments will help relieve it.

Apply a hot fomentation using cayenne (use one part cayenne to eight parts other herbs), chamomile, mullein, and wormwood. Repeat every hour until relief is obtained.

Massage the painful nerve or joint with infused oil of St John's wort.

Zostrix is a cream available in pharmacies. It contains capsaicin, an extract form of chilies, and is helpful in temporarily relieving the pain of neuralgia, arthritis, and the after-pain associated with shingles.

Take two willow bark capsules according to packet directions or two droppers full of tincture to ease pain and relax the nerves.

Make a hot tea of lavender, vervain, and rosemary, and drink three times daily. If you don't have all the herbs, just use what you have.

Fill a hot water bottle with boiling water. Put enough frozen peas in a plastic bag until about the size of a tennis ball; fasten with a rubber band. Hold the ball with a cloth or wear a glove, and massage the painful nerve or joint with the icy-cold bag for a minute or two. Now hold the hot water bottle on the area for the same length of time. Keep alternating the two for 10–15 minutes. This treatment often brings dramatic relief.

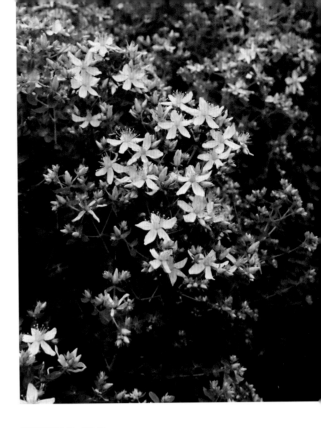

ESSENTIAL OILS
Chamomile, clove, lavender, marjoram
St John's wort infused oil

NEURALGIA MASSAGE OIL BLEND
4 teaspoons St John's wort infused oil or grape seed oil
6 drops lavender essential oil
6 drops chamomile essential oil
4 drops clove or marjoram essential oil

To make and use
Mix in a small bottle. Shake to blend.
Massage a few drops along the affected nerve.
Apply to a cold compress or hot fomentation using one drop of each oil, whichever works best for you.

Hangover

I don't suppose that there are many people reading this book who haven't experienced the pain and misery of a hangover at least once in their lives. My first (and last!) hangover occurred when I was 12 and was keeping my friend company while her parents when out to dinner.

The extremely well-stocked cocktail cabinet had always been a source of interest to us and this was the chance for which we had waited. We thought it safest to take a

St John's wort in flower. This is usually used as an infused oil.

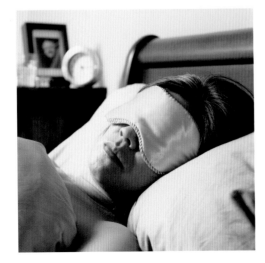

Shutting out the world and the light for a short while can often help overcome aches and pains.

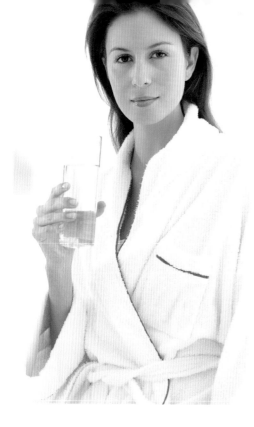

Water helps to combat the dehydration caused by the excess consumption of alcohol.

Sunstroke and heatstroke

Treat sunstroke as an emergency because it means that the body's heat regulation system isn't working. This causes the temperature to rise. The point of treatment is to cool the patient as quickly as possible.

ESSENTIAL OILS

Lavender, eucalyptus, lemon

TREATMENT

Reduce the patient's temperature in a bath of cool (not cold) water with:

6 drops lavender essential oil
2 drops eucalyptus essential oil
2 drops lemon essential oil
1 teaspoon vegetable oil

Mix together the essential oils then add the vegetable oil. Combine well.

Place very wet, cold compresses on the entire head during bathing, changing the compresses frequently to keep them cold.

Continue frequent cool showers or body sponging for up to 48 hours. Restore circulation, rubbing the arms and legs.

Encourage the patient to drink plenty of cool water (not iced) to replace lost body fluids. Add a tiny pinch of salt to each glass of water.

The fields of Provence, France, are a visual feast of lavender blooms in June every year.

little from each of the 20 or so bottles so that a lowered level wouldn't be detected. We each dressed in one of her mother's evening gowns and were complete with fur capes, boas, and her heirloom jewellery. We sat and drank as much of this terrible concoction as we could before we fell unconscious and fully dressed into bed. The following morning we were ill beyond belief, but then my mother discovered what we had done, and we were justly punished and sent to school.

A hangover is virtually a symptom of poisoning and the body needs to get rid of the offending material as soon as possible.

ESSENTIAL OILS

Juniper, grapefruit, rosemary

TREATMENT

If you think that you are in for a festive night, drink lots of water and eat a slice or two of dry bread before going out. When you return, drink more water (alcohol causes dehydration); take a vitamin C and multi-B vitamin capsule according to packet directions. If you still feel terrible in the morning, repeat the vitamin treatment and have a bath containing four drops juniper, four drops grapefruit, and two drops rosemary essential oils.

Alternatively, sprinkle one drop of each of these oils on a wet washcloth and rub briskly over your entire body after showering.

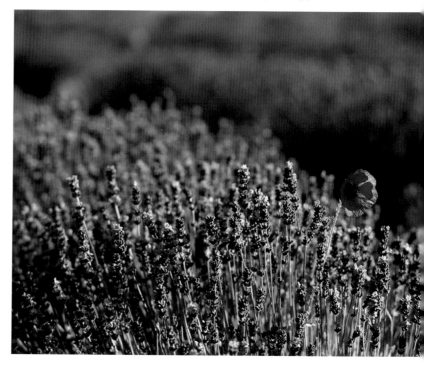

Muscles and joints

Arthritis and rheumatism

Both osteoarthritis and rheumatoid arthritis are characterized by pain, stiffness, and inflammation. Being overweight puts an extra load on joints and makes the symptoms worse.

Osteoarthritis is called a "wear and tear" disease because it usually occurs with ageing. It affects mainly the weight-bearing joints (knee, hip, lower back, neck) and the hands (fingers and thumbs). But it may also affect a shoulder or even your big toe!

Rheumatoid arthritis is an autoimmune disease and is quite distinct from osteoarthritis although the symptoms may appear similar. The following treatments are suitable for both types of arthritis, but I would advise rheumatoid arthritis sufferers to seek professional treatment as well as using natural therapies.

Our muscles and joints should be cared for, even in our youth.

The treatment for arthritis and rheumatism is basically the same. The primary aim of treatment is to cleanse the whole system, and herbs can play a valuable role in this.

* **Bromelian** and **boswellia**: Take as recommended on containers to help reduce tension pain and inflammation.
* **Devil's claw**: 750 mg capsule three times daily.
* **Gotu kola**: Eat two to three leaves fresh in a sandwich or chopped finely into a salad once a day.
* **Willow bark**, **curcumin** and **meadowsweet**: Proven to be anti-inflammatory, and after consultation with your health professional may be a good substitute for the more damaging aspirin.
* **Valerian** and/or **passionflower**: May be taken at night to help ease pain and encourage sleep.

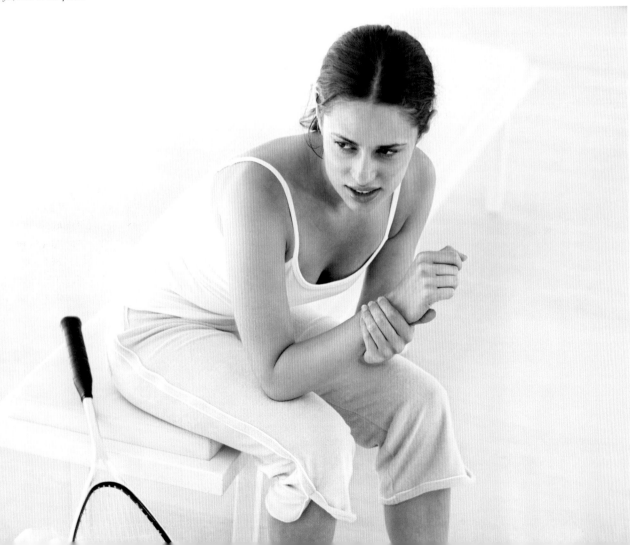

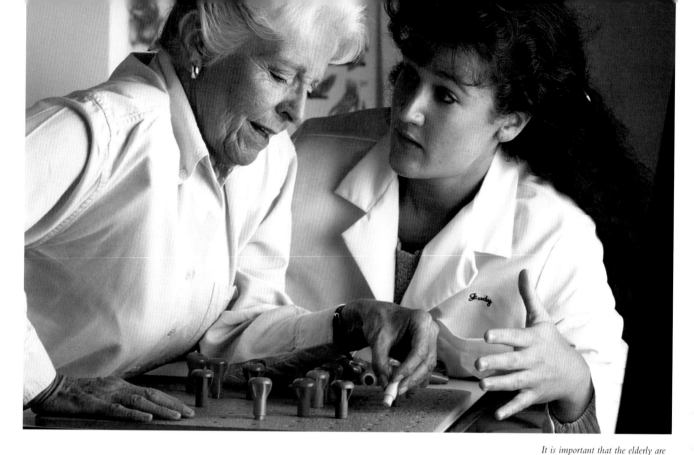

ESSENTIAL OILS

Bergamot, benzoin, black pepper, frankincense, ginger, juniper, rosemary

ARTHRITIS OIL BLEND

1 teaspoon benzoin essential oil
1 teaspoon juniper essential oil
$^1/_2$ teaspoon black pepper essential oil
$^1/_4$ teaspoon ginger essential oil
$1/_4$ teaspoon rosemary essential oil

To make and use

Mix all the oils together in a dropper bottle, and shake to blend.

Leave for four days before using, so that the oils have time to synergize or combine well.

Add 10 drops of the blend to one cup Epsom salts, stir well and add to a warm bath. Agitate the water to disperse the oils, and then soak in the bath for 15–30 minutes, massaging your limbs gently.

Add 14 drops of the blend to four teaspoons grape seed or sweet almond oil and use mixture for a gentle massage.

Use 10 drops of the blend in half a cup of very hot water for a fomentation.

ARTHRITIS TINCTURE

1 part yellow dock root, finely crushed
1 part burdock root, finely crushed
3 parts nettle leaf
1 part yarrow leaf
2 parts celery seed, bruised
2 parts meadowsweet leaves and flowers
1 part cayenne
cider vinegar

To make and use

Place all the herb ingredients in a jar, and pour in apple cider vinegar to about 4 in (10 cm) above the herbs if using dried herbs, or 1 in (2.5 cm) if fresh.

Cover with a non-metallic lid, and leave for two weeks, shaking several times daily.

Strain through a sieve, and then through coffee filter paper. Pour into a labeled bottle.

Take four teaspoons in water (sweetened with honey if liked) twice daily, half an hour before meals.

It is important that the elderly are carefully monitored when suffering from arthritis.

TIP THE ROOT OF THE HERB DEVIL'S CLAW (*HARPAGOPHYTUM PROCUMBENS*) HAS BEEN USED FOR YEARS FOR ITS REMARKABLE ANTI-INFLAMMATORY PROPERTIES. IT IS SAID TO REDUCE INFLAMMATION IN THE JOINTS AND MAY HELP TO EASE THE SYMPTOMS OF ARTHRITIS, GOUT, NEURALGIA, FIBROSITIS, LUMBAGO, AND RHEUMATISM.

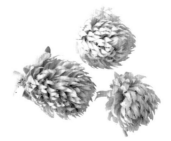

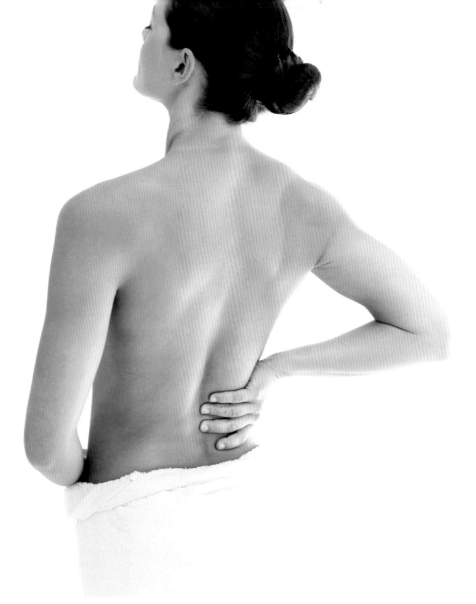

Back pain from exercise and sport can be effectively treated with an essential oil bath.

Back Pain

Here, I am talking about the good old backache you get after a day in the garden, or other manual labor that involves bending. It almost feels satisfying that your body tells you that you've done a good day's work and are now entitled to soak in a bath and, with luck, enjoy a massage afterwards.

ESSENTIAL OILS

Cypress, eucalyptus, geranium, ginger, lavender, nutmeg, peppermint, rosemary

BACKACHE BATH BLEND

1 teaspoon sweet almond oil
4 drops geranium or lavender essential oil
2 drops eucalyptus or cypress essential oil
2 drops peppermint essential oil
2 drops nutmeg or ginger essential oil

Mix all the oils together in a small, labeled bottle and shake to blend.

TREATMENT

Pour the blend into a deep warm to hot bath. Sink into the water with a sigh, and enjoy massaging the floating droplets into your sore muscles for as long as the water is nice and warm.

BACKACHE OIL

1 teaspoon sweet almond oil
2 drops rosemary essential oil
1 drop black pepper essential oil
1 drop eucalyptus essential oil

Mix all the oils together in a small, labeled bottle, and shake to blend. Pour on a small bowl of warm water.

Use Backache Oil Blend to massage the whole body, paying special attention to the upper and lower back.

Bursitis

Bursitis is characterized by severe pain in a joint (usually the shoulder, knee, or elbow) especially on movement, skin that is hot to the touch, and swelling. It is often known by names such as "housemaid knee" or "tennis elbow" indicating an occupation or sport where the joint has been overused. It is sometimes the result of an inflammatory joint disease.

ESSENTIAL OILS

Chamomile, clary sage, cypress, eucalyptus, hyssop, juniper, rosemary
St John's wort (*hypericum*) infused oil. You can make your own or buy it from a health food store.

TREATMENT

Rest the joint as soon as the damage becomes apparent. Eliminate as far as possible, the cause of the condition. Elevate the joint above the head as much as possible.

Massage gently and lightly three times a day with Bursitis Massage Blend.

Apply cold packs and compresses three times a day using Bursitis Compress Blend.

Acupuncture is often a very successful treatment for this condition.

BURSITIS MASSAGE BLEND

3 tablespoons (45 ml) grape seed oil
3 tablespoons (45 ml) St John's wort oil
20 drops rosemary essential oil
15 drops eucalyptus essential oil
15 drops chamomile essential oil
15 drops juniper essential oil

Mix all the oils together in a small, labeled bottle, and shake to blend. Leave for four days before using, so that the oils have time to synergize or combine well.

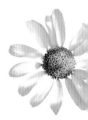

BURSITIS COMPRESS BLEND

$3\frac{1}{2}$ fl oz (100 ml) ice water
5 drops cypress essential oil
3 drops clary sage essential oil
2 drops hyssop essential oil

To make and use
Mix the oils thoroughly together in a small bowl. Make a compress and apply as often as required.

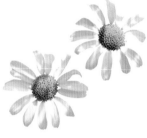

A firm pressure on the "hot spot" can ease bursitis.

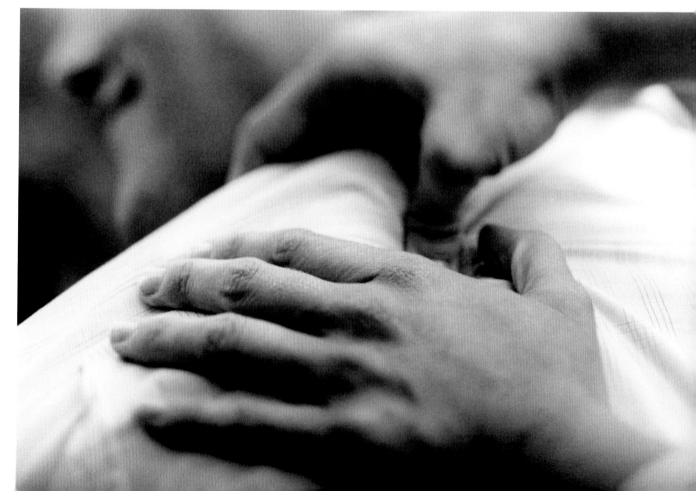

Carpal tunnel syndrome

Carpal tunnel syndrome seems to be most common in middle-aged and pregnant women, arthritis sufferers, and those who use computer keyboards constantly, although the actual cause is often uncertain. I once developed it myself thanks to overlong hours on the computer.

ESSENTIAL OILS
Chamomile
Arnica infused oil

TREATMENT
Use a wrist and thumb brace to immobilize the area for much of the day.

Four to six times a day, massage the wrist, thumb and forearm up to the elbow with alternated three drops arnica infused oil (not to be used on broken skin) in one teaspoon grape seed oil; then four drops chamomile essential oil in one teaspoon grape seed oil. If you have St John's wort infused oil, use it instead of grape seed oil.

Cramps

Cramp is a painful contraction of the muscles, usually in the feet, or the calves of the legs. Cramps often occur at night. Keep a bottle of the following blend on your bedside table ready for emergencies! If the cramps are a regular part of your life you need to find the cause and/or visit a health practitioner for further investigation of the problem.

ESSENTIAL OILS
Lavender, rosemary, marjoram, black pepper

CRAMP MASSAGE OIL
4 teaspoons St John's wort infused oil
$^1/_4$ cup (60 ml) grape seed oil
15 drops lavender essential oil
15 drops rosemary essential oil
10 drops marjoram essential oil
5 drops black pepper essential oil

TIP WHEN THE PAIN LESSENS IT IS IMPORTANT TO EXERCISE THE HAND AND FINGERS REGULARLY UNTIL CURED. IT IS A GOOD IDEA TO CONTINUE WITH THESE EXERCISES TO HELP PREVENT THE PROBLEM RECURRING. FIRST OPEN YOUR HAND RIGHT OUT, AND THEN CLENCH TO MAKE FISTS 10–12 TIMES. STRETCH OUT YOUR ARMS ROTATING YOUR HANDS (FINGERS OPEN) FROM THE WRISTS 10 TIMES IN ONE DIRECTION THEN 10 TIMES THE OTHER WAY.

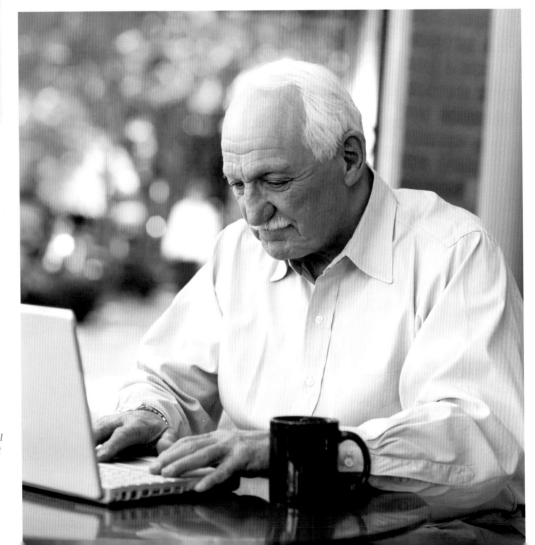

Repetitive movements like typing are often a cause of Carpal Tunnel Syndrome. Support for wrists and arms often helps.

To make and use

Mix all the oils together in a small, labeled bottle, and shake to blend.

Leave for four days before using, so that the oils have time to synergize or combine well.

Massage a little of this blend into the muscles. Walking and stretching the muscle will help.

Sometimes cramps occur at night because your legs and feet are cold. Try wearing woolen socks, or sleeping with your lower body in a sleeping bag.

To help reduce the incidence of cramp, take calcium nitrate and zinc capsules, according to packet directions, at bedtime.

Fibrositis

ESSENTIAL OILS

Black pepper, cypress, juniper, lavender, marjoram, peppermint, rosemary

FIBROSITIS OIL BLEND FOR COMPRESSES AND FOMENTATIONS

1 teaspoon rosemary essential oil
50 drops lavender essential oil
50 drops marjoram essential oil

To make and use

Mix all the oils together in a small, labeled bottle, and shake to blend.

Leave for four days before using, so the oils have time to synergize or combine well.

Apply a cabbage compress followed by a compress or fomentation made with five to eight drops of the recommended essential oils.

Try both the hot and cold treatments to see which gives you relief. Treat as often as needed.

See also Rheumatism.

FIBROSITIS OIL BLEND FOR BATH

1 teaspoon grape seed oil
6 drops juniper essential oil
2 drops cypress essential oil
2 drops black pepper essential oil

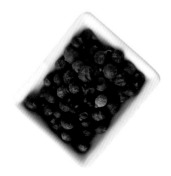

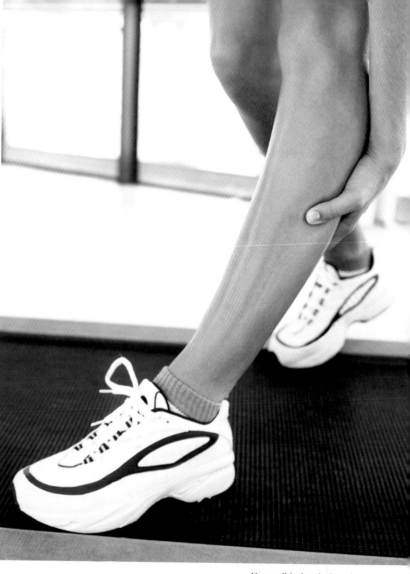

Keep well hydrated when playing sport. It helps prevent cramp.

To make and use

Mix all the oils together thoroughly.

Pour the blend into a warm bath and agitate water to disperse the oils. Massage the sore muscles, (or it you can't reach, ask a friend or partner to help), with the little blobs of oil that will be floating on the water.

FIBROSITIS OIL BLEND FOR MASSAGE

1 teaspoon grape seed oil
2 drops lavender essential oil
1 drop juniper essential oil
1 drop peppermint essential oil

To make and use

Mix the oils together well.

Float the blend on a small bowl of warm water. Use for a gentle massage twice daily to relieve pain and release toxins.

TIP ALSO HELPFUL IS A DECOCTION OF FIVE PARTS CRAMP BARK TO ONE PART GRATED FRESH GINGER ROOT TAKEN THREE TIMES A DAY, OR CRAMP BARK CAPSULES AS DIRECTED ON THE CONTAINER, AND FRESH GINGER ROOT TEA, TWICE OR THREE TIMES A DAY.

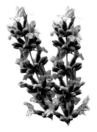

Frozen shoulder

Also know as capsulitis, this is an extremely painful condition caused by inflammation of the muscle or joint fibers. The condition is found mainly in middle-aged women, but the reason for this is not known. In some cases there are deposits of calcium that worsen the condition. Acupuncture, massage, and physiotherapy are suitable treatments.

Willow bark tincture or tablets will help ease the pain. Be sure to take as directed on the container.

Heat a cabbage leaf in the oven until hot and soft (or you can iron it), apply to the shoulder, and slip on a shirt or blouse to hold in place. Leave until cold. Follow with a deep massage, using the massage oil that follows.

Another option is to alternate hot fomentations and cold compresses using very strong teas of chamomile and lavender. Again follow with a deep massage, using the massage oil that follows.

MASSAGE OIL

Make an infused oil of as many of the following dried herbs: Chamomile flowers, rosemary leaves, marjoram leaves, peppermint leaves.

To each 100 ml of the finished infused oil, add 20 drops of oil of cloves. Warm the oil, before using to massage the shoulder.

Although the reasons are unknown, frozen shoulder is most common in middle-aged women.

Lumbago

ESSENTIAL OILS

Chamomile, ginger, lavender, eucalyptus, marjoram, rosemary

LUMBAGO BATH AND MASSAGE OIL

3 tablespoons (45 ml) grape seed oil
10 drops lavender essential oil
10 drops ginger essential oil
5 drops marjoram essential oil
5 drops rosemary essential oil

To make and use

Mix all the oils together in a small, labeled bottle, and shake to blend.

Leave for four days before using, so that the oils have time to synergize or combine well.

Apply cold compresses to any area that feels inflamed, using lavender and chamomile oils. Use cold packs in between compresses.

Float one teaspoon of Lumbago Bath and Massage Oil on warm water in a small bowl, and use for a gentle back massage, after inflammation has receded.

Pour two teaspoons of the blend into a bath, agitate to dispense, and soak in the bath for 10–15 minutes, and massage any floating oil droplets into the skin.

Restless leg syndrome

The symptoms of this distressing complaint, which usually starts about an hour after going to bed, include involuntary jerking leg muscles, an irresistible urge to move the legs, muscle contractions, aching legs or joints.

Taking calcium citrate according to packet directions, half an hour before bed, as a muscle relaxant.

Taking one teaspoon of fluid extract of ginko biloba three times daily can improve peripheral circulation.

A daily dose of hawthorn in capsule form, taken according to packet directions, or 30 drops of tincture three times daily, can improve poor circulation.

Take one valerian capsule according to packet directions, and a cup of the following tea at bed-time, to relax muscles and help sleep.

RELAXING TEA

2 parts skullcap
1 part passionflower
1 part chamomile

To make

Mix the finely chopped herbs together. Use one teaspoon to one cup of boiling water. Cover and steep for 10 minutes. Can be sweetened with honey.

ESSENTIAL OILS

Black pepper, ginger, lavender, marjoram, nutmeg, rosemary

MASSAGE BLEND FOR RESTLESS LEGS

$1/3$ cup (80 ml) grape seed oil
30 drops rosemary essential oil
20 drops marjoram essential oil
10 drops lavender or nutmeg essential oil
10 drops black pepper or ginger essential oil

To make and use

Mix all the oils together in a small, labeled bottle, and shake to blend.

Leave for four days before using, so the oils have time to synergize or combine well.

Pour one teaspoon of the blend into a hot spoon to warm the oil. Use the warmed oil last thing at night, after showering or bathing, to massage the legs using firm, upwards strokes.

Deep massage using the oils, often provides relief and in some cases effects a cure.

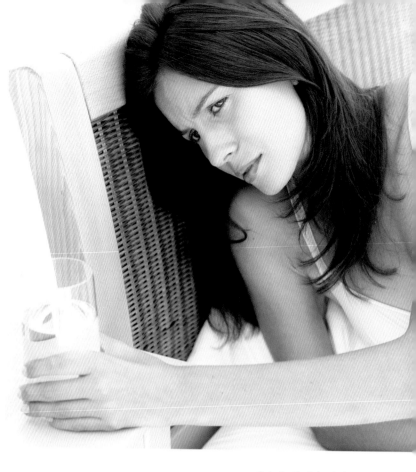

Relaxing Tea before bed can help Restless Leg Syndrome.

Rheumatism, muscular

Rheumatism is a general term that covers an inflammatory disorder, involving pain and inflammation in the joints and muscles.

ESSENTIAL OILS

Cypress, juniper, lavender, marjoram, rosemary

RHEUMATISM OIL BLEND FOR COMPRESSES AND FOMENTATIONS

100 drops rosemary essential oil
50 drops lavender essential oil
50 drops marjoram essential oil

To make and use

Mix all the oils together in a small, labeled bottle, and shake to blend.

Leave for four days before using, so the oils have time to synergize or combine well.

Apply a compress or fomentation using five to eight drops of the mixed essential oils. Try both hot and cold treatments to see which one gives the greatest relief. Treat as often as needed.

RHEUMATISM OIL BLEND FOR BATH OR MASSAGE

$\frac{1}{3}$ cup (80 ml) grape seed oil
12 drops juniper essential oil
12 drops chamomile essential oil
24 drops cypress essential oil
15 drops rosemary essential oil

To make and use

Mix all the oils together in a small, labeled bottle, and shake to blend

Leave for four days before using, so the oils have time to synergize or combine well.

Pour two teaspoons of the blend into the bath after it has been drawn, agitate water to disperse. Massage the sore muscles with the little blobs of oil that will float on the water.

Massage the blend into sore, aching areas as often as needed.

Sciatica

Sciatica describes pain at any joint along the sciatic nerve, and may be felt in the buttocks, behind the hip joint, down the back (or sometimes the front) of the thigh, down the calf, and into the foot. The cause of sciatica (poor sitting posture or pressure on a disk) needs to be found before a cure can be affected. A visit to a chiropractor is usually beneficial for this condition.

Sciatica can recur after sport and even at rest.

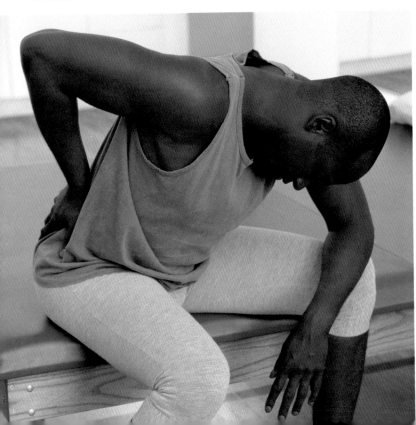

ESSENTIAL OILS

Chamomile, lavender, marjoram, rosemary

SCIATICA MASSAGE BLEND

3 tablespoons (45 ml) grape seed oil or infused calendula oil
12 drops lavender essential oil
10 drops rosemary essential oil
10 drops marjoram essential oil

To make and use

Mix all the oils together in a small, labeled bottle, and shake to blend.

Leave for four days before using, so that the oils have time to synergize to combine well.

While the pain is severe, there may be inflammation, and massage is not indicated. Cold packs, and lavender and chamomile compresses, will reduce the inflammation. Float one teaspoon of the blend on warm water in a small bowl, and use for a massage after the heat of inflammation has gone.

Pour two teaspoons into a warm (not hot) bath, agitate to disperse, and soak in the bath for 10-15 minutes; gently massage any floating oil droplets into the painful areas.

Pour a little of the blend into the palm of your hand and massage over the sciatic nerve after showering.

Sore Muscles

Muscles that aren't regularly exercised can punish us dreadfully, if we suddenly spend a lot of time gardening, playing sport, walking for hours, or doing anything strenuous that they aren't used to. There is a real danger of muscle strain under these conditions so, once again, we need to learn to listen to our bodies.

ESSENTIAL OILS

Black pepper, juniper, lavender, marjoram, peppermint, rosemary
Arnica infused oil

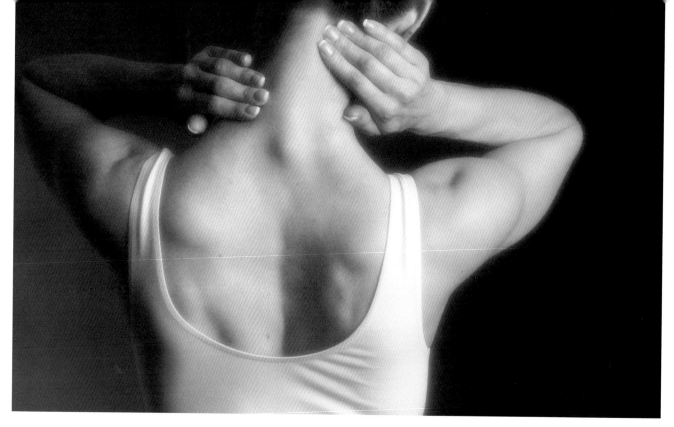

SORE MUSCLE SOAK

1 cup (250 ml) Epsom salts
3 drops lavender essential oil
3 drops juniper essential oil
2 drops peppermint essential oil
2 drops black pepper essential oil

To make and use

Mix the oils a drop at a time into the Epsom salts. Stir well.

Sprinkle the salts into a deep bath of warm water, stir to dissolve.

Soak for 30 minutes or as long as you like, gently massaging the sore muscles under the water.

MUSCLE RELIEF MASSAGE OIL

$1/4$ cup (60 ml) grape seed oil
15 drops juniper essential oil
15 drops marjoram essential oil
10 drops rosemary essential oil
5 drops black pepper essential oil

To make and use

Mix all the oils together in a small, labeled bottle. Shake to blend.

If the muscles are extremely sore, don't expect the pain to subside after a single treatment. You might have to give yourself "the bath and massage" treatment, for two to three days, before the muscles are completely recovered.

Add one teaspoon of the blend to a small bowl of warm water, and use the above oil blend for a massage after the bath, or at any time your muscles are sore and tired.

Infused arnica oil may be used for small areas that are particularly sore, but not if the skin is broken.

Varicose Veins

Eat a diet rich in fiber. When cooking, use spices that stimulate the circulatory system, such as ginger and cayenne. Eat buckwheat porridge every morning for its rutin content.

Relief from varicose veins can be achieved with any of the following treatments.

* Take horse chestnut extract or capsules as directed on the container.
* Eat two to three gotu kola leaves daily in a sandwich or salad.
* Take 500–750 mg of bromelain three times daily between meals.
* Ice-cold compresses using calendula and plantain as a triple strength tea, can also be helpful. Add an equal amount of distilled witch hazel to the tea, and apply two or three times daily, while the leg is elevated.

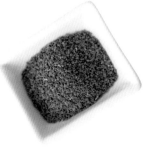

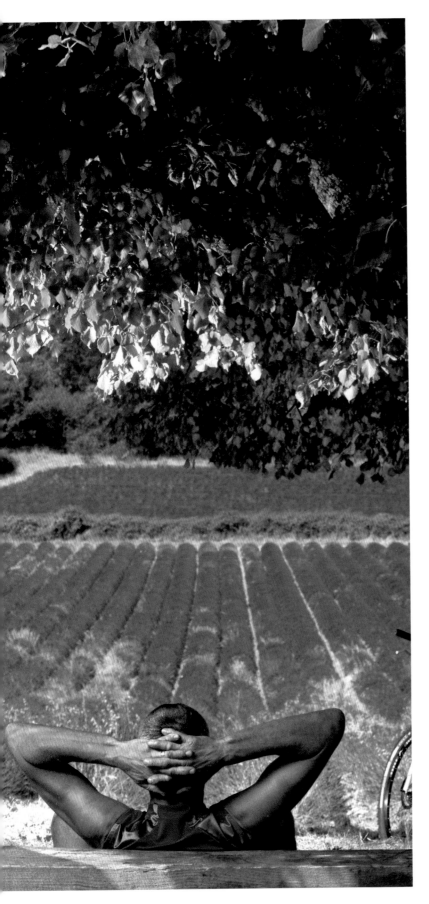

Sports injuries

Achilles tendonitis

This is inflammation of the Achilles tendon, that is situated behind the ankle. The injury can be caused by overuse or by straining the tendon, and the area is often hot, painful and has restricted movement.

ESSENTIAL OILS

Chamomile, lavender, ginger

TREATMENT

Rest to avoid further injury, elevating the foot above the level of the heart.

Apply ice cold compresses using chamomile and lavender essential oils. Repeat every 30 minutes for three hours, then decrease to four compresses a day for two days.

ACHILLES TENDONITIS MASSAGE OIL

After completing the cold compress treatment, use a cabbage poultice, and massage, using a little of this blend, several times a day. Treatment is often lengthy, but unless you persevere it will be even lengthier!

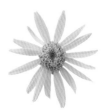

$1/_4$ cup (60 ml) olive oil
20 drops chamomile essential oil
15 drops lavender essential oil
15 drops ginger essential oil

To make and use

Mix all the oils together in a small, labeled bottle, and shake to blend.

Leave for four days before using, so the oils have time to synergize or combine well.

CABBAGE POULTICE

After two to three days of icepack treatment, use the following poultice. Pour boiling water over a cabbage leaf, and leave for a few minutes until hot and wilted. Apply to the ankle while still hot, but cool enough to bear. Bind in place. Replace when cool.

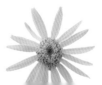

Pre-sport treatment

This massage oil will tone your muscles so that they are ready for the football game, marathon walk, triathlon, or whatever. It will also help you achieve a calm, positive frame of mind.

"UP AND AT 'EM" OIL

$^1/_3$ cup (80 ml) sweet almond oil
20 drops rosemary essential oil
20 drops cypress essential oil
15 drops lavender essential oil
10 drops juniper essential oil

To make and use

Mix all the oils together in a small, labeled bottle, and shake to blend.

Leave for four days before using, so the oils have time to synergize or combine well.

Massage into muscles before strenuous or competitive sport.

After sport treatment

The following massage oil will help to prevent, or ease, muscle soreness.

HERO'S BATH AND MASSAGE OIL

$3^1/_2$ fl oz (100 ml) sweet almond oil
25 drops rosemary essential oil
25 drops lemon essential oil
20 drops clary sage essential oil
10 drops orange essential oil

To make and use

Mix all the oils together in a small, labeled bottle, and shake to blend.

Leave for four days before using, so the oils have time to synergize or combine well.

Use this treatment as soon a possible after getting home. Add two teaspoons to a deep warm bath. Soak for at least three minutes. Massage floating drops of oil into the muscles.

Massage a little of the oil blend into the muscles, after the bath or shower.

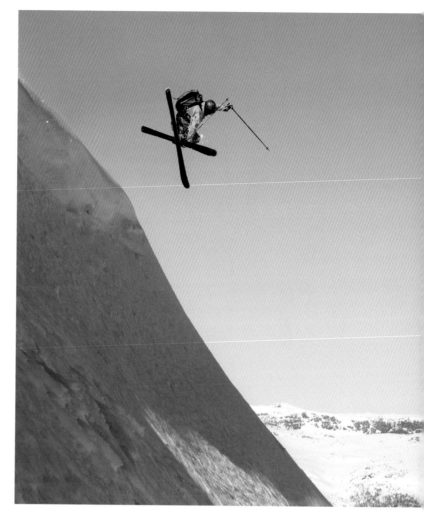

Skiing, and particularly mogul skiing, is a sport where cartilage injury is common. Seek medical advice if you feel any pain.

Cartilage injury

ESSENTIAL OILS

Clove, ginger, black pepper

CARTILAGE MASSAGE BLEND

3 tablespoons (45 ml) grape seed oil
16 drops ginger essential oil
10 drops black pepper essential oil
8 drops clove essential oil

To make and use

Mix all the oils together in a small, labeled bottle, and shake to blend.

Leave for four days before using, so the oils have time to synergize or combine well.

Keep the injured leg elevated, and apply alternate ice packs, and towels or wash cloths, wrung out in very hot water.

Wear a knee brace or bandage until the damage is repaired.

Massage the knee with the massage blend two to three times a day.

Opposite: When exercising, make sure you take the time to enjoy the scenery. Here a cyclist enjoys a lavender field in Provence, France.

Strains and sprains

Sprains are damage to a ligament supporting a joint. Strains are injuries to muscles. The injured area shouldn't be massaged until the initial inflammation, and swelling have receded.

ESSENTIAL OILS

Lavender, chamomile, marjoram, clove, ginger, black pepper

TREATMENT

Apply ice packs to reduce swelling and inflammation. Use cold compresses with lavender, chamomile, and marjoram essential oils every two to three hours, until relief from the initial pain is obtained. After the cold treatments have done their work and the initial heat and swelling has subsided, the area may be massages twice a day using arnica ointment (not if the skin is broken), or the massage blend for cartilage injury on the previous page.

Sprains

Provided the skin isn't broken, arnica oil or ointment massaged in gently twice a day, can relieve pain and swelling. Also try a very cold, crushed comfrey poultice, or a very cold compress of triple-strength comfrey tea.

After 24 hours, gently massage comfrey ointment, or the following liniment, into the sprain.

SPRAIN LINIMENT

This liniment is useful also for rheumatic pain and bruises.

4 parts powdered myrrh
2 parts powdered goldenseal
2 parts echinacea root powder
2 parts dried St John's wort
1 part cayenne

To make and use

Cover the herbs with alcohol and follow the instructions for liniments and tinctures in Practicalities.

Surfing puts great strain on the body which can lead to sprains.

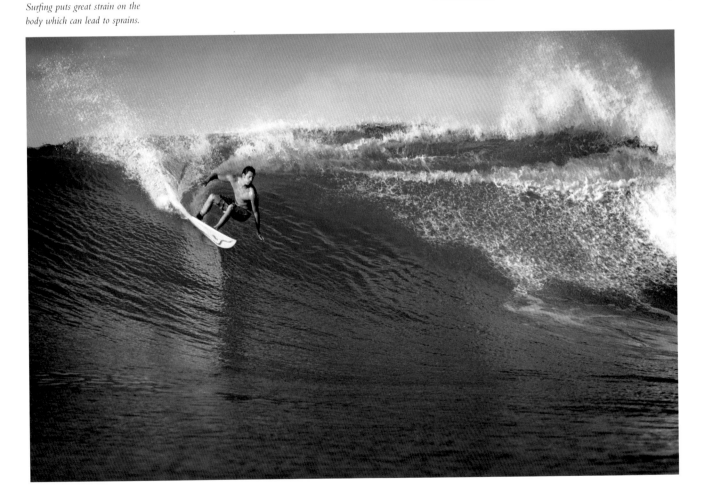

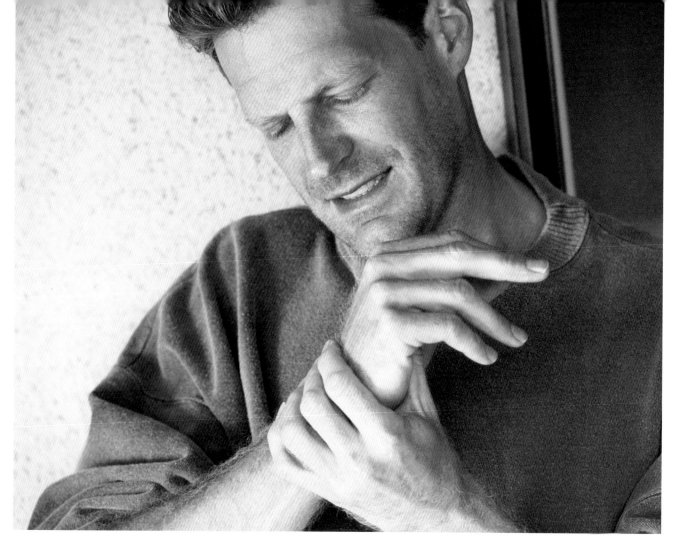

Liniment made with cayenne helps relieve swelling.

Swellings

To treat swellings caused by damage to soft tissue, make a triple-strength tea of as many of the following as possible: Calendula, chamomile, comfrey leaf and root, ginger, mallow, tansy, wormwood. Cool the tea in the refrigerator, and use to make a compress. Sprinkle witch hazel on the compress, and apply as cold as possible. Renew as the compress warms up.

Sports stress

Never underestimate the stress created by sport, particularly competitive sport. There is the pre-game stress, with all the worries about being a worthwhile part of the team, and the unresolved stress after the game if you feel that you have failed, or could have achieved more. And a plea to parents with children playing sport—remember, games are supposed to be fun!

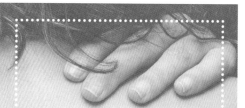

A liniment is an external application that is easily absorbed into the skin. It is generally used for soothing strained muscles and ligaments. Liniments may have cider vinegar, or alcohol (ethanol or vodka), as a carrier for the herbs. Essential oils can also be added to increase the product's potency.

Liniments and tinctures are made in exactly the same way, the only difference being that tinctures are taken internally and liniments are for external use. Cayenne is an ingredient in most liniments, as it brings blood to the area being massaged.

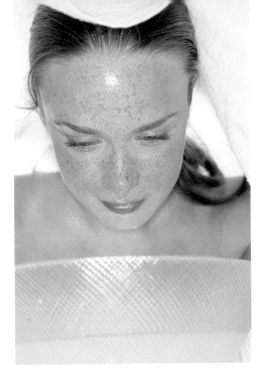

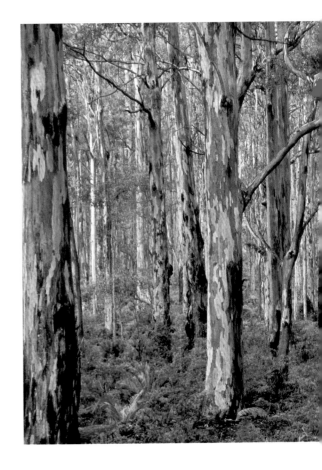

Clear Air Blend used as an inhalation will quickly clear a blocked nose.

Forest of eucalyptus trees. Eucalyptus is one of the most beneficial essential oils for clearing respiratory problems.

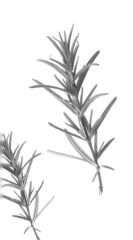

Respiratory problems

Blocked nose and catarrh

Catarrh is inflammation of a mucous membrane, especially of the respiratory tract, accompanied by excessive secretions. Production of excessive mucus can be caused by an infection, hay fever, irritants such as tobacco smoke, chemical fumes, cat fur, pollens, or food allergies.

To help treat it, eat garlic and onions, and plenty of spicy foods such as horseradish, curries, black pepper, and cayenne.

* Take a 1,000 mg garlic oil capsule three times daily.
* Take echinacea, either as a tea three times daily, or an extract taken as directed.
* Drink one cup of mullein leaf tea three times daily (sweeten with honey if liked), or drink 20 drops of mullein leaf tincture in four teaspoons of water, three times daily.

ESSENTIAL OILS FOR CATARRH

Black pepper, peppermint, rosemary, tea tree, pine, eucalyptus

ESSENTIAL OILS FOR A BLOCKED NOSE

Cajuput, clove, eucalyptus, peppermint, rosemary, tea tree, thyme, black pepper, pine

CLEAR AIR BLEND FOR BLOCKED NOSES

50 drops cajuput essential oil
50 drops eucalyptus essential oil
25 drops peppermint essential oil
15 drops clove essential oil
10 drops thyme essential oil

To make and use

Mix all the oils together in a small, labeled bottle, and shake to blend.

Leave for four days before using so the oils have time to synergize or combine well.

Sprinkle a few drops on a tissue and sniff the aroma.

Use 10 drops in an inhalation.

If you substitute oils, remember to keep the proportions the same.

Alternatively, just blend the essential oils together to use as an air spray or in an oil burner.

CHEST MASSAGE BLEND FOR CATARRH

Blend a total of six drops of peppermint, eucalyptus, tea tree, and rosemary oil, in four teaspoons of vegetable oil. Massage into the chest and throat.

Alternatively, an inhalation using two drops of these oils can be made.

CHEST MASSAGE CREAM FOR CATARRH

3 tablespoons (45 ml) coconut oil
2 teaspoons grape seed oil
10 drops tea tree or eucalyptus essential oil
15 drops rosemary or pine essential oil
5 drops peppermint essential oil

To make and use

Melt the coconut oil and grape seed oil until liquefied, by placing in a 2 fl oz (60 ml) labeled jar, standing in warm water. Don't allow the oils to get too hot.

Add the essential oils and mix together well in the jar. Cover quickly with a cap. Shake occasionally until it is cold. Store in the refrigerator.

Massage the chest and upper back twice daily with Chest Massage Cream.

Use two drops of each of recommended essential oils in an inhalation.

Use some or all the essential oils in a room spray or oil burner.

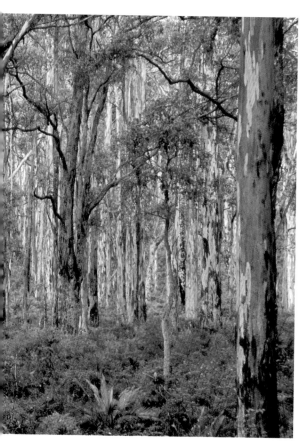

Bronchitis

Bronchitis is best described as an acute or chronic inflammation of the lining of the bronchial tubes, and needs careful treatment. Chronic bronchitis needs the attention of a health-care professional.

ESSENTIAL OILS

Benzoin, cedarwood, eucalyptus, frankincense, lemon, marjoram, peppermint

TREATMENT

Inhalation using some or all of the recommended essential oil.

Massage chest with Bronchitis Chest Massage Oil.

Add 10 drops in total, of the suggested essential oils, to one teaspoon grape seed oil and add to a warm bath, agitate the water to disperse.

Soak for 30 minutes, massaging the floating droplets of oil into the throat and chest.

Use a mixture of the essential oils in an oil burner and/or room spray.

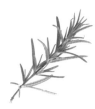

BRONCHITIS CHEST MASSAGE OIL

3 tablespoons (45 ml) olive oil
15 drops eucalyptus essential oil
10 drops cedarwood essential oil
8 drops peppermint essential oil

To make and use

Mix all the oils together in a small, labeled bottle, and shake to blend.

Leave for four days before using, so the oils have time to synergize or combine well.

Use to massage the chest and throat three times daily.

An alternative is just blending the essential oils together to use as an air spray or in an oil burner.

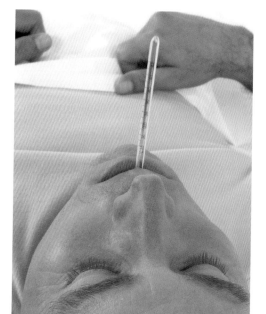

If a fever develops with a cold, see a doctor.

Colds and influenza

If you take notice of the first subtle symptoms of colds or influenza and take action, it is possible to alleviate some of the attendant miseries. I also believe you should mix as little as possible with others when you have a cold or the flu, to try to prevent the disease spreading.

Spray the house regularly with a blend of the essential oils to help prevent the infection from spreading.

Take one teaspoon (5 ml) fluid extract of echinacea three times daily for three days, then $^1/_2$ teaspoon (2.5 ml) three times daily, until all symptoms have gone.

Take a 1,000 mg garlic oil capsule three times daily.

The age-old standby of hot herb teas of equal parts of elder flower, peppermint, yarrow, and a pinch of cayenne, cannot be beaten. (It's a good idea to make a blend of the dried herbs ahead of winter and store it in a jar in the refrigerator or freezer.) Have a hot bath while sipping the hot tea. Go straight to bed with another mug of this herb tea and sweat!

If you can't have a bath, a footbath is a good substitute. The footbath recipe following can help to ward off a cold or influenza as well as easing the symptoms if you've already contracted the disease.

ESSENTIAL OILS

Eucalyptus, tea tree, cinnamon, thyme

ANTI-INFLUENZA BLEND

80 drops eucalyptus essential oil
60 drops tea tree essential oil
40 drops cinnamon essential oil
20 drops thyme essential oil

To make and use

Mix all the oils together in a small, labeled bottle, and shake to blend.

Leave for four days before using, so the oils have time to synergize or combine well.

Mix 10 drops of the blend with one teaspoon grape seed oil, and pour into a hot bath. Agitate well to disperse. Lie in the bath for 30 minutes breathing in the aroma, and massaging any floating oil droplets into the skin.

Pour two to three drops of the blend on a warm wet wash cloth, and rub briskly over the whole body after showering. While sitting in the bath, drink a glass of piping hot ginger and lemon tea.

Add five drops of the blend to one teaspoon grape seed oil, float on a little warm water in a bowl, and massage the whole body, in particular the chest.

Sniff the contents of the bottle containing this blend frequently, to help keep the head clear.

Alternatively, you can simply blend the essential oils together to use as an air spray, or in an oil burner.

COLD AND INFLUENZA FOOTBATH

Mix one teaspoon of chili powder or two teaspoons of mustard powder with a little water and stir thoroughly into a footbath of very hot water. Drink a herb tea (see above) while soaking the feet for 15 minutes. Go directly to bed after the treatment.

A mustard field dotted with apple trees, California, USA. A mustard powder footbath is beneficial for colds and influenza.

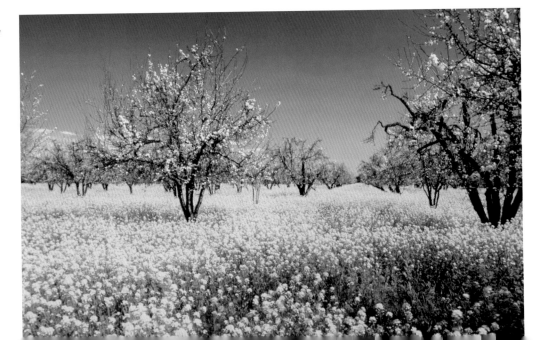

Coughs

The following treatments aim at loosening, lessening, and expelling mucus, as well as strengthening the lungs. If the cough is persistent, and of long duration, it would be advisable to consult a health-care professional.

Take garlic oil capsules according to packet directions.

You can also sip $1/2$ cup (125 ml) of very hot decoction of ginger root, and/or mullein leaves, sweetened with honey every one to two hours.

Taking $1/2$ teaspoon (2.5 ml) fluid extract of echinacea in 3 tablespoons (45 ml) of water, taken three times daily can also help.

A twice daily inhalation using crushed thyme, lavender, and eucalyptus leaves, in boiled water can be helpful.

Another remedy is to prepare a footbath using water as hot as can be borne. Add two drops each of peppermint, thyme, and tea-tree essential oils. Agitate the water to disperse the oils. Immerse the feet for 10–15 minutes, topping up with more hot water if necessary.

ESSENTIAL OILS

Benzoin, cedarwood, eucalyptus, lavender, marjoram, pine, thyme

INHALATION BLEND FOR COUGHS

3 drops marjoram essential oil
2 drops benzoin essential oil
1 drop thyme essential oil

To make and use

Mix the oils well together in a small bowl. Use for inhalation or in an air spray or oil burner.

MASSAGE BLEND FOR COUGHS

3 tablespoons (45 ml) grape seed oil
15 drops eucalyptus essential oil
10 drops cedarwood essential oil
5 drops pine essential oil
3 drops thyme essential oil

To make and use

Mix all the oils together in a small, labeled bottle, and shake to blend. Leave for four days before using, so the oils have time to synergize or combine well. Massage the chest, throat, and back with the blend.

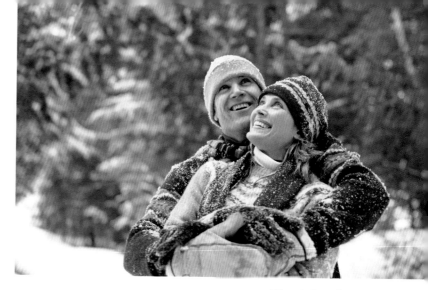

Add two teaspoons of the blend to a warm bath. Agitate the water to disperse. Soak for 30 minutes and use the floating drops of oil to massage the chest and throat.

Winter is always the worst time for coughs and colds. Keep them at bay by the use of essential oils.

Laryngitis and hoarseness

Laryngitis is inflammation of the larynx (voice box), or the vocal chords. This can lead to hoarseness, or temporary loss of voice. Try to rest the voice completely as long as the condition persists, and try the following treatments.

Drink $1/2$ teaspoon (2.5ml) of fluid extract of echinacea in 3 tablespoons (45 ml) of water three times a day.

Take garlic oil capsules according to the packet directions.

Suck zinc lozenges as directed.

Make a strong tea of sage, add 4 teaspoons (20 ml) cider vinegar, alternate with half a teaspoon of salt in one glass of lukewarm water, and use to gargle six times daily. Do not swallow.

ESSENTIAL OILS

Benzoin, chamomile, cypress, lavender, lemon, sandalwood, thyme

LARYNGITIS INHALATION BLEND

3 drops lavender essential oil
2 drops benzoin essential oil
1 drop thyme essential oil

To make and use

Mix all the oils together in a small, labeled bottle, and shake to blend.

Leave for four days before using, so the oils have time to synergize or combine well.

Use as an inhalation three times daily.

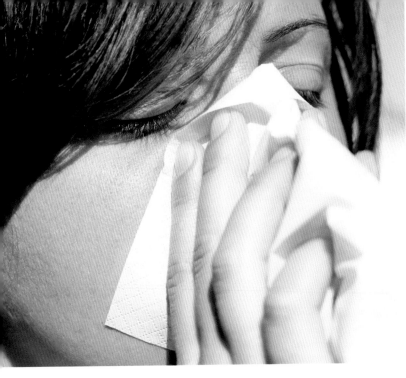

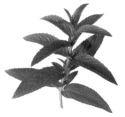

Try to stay clear of others when you have a cold.

Sinusitis

During an allergic reaction, or a cold, the membranes may swell, and produce excessive mucus. The openings from the nose into the sinuses are very narrow and quickly become blocked by the build-up of mucus. This, and the pressure of air in the now constricted space, can cause moderate to severe pain. This is called "sinus congestion."

If, however, there is a bacterial infection, the face feels tender to touch, a colored, thick, nasal discharge is produced, there is fever, and sometimes a frontal headache, and the person can become very sick. In the case of bacterial infection, it's best to seek professional help, as well as using the following treatments.

Drink plenty of fluid, such as diluted fruit and vegetable juices, and herb teas.

Take 500 mg of goldenseal three times daily, or as recommended on the container.

Take $1/2$ teaspoon (2.5 ml) of liquid extract of echinacea three times daily.

Take a 1,000 mg garlic oil capsule three times daily.

Use fomentations and compresses of eucalyptus essential oil, or crushed eucalyptus leaves, over the sinuses, every two or three hours.

Inhale crushed tea tree, eucalyptus and peppermint leaves every two or three hours.

SINUS TEA

1 part sage
1 part elder flower
1 part marshmallow leaf
1 part peppermint

To make and use

Mix the dried herbs in a small, labeled jar. Add one teaspoon of the blend to 1 cup (250 ml) of boiling water.

Cover and steep for five minutes. Drink one cup three times daily.

Sinusitis can be either acute or chronic and both types need prompt attention, as there is a danger that the infection will travel upwards causing meningitis. You will need to persevere with the treatment outlined below, for some time, but believe me, the perseverance will be rewarded by a clear, pain-free head.

ESSENTIAL OILS

Eucalyptus, lavender, peppermint, pine, tea tree

TREATMENT

If the pain or discomfort is bad, a fomentation may bring very fast relief. Use 10 drops of the mixed essential oils for a fomentation. Be careful not to get any of the mixture into the eyes.

During an attack, use one drop of each of the essential oils, in an inhalation, up to five times a day.

Sore throats

Many sore throats are bacterial or viral in origin. They are also the result of what I call irritants—talking too much or too loudly too long, hay fever, open-mouth breathing, dust, cigarette smoke, air-borne chemical fumes, or air conditioning. Gargles work well where irritants have caused the sore throat.

TREATMENT

Gargle with one to two drops clary sage, geranium, or lavender essential oils, and $1/2$ teaspoon salt added to one cup water. Do not swallow. Make an inhalation using benzoin or tea tree essential oils.

Take $1/2$ teaspoon (2.5ml) of liquid extract of echinacea three times a day.

Take garlic oil capsules according to packet directions.

Use an inhalation of benzoin and/or thyme oil.

Gargles are indicated in cases where irritants cause the sore throat. Gargle every two hours with, alternately, a strong tea of sage to which 4 teaspoons (20 ml) of cider vinegar and one teaspoon of honey has been added, and then with half a teaspoon of salt in one cup of warm water.

ESSENTIAL OILS

Bergamot, eucalyptus, hyssop, myrrh, tea tree, thyme

THROAT OIL

4 teaspoons grape seed oil
6 drops bergamot essential oil
6 drops tea tree essential oil
4 drops hyssop or myrrh essential oil

To make and use

Mix all the oils together in a small, labeled bottle, and shake to blend.

Leave for four days before using, so the oils have time to synergize or combine well.

Add one teaspoon of the oil blend to a hot spoon to warm the oil.

Massage the oil over the throat. Cover the entire area with a scarf or warm cloth. Gargle with one drop tea tree essential oil in one cup warm water. Stir water briskly before using.

Tonsillitis

Treat inflammation of the tonsils with the following remedies.

Take $^1/_4$–$^1/_2$ teaspoon (1.25-2.5 ml), depending on age, of echinacea liquid extract three times daily.

Take garlic oil capsules (not for young children) according to packet directions.

Inhale fresh crushed leaves of eucalyptus, myrrh, tea tree, or thyme, or six drops of these mixed essential oils.

Gargle using one dropper of tincture of myrrh in half a glass of warm water, or triple-strength tea of sage, or thyme.

Another effective gargle is half a teaspoon of salt in a glass of lukewarm water.

ESSENTIAL OILS

Lavender, chamomile

Caution *Steam inhalation isn't recommended for asthma sufferers. In between attacks, massage the chest twice daily.*

ASTHMA

Asthma is often an allergic reaction to such things as dust mites, mold, cigarette smoke, car and other chemical fumes, animal fur/feathers, or certain foods. It's wise to conduct a patch test before using essential oils on an asthma sufferer as they may be more sensitive to the oils than the average person.

Asthma is potentially a very serious condition and aromatherapy treatment should be considered an adjunct to, not a substitute for, professional treatment.

Asthma

ASTHMA INHALATION AND MASSAGE BLEND

20 drops lavender essential oil
20 drops chamomile essential oil
$^1/_4$ cup (60 ml) grape seed oil

To make and use

Mix all the oils together in a small, labeled bottle, and shake to blend.

Leave for four days before using, so the oils have times to synergize or combine well.

During an attack, allow the patient to sniff the contents of the bottle.

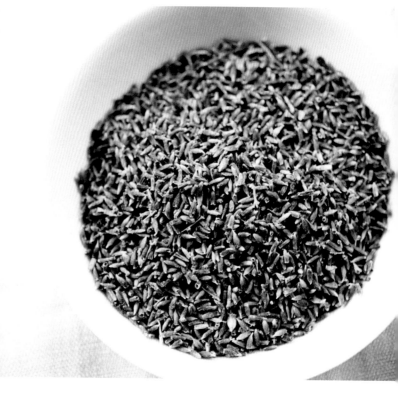

Lavender seeds and flowers ready for distilling into essential oil.

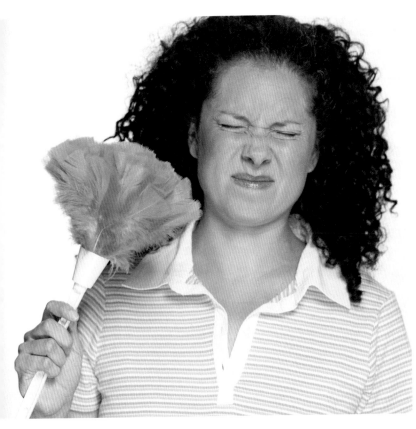

Allergy sufferers should avoid situations that bring on sneezing or coughing. Using a damp cloth to dust will avoid airborne particles..

Allergy

Many complaints are now considered to be allergy related. Essential oils can be of immense help to allergy sufferers, but because of heightened sensitivity it is important to carry out a patch test before trying a new oil. The following oils are of general use to purify the air, control airborne bacterial and viruses, and promote relaxation.

ESSENTIAL OILS

Bergamot, chamomile, juniper, lavender, lemon, peppermint

ALLERGY BLEND

$3^1/_2$ fl oz (100 ml) grape seed oil
30 drops bergamot essential oil
20 drops lavender essential oil
20 drops juniper essential oil
10 drops peppermint essential oil

To make and use

Mix all the oils together in a small bottle, and shake to blend.

Leave for four days before using, so the oils have time to synergize or combine well.

Float one teaspoon of the blend on a little warm water in a bowl, and use for massage. Pour two teaspoons of the blend into a bath, or footbath, agitate to disperse, and soak in the bath for 30 minutes, massaging any floating oil droplets into the skin.

Pour a little of the blend into the palm of your hand, and massage over your body after showering, and while your skin is still damp.

Alternatively, blend the essential oils together, (without the grape seed oil), to use as an air spray or in an oil burner.

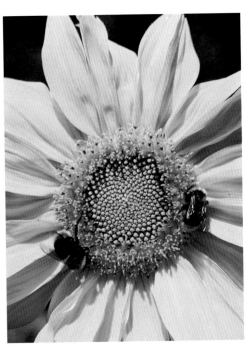

Airborne pollens are a leading cause of allergies.

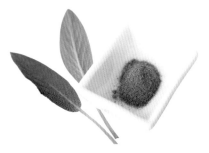

Dust, pollens, and grain crops should be avoided by those suffering hayfever.

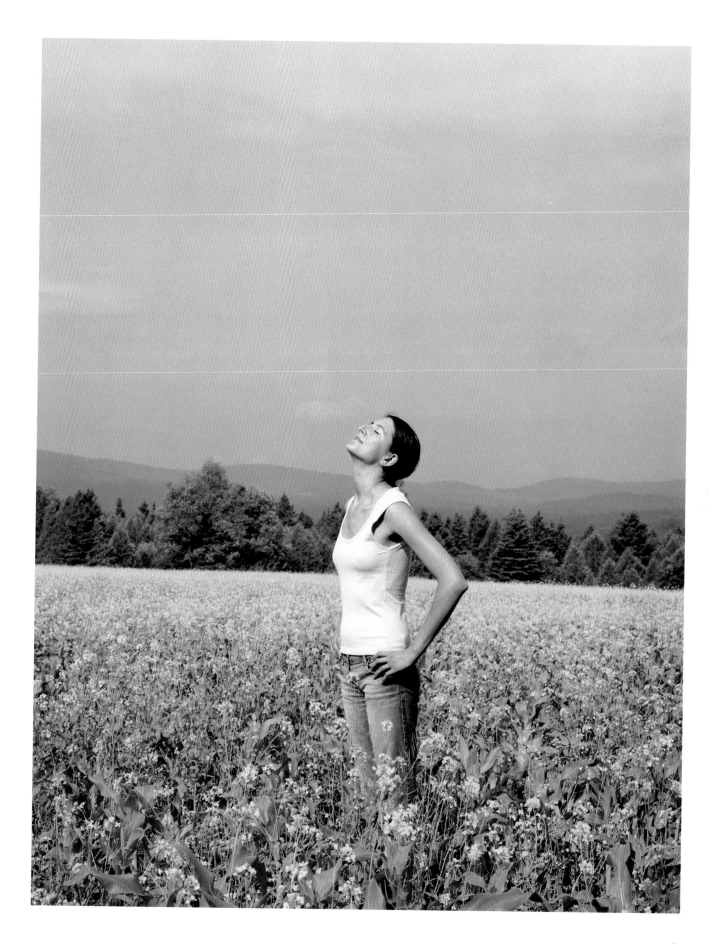

Hayfever

The majority of people suffering from hay-fever are reacting to grass, flower and tree pollens, and spend months of every year, (usually spring), in a misery of sneezing, streaming nose, sore throat, and itchy eyes and ears. Dust mites, mold spores, chemicals, and animal fur are also problems for many people.

Reduce the symptoms of sneezing, a streaming nose, sore throat, and itchy eyes and ears, with dong quai extract or capsules, and take as recommended on the container.

Taking a 1,000 mg garlic oil capsule three times daily is also helpful.

Make chamomile tea using chamomile tea bags. Save the used bags and pop in the fridge to get really cold. Drink three cups of the tea daily, and place the cold bags over the eyes to soothe itching and inflammation.

Fresh air and exercise are essential for all children, even those with allergies.

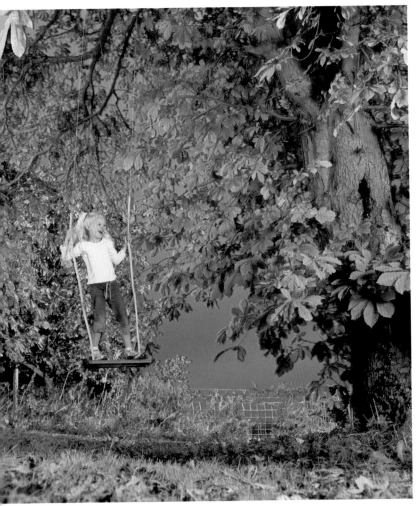

HAYFEVER TEA OR TINCTURE BLEND

1 part sage leaves
1 part elder flowers
1 part eyebright herb
1 part nettle

To make and use

Make a blend of the dried, crumbled herbs, and store it in a labeled jar in the refrigerator, or freezer.

To make a tea, pour 1 cup (250 ml) boiling water over one heaped teaspoon of the herbs, in a warmed cup or pot.

Cover and stand for 5–10 minutes, then strain and sweeten with honey if you wish.

Drink one cup of the tea, or 20 drops of tincture in water, three times daily.

ESSENTIAL OILS

Chamomile, eucalyptus, lavender, lemon, geranium, tea tree

HAYFEVER SALT INHALER 1

20 drops chamomile essential oil
20 drops eucalyptus essential oil
20 drops lemon essential oil
sea salt crystals

HAYFEVER SALT INHALER 2

20 drops lavender essential oil
10 drops geranium essential oil
20 drops tea tree essential oil
10 drops lemon essential oil
sea salt crystals

To make and use

Sprinkle essential oils onto sea salt crystals in a small jar, or on small pieces of cloth in a container, as often as necessary to keep the oils fresh. Inhale the vapors.

Make both inhalers and use alternately for maximum effect.

A steam inhalation using recommended essential oils offers relief.

HAYFEVER MASSAGE BLEND

4 teaspoons grape seed oil
10 drops chamomile essential oil
4 drops lemon essential oil
2 drops tea tree essential oil

To make and use

Mix all the oils together in a small, labeled bottle and shake to blend.

Leave for four days before using so the oils have time to synergize or combine well.

Massage chest and upper back.

Eczema

This is an inflammatory condition of the skin that can be difficult to treat unless the cause is found and treated. Search for the causes from any of the following: allergies, low stomach acid, stress.

The following decoction and tea are excellent internal remedies, but it is important that a cup is drunk three times daily for an extended period.

1 would suggest that you alternate the decoction and tea, using each for a week at a time. If you want to combine the two recipes this can be done by making them separately (in the same quantities) and combining after straining.

ECZEMA DECOCTION

1 part burdock root
1 part dandelion root
1 part yellow dock

To make and Use

Grind the dried roots finely, and store in a labeled glass jar.

Make a decoction using one teaspoon to one cup of water.

It's time saving to make a three-day supply and store it the refrigerator.

ECZEMA TEA

1 part chickweed
1 part red clover
1 part nettle

To make and use

Rub to dried herbs until they resemble tea leaves.

Store in a labeled glass jar.

Use one teaspoon to one cup of boiling water.

ECZEMA HERB BLEND

Make an infused oil including as many possible of the following herbs: calendula, chickweed, mallow, nettle. Use to make an ointment.

The mixed herbs may also be used as a tea to apply as a compress or lotion.

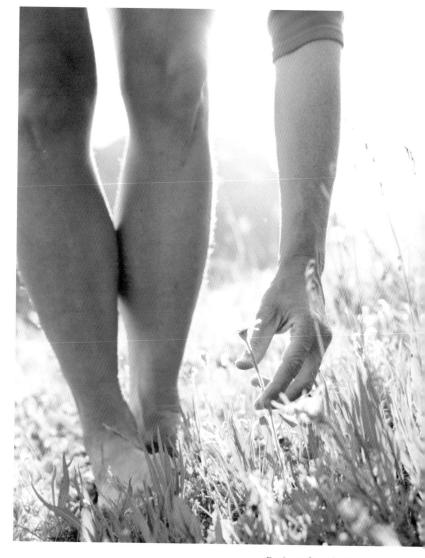

Don't ever forget the pleasure of walking barefoot. Early morning is the best time for allergy sufferers, when dew keeps the pollens and dust settled.

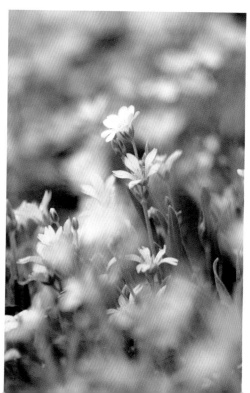

Chickweed, along with red clover and nettle, is used to make Eczema Tea.

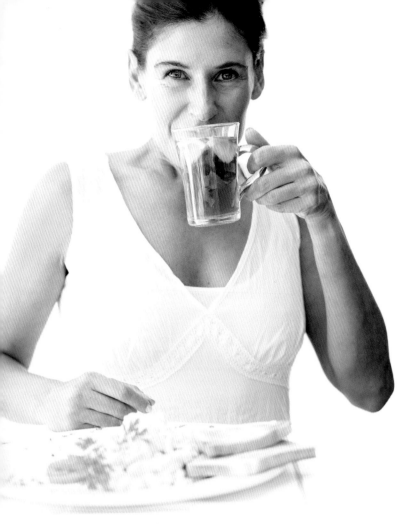

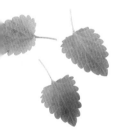

A good healthy diet with plenty of leafy greens will keep your tummy in good condition.

COLIC TEA

1 tablespoon dried passionflower leaves and flowers
1 tablespoon dried peppermint leaves
1 tablespoon dried chamomile flowers
1 tablespoon dried, bruised fennel seed
1 tablespoon dried, bruised anise seed

To make and use

Mix all the ingredients together, and store in a jar in the refrigerator.

Use one teaspoon of the mixture to one cup of boiling water. Steep, covered, for 10 minutes.

Drink $1/4$–$1/2$ cup every hour.

ESSENTIAL OILS

Chamomile, ginger, peppermint

COLIC MASSAGE BLEND

1 teaspoon grape seed oil
3 drops chamomile essential oil
1 drop peppermint or ginger essential oil

To make and use

Mix the oils together and add to a small bowl of warm water.

Massage abdomen with the blend in a clockwise direction as needed.

For colic in babies, see Children and Babies section, page 392.

Tummy troubles

Colic—adults only

Colic is usually caused by gas trapped in the intestines. Avoid fatty and indigestible foods, and try to work out which foods cause the most problems.

You can also try taking one dropper of tincture of passionflower, in water, three times daily, to act as an antispasmodic.

Fresh, grated, ginger tea sipped after a meal can either avert a colic attack, or cure an existing attack.

Heartburn, indigestion, and acidity

Continual problems with the digestive system need to be properly assessed by a health care professional, and the causes found.

The causes may be as simple as overeating, eating the wrong foods, or eating while stressed. By addressing one's lifestyle, the problem may be easily avoided.

To heal and soothe the stomach lining, take two to four slippery elm tablets half an hour before a meal.

To assist digestion, take bromelain and/or papain as directed on the container, and/or gentian tablets, or herbal bitters (available from health food stores), half an hour before a meal.

If there is flatulence, follow a meal with one cup of peppermint, ginger, or meadowsweet tea.

The following herbal vinegar contains digestive herbs.

HERBAL VINEGAR

3 teaspoons crushed ginger root
2 teaspoons ground turmeric
3 teaspoons crushed fennel or caraway seeds
3 tablespoons chopped peppermint leaves
3 tablespoons chopped chamomile flowers
3 tablespoons meadowsweet flowers
3 tablespoons chopped oregano leaves
cider vinegar

To make and use

Place all the herbs in a jar, and cover with cider vinegar to 2 in (5 cm) above the herbs.

Seal with a non-metallic lid, and shake well several times a day for a week.

Strain through a sieve, and then through a coffee filter paper.

Take one tablespoon of the vinegar in a glass of warm water, half an hour before a meal. Sweeten with honey if liked.

Note to those using metric measure: Use two metric tablespoons.

ESSENTIAL OILS FOR HEARTBURN

Peppermint

TREATMENT

Combine one drop peppermint oil with one teaspoon honey in a glass, then top up with lukewarm water, and sip slowly.

ESSENTIAL OILS FOR INDIGESTION AND FLATULENCE

Peppermint, ginger, chamomile, lavender

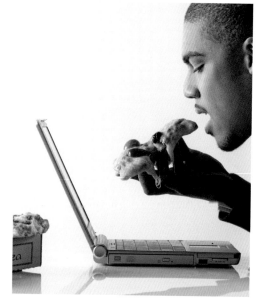

To relieve heartburn, try taking one tablespoon of Herbal Vinegar half an hour before a meal.

TREATMENT

Mix one drop of either peppermint or ginger essential oils, with one teaspoon honey in a glass, then top up with lukewarm water, and sip slowly.

INDIGESTION BLEND FOR MASSAGE

1 teaspoon grape seed oil
2 drops chamomile essential oil
1 drop ginger essential oil
1 drop peppermint essential oil

To make and use

Combine the oils, and warm them in a hot spoon. Massage the blend over the stomach and abdomen.

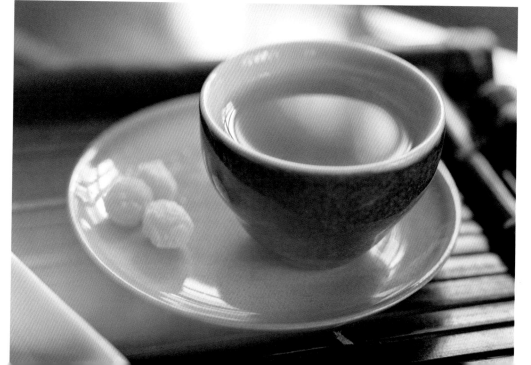

Ginger tea gives relief from colic and other tummy disturbances.

Constipation

Sprinkle two teaspoons of either linseed or ground psyllium husks on cereal, or stir into one glass of water. Drink, and immediately follow with another glass of water, (this is important to prevent the seed husks swelling before it reaches the stomach and intestines). This amount of seed can be varied to your individual requirements, after you find what works best for you.

Substitute chamomile and lemon balm tea for ordinary tea.

Drink at least eight glasses of filtered water every day. (The commonest reason for constipation is insufficient fluid intake).

ESSENTIAL OILS

Black pepper, peppermint

TREATMENT

Add two drops each of black pepper and peppermint essential oils to one teaspoon warmed grape seed oil. Massage the abdomen with this blend two to three times daily, in a clockwise direction.

Diarrhea

The following treatment is for acute (as opposed to chronic) diarrhea. Mild and short-term diarrhea can be nature's way of ridding the body of infection, or contaminated, or unfamiliar food. This cleansing action is beneficial and shouldn't be discouraged in the short term (that is, within 24 hours). If the diarrhea persists, professional help needs to be sought.

One of the dangers of diarrhea is dehydration, so ensure a plentiful supply of liquids. Filtered, bottled, or mineral water, or diluted fruit juices, are ideal.

Drink $^1/_2$ cup (125 ml) of meadowsweet tea every two hours.

Eat only grated raw apple with plain "live" yogurt, and boiled white rice, until the attack has passed.

The following drink will replace lost electrolytes and rehydrate the body. Use for one day only.

Herbal tea is a good substitute when you get bored with drinking water. However, it's still important to maintain a good intake of water.

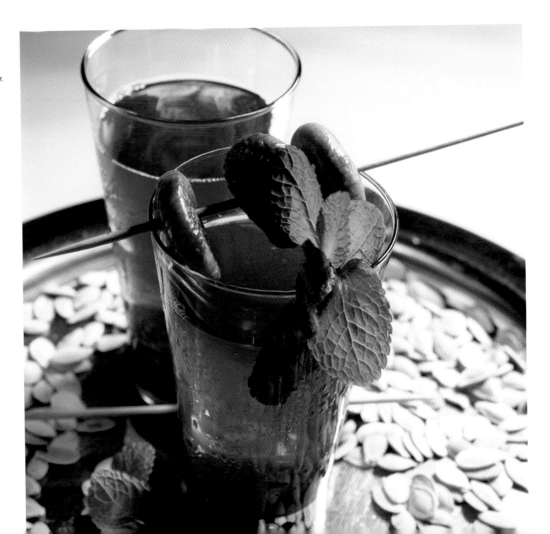

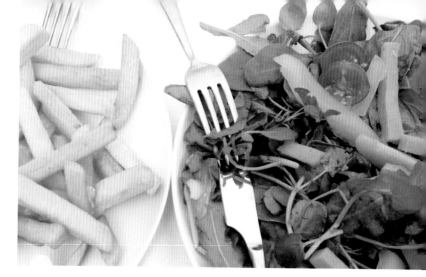

ELECTROLYTE DRINK

1 cup (250 ml) apple juice

1 cup (250 ml) mineral water

3 teaspoons honey

$1/4$ teaspoon salt

$1/4$ teaspoon bicarbonate of soda

To make and use

Combine all the ingredients in a jug, and drink in half-cup doses during the day.

ESSENTIAL OILS

Chamomile, ginger, eucalyptus, tea tree, lavender, lemon, geranium

MASSAGE OIL FOR FOOD-RELATED DIARRHEA

1 teaspoon grape seed oil

2 drops chamomile essential oil

1 drop eucalyptus essential oil

1 drop lemon essential oil

To make and use

Mix the oils together in a warm spoon.

Use to massage the whole abdomen two or three times a day.

MASSAGE OIL FOR VIRUS-RELATED DIARRHEA

1 teaspoon grape seed oil

2 drops chamomile essential oil

1 drop geranium essential oil

1 drop lavender essential oil

To make and use

Mix the oils together in a warm spoon.

Use to massage the whole abdomen two to three times a day.

Irritable bowel syndrome

Irritable bowel syndrome (IBS) has a variety of symptoms, including a colicky pain in the lower abdomen, abdominal bloating, and cramping, constipation, diarrhea, flatulence, and sometimes heartburn. Stress and lack of fiber are both possible causes, which means that you need a professional assessment of your diet and stress levels, before you begin any home treatment.

ESSENTIAL OILS

Chamomile, marjoram, peppermint

IBS MASSAGE BLEND

$1/4$ cup (60 ml) grape seed oil

18 drops chamomile essential oil

18 drops marjoram essential oil

12 drops peppermint essential oil

To make and use

Mix all the oils together in a small bottle, and shake to blend.

If there's time, leave for four days before using, so the oils have time to synergize or combine well.

Use the blend to massage the abdomen in a clockwise direction, two to three times daily.

People who use a combination of one or two enteric-coated, peppermint oil capsules (0.2 ml each, available from pharmacies), and one cup of caraway tea between meals, for irritable bowel syndrome, experience less pain, and note an improvement in symptoms.

Also of help, are garlic oil capsules taken according to packet directions.

Try also 1 cup (250 ml) of milk thistle tea three times daily, or 15–20 drops of tincture three times daily. This herb can also be purchased in capsule form.

Take one valerian or skullcap tablet, or tincture, two or three times a day according to packet directions, if you feel that the problem is stress-related. Continue for one month only; discontinue for one week before resuming.

Make a double-strength infused oil of chamomile, marjoram, and peppermint, and use to massage the abdomen daily, in an anti-clockwise direction.

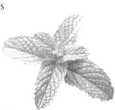

Despite the temptation, it's best to stick to the fresh options and limit your intake of fried food.

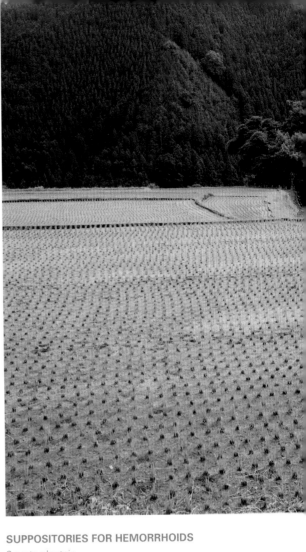

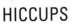

HICCUPS

There are as many "cures" for hiccups as there are for warts!

Essential Oils
Lavender, chamomile

Treatment
Put one drop of lavender, or chamomile essential oil, on either a cube or ¹/₂ teaspoon sugar, and suck it slowly.

Put one drop of either of these oils in a paper bag, hold the bag over the nose and mouth, and breathe in and out slowly.

Fill a glass with water to the brim, lean over, and drink as much as you can (while holding your breath) from the far side of the glass.

Rice plants growing on a terraced landscape in Japan. White rice is an essential part of the diet when recovering from diarrhea.

Hemorrhoids (piles)

These are varicose veins in the rectum, just above the anus.

Cold compresses of distilled witch hazel can help hemorrhoids, particularly if there is discomfort and bleeding after a bowel movement.

An ointment or infused oil of calendula, plantain, St John's wort, and/or goldenseal, massaged onto the affected area three times a day works very well, especially when followed by a witch hazel compress.

SUPPOSITORIES FOR HEMORRHOIDS
2 parts plantain
1 part St John's wort
1 part slippery elm bark
1 part calendula
1 part comfrey or mallow root

To make and use
All the herbs should be dried and ground to a fine powder. See box.

These are most effective when inserted at night.

ESSENTIAL OILS
Cypress, juniper, geranium

Far right: There are many different forms of ginger. Here is a Long Tailed Ginger Plant.

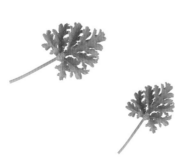

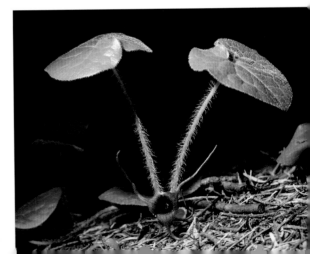

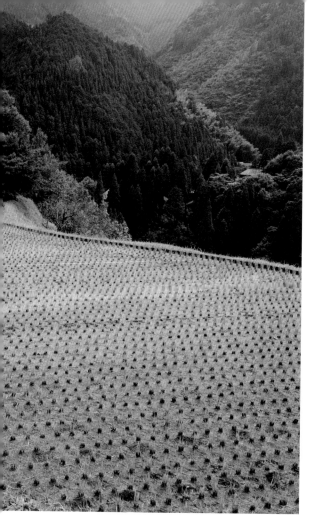

TO MAKE A SUPPOSITORY

Melt about 1 cup (250 ml) of the base of your choice (cocoa butter, beeswax, or coconut oil) in a small saucepan, over low heat. Heat only enough to melt the base. If you are using glycerine as the base, you won't need to do this.

Remove from the heat, and add enough powdered dried herbs to make a thick paste. Incorporate the herbs thoroughly. Tinctures may be added in small amounts, to strengthen the effect. As the dried herbs absorb the base, the mixture will thicken.

Working quickly, form the mixture into a torpedo shapes $\frac{1}{2}$ x 1 in (1.25 x 2.5 cm), or to a size that suits you.

Place the suppositories in single layers, separated by baking parchment, or greaseproof paper, in a moisture-proof box. Store in the refrigerator.

During use, wear sanitary pads to protect undergarments.

Anal fistula

ESSENTIAL OILS
Lavender, tea tree, geranium

ANAL FISTULA MASSAGE CREAM
4 teaspoons unscented gel or grape seed oil
5 drops lavender essential oil
3 drops tea tree essential oil
4 drops geranium essential oil

To make and use
Mix the essential oils thoroughly into the gel, or oil.

First bathe the area with warm water, to which you have added two drops tea tree oil. Massage the cream around the anal area twice daily.

HEMORRHOID GEL
3 tablespoons (45 ml) unscented gel
1 teaspoon distilled witch hazel
2 drops cypress essential oil
2 drops juniper essential oil
2 drops geranium essential oil

To make and use
Mix the oils and witch hazel very thoroughly into the gel, and put in a small, labeled jar. Stir well before each application.

First bathe the area for 10–15 minutes with warm water, to which you have added two drops of each of cypress, juniper, geranium essential oils, to one teaspoon of full cream milk, or milk powder. Add the mixture to half a bowl, (large enough to sit in), of warm water. If you don't have a suitable bowl, use the bath. Fill it with just enough water to cover your bottom. Agitate the water to disperse the oils.

Now gently massage the hemorrhoids with Hemorrhoid Gel. If the blend stings, dilute the mixture with more gel.

Use witch hazel mixed with equal amounts of water, on a pad of absorbent cotton (cottonwool), instead of toilet paper, to wipe the anus after going to the toilet.

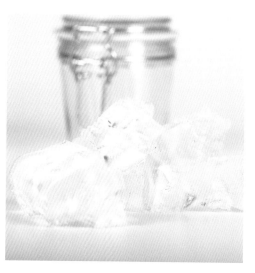

Unscented gel is a perfect base for making firm creams and gels.

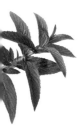

Fatigue and exhaustion

Exhaustion

PHYSICAL EXHAUSTION
Geranium, lavender, peppermint

ESSENTIAL OILS FOR NERVOUS EXHAUSTION
Clary sage, frankincense, peppermint

PHYSICAL EXHAUSTION BLEND
4 teaspoons grape seed oil
10 drops geranium essential oil
3 drops lavender essential oil
3 drops peppermint essential oil

To make and use
Mix all the oils together in a small, labeled bottle, and shake to blend. If there's time, leave for four days before using, so the oils have time to synergize or combine well. Use immediately if necessary.

Float one teaspoon of the blend on a little warm water in a bowl, and use for a massage. If the patient doesn't feel up to a full massage, the hands and/or feet may be the easiest to do—the oils will still enter the bloodstream to do their work.

Pour two teaspoons into a bath or foot bath, agitate to disperse well, and soak in the bath for 10–15 minutes, massaging any floating oil droplets into the skin.

Pour a little of the blend into the palm of your hand, and massage over your body after showering, while the skin is still damp.

Alternatively, just blend the essential oils together to use as an air spray or in an oil burner.

A fabulous foot massage is great for anyone suffering fatigue.

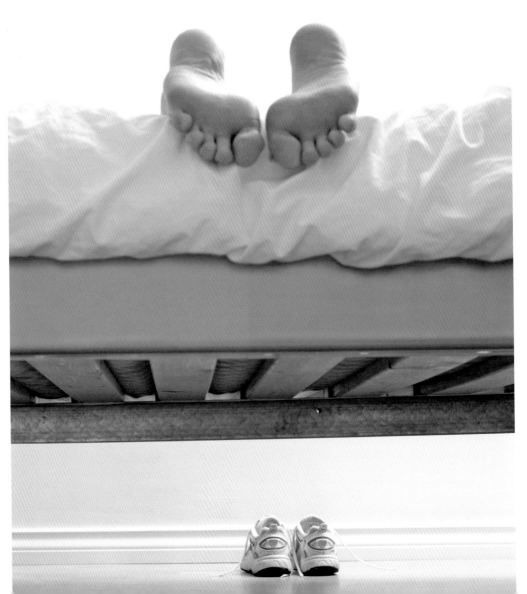

NERVOUS EXHAUSTION BLEND

4 teaspoons grape seed oil
10 drops clary sage essential oil
3 drops frankincense essential oil
3 drops peppermint essential oil

To make and use

Mix all the oils together in a small, labeled bottle, and shake to blend.

If there's time, leave for four days before using, so the oils have time to synergize or combine well.

Float one teaspoon of the blend on a little warm water in a bowl, and use for a massage. If the patient doesn't feel up to a full massage, the hands and/or feet may be the easiest to do—the oils will still enter the bloodstream to do their work.

Pour two teaspoons into a bath or foot bath, agitate to disperse, and soak for 10–15 minutes, massaging any floating oil droplets into the skin.

Pour a little of the blend into the palm of your hand, and massage over your body after showering, while the skin is still damp.

Alternatively, just blend the essential oils together to use as an air spray or in an oil burner.

Fatigue

ESSENTIAL OILS FOR PHYSICAL FATIGUE

Lavender, lemon, clary sage, grapefruit

ESSENTIAL OILS FOR MENTAL FATIGUE

Geranium, lavender, rosemary, peppermint

PHYSICAL FATIGUE MASSAGE BLEND

4 teaspoons grape seed oil
10 drops lavender essential oil
3 drops lemon essential oil
3 drops clary sage essential oil

To make and use

Mix all the oils together in a small, labeled bottle, and shake to blend. If there's time, leave for four days before using, so the oils have time to synergize or combine well. If necessary, this mixture can be used immediately.

First have a bath into which you add five drops lavender, three drops lemon, and two drops grapefruit essential oils, to one cup Epsom salts. Mix well and pour into a warm bath. Stir the water well to dissolve the salts. Soak in the bath for as long as you like.

Next, float one teaspoon of the blend on a little warm water in a bowl, and use for a massage directly after the bath.

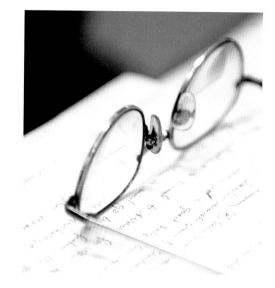

Overwork can cause physical, as well as mental fatigue. Use aromatherapy massage to relieve both.

If there is no one to give you a full massage, you can massage the oils into your feet, legs, hands, and arms; the oils will still enter the blood stream to do their work.

If you prefer to shower, pour a little of the blend into the palm of your hand, and massage over your body afterwards while your skin is still damp.

An aromatherapy foot bath is wonderful for relieving fatigue. Add a total of eight drops of a mixture of the recommended essential oils to the footbath.

Alternatively, just blend the essential oils together to use as an air spray or in an oil burner.

Add petals to your aromatherapy footbath for that touch of luxury.

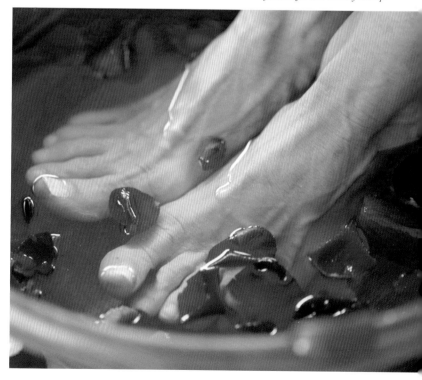

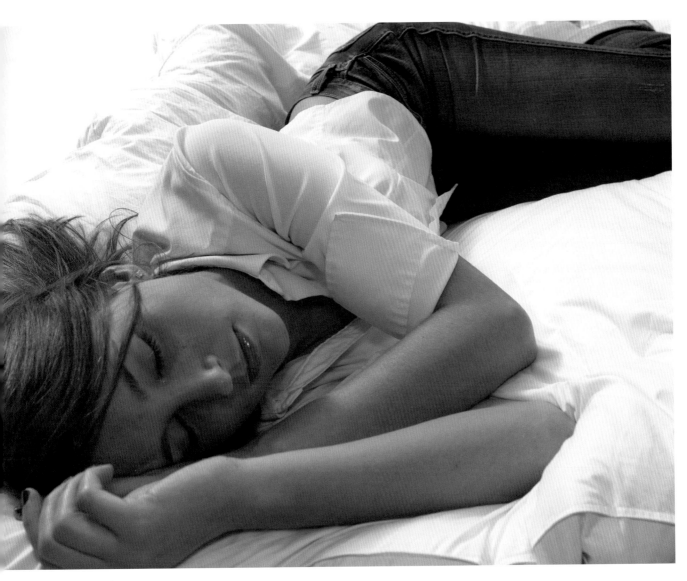

Sleep is the ultimate relaxant.
Try to get six to eight hours a night.

MENTAL FATIGUE MASSAGE BLEND

4 teaspoons grape seed essential oil
5 drops geranium essential oil
5 drops lavender essential oil
3 drops rosemary essential oil
3 drops peppermint essential oil

To make and use

Mix all the oils together in a small, labeled bottle and shake to blend. If there's time, leave for four days before using, so the oils have time to synergize or combine well. Use immediately if necessary.

First have a bath into which you add five drops lavender, three drops lemon, and two drops grapefruit essential oils, to one cup Epsom salts. Mix well and pour into a warm bath. Stir the water well to dissolve the salts. Soak in the bath for as long as you like.

Next, float one teaspoon of the blend on a little warm water in a bowl, and use for a massage directly after the bath.

If there is no one to give you a full massage you can massage the oils into your feet, legs, hands, and arms; the oils will still enter the blood stream to do their work.

If you prefer to shower, pour a little of the blend into the palm of your hand, and massage over your body afterwards while your skin is still damp.

An aromatherapy footbath is wonderful for relieving fatigue. Add a total of eight drops of a mixture of the recommended essential oils to the footbath.

Alternatively, just blend the essential oils together to use as an air spray or in an oil burner.

Chronic fatigue syndrome

This is also known as ME (myalgic encephalomyelitis or "yuppie flu"). But whatever you call it, the result is the same, the sufferer is chronically tired. It is a debilitating and depressing disorder, causing profound weariness and muscle fatigue that has really only been diagnosed by the medical profession since the 1980s. There is some uncertainty as to its cause; however it is probably a post-viral complaint that can last for years, with the symptoms becoming less acute with the passing of time. Treatment is based largely on improving general health, and that of the immune system.

Rest, rest, and more rest is needed, along with the following herbs:

* 1,000–2,000 mg borage (starflower) oil, or evening primrose oil.
* 1,000 mg garlic capsules taken three times daily.
* Skullcap and passionflower tea, or tincture, for depression
* Siberian ginseng to strengthen the system, when the worst stage has passed, and the patient is convalescent.
* Astragalus, (extract is preferred to tablets), to strengthen the immune system (one teaspoon daily in water).
* One cup of cat's claw tea, or 20 drops of tincture in water, three times daily.
* Chamomile tea in place of regular tea, or coffee.

It also pays to fill a large pitcher with filtered water, add two sliced lemons, and drink this lemon water throughout the day. This is one day's supply (the water needs to be freshly made daily or it will becomes bitter). It has a gently cleansing action.

Hot packs, and hot showers or baths, often help to ease the pain in the muscles.

Aromatherapy has a role to play in treating chronic fatigue, by helping ease muscular pain with massage, lifting spirits when depressed, and helping stimulate the immune system. Make up a bottle of each of the following essential oil blends, and use them at appropriate times.

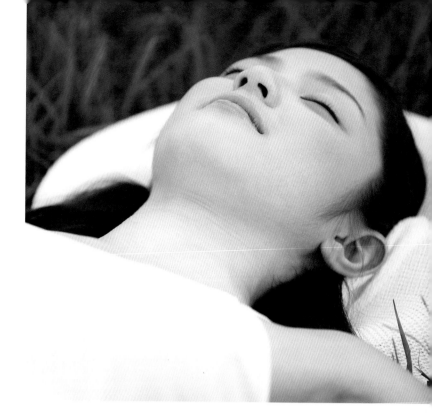

ESSENTIAL OILS FOR DEPRESSION
Lavender, grapefruit, sandalwood, ylang-ylang

ESSENTIAL OILS FOR MUSCULAR PAIN
Bergamot, marjoram, ginger, black pepper

ANTI-VIRAL AND IMMUNOSTIMULANT ESSENTIAL OILS
Rosewood, thyme, tea tree, cinnamon

The causes of Chronic Fatigue Syndrome are largely unknown, but successful treatment seems to rely on rest first, followed by treatment to the immune system.

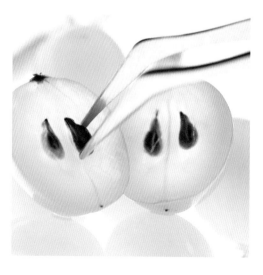

Grape seed essential oil is used in Mental Fatigue Massage Blend.

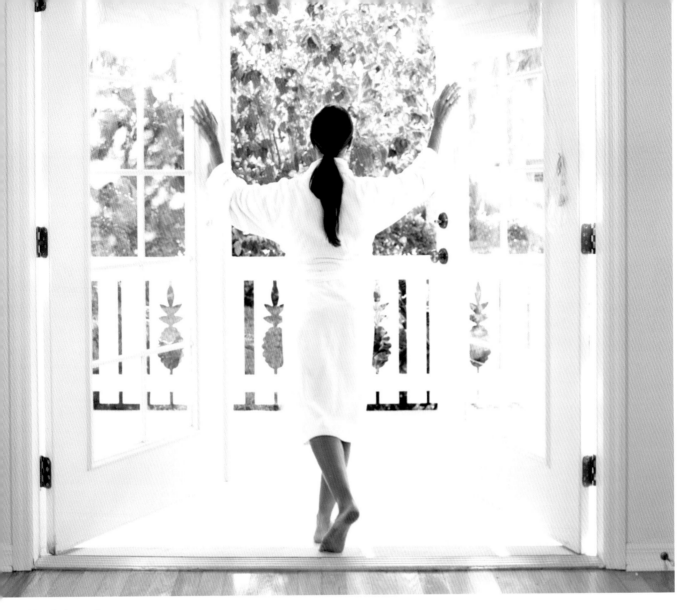

Try to begin your day on a positive note with deep breathing and stretching as soon as you get out of bed.

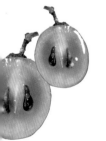

CHRONIC FATIGUE SPIRIT LIFTER

$\frac{1}{4}$ cup (60 ml) grape seed oil
20 drops bergamot or lavender essential oil
15 drops grapefruit essential oil
15 drops ylang-ylang or sandalwood essential oil

To make and use

Mix all the oils together in a small, labeled bottle, and shake to blend.

If there's time, leave for four days before using, so the oils have time to synergize or combine well.

Float one teaspoon of the blend on a little warm water in a bowl, and use for a massage.

Pour two teaspoons of the blend into a bath or foot bath, agitate to disperse, and soak into the skin.

Pour a little of the blend into the palm of the hand and massage over the body after showering, while the skin is still damp.

Alternatively, just blend the essential oils together to use as an air spray or in an oil burner.

CHRONIC FATIGUE MUSCULAR PAIN OIL

$\frac{1}{4}$ cup (60 ml) grape seed oil
20 drops borage seed oil
20 drops bergamot essential oil
15 drops marjoram essential oil
10 drops ginger essential oil
5 drops black pepper essential oil

To make and use

Mix all the oils together in a small, labeled bottle, and shake to blend.

If there's time, leave for four days before using, so the oils have time to synergize or combine well.

Float one teaspoon of the blend in a little warm water in bowl, and use for a full body massage.

Pour two teaspoons of the blend in a bath or foot bath, agitate to disperse, and soak in the bath for 10-15 minutes, and massage any floating oil droplets into the skin.

Pour a little of the blend into the palm of your hand, and massage over your body after showering, while the skin is still damp.

Hot packs and hot showers or baths often help to ease the pain in the muscles.

Alternatively, just blend the essential oils together to use as an air spray or in an oil burner.

CHRONIC FATIGUE IMMUNOSTIMULANT AND ANTI-VIRAL OIL

$1/4$ cup (60 ml) grape seed oil
20 drops borage seed oil
20 drops rosewood essential oil
10 drops thyme essential oil
10 drops tea tree essential oil
1 drop cinnamon essential oil

To make and use

Mix all the oils together in a small, labeled bottle, and shake to blend. If there's time, leave for four days before using, so the oils have time to synergize or combine well.

Float one teaspoon of the blend in a little warm water in a bowl, and use for a full body massage.

Pour two teaspoons of the blend into a bath, or foot bath, agitate to disperse, and soak in the bath for 10-15 minutes, and massage any floating oil droplets into the skin.

Pour a little of the blend into the palm of your hand, and massage over your body after showering, while the skin is still damp.

Alternatively, just blend the essential oils together to use as an air spray or in an oil burner.

Stress

Stress is a constant part of our lives, and without it we would be walking cabbages. There are two main types of stress—eustress and distress.

Eustress is the healthy one that adds sparkle to our lives. We need eustress in order to function, and to be alert. It has a beginning, a middle, and, most importantly, an end.

Dystress (distress) is unresolved stress that is emotionally, and physically, exhausting. The chemicals which our bodies produce in stressful situations, such as adrenalin, are not dispersed, and can contribute to high blood pressure, heart problems, and digestive problems, cancer, migraine, back problems, depression, and nervous breakdowns.

If you have the following symptoms, your stress and tension levels need to be addressed before you "burn out."
- No enthusiasm for work, play, family, or friends,
- Finding it difficult to laugh, and getting upset and irritable easily.
- A feeling of impending doom.
- Constant backaches, headaches, or stomach aches.
- An inability to sleep, or waking up in the morning feeling just as anxious, and as tired, as when you went to bed.

Essential oils used in massage, baths, and oil burners, can help you learn to relax. If you do not have one of the essential oils specified, you may substitute another that feels appropriate. Make up your own blends, using the emotions and conditions detailed on the next page as a guide.

It's not always very satisfactory to use all the essential oils suggested for one condition. Instead, try to choose just one or two for the main problem, along with another one or two which balance the blend.

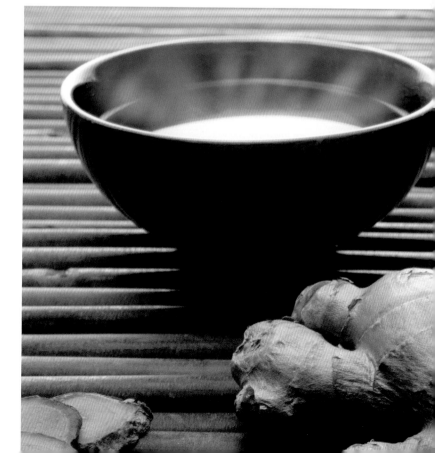

Ginger tea and ginger root. Ginger essential oil helps relieve tired muscles.

Aromatic baths are an ideal way of using essential oils to alleviate stress, insomnia, depression, and other stress–related problems. In fact, it is very difficult to lie in warm, beautifully scented water and remain miserable or tense! Breathe slowly and gently. As you breathe in, feel the aromatic vapors entering every cell of your body and mind, collecting all negative, tense, tired feelings into a gray mist. As you breathe out, imagine the gray mist being breathed out.

You could also use the "One" meditation at this time. Remain in the bath for at least 30 minutes, and top up with more warm water, if necessary. After the bath, imagine all the tension and negative feelings running down the drain with the bath water.

Some of the suggestions below may help you to cope with various tensions until a long term solution is found. If you have depression you really need the help of a trained therapist, especially if the depression is of long duration or profound. Essential oils can help to raise the spirits at this time.

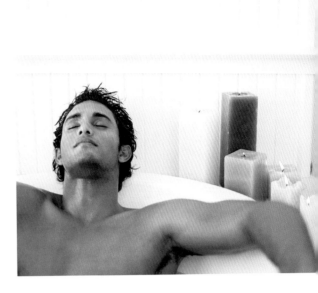

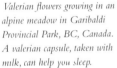

Valerian flowers growing in an alpine meadow in Garibaldi Provincial Park, BC, Canada. A valerian capsule, taken with milk, can help you sleep.

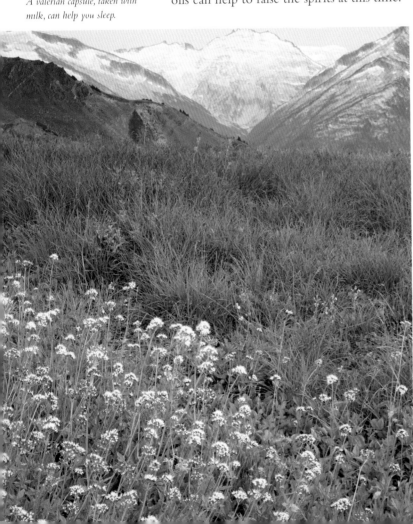

BASIC OIL BLEND

$1/_4$ cup (60 ml) sweet almond oil
50 drops mixed essential oils from the
    following list (page 480)

To make and use

Mix all the oils together in a small, labeled bottle, and shake to blend.

If there's time, leave for four days before using, so the oils have time to synergize or combine well.

Massage a few drops of the blend on pulse points, such as the throat, and the inside of the wrists. Carry the bottle of the blend and sniff occasionally.

Add two teaspoons of the blend to warm bath just before entering, and then agitate the water to disperse the oil.

Shower frequently, as the water removes depressing positive ions, and replaces them with energy-raising negative ions. Put one drop of each essential oil on a wet wash cloth, and use to rub over the body after a shower.

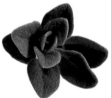

Use essential oils in air sprays and oil burners.

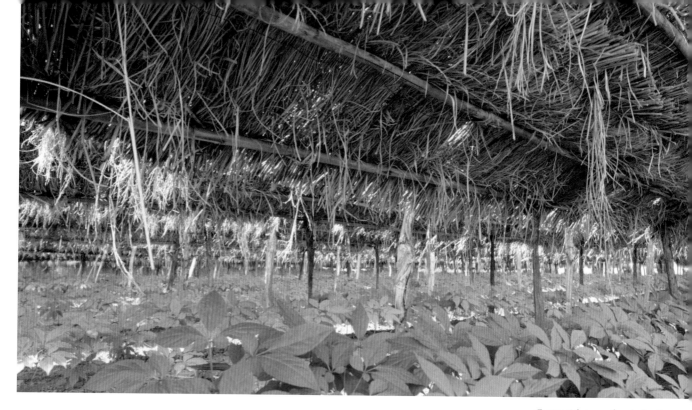

Commercial ginseng farm in South Korea. The plants are protected from the weather by straw roofing.

Insomnia—adults only

True insomnia is the habitual loss of sleep on a regular basis. The occasional "bad night" doesn't qualify. If you can't sleep, don't lie there tossing and turning, get up and do something relatively relaxing, like reading a book, or having a warm milky drink.

Take a warm, (not hot), shower half an hour before going to bed, or, if you have a lawn, walk barefoot on the grass before going to bed to rid of positive ions.

The use of the herbs on page 480 will greatly increase your chances of having a sweet sleep.

Try taking one skullcap or valerian capsule, and two calcium citrate tablets, with a milk drink 20–30 minutes before retiring for the night. Don't use valerian continuously for more than three weeks; have a break of one week before recommencing.

Make a small herb pillow containing crushed hops and lavender, and slip it into your pillowcase with your pillow.

Essential oils used for massaging, as bath blends, or in an oil burner, or air spray, are an easy and pleasurable way to enhance your chances of getting a good night's sleep.

ESSENTIAL OILS

Chamomile, clary sage, lavender, marjoram

SLEEP EASY OIL

4 teaspoons grape seed oil
6 drops lavender essential oil
6 drops clary sage essential oil
4 drops marjoram or chamomile essential oil

To make and use

Mix all the oils together in a small, labeled bottle, and shake to blend.

If there's time, leave for four days before using, so the oils have time to synergize or combine well.

Massage a few drops of the blend on the temples, and the back of the neck.

Sip a cup of chamomile tea while having a warm, (not hot), bath with two teaspoons of the blend added. Agitate to disperse the blend, and soak in the bath for 30 minutes, massaging any floating oil droplets into the skin.

Pour a little of the blend into the palm of your hand, and massage over your body after showering while the skin is still damp.

Alternatively, just blend the essential oils together to use as an air spray or in an oil burner.

TIP FOR CHILDREN WHO CAN'T SLEEP SEE CHILDREN AND BABIES ON PAGE 396.

Essential oils for stress and relaxation

Condition	Oils
Anger	Bergamot, chamomile, cypress, peppermint, ylang-ylang
Anxiety	Bergamot, chamomile, clary sage, frankincense geranium, lavender, mandarin, marjoram, sandalwood
Apathy	Grapefruit, jasmine, lavender, lemon, rosemary
Balancer (moods)	Lavender, geranium, jasmine
Burn out	Grapefruit, jasmine, lavender, lemon, sandalwood
Calming	Bergamot, cedarwood, clary sage, frankincense, jasmine, lavender, mandarin, marjoram, sandalwood, ylang-ylang
Long-term depression	Bergamot, orange, chamomile
Loss of interest in life	Orange, rosemary, ylang-ylang
Emotional stress	Ylang-ylang
Excitability	Cedarwood, chamomile, lavender, mandarin, marjoram, ylang-ylang
Fainting	Lavender, marjoram, peppermint
Frigidity	Clary sage, ylang-ylang
Frustration	Bergamot, lavender
Grief	Cypress, marjoram, sandalwood
Guilt	Chamomile, clary sage, sandalwood
Hysteria	Clary sage, peppermint
Insomnia	Cedarwood, chamomile, lavender, mandarin, marjoram, sandalwood
Irritability	Cypress
Listlessness	Geranium, jasmine, lavender
Manic depression	Geranium, grapefruit, lavender
Meditation	Cedarwood frankincense, sandalwood
Mental dullness	Lemon, peppermint, rosemary
Mental stress	Cedarwood, chamomile, rosemary
Migraine	Grapefruit, marjoram
Negative thoughts	Orange, peppermint
Nervous exhaustion	Grapefruit, lavender, rosemary, ylang-ylang
Nervous headache	Grapefruit, lavender, marjoram
Nervousness (jitters)	Bergamot, frankincense, geranium, lavender
Obsessiveness	Frankincense, sandalwood
Panic attack	Clary sage, Rescue Remedy, ylang-ylang
Paranoia	Clary sage
Pre-exam or interview stress	Bergamot, grapefruit, lemon, lavender, rosemary

Essential oils for stress and relaxation [cont.]

Condition	Oils
Pre-operative stress	Lavender, clary sage, ylang-ylang, chamomile, Rescue Remedy
Post-operative stress	Lavender, grapefruit, mandarin, peppermint, Rescue Remedy
Sexuality (insecurity)	Clary sage, jasmine, sandalwood, ylang-ylang
Shock	Lavender, peppermint, Rescue Remedy
Sluggishness (mental)	Basil, lemon, grapefruit
Trauma	Lavender, marjoram, Rescue Remedy
Vertigo	Lavender, peppermint

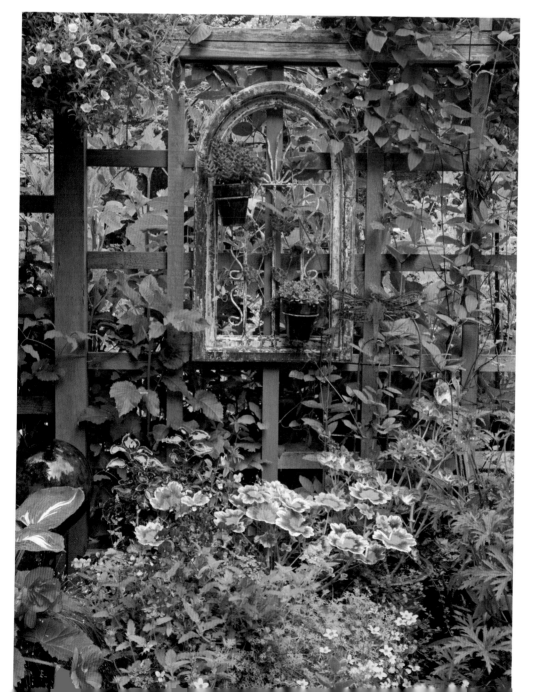

Geraniums grow well mixed in with other flowers. Here they sit happily with clematis and begonias. Geranium oil is an ingredient in most essential oil blends.

Mouth and teeth

We all clean our teeth, and most of us use floss. But that's it when it comes to our mouths and teeth. Unless we get a reminder from the dentist, we expect them to perform their tasks with no problems. The supermarket is full of all sorts of chemically-based products to fix something that does go wrong, but they have strong tastes to hide what's in them. Most are so strong that they often strip the mouth of its natural saliva. The best way to keep our mouths fresh and infection free is to use remedies made from natural products. If mouth ulcers persist you should consult a health professional, as it may be diet or vitamin related. Mouth ulcers and sores are common in chemotherapy patients and these remedies may help to relieve the discomfort.

Some of the recipes contain alcohol but it is not swallowed. It's there as a preservative. Without it the mixture would not last.

Myrrh Mouthwash is excellent for healing mouth ulcers and sweetening the breath. It should not be swallowed.

Breath, bad

A dental check is recommended, as bad teeth are a common source of bad breath. Stomach upsets, and also insufficient gastric acids, can cause bad breath. Depending on the formulation, mouthwashes can be used to sweeten the breath, keep bacteria and fungus infections at bay, and ensure healthy gums. Brush the tongue gently with toothpaste when brushing your teeth.

MYRRH MOUTHWASH
Myrrh helps to heal mouth ulcers.

$1/_3$ cup (80 ml) sherry or brandy
3 tablespoons (45 ml) cider vinegar
1 teaspoon honey
10 drops peppermint essential oil
3 drops clove essential oil
1 teaspoon tincture of myrrh, or 5 drops myrrh
   essential oil
1 teaspoon glycerine

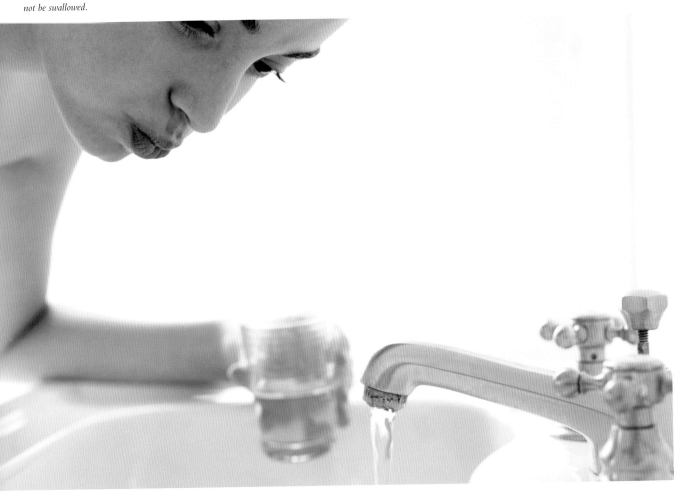

To make and use

Mix all the ingredients in a jar; leave to stand for one week, shaking the jar often. Strain the mixture through coffee paper before using.

Add one teaspoon of the mouthwash to $^1/_2$ glass warm water, and rinse mouth several times with the mixture; spit out. Do not swallow the mixture.

LEMON AND MINT MOUTHWASH

This mouthwash will keep the mouth healthy, and sweet smelling. It will also help to cure sore, or ulcerated mouths.

$^1/_2$ cup (125 ml) vodka or brandy
1 drop thyme essential oil
5 drops lemon essential oil
5 drops peppermint essential oil
2 drops lavender essential oil
2 drops tea tree essential oil
1 teaspoon glycerine

To make and use

Mix all the ingredients in a jar; leave to stand for one week, shaking the jar often. Strain the mixture through coffee paper before using.

Add one teaspoon of the mouthwash to $^1/_2$ glass warm water, and rinse mouth several times with the mixture; spit out. Do not swallow the mixture.

HERBAL MOUTHWASH

1 cup (250 ml) brandy, sherry, or cider vinegar
4 teaspoons crushed anise seeds
4 teaspoons finely chopped peppermint leaves
4 cloves, bruised
$^1/_2$ teaspoon (2.5 ml) tincture of myrrh

To make and use

Mix all ingredients together in a jar with a well-fitting lid. Leave for one week, shaking daily.

Strain through a sieve and then through coffee filter paper. Shake the bottle before use.

Add 2 teaspoons (10 ml) to 2 tablespoons (40 ml) of warm water, rinse mouth and spit out.

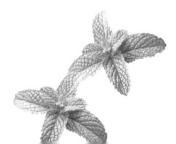

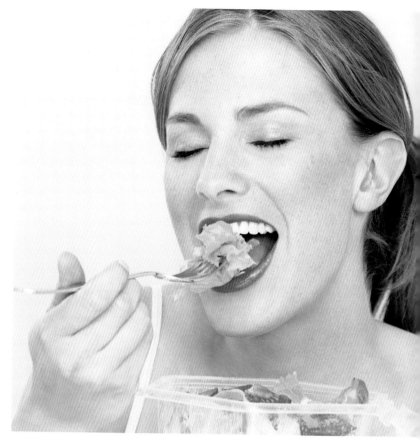

Fresh uncooked food is essential for healthy gums and teeth.

Toothache

There really is nothing worse than toothache. Whether it's because the mouth is so close to the brain or not, I don't know. All I do know is that nothing hurts more. Here are a few quick remedies to try until you can get to a dentist.

Pressing hard on the root of the aching tooth from the outside of the face, often eases the pain. An ice cube held in the same area also helps to numb the nerve.

Using a cotton bud, apply one drop of clove oil onto the aching tooth, and use the residue on the bud to gently massage the gum surrounding the offending tooth.

Gently massage the cheek over the aching tooth, and along the jaw, with three drops of chamomile oil in one teaspoon of warm vegetable oil.

A strong tea made of ground cloves held in the mouth and spit out, will often ease toothache. Whether to use the tea warm or cold is a matter of what eases your particular toothache best—test to see which works.

TIP TO PREVENT THE GROWTH OF BACTERIA ON TOOTHBRUSHES, DIP THEM IN A SOLUTION OF TWO DROPS OF TEA TREE OIL IN A TUMBLER OF WATER. RINSE THOROUGHLY AND ALWAYS STORE IN A PLACE WHERE THERE IS GOOD AIR CIRCULATION.

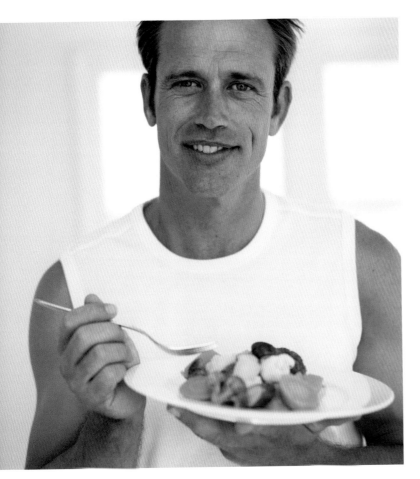

To prevent gum disease it is important to exercise your teeth and jaws by eating crunchy and leafy fruit and vegetables.

GINGIVITIS MOUTHWASH

$\frac{1}{4}$ cup (60 ml) sherry
3 tablespoons (45 ml) brandy
1 teaspoon glycerine
8 drops peppermint essential oil
6 drops thyme essential oil
4 drops myrrh essential oil or 1 teaspoon tincture of myrrh

To make and use

Mix all ingredients together in a labeled jar.

Leave for four days to synergize, shaking frequently. Strain through coffee filter paper. Store in a dark bottle with a stopper.

Add one teaspoon mouthwash to $\frac{1}{2}$ glass warm water, rinse mouth several times with the mixture, and spit out. Do not swallow the mixture.

Repeat several times daily.

Gum infections

ESSENTIAL OILS

Tea tree, myrrh

TREATMENT

Mouthwash using either, or both, essential oils.

Mouth ulcers

If you have frequent recurrent of mouth ulcers, you will continue to be plagued with them until you search for, and find, the cause.

Some of the causes might be poor diet low in vitamins B and C, stress, ill-fitting dentures, a rough edge on a tooth, biting the tongue or the inside of the cheek, food allergy.

Teeth and gum problems

Dental check-ups, brushing with a medium bristle, brush after eating, are all very important treatments. Flossing, eating foods such as fruit and raw vegetables that give teeth and jaws good exercise, will all help to keep your teeth and gums strong and healthy. The following recipes will help to prevent mouth infections.

Gingivitis

Gingivitis is an inflammation and bleeding of the gums, caused largely by bacterial plaque, and a poor brushing technique. In other words, we can prevent this. Check with your dentist if the problem has been long term. To prevent or treat gingivitis, brush teeth regularly and properly with a medium or soft bristle toothbrush. Thorough rinsing of the mouth several times a day with the Gingivitis Mouthwash can be helpful.

Inexpensive coffee filter papers are ideal for straining herbal remedies as they are fine enough to remove any hairs that may irritate the mouth and throat.

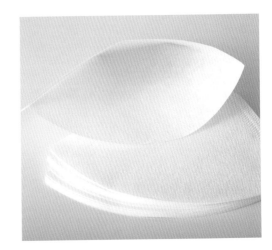

ESSENTIAL OIL
Myrrh

TREATMENT
Add one drop of myrrh oil (or $\frac{1}{4}$ teaspoon tincture of myrrh), and $\frac{1}{4}$ teaspoon Epsom salts to a glass of warm water. Swoosh around your mouth as vigorously as possible. Spit the mixture out. Repeat until all is used. Do not swallow the mixture.

The following is the best method I have found for treating mouth ulcers. Dissolve one teaspoon of Epsom salts in a one glass of warm water. Take a mouthful of the mixture, and "swoosh" it around the mouth as vigorously as possible, then spit out. Repeat with all the mixture. Continue the treatment as long as needed.

If you prefer to use herbs, a tea made from fresh leaves of sage, or one teaspoon tincture of myrrh, added to two teaspoons of water and used as a mouthwash is effective.

Freeze triple-strength sage tea in ice-cube trays, smash a cube to bits and suck the small pieces. The ice numbs the pain, and the sage helps to heal the ulcers.

THREE-WEEK MOUTH ULCER TREATMENT
Mix three parts nettle, and three parts chicory, to one part sage. Add three tablespoons to 1 quart (1 liter) cold water, and leave overnight. Next morning bring the mixture to a boil, then remove from the heat, and leave to steep for five minutes. Strain well through coffee filter paper.

Drink one cup three times daily.

MOUTH ULCERS

The following remedies will assist in the treatment of mouth ulcers.

- Calendula tea or goldenseal tea. Gargle as a mouthwash, three or four times daily.
- Myrrh capsules. Open a capsule and dab a little of the contents directly on the sore.
- Tea. Place a wet tea bag directly on the ulcer. This also helps with toothache and tooth extraction.
- Sage. Gargle with a strong sage tea, once or twice a day. Make sure you do not swallow.
- Echinacea. Echinacea tea in small amounts can be swished in the mouth for two to three minutes, then swallowed, three times a day. Tablets and capsules are also helpful.
- Chamomile. Strong tea can be swished in the mouth three times a day.
- Tea tree oil. Add three drops of tea tree oil to 1 cup (250 ml) water. Rinse twice daily.

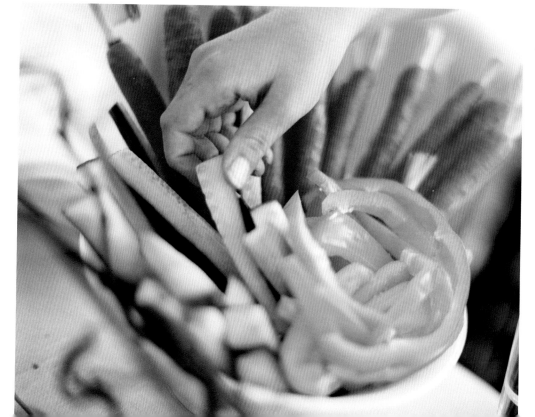

Carrots, cucumber, and celery make colorful and tempting nibbles for family and friends, and also contribute to good dental care.

Eyes and ears

It's normal for our vision and hearing to deteriorate through the years. That doesn't mean we shouldn't take care of our eyes and ears all through our lives.

Infections, allergies, and other eye complaints, cause us to rub our eyes which could cause damage. Extreme sports can also be detrimental, as jarring can tear the retina from the eye and cause blindness. And we have all heard of famous people losing their sight through glaucoma.

And then there is the damage that most of us did to our ears during our early music years. Attending concerts with overloud music, using our iPods too much and too loud, and just generally abusing our hearing, will no doubt cause us problems later on.

Eye problems in particular can be very serious and if any condition is painful or prolonged, it's necessary to see a health professional immediately. Also a serious ear infection can go to the brain (particularly in young children), so take care, and don't wait for things to get better. If you feel severe pain in your ears, or any clouding or loss of vision in your eyes, see a doctor immediately.

Eye problems

Here are a few simple remedies for irritable eyes. Any painful, or serious condition should be treated by a health professional immediately.

Studies have shown that bilberry fruit can provide a rich source of flavonoids that are helpful for easing poor night vision and eyestrain.

Eyebright or goldenseal teas, well strained through coffee filter paper, are premium treatments for eye infections and irritations.

Small pieces of sand, grit, or dust may be removed by placing a linseed under the outer corner of the bottom eyelid and leaving it there. The seed will swell to a jelly, collect the irritant, and take it to the inner corner of the eye where it can be removed.

The tannin in tea is good for soothing sore, tired eyes. Put used tea bags in the fridge, and then lay them, deliciously cold and wonderfully soothing, on your eyes for five minutes. Chamomile tea bags may be used the same way.

Slices of cold cucumber or potato help to reduce under-eye puffiness caused by eyestrain.

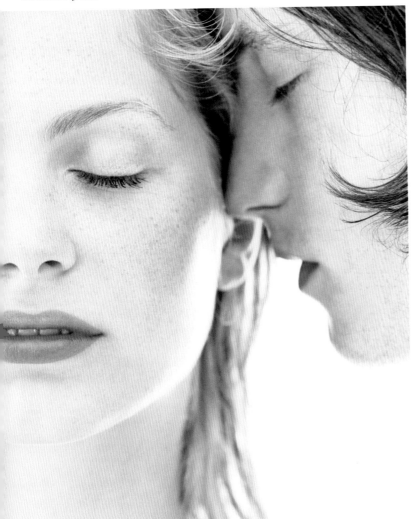

Our eyes and ears provide two of our most important senses. Take extreme care of both.

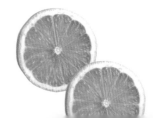

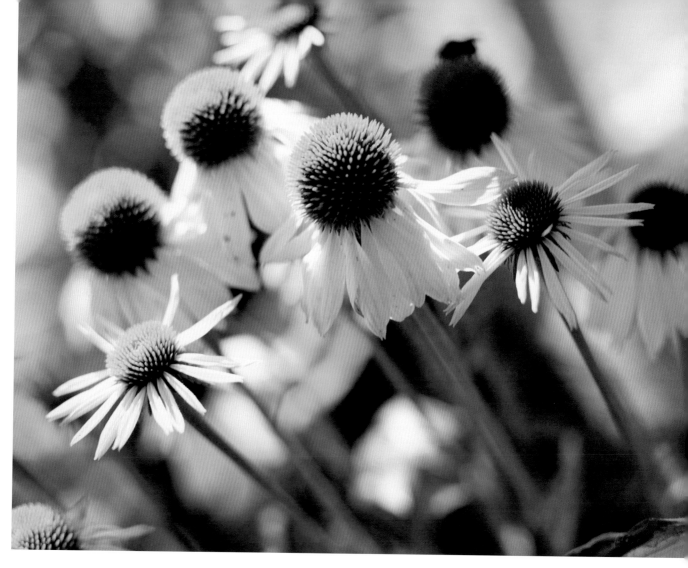

Conjunctivitis

Conjunctivitis is highly contagious and is common in children who rub their eyes and touch each other. It's almost impossible to keep conjunctivitis from spreading to both eyes.

The symptoms of conjunctivitis are a yellow discharge, sore, red, and itchy eyes and inflamed eyelids. It isn't a serious problem except in newborn babies, when medical attention should be sought.

Take half a teaspoon of fluid extract of echinacea in two tablespoons of water, three times daily for two weeks to strengthen the immune system.

ESSENTIAL OILS

Chamomile, lemon

TREATMENT

Make a compress using one drop of chamomile and lemon essential oils, mixed well into a combination of one tablespoon of ice cold witch hazel and two teaspoons of ice cold water. Squeeze as much of the moisture out of the compress cloth as you can. Use the compress over the entire eye area, keeping the eye closed during treatment.

Caution *Do not let any oil get into the eye.*

Chamomile flowers are dried and used to make chamomile tea.

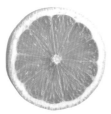

Swimming at Chankanaab National Park, Cozumel, Mexico. Unfortunately, not all swimming holes have water this clean.

TIP REMEMBER, THE SMALLEST THING YOU SHOULD EVER PUT IN YOUR EAR IS YOUR ELBOW!

Knobs of garlic hanging on a window in Provence, France. Garlic essential oil is helpful in the treatment of earache.

Earache

Ear pain must always be taken very seriously, especially in a child. It can be a symptom of middle-ear infection, mastoiditis, or other complaints that need treatment by a professional.

The following suggestions are to be used to treat simple earache caused by draughts or mild infections. If earache persists, seek the help of a professional.

Dry eczema, excess wax, and outer-ear infections are some of the problems that can be dealt with very effectively by the use of garlic oil. It's an easy process to make your own garlic oil. It won't be as strong as the oil in capsules, but is an advantage for children, as they cannot tolerate the full-strength garlic oil. Just place $\frac{1}{2}$ peeled garlic clove in 2 cups vegetable oil. Place in a sealed jar in the refrigerator for at least four days. This is a very mild solution.

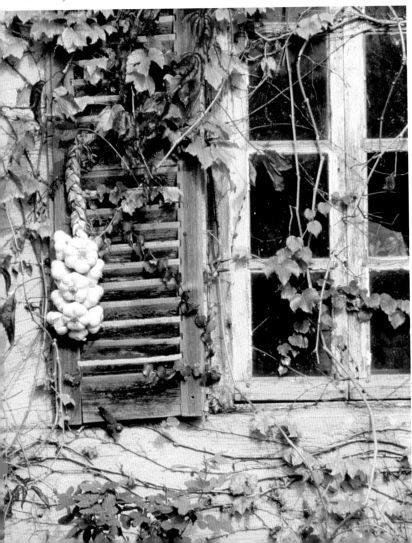

ESSENTIAL OILS
Tea tree, garlic

TREATMENT
Put three drops of tea tree or garlic oil in one teaspoon olive oil warmed to blood heat (no hotter), drip a few drops into the ear. Plug the external opening of the ear with absorbent cotton (cottonwool). Repeat as needed.

Other remedies

Infused mullein flower oil is also very soothing and healing for simple earache.

The "grandmother remedy" that works really well is the cooked onion! Cut an onion in half and wrap one half in foil. Bake or grill until soft. Fold back the foil, leaving it under the onion as a holder. Hold the onion to the sore ear where the steam, heat, and fumes will enter the ear (not touching until cool enough so that it won't burn the skin). Keep the ear warm after the treatment by resting on a hot water bottle, or by wrapping a scarf around the head.

Treat earaches seriously as any infection can spread to the middle, and inner, ear. The following suggestions are for simple earaches cause by draughts or mild infections. See your doctor if an earache is regular, persistent, or severe. Never poke around in the ear.

There are a number of prepared natural remedies on the market for treating mild ear problems. Aloe is particularly effective and comes in drops, especially for ears.

Swimmer's Ear

The symptoms of swimmer's ear vary slightly but usually appear as a low ache which accelerates quickly. It often occurs after swimming in a pool that may have bacteria, or from residual water left in the ear. Make sure to lie your head on each side for a short while after swimming, to allow any water to run out. You can usually hear the "crackle" as it comes. The remedies below will assist if the condition continues. But don't wait too long before seeing a professional. Persistent earache could be serious.

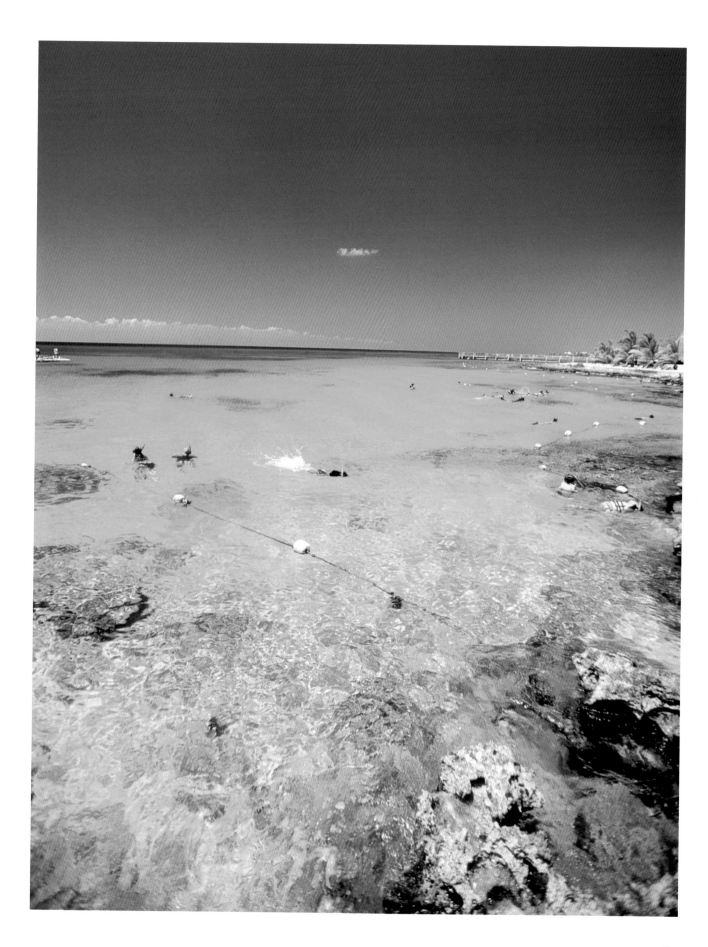

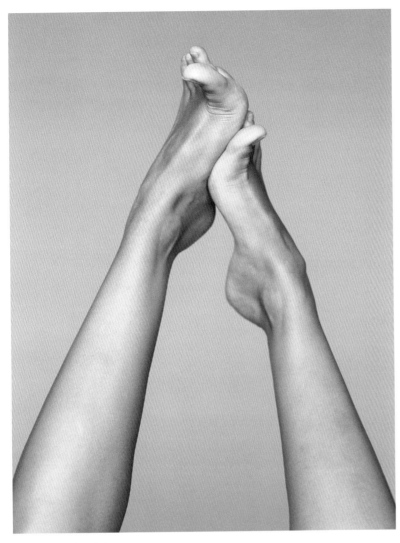

Let's face it, we don't look after our feet well enough. Take care of them by massaging with essential oils.

Foot work

Feet are the unsung heroes who carry us, more or less uncomplainingly, on our journey through three score years and ten, and much more these days. We usually give them attention only if they ache or grow corns. We abuse our feet with ill-fitting shoes, synthetic shoes, stockings, tights or socks, by cutting toe nails incorrectly, weighing too much, and standing for too long. Let's give a thought and a cheer to the feet, and promise them a bit of loving care.

Aching feet

ESSENTIAL OILS
Benzoin, cypress, lavender, lemon grass, peppermint, rosemary

TREATMENT
A foot bath is a soothing treatment for aching feet. Try to relax as much as possible while enjoying this experience; listen to music or read a book.

Fill two bowls (each large enough to fit both feet) with water—one cold and one hot. Sprinkle four to six drops cypress, rosemary, or lavender essential oil, or two drops of each oil, in the cold foot bath, and agitate well to disperse the oil. Soak the feet for a few minutes, first in the hot foot bath, and then in the cold. Repeat for about 15 minutes.

Follow with a foot massage using Foot-ease Oil.

If your work involves a lot of standing, your feet are probably aching and swollen when you get home. Make the following herbal vinegar, and use very cold for the most soothing effect.

VINEGAR FOOT SOOTHER
1 cup (250 ml) white vinegar
20 drops grapefruit essential oil
20 drops lavender essential oil
20 drops black pepper essential oil
10 drops thyme essential oil
20 drops rosemary essential oil

To make and use
Mix all the oils and vinegar together in a labeled bottle, and shake to blend.

Leave for four days before using, so the oils have time to synergize or combine well.

Shake well before use. Store in the refrigerator
Dab on the feet and air dry.

FOOT-EASE OIL
4 teaspoons sweet almond oil
2 teaspoons avocado oil
1 teaspoon wheat germ oil
2 teaspoons jojoba oil
10 drops rosemary essential oil
10 drops lavender essential oil
5 drops benzoin essential oil
1 teaspoon vodka

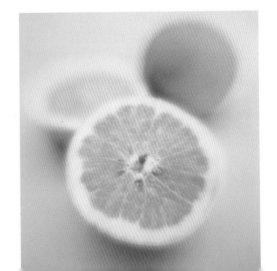

To make and use

Mix all the ingredients together in a labeled bottle, and shake to blend.

Leave for four days before using, so the oils have time to synergize or combine well.

Shake well before use. Store in the refrigerator.

Follow that foot bath with a foot massage.

FOOT AND LEG GEL

Because this gel isn't greasy it can be used anywhere, any time. It is a lovely, soothing treatment for those times when your legs ache and you can't have a foot bath, and don't want to use oil.

4 teaspoons unscented gel
5 drops peppermint essential oil

To make and use

Combine ingredients in a bowl and mix together really well. Pot and label.

Keep a little pot with you in your pocket or handbag. Smooth it gently over the feet and legs.

Swollen feet and ankles

Feet can swell for many reasons, and most of these are not serious conditions and are easily treated. If your feet and legs swell often, it may be an indication of either a heart or kidney problem, and you should seek professional help.

Not serious causes include standing for long periods of time, arthritis, rheumatism, varicose veins, constipation, hot weather, long flights.

Elevating the feet, avoiding sitting or standing without movement for lengthy periods, and addressing the problem of constipation, can all help to avoid or cure this condition. Ice-cold compresses containing lavender, cypress, and lavender essential oils, laid on the ankles and feet will reduce the swelling, while the above massage blend will reduce the feeling of "fullness" and discomfort.

ESSENTIAL OILS

Cypress, eucalyptus, lavender

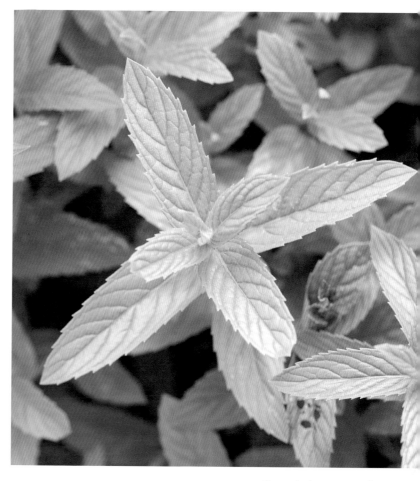

Peppermint leaves are ground and distilled to make peppermint essential oil used in Foot and Leg Gel.

MASSAGE BLEND FOR SWOLLEN FEET AND ANKLES

1 teaspoon grape seed oil
2 drops cypress essential oil
1 drop eucalyptus essential oil
1 drop lavender essential oil

To make and use

Mix all the ingredients together in a small, labeled bottle, and shake to blend.

Leave for four days before using, so the oils have time to synergize or combine well.

Float the oil blend on a little warm water in a bowl. Massage firmly into the feet, ankles and calves of the legs, using sweeping movements. Draw the knuckles of the hand firmly across the soles of the feet from the big toe to the heel. Repeat several times.

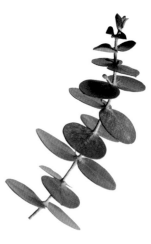

A firm massage on the balls of the feet can relieve pressure on toes and bunions.

Bunions

Bunions are a swelling, thickening, and deformity of the joint of the big toe nearest to the foot. Pain and discomfort is created by the chafing caused by shoes.

ESSENTIAL OILS
Carrot, chamomile
Calendula infused oil, French marigold infused oil

MASSAGE BLEND FOR BUNIONS
4 teaspoons calendula infused oil
4 teaspoons French marigold infused oil
15 drops chamomile essential oil
15 drops carrot seed essential oil

To make and use
Mix all the ingredients together in a small, labeled bottle, and shake to blend.

Leave for four days before using, so the oils have time to synergize or combine well.

Gently massage the whole foot with the blend paying special attention to the bunion itself. Repeat twice daily.

TIP FIND SHOES THAT FIT AND VISIT A QUALIFIED PODIATRIST WHO CAN MAKE SPECIAL PADS TO PROTECT THE BUNION. GO BAREFOOT AS MUCH AS POSSIBLE OR FIND SANDALS WITH STRAPS THAT DON'T TOUCH THE SORE AREA.

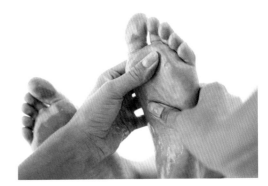

Corns

ESSENTIAL OILS
Calendula infused oil

TREATMENT
It is possible to buy a hard black pumice-like treatment called a "chiropody sponge." If the corn is not too painful, it may be removed by following the instructions on the packet. After treatment, apply calendula infused oil to the area, and either bandage, or use a non-stick dressing.

If the corn is too painful for the abrasive treatment, massage it with calendula infused oil morning and night, cover with a dressing and when soft enough, lift out the core. Shoes are almost invariably the cause of corns, so find the culprits and bin them!

Marigold infused oil helps bunions. Here a small girl carries a box of marigold plants on her head.

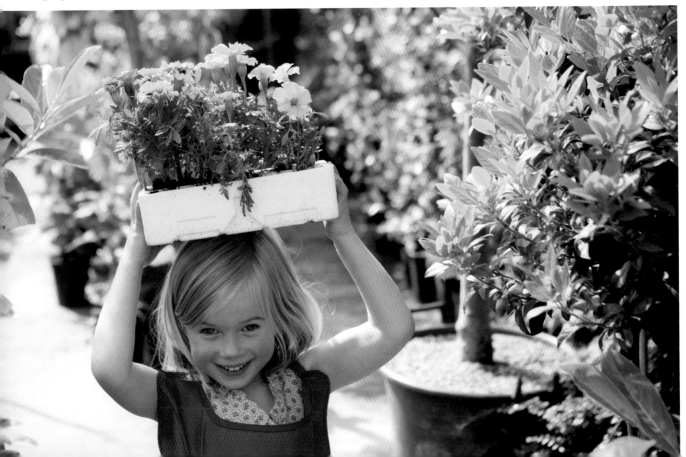

Athlete's Foot

Athlete's foot or tinea is caused by infectious fungi that are rife in gymnasiums and swimming pools. The skin is itchy and flaky and the areas between the toes become spongy and white.

* Wear cotton or woolen socks and non-synthetic shoes.
* Dry the feet very thoroughly after washing.
* Wash the socks and towels separately using a few drops of tea tree oil in the final rinse to prevent the infection spreading to others.

ESSENTIAL OILS

Cypress, tea tree, lavender, manuka, rosemary

TREATMENT

Add four drops tea tree or manuka essential oil, and four drops lavender essential oil, to one teaspoon vegetable oil. Add to a bowl of warm water large enough for the feet. Stir to disperse the oils, and soak the feet for five minutes, dry gently but well, particularly between the toes. Dust with Herb Oil Foot Powder, which is antiviral, and a deodorant.

HERB OIL FOOT POWDER

1 cup (150 g) cornstarch (cornflour)
6 drops tea tree essential oil
6 drops lavender essential oil
6 drops cypress essential oil
6 drops rosemary essential oil

To make and use

Drip the oils very slowly into the cornstarch, while stirring constantly to prevent lumps. Store in a labeled jar with a well-fitting lid.

Using a fresh piece of absorbent cotton (cottonwool) each time, dust the feet thoroughly, particularly between the toes, and sprinkle in socks. Use after washing and before bed.

Sprinkle this powder inside the socks and shoes if you suffer from sweaty or smelly feet.

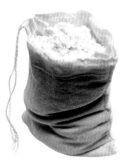

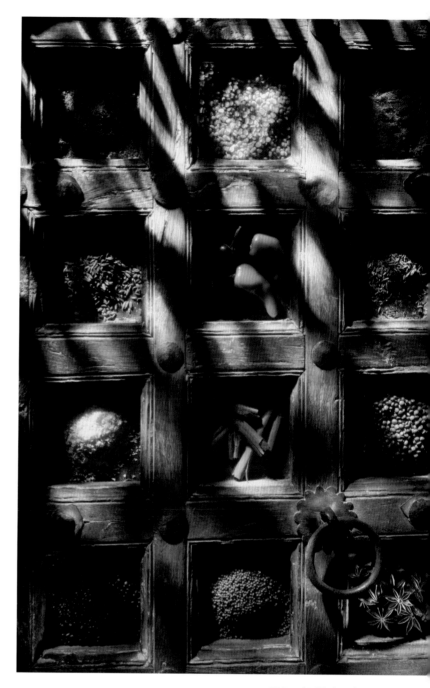

Various dried herbs and spices in an ancient wooden display box.

SMELLY FEET

The embarrassing condition is often worse during puberty, but also can be the result of a poor diet with too many "indulgences." Follow the suggestions for Athlete's Foot.

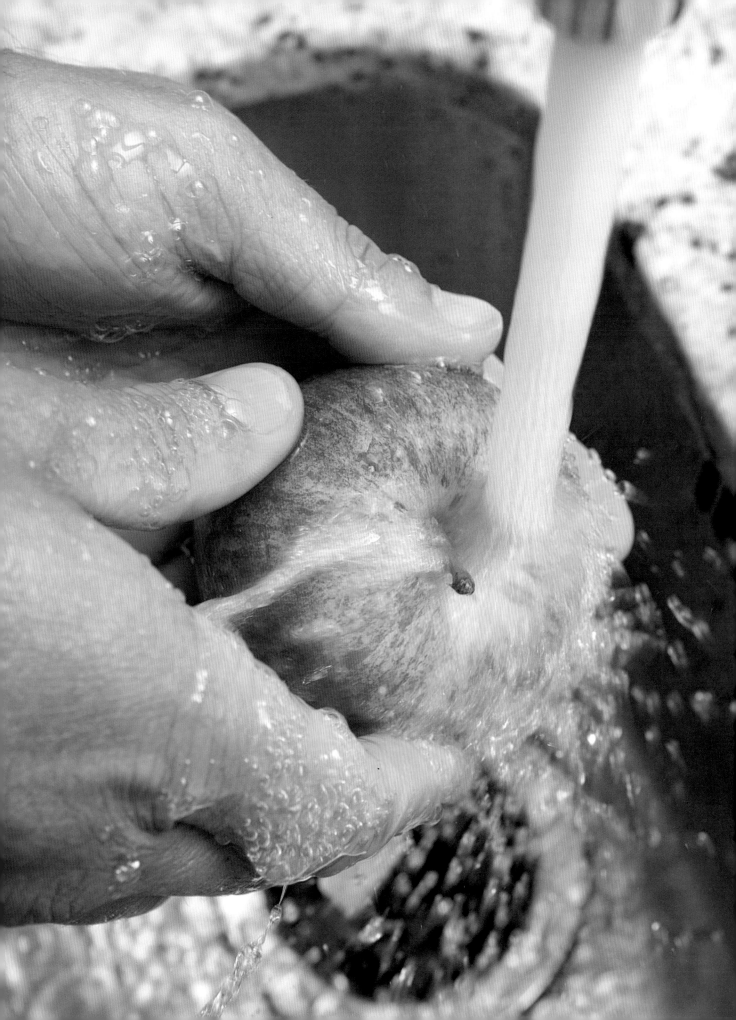

Common infections and complaints

In these days of commuting, cramped offices and greater populations, we are increasingly being exposed to various infections and complaints from others. It's impossible to avoid all the bugs around us, and it's been shown that being too careful with antibacterial solutions can make us sicker by reducing our natural immunity to everyday bugs.

The secret is common sense. Wipe down the kitchen benches and don't use the cloth for other tasks. Wash and dry it regularly. Make sure your cutting board is spotless, and use different cutting boards for raw meat and vegetables. I have three or four that I keep for special tasks. You can now buy colored boards for different jobs.

Teach children to wash their hands regularly, not just in the bathroom, and don't go to work or school if you have a bad cold. You'll only make others around you sick and continue the infection.

Additional essential oil treatments

Candidiasis
Candid albicans is a harmless yeast (fungus), present in our bodies from birth. Occasionally it grows excessively, and causes health problems. It is sometimes considered a stress-related condition which affects the immune system. It lives quite happily in our bodies for years, but when our immune system is compromised or reduced, candida can begin to multiply quickly, and can enter the bloodstream.

It presents itself in various ways, often as a yeast infection in the vagina. The most common reason for this is antibiotic treatment, which upsets the chemical balance of the body.

Thrush, an infection of the mucous membranes, is the most common symptom. It sometimes affects the mouth (especially in babies), but is more usually found in the vagina.

Men can transmit thrush even though they may show no symptoms, so it is important to treat both partners to prevent reinfection. As well as using the following blends it is important to eat three cups of yoghurt, and take multi-B vitamin tablet daily. This re-establishes the correct chemical balance in the body.

Thrush in a baby's mouth can be treated with yoghurt and gentle swabbing with chamomile tea.

ESSENTIAL OILS
Cedarwood, lavender, tea tree

TREATMENT
Add one drop of cedarwood, lavender, or tea tree essential oils, to one tablespoon of plain yoghurt and one teaspoon of water, and use as a douche. Dissolve four tablespoons bicarbonate of soda in 4 quarts (4 liters) of warm water, in a bowl big enough to sit in. Sit in the bowl, and holding the vagina open with one hand "swoosh" the water as far inside as possible. Stay in the water for about 10 minutes.

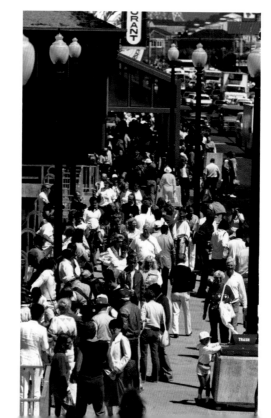

Unfortunately, most of our infections come from others.

AVOIDING EPIDEMICS

Handling money, and shaking hands, are easy ways of picking up what's laying everyone else low. This is because you transfer the infection or virus to your mouth, or nose, when you touch your face—and most of us are aware how often we do that. Wiping fingers or hands, (discreetly), with Anti-infection Hand Wipes after contact can help protect you from what's going around.

Essential oils
Lavender, tea tree, manuka, bergamot, citronella

Anti-infection hand wipes
$^1/_4$ cup (60 ml) vodka
20 drops lavender or manuka essential oil
20 drops bergamot essential oil
20 drops tea tree essential oil
10 drops lemon tea tree essential oil

To make and use
Mix all the ingredients together in a small, labeled bottle, and shake to blend.

Leave for four days before using, so the oils have time to synergize or combine well.

Make hand wipes out of pieces of suitable fabric, such as kitchen cloths or wipes, and sized to fit a small (waterproof) container that will fit in your pocket or bag.

Spray them with the blend as often as necessary to keep the oil fresh. Use as required.

Alternatively, just blend the essential oils together to use as an air spray or in an oil burner.

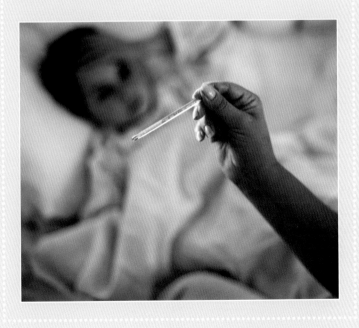

Chickenpox

Chickenpox is a highly infectious viral disease. It starts off as a feverish cold before the red, spotty rash that looks like insect bites, and then develops into blisters that are often intensely itchy.

Chickenpox, which occurs most often in late winter and early spring, is very contagious—most of those in a household who haven't had chickenpox will get it. However, immunization is now available for children, and mass treatment of young children is expected to decrease cases dramatically over the next few years.

Although it's more common in those under the 15, anyone can get chickenpox. However, we usually only get one episode in our lifetime. The virus that causes chickenpox can lie dormant within the body and can cause a different type of skin eruption later in life called shingles.

See Shingles, page 501.

Essential oils are useful in soothing the itchy spots and the child! And the adult if he or she is unlucky enough to catch it.

ESSENTIAL OILS
Lavender, tea tree

TREATMENT
Add 20 drops lavender essential oil (a drop at a time to prevent lumping) to two cups bicarbonate of soda. Stir constantly. Mix one or two teaspoons of this paste with enough cold water to make a milky lotion. Dab the lotion on the spots with absorbent cotton (cottonwool), or add enough water to make a very thin lotion. Pour the mixture into a spray bottle and spray the spotty areas. Shake well before use, and repeat as often as needed.

Add two drops lavender essential oil and two drops tea tree oil to $^1/_2$ cup bicarbonate of soda, stir well and sprinkle into a warm bath. Stir the water well to dissolve the salts. This bath will soothe the itching (and has the added advantage of making the little patient calmer).

See also Children and Babies section, page 399.

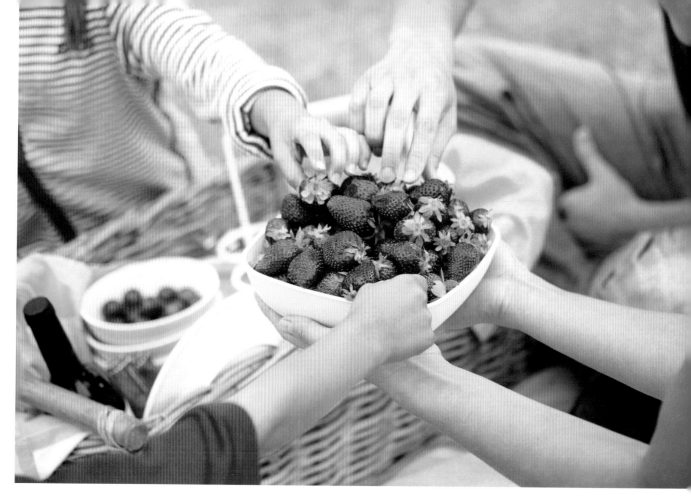

Try to get all the family to wash their hands before eating.

Intertrigo

This is a bacterial infection that develops in places like the groin, and under the breasts, where skin is in contact with skin. It often occurs in athletes when sweat occurs on parts of the body that continually come in contact with other parts.

It is most often due to chafing together of the warm, moist skin, more especially in those who are overweight, or diabetic. Infection with bacteria or yeast may then develop in the broken skin.

ESSENTIAL OILS

Lavender, rosemary, tea tree

INTERTRIGO POWDER

1 cup cornstarch (cornflour)
20 drops tea tree essential oil
20 drops lavender essential oil
20 drops rosemary essential oil

To make and use

Place the cornstarch in a bowl, then add the oils a few drops at a time, stirring constantly to prevent lumping. Store in an airtight container.

First wash the area (two to three times a day) using absorbent cotton (cottonwool) dipped in a small bowl of lukewarm water, to which four drops of tea tree essential oil have been added. Gently pat the skin dry with a very soft towel.

Now, dust the skin lightly with the Intertrigo Powder blend, using fresh absorbent cotton (cottonwool) each time.

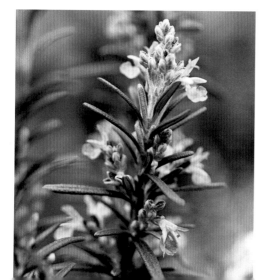

Rosemary in flower. The oil is used in powders.

Measles

Measles is caused by a virus. The infection is spread by contact with droplets from the nose, mouth, or throat, of an infected person. The incubation period is 8 to 12 days before symptoms generally appear. Immunization is available in most countries, and is considered necessary as measles can have very serious complications, particularly in young children.

The period between the appearance of the earliest symptoms and the appearance of a rash or fever is usually three to five days.

Measles should never be treated lightly and can lead to secondary infections of the eyes, ears, and chest. It is best to confine the patient during the contagious period. Complete bed rest is essential to help to avoid complications. Give body sponges to reduce high temperature, keep both the bedroom and the house sprayed with the following blend to help prevent the spread of infection.

It is important to consult your doctor if anyone in your household has measles, but there are also things you can do to reduce the discomfort of the symptoms.

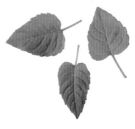

Measles, mumps and other contagious childhood diseases are spread through direct contact.

ESSENTIAL OILS

Cypress, eucalyptus, lavender, rosemary, tea tree

To make and use

Add two drops of lavender oil (one drop at a time to prevent lumping) to one cup bicarbonate of soda. Mix one or two teaspoons of this blend with enough cold water to make a milky lotion. Dab the lotion with absorbent cotton (cottonwool) on the itchy spots as often as needed.

Add four drops lavender essential oil to $1/2$ cup bicarbonate of soda, stir well, and add to a warm bath. Agitate the water to dissolve the powder. This bath will soothe the itching and has the added advantage of making patients calmer as well.

ANTI-INFECTION AIR SPRAY FOR MEASLES

1 teaspoon lavender essential oil
$1/2$ teaspoon cypress essential oil
$1/2$ teaspoon rosemary essential oil
$1/2$ teaspoon eucalyptus or tea tree essential oil

To make and use

Mix all the ingredients together in a small, labeled bottle, and shake to blend.

Leave for four days before using, so the oils have time to synergize or combine well.

Use 50 drops of the blend in an air spray.

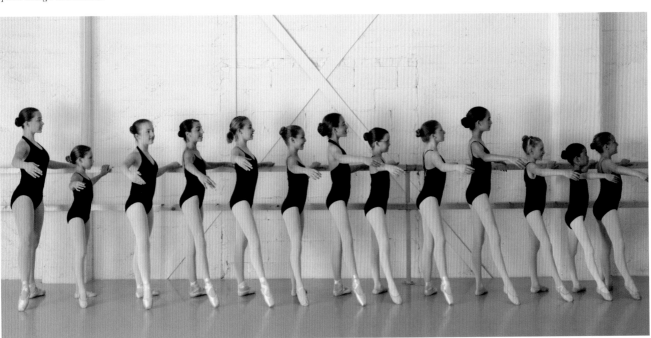

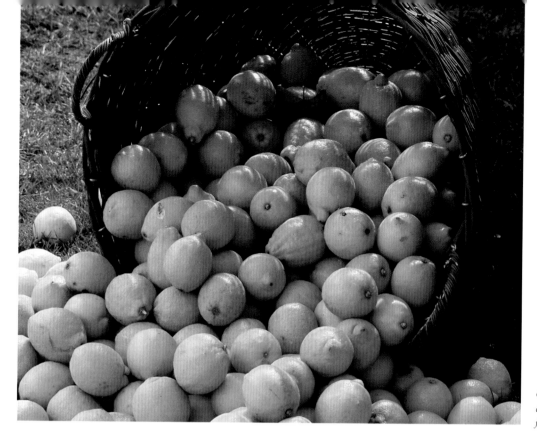

Children always seem to be happy drinking a mild solution of lemon juice and honey.

Mumps

Mumps is caused by a virus that is spread from person-to-person by respiratory droplets, or direct contact with articles that have been contaminated with infected saliva.

It is highly contagious and usually strikes children and adolescents. Mumps vaccine was introduced in 1967 and since then the incidence of the disease has decreased by almost 99 percent in the western world. A person develops life long protection after having the disease once.

Mumps is characterized by swollen glands on one or both sides of the jaw, and possibly earache, mild fever, and headache.

Symptoms usually start 14 to 24 days after infection. Mumps most often occurs in children between five and nine years of age.

The very uncomfortable stage usually lasts for only a few days, but during this time, bed rest is essential to avoid complications.

Mumps is more serious in adults, particularly men, as it usually infects glands in the groin, causing swelling and severe pain.

The swollen glands under the ears may make the patient very miserable, as it becomes painful to eat or swallow.

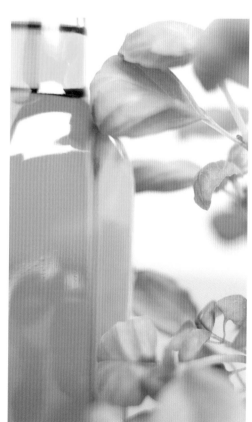

Olive oil is the base of Gland Massage Blend, page 500.

ESSENTIAL OILS

Tea tree, lavender, lemon, niouli

GLAND MASSAGE BLEND

4 teaspoons olive oil
2 drops lavender essential oil
2 drops lemon or niouli essential oil
1 drop tea tree essential oil

Immunization is the best way to prevent the possibly dangerous side effects of the many contagious childhood diseases.

To make and use

Mix all the ingredients together in a small bottle, and shake to blend. Leave for four days before using, so the oils have time to synergize or combine well.

Gently massage the glands and the whole neck area. Spray the bedroom and house with air spray containing these essential oils.

Place cold compresses on the swollen glands to bring relief.

Alternatively, just blend the essential oils together to use as an air spray or in an oil burner.

Rubella (German measles)

Rubella is commonly called German measles or three-day mealses. It is caused by the rubella virus and is not the same as ordinary measles. Rubella is most commonly transmitted by secretions from the nose or throat.

Incubation is 14 to 23 days and total recovery is usually within one week, although adults may take a little longer.

It is an extremely serious disease for pregnant women as it always infects the unborn child, causing severe disease and possible defects in the unborn child, particularly if contracted in the first trimester.

Children who are infected with rubella before birth are at risk for growth retardation, mental retardation, deafness, and sometimes malformations of the eyes and heart. Defects are rare if the infection occurs after the 20th week of pregnancy.

In children and adults, rubella is usually mild, and may even go unnoticed.

Children generally have few symptoms, but adults may experience fever, and some headache before the rash appears. It is only contracted once in our lives, and immunization is readily available in most countries.

Ginger or clove tea is believed to speed up the progress of the disease. Traditional Chinese practitioners often prescribe peppermint (*Mentha piperita*) and distilled witch hazel is said to relieve the itching.

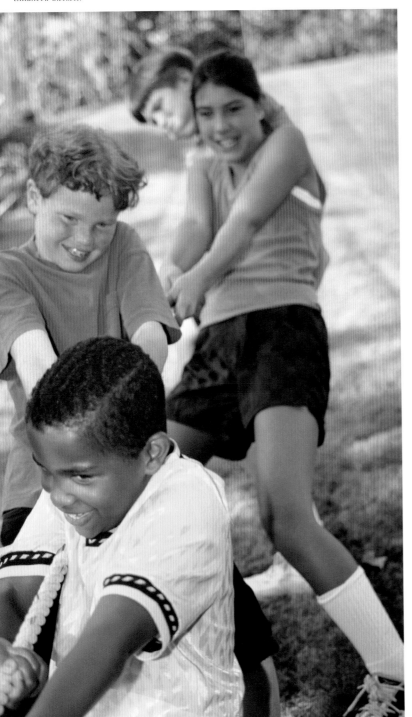

ESSENTIAL OILS
Chamomile, lavender, tea tree

TREATMENT
Add five drops lavender and five drops chamomile essential oils (a drop at a time to prevent lumping), to one cup bicarbonate of soda. Mix one to two teaspoons with enough cold water to make a milky lotion. Use absorbent cotton (cottonwool) to dab the lotion on the itchy spots. Repeat as often as needed.

Add four drops lavender essential oil to ¼ cup bicarbonate of soda. Sprinkle into a deep warm bath, agitate the water to dissolve, and allow the patient to sit in the bath for half an hour or more. Don't leave young children alone in the bath. This bath will soothe the itching, and calm the patient.

Add four drops lavender and four drops chamomile essential oils into two cups water in a spray bottle. Use to spray on the spots to ease itching.

Use tea tree and lavender essential oils in oil burners and air sprays to help to prevent the spread of infection.

Shingles

Shingles is a disease caused by the same virus that causes chickenpox. After an attack of chickenpox, the virus lies dormant in the nerve tissue. As we get older, it is possible for the virus to reappear in the form of shingles.

Although it is most common in people over age 50, if you have had chickenpox, you are at risk for developing shingles. Shingles is also more common in people with weakened immune systems from HIV infection, chemotherapy or radiation treatment, transplant operations, and stress.

Shingles are blisters that look like chicken pox but are usually larger. Because nerve endings are involved there is often severe pain. If the blisters are on, or near, the eyes seek medical help.

ESSENTIAL OILS
Bergamot, chamomile, eucalyptus, lavender, tea tree

TREATMENT
Dab a mixture of equal quantities of neat tea tree, and lavender essential oils, on the blisters. Soothe the blister with a compress of bergamot and chamomile, or eucalyptus, essential oils.

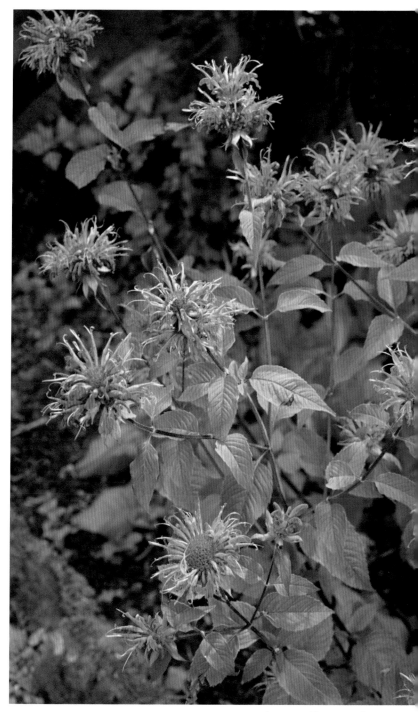

A compress of bergamot and chamomile soothes the blisters associated with shingles.

L-lysine (an amino acid), taken as directed, is important for healing. Vitamin C plus bioflavinoids, taken as directed, helps in destroying the virus and boosts the immune system.

Cayenne capsules (Zovirax) taken as directed on the packet relieve pain and help healing.

Vitamin B complex taken as directed helps to heal herpes and skin lesions.

Vitamin E taken as directed promotes the healing of lesions.

Many organically grown herbs can be found at produce markets, open in most cities and towns.

Combine equal parts tincture of valerian, calendula and St John's wort. Take 30 to 60 drops three to four times per day.

A poultice made from powdered slippery elm, comfrey, and goldenseal, is soothing and aids healing.

Oatmeal baths may provide relief from itching and burning. Place one cup of oats in the foot of a stocking or tights, tie in a knot, and let it soak in the tub. Squeeze the stocking to release the soothing oat milk.

Make a strong calendula and peppermint tea, cool completely, and lay as a compress over the blistered area.

Some people suffer from neuralgia after the blisters have gone. Any of the following treatments will help relieve it.

Apply a hot fomentation using cayenne (use one part cayenne to eight parts other herbs), chamomile, mullein, and wormwood. Repeat every hour until relief is obtained.

Massage the painful nerve or joint with infused oil of St John's wort.

Zostrix is a cream available in pharmacies. It contains capsaicin, an extract form chilies, and is helpful in temporarily relieving the pain of neuralgia, arthritis, and the after-pain associated with shingles.

Herbal Remedies

There has been little or no research into the effects of herbs and herbal medicine on the human condition. In Asia, where it has been in practice for thousands of years, herbal alternatives are offered side by side to Western medicines and no one thinks anything of it. In the US, however, some states still have laws forbidding the practice of herbal medicine, even though most doctors would agree that it definitely has a place in modern society.

If you choose to consult a herbal practitioner, it's probably wise to go with someone who is recommended, rather than just using the telephone directory to locate one. There are many magazines and on-line forums that you can access, which will give you a well-rounded look into your needs, and allow you to make an educated decision.

There are also chain stores selling natural remedies, and this makes it easy to access some of the more obscure herbs and oils. However, read the directions and follow them closely. Don't think that two pills will be better than one. The use of natural remedies is as strict in its dosage as any prescription drug.

Herbal medicine is natural and effective but it is not harmless. Directions must be followed, and you must inform your health professional of any herbal treatments you are taking, as they may very well counter what the doctor is trying to cure. If you find your doctor is opposed to any sort of natural remedy, then maybe it's time to find a doctor who is, as proper management of illness is usually best with a combination of both.

A collection of culinary or medicinal herbs. Although herbs and herbal medicine have been in use for thousands of years, the Western world is still coming to terms with their benefits.

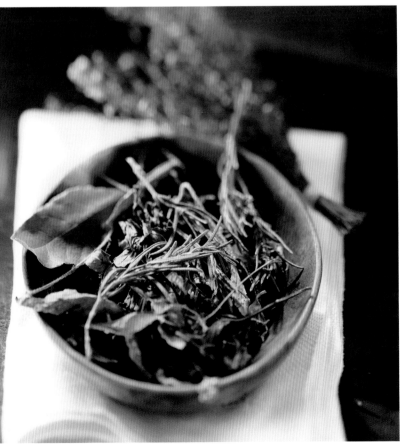

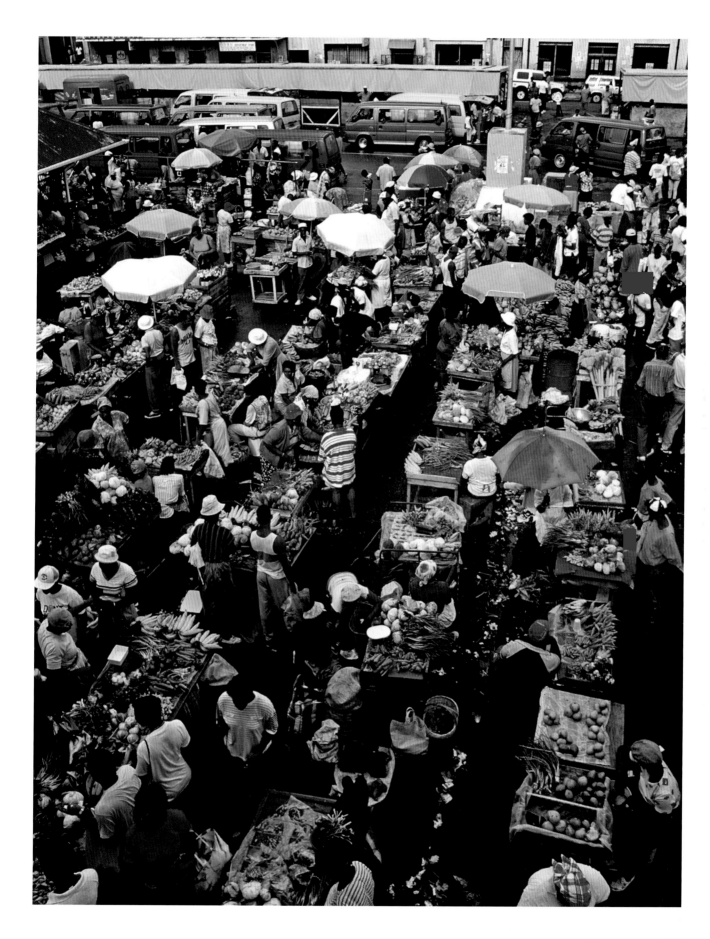

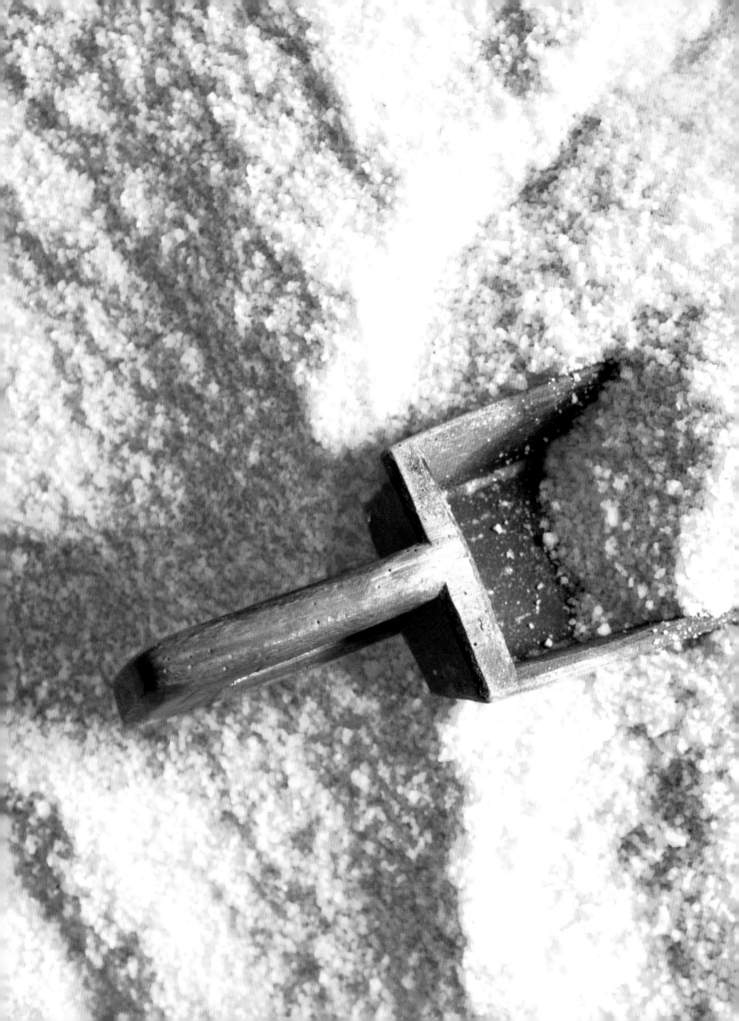

PART FOUR

PRACTICALITIES

All tasks require some planning and here I've listed all the necessary conversion charts, equipment, and essentials required to make the recipes in this book. My genie is the oil, which, when released, will perform all sorts of wonderful magic for me. I hope that you find this book helpful and more importantly, inspirational. The recipes are not at all difficult. They don't take long to make and most of them are quite inexpensive.

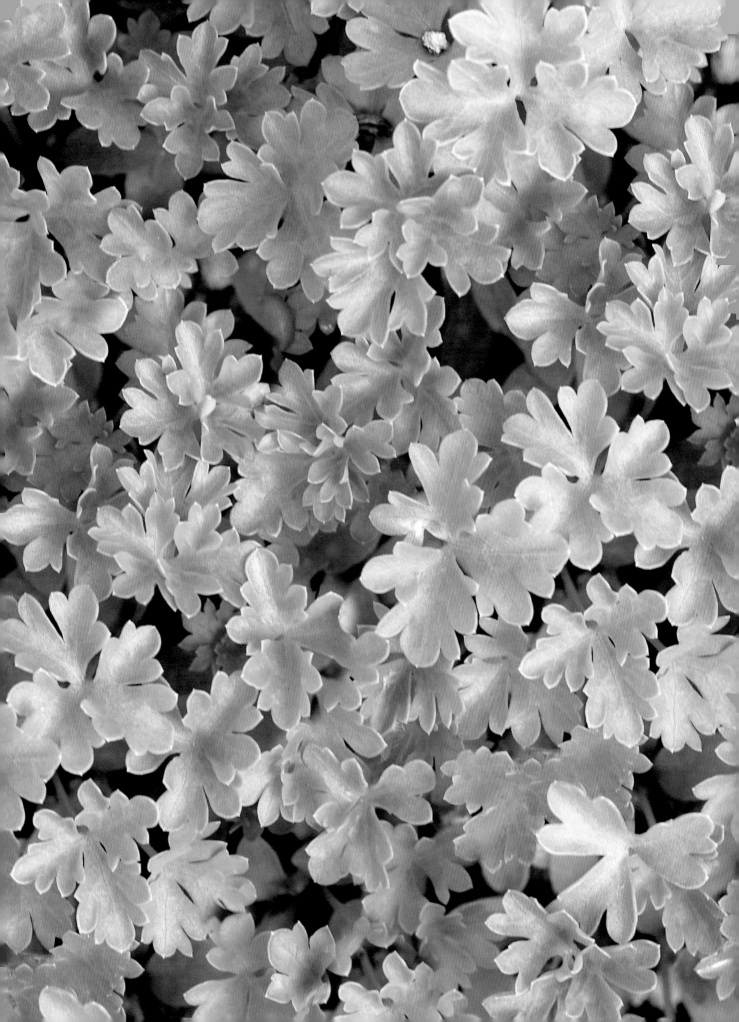

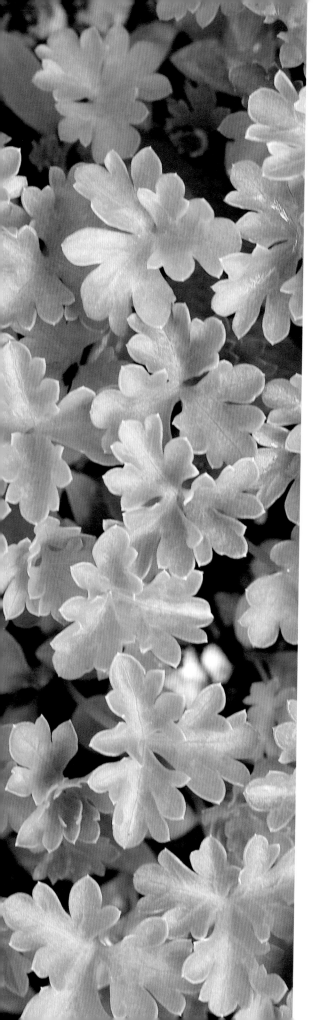
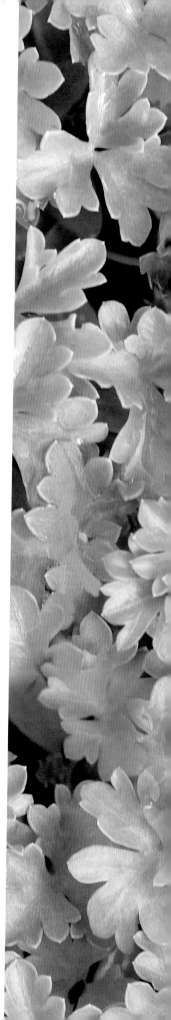

METHODS AND TECHNIQUES

It's all well and good to read pages and

pages of marvelous recipes and teas, but in

the end we have to make them. And here

are the weights and measures, the basic

methods and the tools to use. There are

directions on different kinds of luscious

baths to refresh your mind and body, and

the A-Z Methods makes it easy to find the

right course for each recipe. There is also

a lovely sampling of what herbs to use in

your cooking.

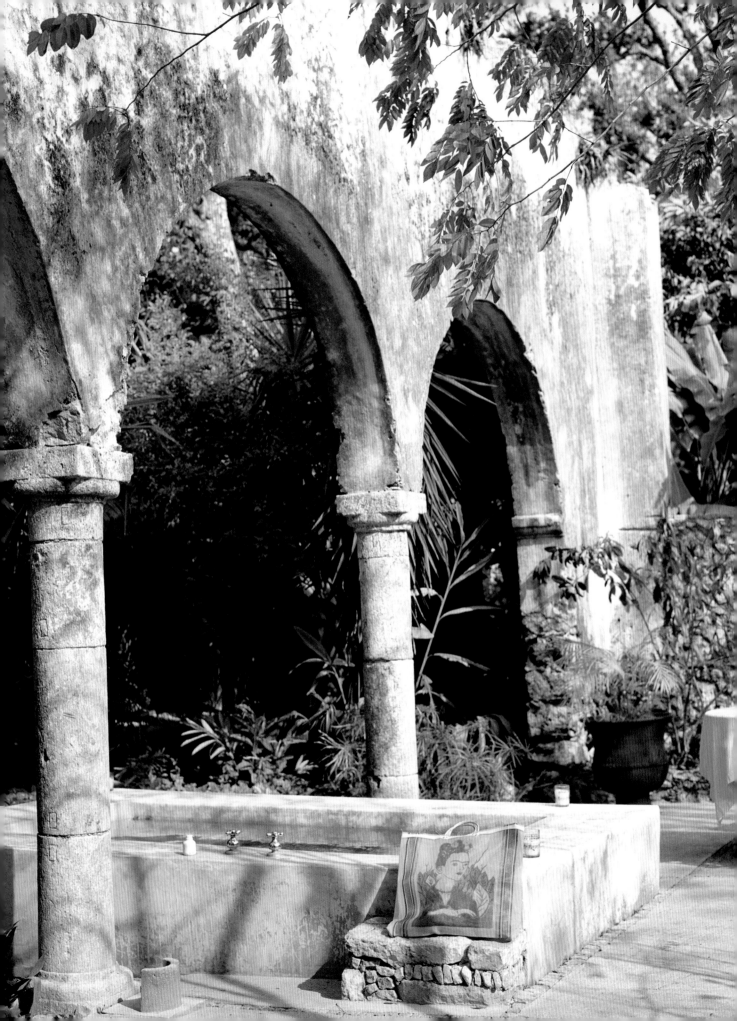

Types of baths

Full body bath

Baths that are too hot or too cold are not relaxing. The temperature should be body heat or very slightly higher, about 95°–100°F (35°–38°C). You can buy special pillows for use in the bath to make yourself as comfortable as possible. You gain most benefit by staying in the water for about 30 minutes.

Bran bath

Anyone who suffers from dry, itchy skin will enjoy the benefits of a bran bath. Throwing a handful of bran in the bath is really messy, so it's better to put a handful in a pan, cover with 3 cups (750 ml) of water, bring to the boil, simmer for a few minutes and strain the water into the bath. Alternatively, tie a handful of bran in a muslin bag, squeeze it under the bath water to release the "milkiness" and then use the bran-filled bag as a washcloth.

Bubble bath

These are fun and have a luxurious feeling, but it's not good to indulge for too long or too often as they are detergent based and can overdry the skin. Use only the amount recommended and apply moisturizer to your skin after the bath.

Epsom salts bath

After a long day in the garden, my soul is flying but my body feels wrecked. An Epsom salts bath seems to take all the weariness away and leaves me feeling refreshed.

Epsom salts can help the body to get rid of toxins and are particularly beneficial for easing joint and muscular pain and stiffness. To make the bath, add one cup of Epsom salts and the herbs of your choice as the bath is running, and make sure the salts are dissolved. Stay in the bath for 20–30 minutes, massaging affected parts of your body while in the bath. Essential oils may be substituted for herbs.

HOT BATH

The temperature should be 100°–104°F (38°–40°C) and you should stay in the water for 10–15 minutes only.

The effects are increased perspiration and rate of breathing; reduction of fevers; elimination of toxins. Wrap up in warm pajamas and blankets after the bath, and drink appropriate hot herb teas both during and after the bath.

WARM BATH

The temperature should be approximately 80°–95°F (27°C–35°C), and you should indulge for 20–60 minutes.

The effects are mild, calming, relaxing.

COLD BATH

The temperature should be 35°C–38°F (21–27ºC) for two to five minutes only.

The effects are improved breathing and muscle tone; decreased fatigue; improved thyroid function and skin tone; as well as relief from constipation.

Footbath

A footbath is, as the name suggests, a bath for the feet. Ideally the bath should be deep enough to cover the calves of the legs as well. Footbaths can ease the pain of aching feet stimulate circulation, ease tension headaches, lessen the symptoms of colds and influenza and relax the nervous system.

Cold footbaths will soothe tired feet and help to stop nosebleeds.

Herb bath

There are many suggestions for herb baths throughout this book. Herbs may be used to heal, hydrate, soothe, stimulate, relax, soften, tighten and much more. There are many ways to introduce the plants to your bath: infusions, decoctions, bath bags, bath mitts, oils, or combined with any of the other treatments in this section.

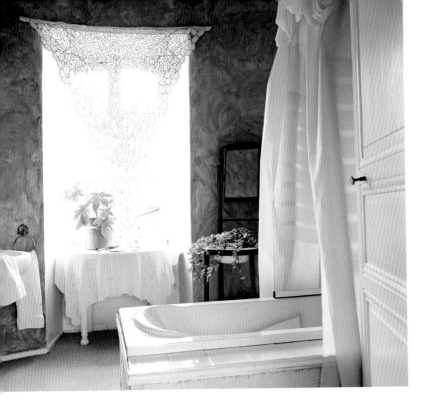

A traditional bath with an old-world touch.

Spring mustard blooms growing in a vineyard in Napa Valley, California, USA.

Honey bath

This is an old, well-tried, and simple skin softener which also helps you to sleep. Mix one tablespoonful of honey with some warm water until it is very runny. Pour into a warm (not hot) bath, swish it around and enjoy!

Milk bath

Unless, like Cleopatra, you have access to an ass, you will have to be content with adding fresh or powdered cow's milk to your bath water. The protein and other contents of the milk leave the skin feeling silky and soft. Yoghurt or buttermilk give a mildly acidic and protein-enriched bath.

Mustard footbath

When you arrive home cold, wet and shivery you can avoid a full-scale cold by having a mustard footbath.

Salt bath

If you feel dirty you might like to have a shower or wash before this bath, as the salt prevents soap lathering. Add two cups of cooking salt to the bath as the water is running. It should be a warm, not hot, bath for the best results. After this bath you will feel fresh, stimulated, and silky skinned.

Sitz bath

This is a bath where the water just covers the hips and abdomen and is used to treat problems in the abdominal area.

Vinegar bath

This is another bath to ease itchy skin. You can either swish around in cider vinegar or an herbal vinegar.

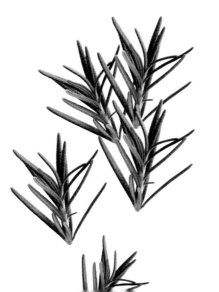

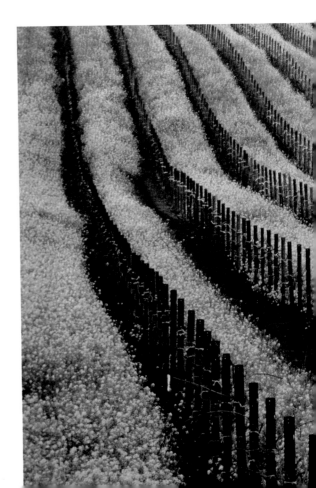

Therapeutic herbal baths

Baths can have more than just a soothing effect. They can help to remedy a variety of ills, as you will see from the chart below. Make either a triple-strength tea and pour the strained liquid into the bath or make as in the Oat Cleanser recipe, but with herbs as the only ingredient. I like the bag method best, as I enjoy scrubbing myself with the bagful of herbs.

Arthritis

Make 1 quart (1 liter) of triple-strength tea of rosemary and thyme. Add 1 cup (220 g) of Epsom salts to the infusion and stir to dissolve. Pour into a deep bath that is a little hotter than usual. Remain in the bath for 30 minutes, massaging affected parts of the body while in the bath.

Chills and colds

Dissolve two tablespoons of dry mustard powder and add to a footbath of hot water. Keep your feet immersed for 15-30 minutes, topping up with more hot water as needed.

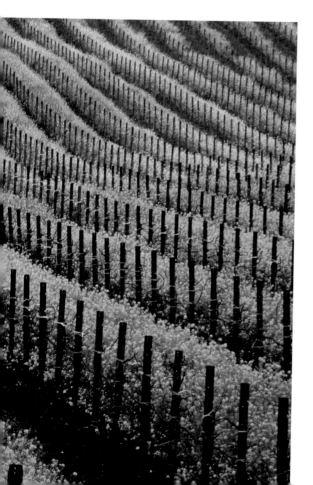

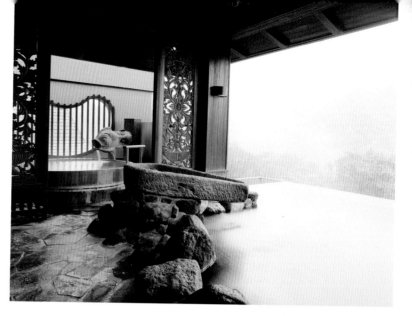

A sublime bathroom overlooking a bay, in Tokyo, Japan.

Alternatively, make 1 quart (1 liter) of triple-strength tea of borage, sage, and thyme, and pour into a hot bath. Soak for 15–25 minutes.

Cramps

Make 1 quart (1 liter) of triple-strength rosemary and thyme tea, dissolve 1 cup (220 g) of Epsom salts into the tea and pour into a hot bath. Soak for 20–25 minutes, massaging the affected limbs.

Dry and/or itchy skin

Make 1 quart (1 liter) of decoction of chopped comfrey root and mallow root. Mix 2 cups (200 g) of dry milk powder into the decoction and pour into a warm bath. Soak for 20 minutes.

See also Eczema. Use a bran and oats bag in place of soap for its cleansing and soothing and non-drying action.

Eczema

Put 1 cup (90g) of mixed bran and oats in a muslin bag and tie the top securely. Put the bag into a saucepan and cover with 1 quart (1 liter) of water. Bring to the boil and barely simmer, covered, for 15 minutes. Pour the liquid into the bath and use the muslin bag as a washcloth. Don't use soap.

Alternatively, make 1 quart (1 liter) of triple-strength tea of calendula, chickweed, and yarrow, and add to a warm bath, making sure that the affected areas are either submerged or sponged repeatedly with the water.

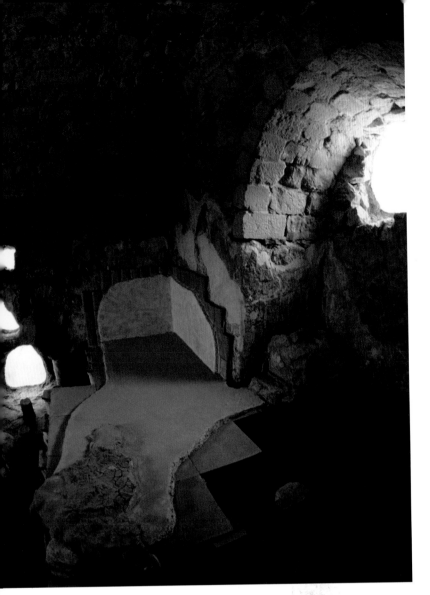

A calidarium or "Turkish bath," commonly known as a steam bath, is the first room in a Roman bathhouse.

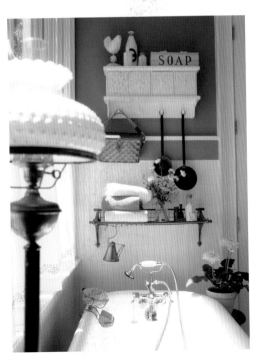

A bathroom with a very Parisian feel.

Fibromyalgia (Fibrositis)
Use the same method as for Arthritis but use thyme and Epsom salts instead.

Headaches
Make 1 quart (1 liter) of triple-strength lavender and rosemary tea. Add to a warm bath. Add 10 drops of lavender essential oil and swirl to distribute. Relax for 20 minutes.

Insomnia
Make 1 quart (1 liter) of triple-strength chamomile, lavender, and lemon balm tea and pour into a warm bath. Relax for 20 minutes while sipping a cup of chamomile tea.

Lumbago
See Arthritis

Nervous Exhaustion and Stress
Make a triple-strength tea of chamomile, lemon balm, thyme and valerian and pour into a warm bath. Soak for 20–30 minutes while sipping a cup of chamomile tea.

Poor circulation
Soak your feet in a mustard footbath.

Alternatively, make 1 quart (1 liter) of triple-strength nettle, pennyroyal, and sage tea and pour into a hot bath. Soak for 15–20 minutes.

Psoriasis
See Bran and Oats recipe under Eczema.

Alternatively, make a 1 quart (1 liter) triple-strength lavender, thyme, and yarrow tea, pour into a warm bath and soak for 15 minutes. Use the infusion as a compress on affected parts between baths.

Sore muscles
Make 1 quart (1 liter) triple-strength rosemary, sage, and thyme tea, add 1 cup (220 g) of Epsom salts and dissolve. Pour into a hot bath. Soak for 20–30 minutes, massaging the sore muscles. Follow with a massage.

General index

Main plant entries and fixed oils have **bold** page numbers.

Major ailments and treatments are indicated by **bold entries**.

Recipes begin with a Capital letter.

An alphabetical index of recipes can be found on page 573.

For major sections, refer to Contents

Recipe index

Photographic credits